The Psychiatrist's Guide to Diseases of the Nervous System

The Psychiatrist's Guide to Diseases of the Nervous System

RICHARD LECHTENBERG, M.D.
Assistant Professor of Neurology
Downstate Medical Center of the
State University of New York
Brooklyn, New York

1807 1982
175 YEARS OF PUBLISHING

A WILEY MEDICAL PUBLICATION
JOHN WILEY & SONS
New York • Chichester • Brisbane • Toronto • Singapore

Library of Congress Cataloging in Publication Data:

Lechtenberg, Richard.
The psychiatrist's guide to diseases of the nervous system.

(A Wiley medical publication)
Includes index.
1. Nervous system— —Diseases. 2. Neuropsychiatry.
I. Title. II. Series. [DNLM: 1. Nervous system diseases. WL 100 L459]
RC346.L43 616.8 82-2792
ISBN 0-471-08727-0 AACR2

Printed in the United States of America

10 9 8 7 6 5 4 3 2 1

To
Dr. Norman Geschwind
and
Dr. George Vaillant

Preface

The Psychiatrist's Guide to Diseases of the Nervous System answers the questions that psychiatrists, psychologists, psychiatric social workers, and other mental health professionals ask neurologists most frequently. To make it a practical guide for persons who care for patients with primarily psychiatric problems, this book is organized around the signs and symptoms that develop in such patients. The attention given a particular sign or symptom reflects the frequency with which it provokes questions. Movement disorders, seizure disorders, intellectual problems, and abnormalities of affect frequently appear in patients cared for by mental health professionals, and so these problems are discussed in detail. Much of the information provided is intended to help in the diagnosis and treatment of conditions routinely encountered by mental health professionals. The characteristic features of diseases easily misdiagnosed as psychiatric, rather than neurologic, problems are discussed in considerable detail. With the information provided, the psychiatrist or psychologist evaluating a patient should be able to determine rapidly the implications of specific signs and symptoms. Diagnostic approaches to a variety of signs and symptoms that often develop in patients with psychiatric problems are provided for the psychiatrist who wishes to expedite the evaluation of his or her patient's neurologic problem.

This book is a guide for clinicians treating patients with apparent psychiatric disorders, psychiatric complications of neurologic disorders, neurologic complications of psychiatric treatment, and psychiatric complications of neurologic treatment. Although psychiatrists may not be the primary physicians directing the treatment of a neurologic disorder, they are still at an advantage in dealing with neurologic patients if they understand the alternatives to and the complications of the therapy that their patients are receiving. Therapeutic approaches to patients with neurologic problems who often have a psychiatrist as their primary physician are discussed in adequate detail to allow the mental health professional to provide the patient and his or her family with a clear picture of what the therapy involves.

R.L.

Acknowledgments

Many people helped in the preparation of this book. Neuroradiologic material was provided by Drs. Michael Tenner, John Loh, Wendy Hotson, and Sharon Kreps. Ms. Luisa Karoly helped prepare the electroencephalograms, and Dr. Philip Duffy provided neuropathologic material. Albert Paglialunga assisted with the photographic work. Russell Madras helped with computer operations. Sarah Hogan, Faith Cardwell, Carolyn MacCarthy, and Carol Brenner assisted in the preparation of the manuscript. Clinical material came from the College of Physicians and Surgeons of Columbia University, Downstate Medical Center of the State University of New York, and Lenox Hill Hospital of New York.

R.L.

Contents

1
Neurologic Problems in Psychiatry

Neurologic disorders affect many patients with psychiatric problems. The neurologic problem may be little more than slowed movements from antipsychotic drugs, or it may be progressive stupor associated with a nervous system infection that presented as a psychosis. In practice, most of the nervous system disturbances faced by psychiatrists and psychologists are side effects of therapies routinely used with patients suffering from affective and cognitive disorders. Lithium carbonate given to the patient with a bipolar psychosis may produce hand tremors and slurred speech. Electroconvulsive therapy in the treatment of a depressive psychosis will produce a transient memory disorder. Allaying the anxiety provoked by these predictable and often treatable effects of therapy is often essential in convincing the patient or his family to continue with the treatment. A much less obvious, but therapeutically more important, problem affecting all individuals working with mentally ill patients is the recognition of neurologic disorders with primarily psychiatric manifestations. Treating a patient with Wilson disease for his depression without recognizing the underlying neurologic disease is both futile and tragic. The patient will not respond to the psychiatric intervention, regardless of how appropriate it is for a conventional psychotic depression, and failure to recognize the neurologic disease early in the course of the illness allows the development of irreversible brain damage, which could have been avoided with appropriate treatment.

Distinguishing between psychiatric and neurologic problems is an increasingly complicated task for both the psychiatrist and the neurologist. Psychiatric problems can cause neurologic signs and symptoms, and neurologic diseases may have psychiatric manifestations. Further undermining the differences between psychiatric and neurologic syndromes is the already mentioned production of neurologic signs by drugs used in psychotherapy and the occasional development of psychiatric reactions to drugs used in treating neurologic disorders. Deciding what caused an affective change, movement disorder, insidious intellectual deterioration, or acute convulsive disorder is important in choosing the treatment for the problem, whether it is evolving or longstanding. If an apparent dementia has developed from depression, then treatment of the depression is of primary importance. If visual and olfactory hallucinations have developed from a psychomotor seizure disorder, then treatment of the convulsive disorder has priority.

Many diagnostic techniques are available to help in the evaluation of patients with neurologic and psychiatric symptoms, but the risks involved in many of these tests require a high level of confidence in the diagnosis before they are used. An arteriogram of the cerebral blood vessels will establish whether or not the patient has an arteriovenous malformation causing his headaches, but the risks associated with an arteriogram include stroke. Subjecting a patient with tension headache to this type of procedure is obviously unjustifiable, but recognizing what is a typical tension headache may be no small feat even for the mental health professional routinely dealing with anxious or depressed patients. A neurologist can help establish the diagnosis, but the physician most familiar with the patient is in the best position to accurately assess the patient's signs and symptoms. Patients with bizarre behavior, vague complaints, apparent emotional problems, unreasonable rage or irritability, or sexual dysfunctions are all frequently referred for psychiatric evaluation or assistance early in the evolution of their problems. Even when the patient is referred by another physician, the burden of assessing the problem falls on the psychotherapist. The information gathered as the therapist becomes familiar with the patient is the most effective tool available for diagnosing the problem correctly or, at least, designing a strategy for diagnosing the problem rationally.

PSYCHIATRIC MANIFESTATIONS OF NEUROLOGIC DISEASES

Psychiatric symptoms occur in many neurologic diseases. Because the psychiatric complaints may be the first or the most prominent signs of a problem, the patient usually seeks or is referred for psychiatric attention initially. If the psychiatrist or psychologist recognizes the neurologic basis for the patient's psychiatric difficulty, early treatment and resolution of the nervous system disease are possible. Protracted delays in the diagnosis of a primarily organic problem can cause irreversible damage. A slowly progressive frontal lobe tumor may be completely resected early in its evolution; but, when an affective disorder is the only manifestation of the tumor, the patient may go untreated long after removal of the tumor is still feasible. Fortunately, this is an unusual situation. A more common problem is a seizure disorder that goes unrecognized until typical convulsions occur. The patient may suffer considerable disability while the seizure disorder is untreated, but he does not face substantial risk of irreversible damage. With anticonvulsant treatment, the patient will be able to return to his usual lifestyle. Despite the stigma still attached to epilepsy, most people affected by the patient's abnormal behavior will accept this diagnosis as an explanation for his problems and will reintegrate the epileptic individual into their lives.

Diagnosis of the neurologic problem does not signal the end of psychiatric support for the individual and those close to him. Fear of the implications of the neurologic disease may be extremely disabling to the patient, his spouse, or his family. The emphasis of the psychiatric assistance may change with the recognition of the organic nature of the problem, but the psychiatric assistance is still often valuable, if not, in fact, indispensable.

Affective disorders develop with structural and metabolic lesions in the brain. Wilson disease and Huntington disease are both degenerative disorders of the brain often causing life-threatening depressive disorders. Suicide is common in both of these diseases. In fact, a suicide attempt may be the first sign of a degenerative central nervous system disease. Although Huntington disease is incurable, Wilson disease can be treated effectively with medication. Without early, appropriate treatment the patient with Wilson disease will develop permanent intellectual problems and movement disorders. Establishing the diagnosis of Huntington disease is also important in a very practical sense because this is a hereditary disorder. Half of the affected individual's children will inherit the gene causing the disease. Early diagnosis will help his or her spouse decide whether or not to have more children with the affected individual.

Cognitive disorders also develop with organic brain disease. Schizophrenia-like syndromes appear with certain rare metabolic and convulsive disorders. Of course, the cognitive problems need not be so severe that the patient is clearly psychotic. Children with frequent, inapparent seizures may have substantial learning problems and often present considerable discipline problems. Adult behavior is also profoundly affected by clinically inapparent seizures or slowly progressive brain damage. The attentive, considerate husband may become indifferent or abusive to his wife. The sexually active woman may abruptly lose sexual interest. Each of these problems demands a critical appraisal by the psychiatrist. He must be aware of when to suspect a neurologic problem and when to dismiss it. Viewing every patient with psychiatric disease as a victim of neurologic disease is just as unproductive as never entertaining the possibility of structural or metabolic disease in psychiatric disorders.

PSYCHIATRIC BASES FOR NEUROLOGIC SIGNS AND SYMPTOMS

Patients with psychiatric problems often have neurologic symptoms. More sophisticated patients may even feign neurologic signs. Psychogenic unresponsiveness is a frequent problem in an emergency room setting.

Patients with psychiatric problems are presented to the emergency room staff with little or no history in a variety of unresponsive states. A patient's behavior often raises concerns that a catastrophic intracranial event has occurred and dramatic measures, such as intubation or arteriography, may be taken before the psychologic basis for the patient's condition is appreciated. Chronic psychogenic complaints can also place the patient at risk of iatrogenic disease. Lumbar spine pain is an especially common cause of surgical intervention in patients with essentially psychiatric problems. When the low back pain provides substantial secondary gain for the disabled patient, recovery from the disability may be virtually impossible. Multiple back operations, regardless of the skill exhibited by the surgeon, commonly produce intractable back pain or weakness; and the patient with unremitting back pain for whatever reason is precisely the individual most at risk for multiple surgical procedures on the back. What starts as a "compensation neurosis" may lead to structural damage to the spine. Damage to body parts also occurs even when the medical or surgical physician does not intervene directly in an effort to relieve the patient's symptoms. A patient intent upon immobilizing a limb because of an alleged disability may soon discover that objective changes are occurring in the limb as the abnormal lack of activity starts taking its toll. The classic example of this is reflex sympathetic dystrophy. Patients with reflex sympathetic dystrophy have abnormal autonomic nervous system activity in the immobilized limb after the inactivity has been enforced for several weeks.

Seizures are frequently contrived, but distinguishing an authentic seizure from a contrived seizure is difficult even for physicians observing seizures every day. Patients with well-documented seizures may be able to feign very convincing epileptic fits. Fortunately, the technology necessary to separate true epilepsy from contrived epilepsy places the patient at no risk.

NEUROLOGIC COMPLICATIONS OF PSYCHIATRIC TREATMENT

Most psychoactive drugs cause neurologic side effects. Patients receiving electroconvulsive therapy rather than or in addition to medication are especially likely to manifest neurologic signs and symptoms. These are accepted consequences of psychiatric treatment, but they must be minimized for the psychiatric treatment of the patient to be truly successful. A mildly anxious patient who develops a permanent movement disorder secondary to the psychoactive drugs used to ameliorate the anxiety does not benefit optimally from the psychiatric intervention. Severe memory disorders after electroconvulsive therapy are unlikely but should be avoided with all the techniques currently available for managing depressed patients. Dealing with these neurologic complications of psychiatric treatment demands some familiarity with what signs and symptoms may arise and some knowledge of what treatments are available for the signs and symptoms once they have occurred. The stereotypy and mannerisms characteristic of some schizophrenic patients should not be confused with the tardive dyskinesias developing with neuroleptic use. Recognizing the precise nature of the movement disorder allows the psychiatrist either to pursue more aggressive treatment of the schizophrenia or to introduce additional drugs to deal with the tardive dyskinesia. Anxiety can produce tremor in the severely depressed patient, but lithium can also elicit this neurologic sign. Identifying what is responsible for the neurologic sign will allow adjustment of the treatment to minimize the side effects.

PSYCHIATRIC COMPLICATIONS OF NEUROLOGIC TREATMENT

Psychiatrists frequently assist in the evaluation and treatment of patients with well-documented neurologic diseases who develop psychiatric signs and symptoms during their treatment. Levodopa and bromocriptine treatment of Parkinson disease often causes acute psychotic disorders with prominent hallucinations and paranoid ideation. Visual hallucinations are a common problem after occipital lobe damage, and auditory hallucinations occasionally confuse the evaluation of patients who have had temporal lobe surgery. Although steroids may ameliorate an organic psychosis secondary to systemic lupus erythematosus, steroid treatment of a central nervous system vasculitis, or of an inflammatory muscle disorder, may also precipitate a schizophreniform psychosis. Dealing with psychiatric complications or features in patients with organic brain disease requires some familiarity with the neurologic condition causing the affective or cognitive disorder. One of the common functions of the psychiatrist is to recommend treatment that will not exacerbate the underlying condition. Substantial phenothiazine or butyrophenone use in psychotic patients with Parkinson disease is generally self-defeating. The psychosis may subside, but the patient will be seriously impaired by the treatment. Using electroconvulsive therapy in a severely depressed patient with poorly controlled epilepsy may simply exacerbate the seizure disorder and precipitate a more profound depression. What is appropriate psychiatric intervention in conventional settings may be totally inappropriate in patients with neurologic disease.

2
Diagnostic Tools

Many different diagnostic tools are available for investigating the structure and function of the nervous system. Clinical, physiologic, radiologic, and histologic approaches to neurologic disorders allow early, accurate diagnosis of most diseases affecting neural tissue and skeletal muscle. Of course, there are still many conditions affecting nerve and muscle tissues that cannot be explained or treated, but, with the diagnostic techniques currently available, they at least can be recognized. This has eliminated much of the mistreatment of patients with untreatable lesions that was unavoidable when one disease could not be differentiated from another. For the patient with signs and symptoms that can be easily contrived, the current assortment of objective tests provides a generally reliable basis for discriminating between victims of neurologic disease and victims of psychiatric disease. Unfortunately, all of the tests used in the evaluation of psychiatric and neurologic problems provide limited information about the patient. The authenticity of a patient's complaints is often more easily determined by a physician familiar with the patient for months or years than by a battery of tests arbitrarily chosen to investigate poorly defined symptoms. Even when the diagnostic studies reveal a lesion, it is ultimately the clinician's job to decide whether the pathology uncovered is responsible for the symptoms that brought the patient to the attention of a psychiatrist or psychologist.

The neurologic examination unassisted by invasive techniques or special apparatus is the oldest and still the most useful tool for establishing the presence or the absence of disease of the nervous system. Most neurologic diagnoses can be arrived at with a clinical examination alone (1). The invasive and noninvasive studies available to the clinician will help to confirm suspicions or dismiss fears, but they will not often reveal unanticipated pathology. Tests routinely used vary from not at all invasive to highly invasive and damaging to the nervous system. The less invasive a diagnostic test, the more likely it is to be used; and so the x-ray films of the skull and the electroencephalogram are commonly employed as adjuncts to the clinical examination with psychiatric or neurologic complaints. Computed tomography of the head is a noninvasive technique for studying densities in and around the brain. It is as safe as an x-ray study of the skull, but its current costs and technical complexity limit its application. Radionuclide studies of the brain and the cerebrospinal fluid are minimally invasive, but the problems involved in handling radioactive materials make radionuclide studies less attractive than computed tomography for routine investigations. Electrical studies of nerve and muscle function, called electromyography and nerve conduction studies, are uncomfortable and necessarily invasive, but little real damage is done to muscle or nerve during these studies. These electrophysiologic techniques are commonly used to investigate patients with peripheral neuropathy or primary muscle disease. Introduction of a needle into the subarachnoid space at the level of the lumbar spine or into the cisterna magna at the base of the skull will yield cerebrospinal fluid. This fluid often provides much information on the status of the central nervous system, but the spinal or cisternal tap is somewhat hazardous in inexperienced hands. Biopsy studies of nerve, muscle, or brain tissue are obviously very invasive; they are employed only when destruction of some of the patient's tissue is essential for establishing a diagnosis. This technique is usually employed when the loss of tissue is inconsequential and the dangers inherent in treating the patient without histologic confirmation of the diagnosis are unacceptable.

Some investigative techniques are useful in evaluating quite specific signs or symptoms. Electronystagmography helps in the investigation of abnormal eye movements or vertigo, and visual evoked potentials help in the assessment of optic nerve function. Other techniques carry substantial risks, but they are routinely used because alternative approaches to certain types of pathology are not currently available. An aneurysm, that is, an outpouching on an intracranial artery, cannot be seen with any of the diagnostic tools already mentioned, but will be apparent on arteriography. The patency of a major artery supplying the brain also can only be established by an arteriogram. Noninvasive blood vessel studies, such as Doppler studies, show some promise, but are still too imprecise to help with clinical decisions. Evoked potential studies using visual or noxious stimuli are also developing into promising techniques; but they currently have little application in routine clinical situations. Proton emission tomography is an entirely experimental technique developed along the lines of computed tomography, and its application to clinical investigations remains to be developed.

The following is a cursory review of the diagnostic tools most commonly used in the investigation of patients with neurologic problems. Their application to specific psychiatric problems will be enlarged upon in the chapters dealing with various symptoms. Familiarity with these techniques is of value for the psychiatrist or psychologist not only because it enables him to apply them when appropriate, but also because it provides him with perspective on their usefulness and their limitations.

NEUROLOGIC EXAMINATION

History

Many neurologic conditions can be diagnosed on the basis of the patient's history alone, but the patient's intellectual function will influence the value of the history (2). In some cases vital details can be provided only by the patient. Even individuals present when a patient loses consciousness cannot describe the sensations experienced by the victim of the altered consciousness. If the patient cannot recall the events surrounding his illness or if he cannot communicate what he can recall, valuable information is lost. Of course an extensive history is not necessarily a reliable history. Regardless of how detailed and convincing the patient's history is, it must always be viewed with a critical eye. Confabulation is prominent in a variety of dementias, including Korsakoff psychosis associated with chronic alcohol abuse. Impaired memory is also an early sign of several progressive degenerative diseases of the brain, such as Alzheimer and Pick disease. More discrete gaps in memory suggest more transient brain dysfunctions. The patient will be unable to account for long periods of time if during that time he had an epileptic fit or a transient ischemic attack. Transient ischemic attacks are episodes of impaired blood flow to the brain that cause neurologic signs that last less than a day. In some patients, the only neurologic sign developing with the transient ischemic attack is a transient global amnesia.

A comprehensive neurologic examination should include an assessment of the patient's consistency and attentiveness (3). This may require little more than an informal discussion of items ordinarily familiar to the patient, such as current political figures, recent changes in the weather, or features of the location in which the examination is being conducted. These topics should elicit no affective reaction in the patient and will provide an indication of the patient's ability to accurately answer questions relating to the history of his illness. A more formal evaluation of the patient's intellectual function is advisable after as much history has been obtained from the patient as possible. Since many diagnoses can be reached on the basis of the history alone, it is important to obtain this information before the patient is fatigued or uncooperative.

Most patients are reluctant to discuss specific items in the history which they find embarrassing, but significant information can usually be gleaned by matter-of-fact questioning of the areas not discussed by the patient. Every examination should include specific questions regarding family problems, sexual behavior, financial concerns, and chronic fears. A family history of psychiatric difficulty may be purposely omitted by the patient concerned about his own mental health; but, when this information is obtained, it may suggest a treatable brain disease that was never considered by physicians treating the other affected family members. Most patients seek professional help after they have decided upon possible causes of their symptoms. They may fear a brain tumor, multiple sclerosis, stroke, or other devastating illness is responsible for their neurologic or psychiatric disease. Reassurance that they do not suffer from these disorders may do more for their illness-related anxiety than actually providing them with a diagnosis. Sexual problems, venereal diseases, and failures in intimate relationships are usually glossed over by the patient, but they may play vital roles in determining the cause of the patient's current problems. Psychiatrists and psychologists are generally more sensitive than most clinicians to what the patient is not saying. This is especially valuable in dealing with patients with neurologic or psychiatric disorders, because the gaps in the history are often where the bulk of the history is.

Some questions will usually not be answered honestly regardless of how direct the physician is. Lawsuits and addictions are especially sensitive areas. Whenever the patient has alluded to an accident or an assault, it is wise to ask if he is involved in litigation. A compensation neurosis may have induced the patient to seek medical advice. A denial of alcoholism in a patient with a syndrome highly suggestive of alcohol abuse should be noted, but not taken as an established fact. Quite often family members will try to conceal the patient's alcohol abuse or past psychiatric history in a misguided attempt to maintain the patient's dignity. Past operations, past illnesses, and past hospitalizations should be specifically questioned, and all the medication that the patient is currently taking must be known. Scars, bruises, and needle marks on the body should be explained, and the explanations should be consistent.

Systemic Examination

Any neurologic exam includes a general physical examination with evaluation of the skin, joints, heart, lungs, abdominal organs, blood pressure, temperature, pulse, and respiratory rate of the patient. Deficits in organ systems separate from the neuromuscular systems may explain the psychiatric or neurologic dysfunction that prompted the patient's initial consultation (2). A purplish (heliotrope) rash about the eyes in a patient with proximal muscle weakness and tenderness indicates dermatomyositis, a collagen vascular disease. Fever and a heart murmur in a child with weakness on one side of the body is fairly specific for a stroke associated with subacute bacterial endocarditis, an infection of the heart valves that discharges emboli to lodge in the brain. An abdominal mass in a child with erratic eye movements (opsoclonus) and a very unsteady gait ("dancing feet") are highly suggestive of cerebellar degeneration in association with a neural tumor, neuroblastoma. Hypertension, arthritis, and an acute psychosis suggest systemic lupus erythematosus. Any abnormal physical finding on the general examination must be viewed as possibly related to the problem prompting the consultation.

Neurologic Signs

The neurologic examination includes a systematic evaluation of mental status, cranial nerve function, sensory function, motor abilities, coordination, and reflexes. The attention given to each of these areas will be determined by the nature of the patient's major complaint (3). If the patient seems unable to communicate, a lengthy speech evaluation is obviously appropriate and an exhaustive evaluation of muscle strength in intrinsic muscles of the hand is inappropriate. Sensory testing with pain, touch, vibration, and joint position stimuli is adequate in most cases, but some patients with confusing patterns of sensory loss or special cognitive dysfunctions may require an evaluation of two-point discrimination, traced figure recognition, temperature comparisons, and tactile recognition of objects (4). The functions requiring special testing are usually determined during the course of the neurologic examination itself.

Mental Status Assessment

Having assessed the course of the patient's illness, its duration and onset, and the instances of past episodes, the examiner has usually reached some conclusions about both the disease and the patient's ability to communicate. Language skill is often related to the extent of the patient's formal education, and so the examiner must know how much and what type of schooling the patient had. Problems with language are important to recognize early in the examination. If the patient cannot understand instructions, his failure to accurately perform tests may be misconstrued as dementia (5). Difficulty with naming items that arise in conversation or with finding the right word to convey a specific idea will force the patient to circumlocute. If there is an abnormal rhythm or impaired clarity inherent in the patient's speech, then family members should be consulted to see if this is a new feature, a slowly evolving deficit, or a feature of speech exhibited by all members of the family. Quite often the patient himself will be unaware of any changes in his speech, even though considerable slurring and slowing of speech may be present. Reading and writing samples will help to further document the patient's language problems, and every patient should be asked to repeat a few simple phrases. Even if the patient has no problems finding the right words for conversational speech, he should be asked the names of several familiar items. If any of these language functions are impaired, that impairment must be considered in assessing any other problems exhibited by the patient during the examination. Errors in performing tests of coordination may be from a misunderstanding of the maneuver requested by the examiner. Failure to look to one side may be because of failure to understand the instruction rather than because of extraocular muscle weakness.

Every language examination should include an assessment of the patient's handedness. Because peculiar patterns of language impairment develop in patient's who are not strictly right-handed, the true handedness of the patient should not be assumed to be the hand with which he writes. Many children are forced to write with their right hand as part of their socialization. These individuals with a tendency to use their left hands may still eat, open locks, point, and throw with their left hands. Some individuals are not strictly right-handed or left-handed. Where there is some question about which hand is dominant it is best to simply note what the patient routinely does with each hand.

That there is an affective disorder or cognitive disorder will usually be obvious although the precise nature of the problem may not be so obvious. A patient with a flat affect, with loose associations, or with delusions about changes in various body parts will usually exhibit these abnormalities while the history is being obtained. If the patient laughs or cries for no apparent reason during the interview, a degenerative brain disease producing labile affect may be responsible. If the patient constantly shifts the focus of the discussion, a metabolic encephalopathy, such as that developing with hyperthyroidism, may be responsible. Patients occasionally try to conceal intellectual problems by inventing complex explanations for their aberrant behavior. If a memory defect is part of the patient's problem, he may have frank confabulation. With confabulation the patient is usually quite inconsistent or contradicts information already obtained from individuals familiar with him. Regardless of how intact the patient's intellectual function appears, specific questions to assess orientation are essential. An intelligent patient may evade the entire issue of orientation without the examiner's being aware of the omission. Whether or not the patient knows who he is, where he is, what the date is, and what his current situation is will help quantify the degree of dementia present.

Tests to evaluate the patient's ability to construct items either with objects or with pencil and paper can be used with patients who have motor, sensory, or visual impairments that interfere with their constructional abilities, but the neurologic defect will affect the results in fairly predictable ways. Patients with visual field cuts will omit the parts of the drawing or construction that fall into their field cuts. Impaired position sense on one side of the body will impair any performance that involves the defective limbs. Construction tests may be quite revealing when the patient has no focal deficits, but still fails to accurately perform the task requested. A clock drawn with all of its numbers on one half of the face may indicate neglect of one visual field, even though there is no visual field cut. Efforts to draw a circle may be frustrated by the patient's inability to connect the beginning and end of the circle. Consequently, his arc spirals in toward the center of his drawing. These types of construction problems often indicate parietal lobe damage that may not be otherwise evident (Figure 2.1).

Memory enters into many aspects of the neurologic examination, and problems with memory may produce confusing signs unless the nature of the defect is recognized early in the evaluation. There are several facets to memory, and each must be assessed separately. Much of what is considered judgment is actually a test of learned responses to specific situations. When asked what they would do with an envelope found on the street, stamped and addressed, some patients will answer that they would mail it and other patients will answer that they would open it. Which answer they choose is more a matter of training and recall than of judgment. Recalling five items after waiting 5 minutes is a more objective test of memory function than the situation presented above, but this is only a test of short-term memory. Similarly, the immediate recall of a list of digits either in order or in reversed sequence requires no special training or specific cultural background to be accurately performed, but only the registration and repetition of uncomplicated material is tested

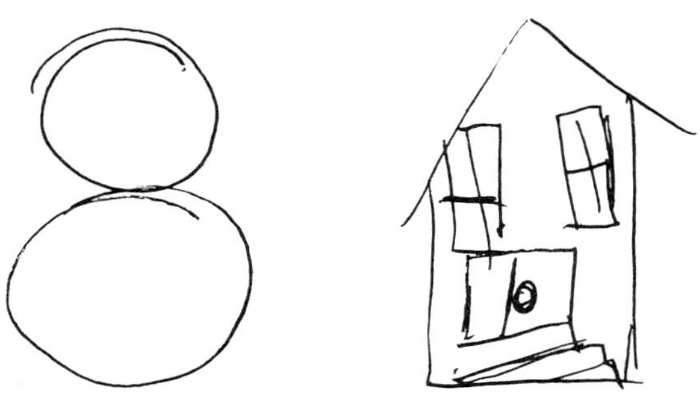

A. B.

Figure 2.1. A 61-year-old, right-handed man drew these circles (A) and this house (B) six years after he had suffered a right parietal lobe stroke. Although the left arm and leg weakness that developed at the time of the stroke had completely resolved, he was still disabled by his inability to deal with spatial relationships. Despite repeated attempts to improve his drawing and three-dimensional construction, he always failed to perform near the level he was capable of before the stroke. Before his illness, this man worked as a highly skilled, custom tailor and drew maps as a hobby. After the stroke, he was no longer able to assemble garments. He put zippers in backward and always failed to end a hem where he started it. On trying to draw circles, he could never complete the circle at the point where he had started it, He explained this as simply losing track of where the beginning was. The angles on the house that he drew were irregular, and many elements in the picture, such as the front door and the stairs, were fragmented. He had no visual field defects, weakness, clumsiness, or impaired sensation.

with this technique. Comparing the history provided by the patient with well-documented facts available to the examiner is the simplest and best method for evaluating long-term memory. There are cognitive problems that will limit the application of many of these tests. If the patient is actively hallucinating, his cooperation may be quite poor; and, if the patient is stuporous, his cooperation will be inconsistent.

Calculations involve memory, but memory alone is not enough to accurately perform mathematical manipulations. Logic and the application of rules are also involved, but how well the patient will perform calculations is largely dependent upon his training. Tests of multiplication, division, subtraction, fractions, and square roots may be appropriate depending upon the extent of the patient's education. The evaluation of a certified public accountant is vastly different from the evaluation of a fourth grade dropout. Quite often the patient will point to the difficulty even when it does not appear on a cursory examination. A bank teller may report that he is miscalculating on a daily basis, when extensive tests of arithmetic abilities fail to turn up any deficits whatsoever.

Subtle changes in behavior often suggest major pathology, but the behavior itself may be very uninformative when considered isolated from the patient. A bank president who arrives at work with unpolished shoes and an unbuttoned shirt arouses much more concern in his fellow employees than does a medical intern arriving in the same unkempt condition. The bank president may have a frontal lobe tumor, whereas the medical intern probably has profound sleep deprivation. The change in behavior and the context of the behavior is often helpful in deciding what types of problems to consider (6).

Cranial Nerve Examination

The cranial nerves supply the head and neck with sensory and motor innervation and are separated into twelve discrete elements by anatomic convention. More than 12 functions are served by these nerves, and, in fact, several of the nerves have several components (7). Because of the intimate relationship between several of these nerves and the brain, abnormalities of cranial nerve function can be very helpful in defining intracranial pathology.

Olfactory Nerve. The first cranial nerve is the olfactory nerve, and it is responsible for smell. Disorders of the olfactory nerve and resulting loss of smell may develop with serious neurologic conditions, such as olfactory groove meningioma, a benign tumor in the lining of the brain overlying the olfactory nerve. Unfortunately, many people lose their ability to smell and to differentiate between various smells as they grow older. This is especially true in heavily industrialized areas with substantial air pollution. Items used in evaluating smells should never be irritating to the nasal mucosa. Bland, but distinctive, odors, such as that from coffee or tobacco, are appropriate for olfactory testing. Taste and smell are intimately related in practice, and so many patients complaining of impaired taste actually have disturbed smell. Olfactory hallucinations are common in both schizophrenic and epileptic disorders. Chronic complaints of an inescapable foul smell occur with some structural lesions in the temporal lobes. This type of hallucination in association with a change in behavior justifies further investigation of the patient's temporal lobe function (8). An electroencephalogram with nasopharyngeal leads and a computed tomogram with contrast enhancement, both of which are discussed below, will demonstrate most of the structural or physiologic problems that could cause this combination of signs.

Optic Nerve. The second cranial nerve is the optic nerve. It is actually an extension of brain tissue rather than a true nerve, which is why many of the abnormalities apparent in the optic nerve provide insight into abnormalities in the brain itself. Increased intracranial pressure will cause swelling of the optic nerve at its entry into the retina. The site exhibiting the swelling is called the optic disc, and the swelling itself is called papilledema. With greatly increased intracranial pressure, papilledema will be accompanied by minor hemorrhages and exudates in the retina. Several conditions produce changes in the optic disc that are difficult to distinguish from papilledema but are not caused by increased intracranial pressure. Inflammation of the optic nerve with infection or demyelinating disease, congenital abnormalities of the nerve including abnormally myelinated retinal fibers, and idiopathic deposits in the optic nerve or at its margins (drusen) can all produce pseudopapilledema (9). Tumors about the optic nerve can produce swelling of the optic disc that is not associated with increased intracranial pressure. Persistent papilledema can produce visual loss, but the principal danger with papilledema is from the lesion responsible for the increased intracranial pressure.

Degenerative diseases of the brain may be associated with degenerative changes in the retina not limited to the optic disc. Pigmentary degeneration and retinal damage develop with some metabolic diseases causing peripheral neuropathy and cerebellar damage. Of course, retinal changes need not always be associated with damage to the central nervous system in diseases with systemic signs. Diabetes mellitus often causes changes in the blood vessels of the retina with no similar damage appearing in the blood vessels of the brain or spinal cord. Infections that affect the brain may affect both the brain and the eye. The retinal damage called chorioretinitis that develops with toxoplasmosis infection may indicate damage to the basal ganglia of the brain from the same agent.

The limits of peripheral vision constitute the visual field. This is mapped out by having the patient stare at one spot and report when a small object can be seen at the periphery. The visual field of each eye is examined separately because the two fields overlap and defects in the visual field of one eye may be compensated for by the extent of vision in the other eye. The lateral half of the field is called the temporal field and the medial half is the nasal field. Quadrants of the field are called superior or inferior. Normal individuals have a small blind spot in their temporal visual fields because there are no photoreceptor cells on the retina at the optic disc. Blind spots are referred to as scotomas, and the blind spot marking the optic disc is called the cecal scotoma. Defects in the visual field and constriction of the visual field can develop with disease in the eye, in the optic nerve, at the juncture of the optic nerves (the optic chiasm), along the optic tract, or in the brain (9,10). A bitemporal field cut, that is, a field cut that affects the lateral half or a lateral quarter of the field in each eye usually develops with a tumor of the pituitary gland or a lesion in the region of the optic chiasm. Binasal field cuts (binasal hemianopias) are most characteristic of glaucoma, an increase in the intraocular pressure. With nutritional diseases, an enlarged blind spot extending into the central field of vision, a so-called centrocecal scotoma, may produce functional blindness without loss of peripheral vision. Most centrocecal scotomas are idiopathic, but tobacco and alcohol have been implicated so often as causes that this type of visual loss is often called tobacco-alcohol amblyopia. In the early ophthalmologic literature sexual excess was considered the most common cause. Sexual activiy is no longer considered a basis for visual loss.

Oculomotor, Trochlear, and Abducens Nerves. The third, fourth, and sixth cranial nerves are responsible for eye movements. The third nerve alone controls pupillary constriction. Examining both the eye movements and the pupils will frequently clarify the cause of a central nervous system problem. An irregular pupil that responds to changes in the distance an object is from the eye, but not to changes in the brightness of a light shining into the eye, is called an Argyll-Robertson pupil. This disorder of pupillary constriction commonly developed with neurosyphilis before the introduction of penicillin. Now it is more typically seen with diabetes mellitus. Unilateral dilatation of a pupil in a conscious patient may develop when an aneurysm is pressing on the third cranial nerve. This sign of a blood vessel abnormality usually occurs when the posterior communicating artery in the circle of Willis has the outpouching. Pupillary responses may be direct, that is, from light shining into the responding eye, or consensual, that is, from light shining into the other eye. Particular patterns of pupillary response may be quite specific for particular disease entities. A brisk consensual response associated with a weak direct response develops with optic neuritis and is most often seen with multiple sclerosis. This type of afferent pupillary defect is called the Marcus-Gunn pupillary reflex. Dilatation of the pupil is controlled by an entirely separate system of nerves, which are part of the sympathetic nervous system. Damage to these nerves may produce a persistently small pupil.

A full range of extraocular movements should be apparent in every patient. The eyes should be able to move smoothly in pursuit of a moving object or briskly in step-like movements in looking from one point to another. The smooth movements are called pursuit or tracking eye movements, and the step-like movements are saccades. Upward gaze is the most commonly limited eye movement. With age, the range of upward movement decreases. Premature impairment of upward gaze may indicate degenerative brain disease, such as Parkinson disease. All eye movements should be coordinated so that the two eyes are moving in step together, that is, conjugately. One eye moving independently of the other is abnormal, and the movement is called dysconjugate. Minor weakness in an extraocular muscle may be made more obvious by covering one eye with a red filter and thereby allowing dysconjugate movements to occur. Since the two eyes are seeing different images, one red and one normal in color, the strongest stimulus for conjugate gaze, the coincidence of the same image in both eyes, is disturbed. Individuals with no problems in coordination of eye movements will still have conjugate gaze, but an imbalance in the activity of any extraocular muscle will be enhanced with this technique. If the red filter is over the eye with the weak muscle, the red image will appear to be where the eye is not moving. In other words, if the patient is looking at a light and the filter is over the right eye, the red light will appear to be to the right of the white light if he has weakness in the muscle abducting the right eye. This would be a lateral rectus muscle palsy. Weakness in abduction often develops from compression of the nerve to the lateral rectus, the abducens nerve, when there is increased intracranial pressure.

Specific eye movement disorders are sought in every patient examined neurologically. One of these is nystagmus, an oscillatory movement of the eyes, often induced by drugs or structural brain disease. Although it is always pathologic when it appears spontaneously, it can be elicited with special maneuvers in any normal individual. Nystagmus appears normally when a striped cloth is drawn in front of the eyes. The patient is asked to count the stripes as they go by the center of his vision, and, with each passing stripe, the patient momentarily follows and then shifts his gaze to the next stripe. This type of nystagmus is called optokinetic nystagmus (11). Both eyes should move with the same speed and amplitude. If movements in the two eyes are not symmetric, the patient may have disease of the parietal lobe. Nystagmus on lateral and upward gaze, but not on downward gaze, commonly occurs with barbiturate or anticonvulsant excess. Some antipsychotic drugs will also produce nystagmus even when the drug is within the therapeutic range.

Damage in the brainstem, rather than higher in the brain in the cerebral cortex, may involve the third, fourth, or sixth cranial nerve nuclei or the nerves themselves (7,12). Because the brainstem has so many motor and sensory pathways passing by each other in such a small space, damage to an ocular motor nucleus is rarely an isolated sign. Facial weakness or a sensory deficit will routinely accompany the ocular motor abnormality. Damage to the nerve as it exits the brainstem or before it reaches the extraocular muscles is more often an isolated event. With head trauma the patient may have damage to the fourth nerve and compensate for the resulting weakness in the superior oblique muscle with a slight head tilt. The superior oblique rotates the eye inward, and so loss of function in this muscle can be compensated for by tilting the head away from the involved eye.

Trigeminal Nerve. The fifth cranial nerve has three divisions, the ophthalmic, maxillary, and mandibular. These monitor facial pain and touch as well as the sensory input for the corneal reflex. Problems with head and facial pain are extremely common in patients with psychiatric problems; this topic is discussed in detail in the chapter on headache and facial pain. While examining the face, the clinician should remember that facial pain can develop without any associated sensory loss over the face. Loss of facial sensitivity to touch or pinprick may indicate damage to a branch of the trigeminal nerve, but it may also be from damage to the brain. Any loss of facial or corneal sensitivity raises the possibility of brainstem damage (13). A destructive lesion of the brainstem, however, usually produces deficits in cranial nerves besides the fifth cranial nerve.

The most objective element in the tests of trigeminal nerve function is the corneal blink reflex. Touching the edge of the cornea with a wisp of cotton will provoke a blink that is difficult to suppress. Both eyes usually blink with stimulation of just one cornea. Even the hysterical patient who claims to have no sensation over one half of his face will exhibit this blink response. Most patients do not realize that the reflex is related to facial pain appreciation, because the stimulus for the blink reflex is not painful. Although the corneal reflex is primarily a brainstem reflex, cerebral cortical strokes will produce asymmetry in the corneal reflex along with facial weakness and hemiplegia if the motor cortex is involved.

Patients with hysterical sensory loss over the face will usually complain of nonanatomic patterns of sensory change. Impaired sensation may stop at the hairline or precisely divide the skin of the nose along the midline. An injured trigeminal nerve will cause loss of sensation well above the hairline if the first division of the nerve is involved. Patients with authentic impairment of facial sensation occasionally consult physicians because they believe they are having sensory hallucinations. After a severe facial injury, the patient may have pins-and-needles or stabbing sensations in the face about the same area as the loss of sensation. These are normal phenomena and are not from anxiety. Most patients do not realize that pain and anesthesia can coexist, and they are often the first to suggest that the disturbing facial sensations developing after a nerve injury are from anxiety.

Facial Nerve. The seventh cranial nerve is primarily responsible for facial strength. A small branch supplies the muscle on the stapedius ossicle in the middle ear. Branches also arise from the taste buds and join the facial nerve in the middle ear, and so with damage to the seventh cranial nerve there may be disturbed taste as well as hearing (14). Facial weakness is a common problem, the cause of the weakness usually not being apparent. This idiopathic facial weakness is called Bell's palsy, and it is often associated with some pain behind the ear, as well as loss of taste and increased sensitivity to noises in the ear on the side affected. Mild facial weakness developing after involvement of the motor cortex in the brain may be apparent by flattening of all the folds on the face on the side of the weakness, but in more subtle cases only a slight widening of the palpebral fissure will be evident. In extreme cases weakness may be experienced by the patient but not be apparent to the examiner except when the patient is talking. Although there is no significant sensory loss with damage to the facial nerve, the patient often complains that his face feels heavy.

Acoustic Nerve. The eighth cranial nerve carries information for hearing and balance. Progressive hearing loss will develop with disease anywhere along this cranial nerve. Obviously most problems with hearing do not result from damage to the nerve, but rather result from damage to the cochlea, the hearing end organ, or to the structural elements of the middle or outer ear (14). Hearing can be easily tested in the cooperative patient by rubbing fingers together close to the ear or by having the patient indicate when he starts hearing a watch moving closer to the ear. Subtle differences between the two sides can be checked by putting a vibrating fork on the middle of the forehead and seeing if the sound is perceived as coming more from one side than the other. This test involves conduction of sound primarily through the bones of the skull, rather than through the external auditory meatus and into the ear by way of the tympanic membrane. Placing a tuning fork beside the ear and asking the patient when the sound is no longer audible will help determine the ear's ability to perceive sounds conducted through air, rather than bone. The normal patient will be more sensitive to sounds transmitted by way of the skull, and when he can no longer hear the vibrating fork near his ear he should still be able to hear it when the fork is in place on the skull behind the ear.

Lesions to be considered in cases of progressive hearing loss or intermittent balance problems include neurofibromas of the eighth cranial nerve, also known as schwannomas, and viral infections of the ear. Intractable balance problems are as often from cerebellar or brainstem damage as they are from damage to the semicircular canals of the ears. Problems related to function of the acoustic nerve are considered in more detail in the chapter on hearing and balance problems.

Glossopharyngeal and Vagus Nerves. The glossopharyngeal and vagus nerves are extremely important in a variety of neurologic disorders, but they rarely cause disorders confused with psychiatric difficulty. On routine examination, these two nerves will be tested by observing voluntary palate retraction and the gag reflex. Sensation and taste from the palate and some of the oropharynx are carried along the ninth or glossopharyngeal nerve. Innervation of the muscles of the soft palate and the adjacent oropharynx is provided by the tenth or vagus nerve. The vagus nerve is an exceptional cranial nerve with branches travelling into the thorax and abdomen to regulate a variety of body functions.

Problems with vomiting are discussed in the chapter on abnormal movements. Questions sometimes arise regarding hyperactivity of the gag reflex in patients with recurrent vomiting, but problems with this reflex are almost always limited to impaired activity, rather than overactivity. Patients with eating disorders induce vomiting by stimulating the gag reflex in most cases, but there are neurologic disorders, such as increased intracranial pressure, that can increase the tendency to vomit.

Spinal Accessory Nerve. The eleventh cranial nerve innervates the sternocleidomastoid and trapezius muscles. The function of this nerve is readily checked by having the patient shrug his shoulders or turn his head to one side. Patients with hysterical weakness usually claim weakness on trying to turn their head towards the side of their arm and leg weakness. With real sternocleidomastoid weakness, the deficit will be on turning the head away from the weak side. This means that with paralysis of the left side of the body the patient will usually be able to turn his head to the left but unable to turn his head forcefully to the right. Weakness in these muscles will cause unstable or abnormal head postures. Although a variety of head tilts and head bobs have psychiatric bases, a spasmodic torticollis, an early myasthenia gravis, or a progressive anterior horn cell disease should not be overlooked as possible explanations for abnormal head postures and movements. These possibilities are discussed in the chapters on weakness and abnormal movements.

Hypoglossal Nerve. The twelfth cranial nerve supplies the muscles of the tongue. Normal tongue protrusion will be disturbed with damage to this nerve. If the nerve is cut, the tongue deviates toward the weak side, and the denervated half of the tongue atrophies. Twitching in the tongue may be the first sign of bulbar amyotrophic lateral sclerosis, a lethal degenerative disease of the motor system. Problems with tongue protrusion will develop in a variety of movement disorders, some of which are induced by antipsychotic drugs. Excessive tongue movements and protrusion are routine problems faced by psychiatrists treating psychotic patients with butyrophenones or phenothiazines.

Sensation

Normal individuals can feel several kinds of sensory stimuli. These sensory perceptions may be grossly divided into touch, pain, position sense, vibration sense, and temperature sense, but normal people are capable of sensory discriminations not suggested by these categories. Superficial and deep pain are distinctly different; a patient who feels pain when stuck with a pin may fail to feel pain when his Achilles' tendon or testicle is squeezed. Deep pain increases in intensity with persistence of the painful stimulus and subsides slowly after the stimulus is removed. Superficial pain is more immediate and transient. This does not mean that individual sensory functions are necessarily impaired independently of each other. In most cases, the opposite is true. Temperature perception is often linked to superficial pain perception. Vibration sense and position sense are both routinely impaired with vitamin B12 deficiency and with traumatic injuries to the dorsal aspect of the spinal cord.

With peripheral nerve damage, sensory functions may be selectively or uniformly disturbed. Position sense is selectively impaired in some patients with diabetes mellitus. If the impairment of position sense is substantial, the patient will be unable to stand with his feet close together when his eyes are closed. He has a positive Romberg sign if he can stand on a narrow base with his eyes open, even though he falls when he closes his eyes. Although this sign usually is positive if the patient has severe peripheral nerve damage from diabetes mellitus, it is not necessarily a sign of diabetes mellitus. It occurs with any disorder impairing position sense. The Romberg sign was initially described in patients with tabes dorsalis, the type of neurosyphilis that causes spinal cord damage.

Special sensory tests that all patients should be able to perform without any difficulty include recognition of numbers traced on their palms or even on their fingertips and recognition of objects placed in their hands. Stereognosis, the recognition of an object by feeling it, may be impaired when light touch or superficial pain is lost. This is also true of discriminating between two points. Two sharp points placed closely together on the skin may be perceived as one point. This test is of value in assessing the difference in sensory perception between two sides of the body. Different surfaces of the body have different capacities for two-point discrimination. The fingertips are especially sensitive and can perceive two points as separate when they are only a few millimeters apart; two points placed a centimeter apart on the back are generally perceived as one point. Some tests of sensory function are only appropriate under special circumstances. Assessing deep pain by pressing on the base of the fingernail or by squeezing the Achilles' tendon is useful in assessing the level of consciousness of a patient in coma but is generally not necessary in assessing the sensory function of an awake patient.

Strength and Tone

Motor function, like sensory function, is multifaceted. Several different elements work together in the motor system, and one element may be disturbed while others are unaffected. Muscles may have good strength and normal tone, but exhibit easy fatigability. Strength may be impaired by the inability of the muscle to relax. The type of problem exhibited by the patient often helps determine where in the neuromuscular system the problem is, but, more often than not, electrical and histologic studies of the muscle are needed to define the site of the problem.

Gait is a very sensitive test of motor function. Weakness in an arm may be manifested by decreased swing of the arm while the patient walks. Minor weakness in the leg may appear through circumduction of the leg at the hip or scuffing of the foot. The resistance that can be felt in a limb when it is moved passively is also quite revealing. Muscle tone in all limbs is normally equal. A stroke may leave the patient with markedly increased tone that produces increased resistance in the limbs on one side of the body when they are moved quickly. This rate-dependent increase in tone is called spasticity. It is quite different from the increased tone felt in the limbs of a parkinsonian patient. In those patients, tone is usually increased to the same extent regardless of the speed of the movement of the limb.

Nerve damage or spinal cord degeneration may be reflected in a muscle by very small contractions underneath the skin called fasciculations. With prolonged disconnection of a muscle from the nerve innervating it, atrophy, that is, a decrease in the mass of the muscle, will develop. Occasionally movement abnormalities developing with changes in strength are at a gross level. Minor weakness can produce tremors; testing the strength in the limb should help to ascertain whether the limb is weak or just poorly coordinated. If the patient has slight weakness in an arm, an apparent drift will develop when the arms are held out in front of the patient with his eyes closed. Patients with factitious weakness routinely allow their allegedly weak limbs to drift, but the authentically weak arm will usually pronate as well as drift.

Strength is often difficult to test because it differs so markedly between different normal patients. What is significant in the individual patient is an asymmetry in strength between limbs on the two sides of the body. A patient claiming to be weak over his entire body need not necessarily be hysterical. There are muscle disorders that result in diffuse weakness. One of these, myasthenia gravis, is usually associated with ocular problems. In these patients diffuse weakness will be associated with complaints of blurred vision or double vision. Older patients may have an arteritis producing diffuse weakness and malaise with no focal neurologic signs. The possible causes of weakness are considered in more detail in the chapter on weakness.

Coordination

Coordination is involved in isolated limb movements and in total body movements. There are several types of deficits that appear with impaired coordination, each type being caused by damage to one of several central or peripheral mechanisms. On routine neurologic examination, many of these coordination functions are tested simply because they are rather nonspecific indicators of nervous system damage. If the patient cannot accurately touch his nose with his eyes closed, this is called dysmetria. If he reaches for a point in space and misses that point, despite having his eyes open, that is usually called pastpointing. These defects in coordination are often associated with poor rapid alternating movements, a disorder known as dysdiadochokinesis. Problems with coordination are likely to be associated with tremors. The tremor may involve one limb, several limbs, the head, or the trunk. When it involves the head it is called titubation.

Starting and stopping movements smoothly and quickly are also aspects of coordination. If the movement is not stopped briskly, the patient has impaired check. If compensatory movements are exaggerated, the patient has excessive rebound. Many of these disorders, the dysmetria, pastpointing, impaired check and rebound, are the result of cerebellar disease (15). There are, of course, other causes for these deficits: marked dysmetria may develop with impaired position sense. The cause of the clumsiness and incoordination is invariably much more difficult to ascertain than the precise character of the coordination problem.

Reflexes

Reflexes normally change as the patient matures, and so any evaluation of reflexes must consider the age of the patient. Reflex muscle contractions on tapping the muscle tendons are normally present at all major joints, but their absence need not indicate significant pathology. Middle-aged women with absent ankle jerks and unreactive pupils have Adie's syndrome, a benign disorder of unknown cause. Stroking the lateral margin of the foot will induce the great toe to dorsiflex in an infant, but it does this in adults only when there is damage to the motor system above the level of the anterior horn cell of the spinal cord. This is called upper motor neuron disease, although that is more of a convenience than an accurate anatomic description of the lesion. Patients with cerebral strokes may have an upgoing or extensor plantar response (positive Babinski sign) in the foot opposite the side of the lesion. Deep tendon reflexes in the limbs are often lost with any disorder causing peripheral nerve damage. The grasp reflex, which is normal in infancy, may reappear in adults with progressive cerebral deterioration. This is also true of the sucking and snout reflexes. Stroking the palm of the hand may elicit a reflex contraction of a facial muscle in the chin on the same side of the body. This is called the palmomental reflex, and, when it is present asymmetrically, it usually indicates central nervous system disease.

ELECTROENCEPHALOGRAPHY

The electroencephalogram is a useful, noninvasive technique for evaluating brain activity. It has the advantage over most other diagnostic techniques of indicating physiologic disorders of the brain, even when there is no apparent structural damage. Structural lesions will usually cause changes in the brain wave activity, but determining the type of structural lesion responsible for the changes on the electroencephalogram will usually require further diagnostic studies. This technique is especially useful for evaluating psychiatric patients with symptoms probably not caused by a structural brain lesion. If the electroencephalogram is abnormal, further appropriate studies can be pursued; and, if it is not abnormal, the patient will be spared more invasive techniques. A patient with episodic confusion can be evaluated for seizure activity or transient ischemic attacks. The elderly patient who has dementia associated with profound depression can be assessed for focal brain damage. An unresponsive patient with a history of psychiatric disease and epilepsy can be evaluated for recurrent epileptic fits, metabolic encephalopathy, and other causes of stupor and coma. The changes in brain wave activity caused by psychoactive drugs are well defined, and so psychiatric patients can be examined with this technique even if they are on relatively high doses of antipsychotics or antidepressants.

Normal Brain Wave Patterns

Wires applied to the scalp at standard locations will normally pick up low amplitude electrical potentials arising largely from the cerebral cortex. Changes in these electrical potentials are registered by the electroencephalograph as deflections of a voltage-sensitive needle. Most machines currently in use have the voltage-sensitive needle connected to a pen, and the deflections are recorded when paper is drawn under the pen at a constant rate. Sets of eight or 16 pens allow several different combinations of electrodes to be monitored simultaneously. Each pen records the changes in electrical potential between only two electrodes on the scalp.

Several patterns of brain wave activity are normal in children and adults. When the patient is relaxed and has his eyes closed, rhythmical oscillations in the electrical potentials arising from the posterior part of the head will appear with a frequency of about 8 to 12 cycles per second. This 8 to 12 hertz activity is called alpha activity, and it will disappear abruptly when the patient opens his eyes or when he attempts complex intellectual tasks, such as multiplication or division (Figure 2.2). In normal adults this alpha activity will be the most apparent rhythmic activity; and the frequency of the alpha activity routinely decreases after the seventh decade of life (16). More anteriorly, the electroencephalogram will consist of irregular combinations of waves at varying frequencies. With drowsiness the overall frequency of the record slows. The various wave forms characteristic of sleep are discussed in the section on sleep disorders.

The significance of slow brain waves in the awake patient varies with the age of the patient. Infants have much slower brain wave activity than adults, and focal slowing is common and often benign in the elderly. Focal slowing of the brain waves to 5 or 6 hertz over one temporal lobe would be a worrisome sign in a 30-year-old individual, but it is usually associated with no significant pathology when it appears in a 70-year-old individual (16).

If a wave is sharply contoured and lasts less than one-fifth of a second, it is called a sharp wave. When a sharply contoured wave is less than 80 milliseconds in duration, it is called a spike. Sharp waves and spikes are often an indication of pathology, but in some situations they are normal. As discussed in the section on sleep, sharp waves may occur over the vertex of the head in various stages of sleep. Sharp waves may also be normal when they arise from the posterior head leads (electrodes) in the elderly. The significance attached to sharp waves and spikes has changed over the past 2 decades. Much of the controversy that arose in the past over whether or not patients behaving abnormally actually had seizure disorders, psychiatric problems, or criminal intentions arose from confusion over what sharp wave and spike forms were actually pathologic. Spikes that appear to be pointing downward and that occur at a frequency of 14 or 6 cycles per second, are called 14 and 6 per second positive spikes. These usually appear to arise in the temporal regions in healthy young adults or adolescents. They may appear during sleep and are not at all correlated with organic brain disease (17). With arousal from sleep, there may be high voltage wave activity with small notches that resemble spike and slow wave activity. These are generally seen in childhood and can easily be mistaken for pathologic activity (18). Prominent occipital sharp waves may appear early in sleep, but these too are normal activity. One of the most confusing normal variants is the so-called psychomotor variant, in which children or young adults have sharp or notched temporal waves. These are occasionally more prominent with drowsiness, but they are not associated with epilepsy or any particular structural lesion. Another unusual, but normal, wave form is the mu rhythm; this appears as a series of sharp waves at a rhythm of about 10 cycles per second. Obviously all of these variants can lead to considerable misinterpretation on the electroencephalogram, especially when a seizure is suspected. A child with a behavior disorder evaluated with an electroencephalogram may well

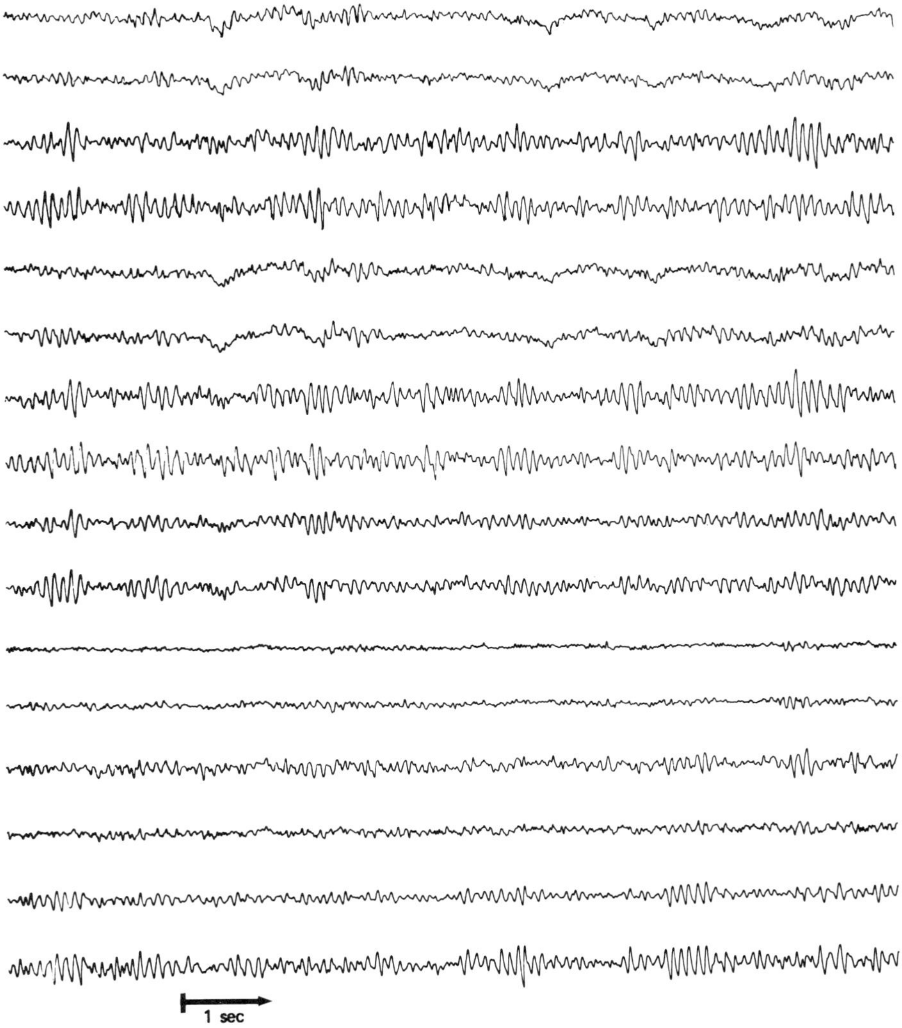

Figure 2.2 This is a page from a standard electroencephalogram recorded from a 38-year-old woman with daily episodes of decreased strength and sensation over the right side of her body. The recording was obtained during a severe episode of weakness and is completely normal. All other investigations on this woman, including computed tomography, metabolic studies, and cardiac monitoring, were also normal. Her neurologic examination revealed an abnormal gait with dragging of the right leg when she walked forward but a completely normal performance when she was asked to perform heel-to-toe (tandem) gait backward. The final diagnosis was conversion reaction triggered by family conflicts. This electroencephalogram displays 16 different electrode combinations (leads) simultaneously, a feature available on most standard electroencephalographs. This feature allows comparison of simultaneous brain wave activity over different parts of the head. The sinusoidal waves with a frequency of 10 cycles per second on this normal electroencephalogram are typical alpha waves. The alpha waves appeared over the posterior part of the head when the patient was awake with her eyes closed.

exhibit one of these normal variants, which in the context of the periodic behavior disorder will be misinterpreted as a seizure focus.

Abnormal Brain Wave Patterns

The electroencephalogram only shows waves, spikes, and electrical silence, but these three elements can be very informative to an experienced interpreter. A variety of pathologic abnormalities are suggested by specific patterns of abnormal brain wave activity. Electroencephalographic abnormalities include continuous slow activity, excessive fast activity, periodic patterns of slow and fast activity, combinations of spike and slow activity, and electrocerebral inactivity. Focal spike activity and focal slow wave activity are the simplest to identify because of the asymmetry they lend to the electroencephalographic pattern (Figure 2.3).

Diffuse slowing of the brain waves occurs with several metabolic disorders, including liver disease, kidney failure, hypothyroidism, and pulmonary insufficiency, which can produce intellectual abnormalities (16). Slow waves with three components, called triphasic waves, develop in 20 percent of the patients with a metabolic encephalopathy from kidney or liver failure (16). If the patient has a severe dementia and the electroencephalogram is largely normal, it is less likely that the problem is metabolic, toxic, neoplastic, or infectious in origin. It is still possible that the patient has a degenerative brain disease or a psychotic reaction producing a pseudodementia, but the information provided by the electroencephalogram will decrease the chances of leaving a treatable cause of dementia untreated. Bilateral frontal slowing of the brain waves that appears intermittently, rather than continuously, is often a sign of damage to deep, subcortical structures. This may be an early sign of hydrocephalus, an increase in the volume or pressure of the cerebrospinal fluid. Slow wave activity need not occur alone with certain organic brain syndromes. In delirium, a reversible organic brain syndrome commonly resulting from a metabolic encephalopathy, the electroencephalogram will reveal diffuse slow wave activity with superimposed fast waves (6,19).

Seizure activity usually appears as spike or slow wave activity. The absence attacks of children with petit mal epilepsy are associated with small spikes followed by single slow waves at a frequency of three per second. When focal abnormalities are not obvious, various maneuvers may make them more apparent. Hyperventilation or sleep may enhance a spike focus that is not prominent in the awake patient breathing at a normal rate. Spike activity arising on the mesial or inner surface of the temporal lobe may require special electrode arrangements for recording. One type of special electrode intended for this type of recording is the nasopharyngeal lead: this electrode is inserted into the nose and set against the lateral aspect of the nasopharynx so that it lies close to the inner face of the temporal lobe.

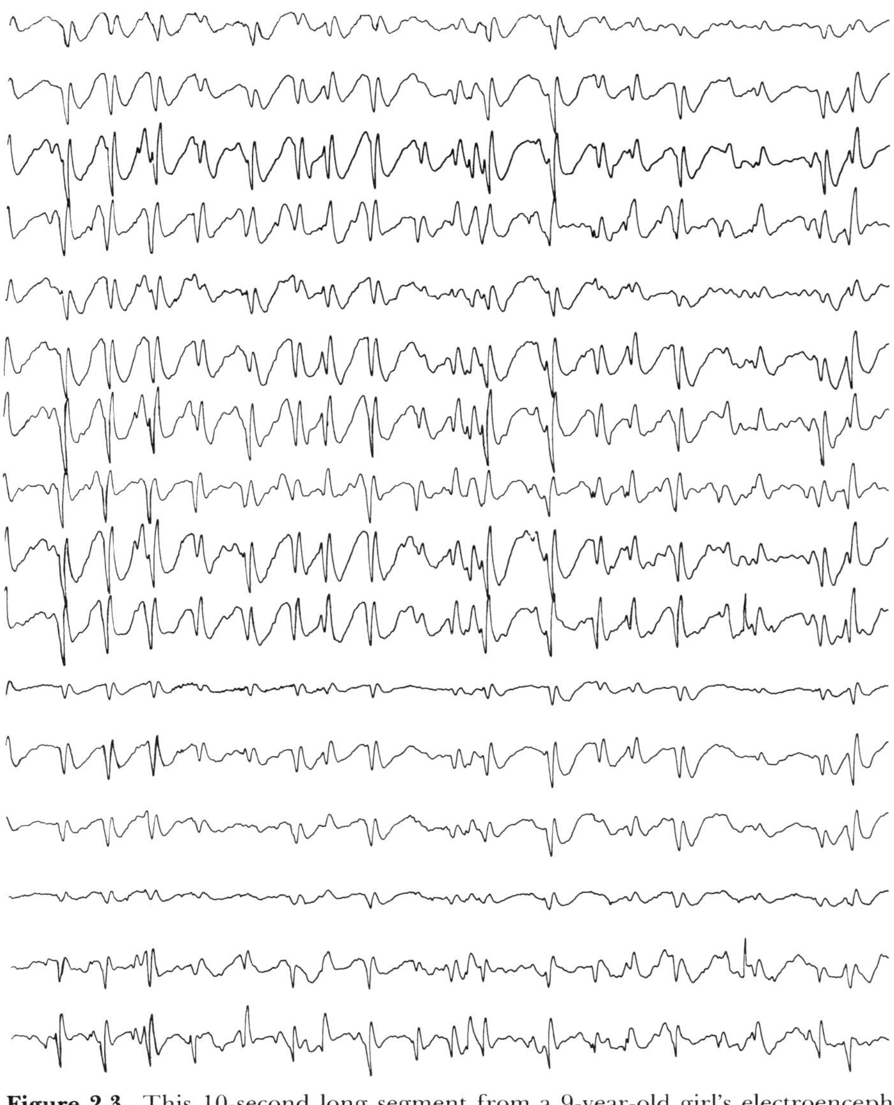

Figure 2.3. This 10-second long segment from a 9-year-old girl's electroencephalogram reveals spikes and slow-wave activity constituting almost all of the brain wave activity present. The child had a long history of seizures and mental retardation, and the electroencephalogram showed this profoundly abnormal pattern just as the child had a generalized convulsion.

Slow wave abnormalities are primarily of two types, delta and theta. These names refer only to the range of frequency of the slow wave. They say nothing about the size or location of the brain waves. Delta waves are the slowest brain waves with a frequency range of 0 to 3 hertz. Theta waves are slow waves at a frequency from 4 to 7 hertz. These are generally pathologic when they appear in the electroencephalogram of an awake adult under 60 years of age. This is not to say that alpha waves are always normal and delta and theta waves are always abnormal. Alpha activity may appear diffusely over the entire head, in which case it is pathologic, but this generally does not occur in a conscious person. Theta and delta activity are normal in sleep, and some slow wave activity may appear in patients with migraine headaches even when there is no evidence of a structural lesion anywhere in the brain. Focal continuous slowing, however, usually arises with an acute or subacute lesion that is causing progressive damage to the brain. Focal slow wave activity also occurs after seizure activity, during the period called the postictal state.

Brain waves can also be unusually fast. When the frequency of brain waves is between 13 and 35 cycles per second, they are called beta waves. This type of brain wave activity usually appears when the patient is taking a sedative. Another common brain wave pattern that is abnormal is an asymmetric record. If the amplitude of the voltages recorded from the two sides of the head are different, the patient will usually have focal brain damage. The side suffering the damage will have the lower amplitude waves. A subdural hematoma will produce asymmetry, and the lower amplitude waves will be on the side of the subdural (Figure 2.4). If the patient has had a craniotomy, however, the defects associated with the surgery usually produce asymmetries in the record with the higher amplitude wave forms on the side of the surgery.

Periodically appearing sharp waves or spikes distributed over the entire head indicate an acute or subacute encephalopathy. This diffuse encephalopathy is invariably severe when such wave forms are apparent. Periodic discharges occurring at a rate of less than one discharge every 4 seconds often develop with subacute sclerosing panencephalitis, a lethal degenerative disease of the brain. When the discharge rate is greater than one discharge every 2 seconds, the underlying brain disease may be Creutzfeldt-Jakob disease, a slow-viral illness causing dementia in adults, or Tay-Sachs disease, an inborn error of metabolism causing dementia in children. With encephalopathies resulting from poisons or anoxia, a periodic pattern in which wave activity is largely absent between discharges occasionally appears. This is called periodic lateralized epileptiform discharges (PLEDS). Tumors, strokes, or other severe, progressive lesions may produce PLEDS, but this pattern also develops with focal lesions which are epileptogenic, but not structurally prominent. Focal seizures often appear in patients with PLEDS.

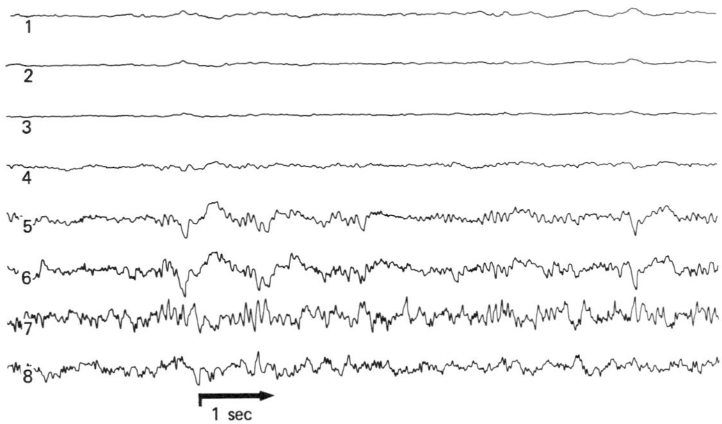

Figure 2.4. Half of this electroencephalogram (first four lines) has markedly depressed voltages, and half (last four lines) has normal wave amplitudes. This asymmetry between the right and left cerebral hemispheres developed in a child after a subdural hematoma had been removed from the side of the head that had the low voltage. The persistence of the voltage asymmetry reflected permanent damage to the injured cerebral hemisphere.

Medication Effects on Brain Wave Activity

The electroencephalogram is affected by a variety of drugs. When a drug overdose is suspected the electroencephalogram may be helpful in confirming the diagnosis and also in narrowing down the range of possible drugs involved. With depressant drug ingestion there is a range of electroencephalographic changes dependent upon the dosage of the drug and the duration of the drug intake. With barbiturate excess the patient usually has excessive fast wave activity. Initially this beta activity may be followed by slowing and even electrocortical silence. With small doses of barbiturate the beta activity will be limited to the anterior head leads, but with higher doses the patient will have generalized beta activity. Extremely high doses will produce generalized delta activity. Some nonbarbiturate sedatives, such as chloral hydrate, produce relatively little beta activity; but other commonly used nonbarbiturate sedatives, such as glutethimide, may increase beta activity substantially. With a phenothiazine overdose, the electroencephalogram will show diffuse slowing and other signs consistent with drowsiness, but this only appears at very high doses. At most doses benzodiazepines, such as chlordiazepoxide, produce generalized fast activity, whereas tricyclic antidepressants produce generalized slow activity. Monoamine oxidase inhibitors produce little effect on the electroencephalogram, but they do affect sleep substantially. These antidepressants suppress rapid eye movement sleep. Drugs related to the poison atropine can cause profound psychiatric problems, including visual hallucinations, and they are readily available in sleep preparations bought over the counter. These atropinic drugs include scopolamine and hyoscamine, both of which can cause rhythmic slowing on the electroencephalogram. The commonly abused hallucinogen lysergic acid diethylamide (LSD) increases the frequency of alpha activity. Morphine will initially produce some slowing of the electroencephalographic activity, but individuals using the drug on a regular basis will exhibit a characteristic pattern of prominent alpha waves that are synchronous. With meperidine and methadone the electroencephalogram will show excessive, random slowing of brain wave activity.

CEREBROSPINAL FLUID STUDIES

Examination of the cerebrospinal fluid is essential in cases of suspected meningitis and is helpful in the diagnosis and treatment of several other neurologic diseases. Tests routinely performed on the fluid include cell counts, cultures, protein and glucose determinations, and flagellated treponemal antigen (FTA) for neurosyphilis. In cases of suspected tumor, cytologic examination is more rigorous. Tumor cells may be found in the fluid, whether the tumor is a primary neoplasm of the central nervous system or a neoplasm spreading from sites outside the central nervous system. Immunoglobulin analysis of the fluid may be helpful when the level of suspicion for multiple sclerosis or neurosyphilis is high. Whether the fluid is obtained by sticking a needle into the lumbar subarachnoid space or into the cisterna magna at the base of the skull, the pressure registered by the initial sample of fluid will reveal much about the forces acting upon the fluid. Collecting cerebrospinal fluid is rarely a therapeutic measure but gaining access to the fluid to introduce medications is becoming increasingly important in the management of recurrent infections and malignant tumors.

The fluid is normally clear and colorless, with a protein content less than 55 milligrams per deciliter and a sugar content approximately two-thirds of the serum glucose concentration. There should be no erythrocytes in this fluid, and, if there are any white cells, they should all be mononuclear cells. The total number of mononuclear cells normally does not exceed 10 per cubic millimeter. The pressure on the fluid should not exceed 170 millimeters of water when the patient is fully relaxed, but relaxation is often difficult to achieve when the patient is aware that a large needle is being stuck into his spine. The two common routes for obtaining fluid are the lumbar and the suboccipital route. In a lumbar puncture, the lumbar sac below the end of the spinal cord (conus medullaris) is entered in the interspace between the second and third, third and fourth, or fourth and fifth lumbar vertebrae. The patient may develop a shooting electric pain down one leg if the needle catches one of the spinal roots (cauda equina) occupying this part of the subarachnoid space. With a suboccipital puncture, the cisterna magna just inferior to the medulla oblongata is entered. The subarachnoid space at the level of the upper cervical spinal cord may also be approached with fluoroscopic guidance. Although the subarachnoid space is the most accessible site for collecting cerebrospinal fluid, this fluid is inside, as well as around, the brain. Cerebrospinal fluid may be obtained from the ventricular system inside the brain as part of an operative procedure or by way of a catheter or shunt left in the ventricles during a neurosurgical procedure. The protein content is slightly lower in fluid collected higher in the craniospinal axis.

Cerebrospinal fluid collection, especially by lumbar puncture, is ill-advised when a mass lesion is suspected in or on the brain. Acute changes in cerebrospinal fluid pressure may allow precipitate shifts in the intracranial contents, and irreversible or lethal damage may occur. Unfortunately, space occupying lesions are often unsuspected in patients with conditions necessitating cerebrospinal fluid analysis, such as meningitis. Papilledema is a useful sign of increased intracranial pressure, but it is present in many cases of meningitis and so is not a strict contraindication to spinal tap (20).

Evaluation of Spinal Fluid Abnormalities

Central nervous system lesions produce a variety of changes in the cerebrospinal fluid. A low sugar in a patient with fever and a stiff neck indicates an infectious meningitis, until proven otherwise. Polymorphonuclear white blood cells in the fluid should also be interpreted as a sign of meningitis, even if only one is present, when there is not a proportionate number of red blood cells associated with the white blood cells. An organism identified in the fluid is an extremely useful aid in choosing the appropriate treatment for an infection. Unfortunately, organisms, whether they be bacterial, fungal, or parasitic, are often quite difficult to identify in the fresh cerebrospinal fluid and may require a day or more in culture or a variety of special stains for accurate identification.

The changes in the cerebrospinal fluid developing with an infection vary with the type of organism responsible for the infection. Patients with viral meningitis or encephalitis may fail to have the glucose content depression characteristically seen with a bacterial meningoencephalitis. Viral infections may, however, produce an elevated white blood cell count in the fluid. Typically, the cerebrospinal fluid in patients with herpes encephalitis, a common infectious cause of acute psychosis, will show an increase in both erythrocytes and leucocytes. Fungal infections may produce little change in the cerebrospinal fluid, even when a lethal infection is present. Cryptococcal meningitis, an infectious cause of progressive cognitive dysfunction, invariably requires special stains for its identification. The India ink preparation, in which a drop of ink is added to the fluid, may help outline the organism, but recently introduced immunologic techniques to detect the cryptococcal antigens are simpler and more reliable.

A large number of red cells in the cerebrospinal fluid indicates subarachnoid hemorrhage or a traumatic tap. Disruption of small vessels on entering the subarachnoid space usually produces transient bleeding into the fluid collected from the puncture site. As fluid is withdrawn, the red cell content falls progressively. If substantial bleeding has occurred in the subarachnoid space, the protein content of the cerebrospinal fluid will be increased simply as a result of the additional serum protein. This means that in a patient with a normal blood count and normal serum protein, about 1 milligram of protein will be added to the cerebrospinal fluid with every 700 red blood cells introduced. Consequently, if a lumbar puncture yields bloody fluid that clears at least partially as the cerebrospinal fluid is withdrawn and the protein content of the cerebrospinal fluid is elevated only 1 or 2 milligrams per deciliter in fluid that has 1400 red cells per cubic millimeter, the blood can be ascribed to trauma at the time of the spinal tap. When blood has been in the cerebrospinal fluid for hours or days, the protein content of the fluid will be elevated greatly in excess of the 1 milligram per 700 cells seen with a traumatic tap. The cerebrospinal fluid protein rises as the erythrocytes break down. Another indication that the erythrocytes are from bleeding that occurred before the diagnostic procedure was performed is xanthochromia. This is a yellowish discoloration of the normally colorless cerebrospinal fluid that develops with pigment collection in the fluid after the breakdown of red cells. Another indication that the blood is from a subarachnoid hemorrhage is that it does not clot. Blood that has been in the subarachnoid space for hours or days will not clot when it is left to stand.

Occasionally the cerebrospinal fluid will be completely normal except for an elevated protein. This may reflect an unsuspected tumor or chronic subdural hematoma, but it is also seen in a number of metabolic problems, such as diabetes mellitus or hypothyroidism. A markedly elevated protein, in excess of 300 miligrams per deciliter, usually indicates obstruction of cerebrospinal fluid flow in the subarachnoid space. This can occur with a tumor in or about the spinal cord.

Elevated Intracranial Pressure

The cerebrospinal fluid pressure may be elevated with subarachnoid bleeding, whether it is from an aneurysm or head trauma, with tumors, whether they are benign or malignant, with infections, regardless of the organism responsible, or idiopathically. An elevated cerebrospinal fluid pressure is usually the only apparent abnormality in the syndrome called pseudotumor cerebri. Patients with this disorder complain of headache, have papilledema, and may develop progressive visual loss as a result of the chronic elevation of cerebrospinal fluid pressure. Obese young women are especially susceptible to this idiopathic cerebrospinal fluid hypertension. Characteristically, they have spinal fluid pressures in excess of 200 millimeters of water on repeated spinal taps. Pseudotumor cerebri does not produce intellectual deterioration, but other conditions involving increased intracranial pressure do. If the flow of spinal fluid is obstructed in the head or the reabsorption of spinal fluid into the venous system around the brain is impaired, the intracranial pressure may increase tremendously and produce brain damage as a direct effect of the increased pressure. Relieving this pressure with a tube introduced directly into the ventricles of the brain may be the only way to avoid progressive intellectual deterioration resulting from the cerebrospinal fluid disorder.

Therapeutic Applications of the Spinal Tap

Repeated lumbar puncture to treat pseudotumor cerebri is only one of several therapeutic applications of the spinal tap. Chemotherapy to treat tumors metastatic to the nervous system and antibiotics to eradicate organisms causing recurrent meningitis are occasionally introduced into the cerebrospinal fluid by lumbar puncture or direct ventricular puncture. A tube is permanently left in the ventricle when ventricular instillation of drugs is appropriate, this tube being connected to a reservoir left under the scalp.

Myelography

The most common radiographic procedure utilizing a spinal tap is myelography. In this test, contrast material is introduced into the subarachnoid space to demonstrate lesions protruding into this space or blocking it. Radiopaque materials are most often used (Figure 2.5). Lipid-soluble dyes were generally used for all studies until water-soluble dyes were developed that did not irritate the nervous system. The advantage of a water-soluble material is that the dye will be absorbed into the blood and excreted by the kidney. Lipid-soluble materials must be removed from the subarachnoid space at the end of the study or the material will stay in the space for the remainder of the patient's life. Air is occasionally used instead of a radiopaque dye; the main advantage of air is that it rises rather than falls. Cysts in the spinal cord that appear swollen when the patient is head down will collapse when the patient is head up. Although air provides little contrast with the spinal cord, it provides enough to reveal this characteristic behavior of intraspinal cysts. Myelograms will also reveal tumors enlarging the spinal cord, discs pressing on spinal roots, and masses obstructing the subarachnoid space. This procedure is usually reserved for patients with lesions thought to be surgically correctable.

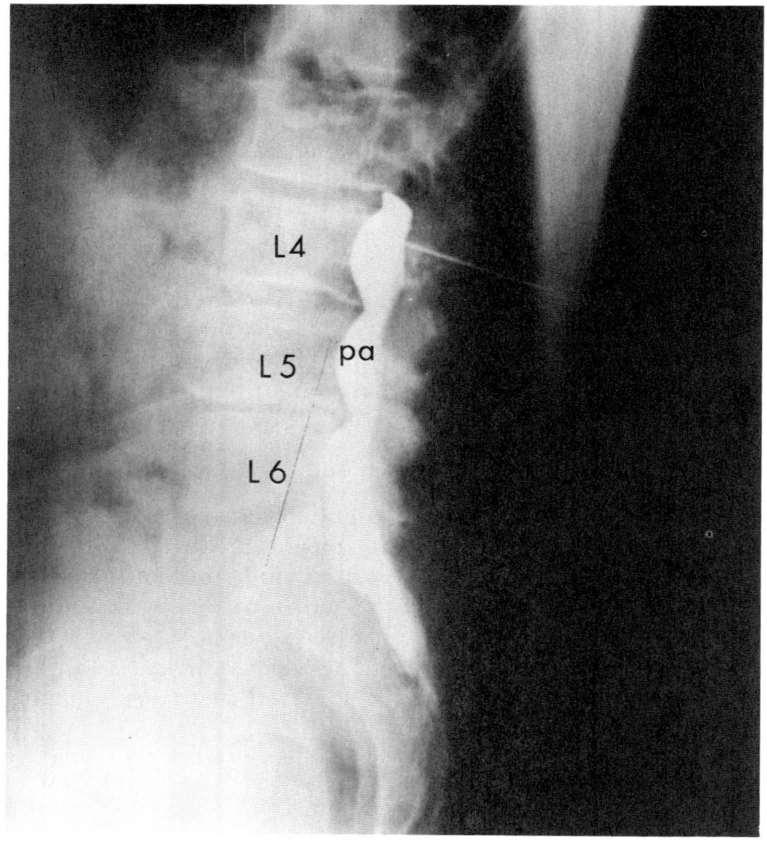

Figure 2.5. This 65-year-old man with multiple myeloma had a myelogram performed to investigate leg pain. His lower spine was abnormal because of severe degenerative disease of the vertebral bodies and because of a sacral vertebra (L6) that was not fused with the sacrum. The lumbar vertebrae are labeled L4, L5. The column of lipid-soluble, radiopaque dye (pa) flowed freely in the subarachnoid space up to the twelfth thoracic vertebra, where it was blocked by an extradural tumor mass.

X-RAY STUDIES OF THE SKULL

Radiograms of the skull are a valuable noninvasive step in the initial evaluation of patients thought to have structural lesions in the head. Although the x-ray film of the skull only shows changes in the bony structures of the head, many conditions produce noticeable changes in these structures, even though they are not primarily disorders of the bone. Chronic headache, indistinguishable from tension headache, may develop with a meningioma, a neoplastic lesion that commonly produces local thickening of bone or blistering of bone on the plain x-ray film of the skull. Other unsuspected tumors often have flecks of calcium in the tumor mass which appear on routine views of the skull. A tumor in the area of the eighth cranial nerve usually produces widening of the internal auditory meatus. Metastatic disease to the head may be suggested by punched-out lesions in the skull, and a lesion on the optic nerve is often reflected in widening of the optic foramen. An enlarged sella turcica from a pituitary lesion would help explain complaints of visual change that develop as the nearby optic chiasm is compressed. Even foreign objects, such as bullets, may be revealed on skull radiography when the patient has no recall of incidents to explain this finding.

After head trauma, skull films can give the physician a better sense of the complications likely to be faced by the patient. A fracture crossing the groove on the lateral aspect of the skull for the middle meningeal artery increases the likelihood that an epidural hematoma will develop. Air about the brain indicates a cerebrospinal fluid leak and an easy route of entry for organisms that can cause meningitis (Figure 2.6). Since depression commonly develops after severe head trauma, it is valuable to know how vulnerable the patient is to a meningoencephalitis that could also cause the depression before more serious neurologic signs develop.

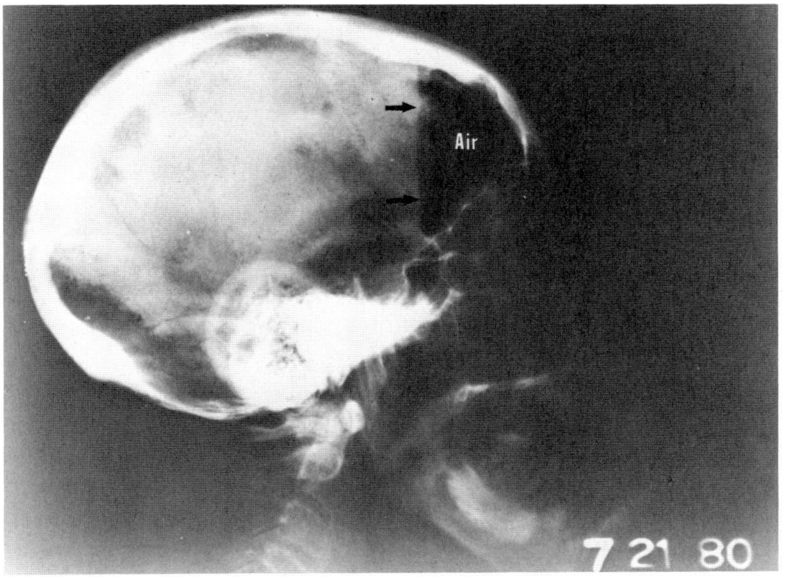

Figure 2.6. An elderly woman was struck by a taxicab while crossing the street. Although she did not lose consciousness, she was mildly confused and irritable when first examined in the emergency room. There were no focal neurologic deficits, but clear fluid was dripping from her nose. She was urged to stay for observation, but she refused and left after x-ray films of her skull were obtained. These films revealed air in the head (pneumocephaly), which gained entry through an inapparent skull fracture. The skull fracture was also responsible for the discharge of cerebrospinal fluid (cerebrospinal fluid rhinorrhea) through her nose.

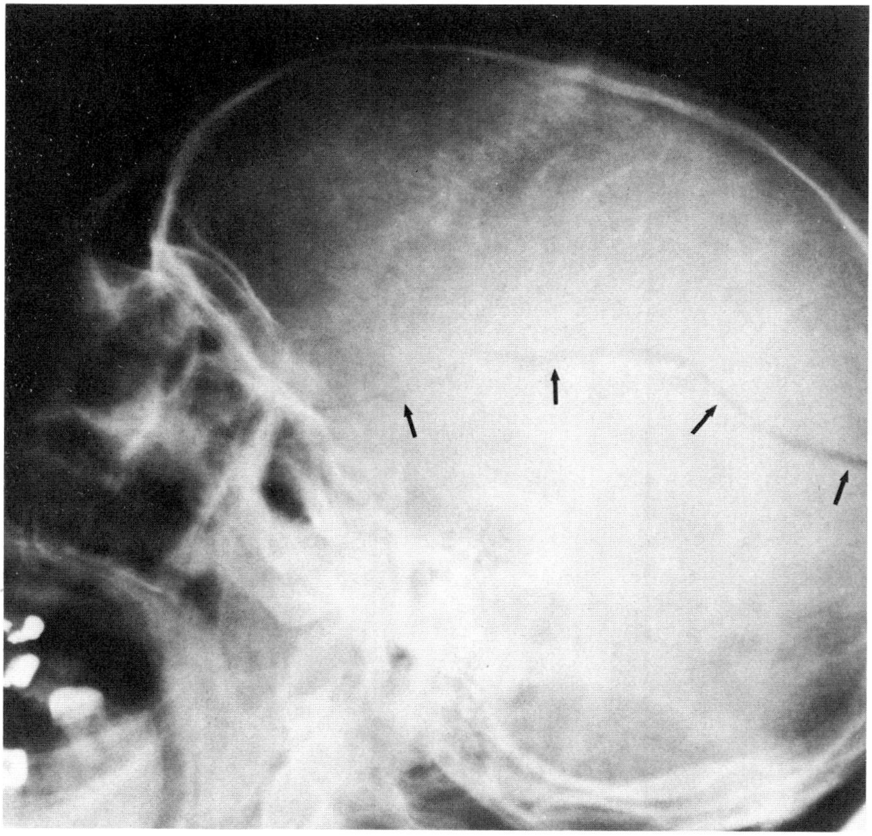

Figure 2.7. Massive head trauma produced these obvious fractures (arrows) passing through the frontal and parietal bones. A patient with this much evidence of trauma will often develop a subdural or epidural hematoma (courtesy of Drs. J. Loh and W. Hotson).

Like the electroencephalogram, the skull radiogram is a useful screening test. If it is normal, it does not guarantee that there is no structural disease, but it decreases the likelihood of overlooking an obvious structural lesion in the head (Figure 2.7). Many sophisticated techniques have developed from skull radiography, but they have not eliminated the usefulness of the x-ray film. One of the most useful radiologic techniques developed in the past 3 decades is the computed tomogram of the head.

COMPUTED TOMOGRAPHY OF THE HEAD

Computed tomography combines conventional radiographic techniques with computer analysis of the information obtained. The technique allows

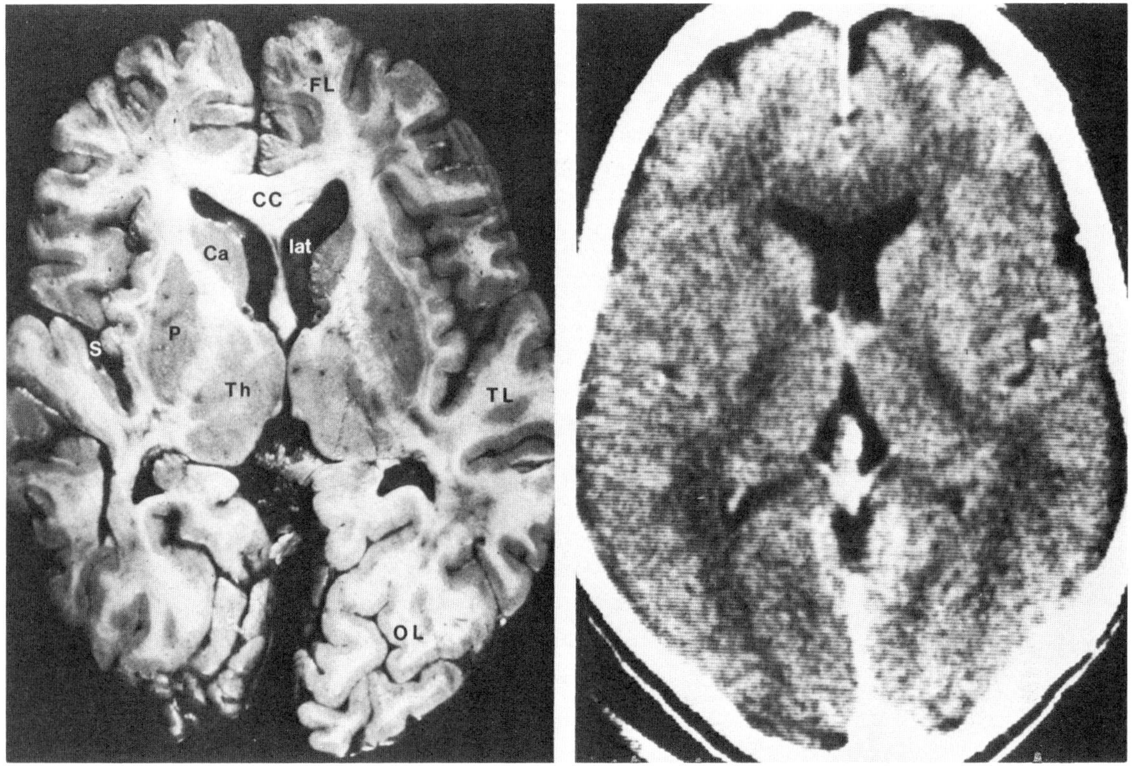

Figure 2.8. The computed tomogram (right) in this illustration was obtained at about the same level in the brain as the horizontal section shown through a normal brain (left). Structures obvious on both the computed tomogram and the formalin-fixed brain include the lateral ventricle (lat), the Sylvian fissure (S), the putamen (P), the caudate nucleus (Ca), part of the thalamus (Th), the corpus callosum (CC), the temporal lobe (TL), the occipital lobe (OL), and the frontal lobe (FL).

densities at thousands of points in the head to be measured and assembled into a picture of the cranial contents and extracranial structures. X-rays are generated in a standard x-ray tube and are directed as a thin beam through the head to a detector or system of detectors on the other side of the head. Absorption of x-rays is measured at many points as the beam sweeps across the head in a single plane. The position of the x-ray tube is rotated about the head after each scan from one position. The computer analyzes x-ray absorption values for points inside the head and calculates what the density of each point must be to produce the observed level of absorption (Figure 2.8). With this information it can reconstruct the appearance of the intracranial contents. The differing densities of normal and abnormal intracranial tissues provide a picture that resembles a section cut through the brain in the plane of the tomographic study. Fresh blood is denser than brain, brain is denser than cerebrospinal fluid, and cerebrospinal fluid is denser than air (Figure 2.9). Abnormal structures can be enhanced with the addition of radiodense materials into the blood or cerebrospinal fluid. An iodinated dye is routinely injected intravenously during the examination to delineate breakdowns in the blood-brain barrier and to better define large vascular structures. A water soluble dye added

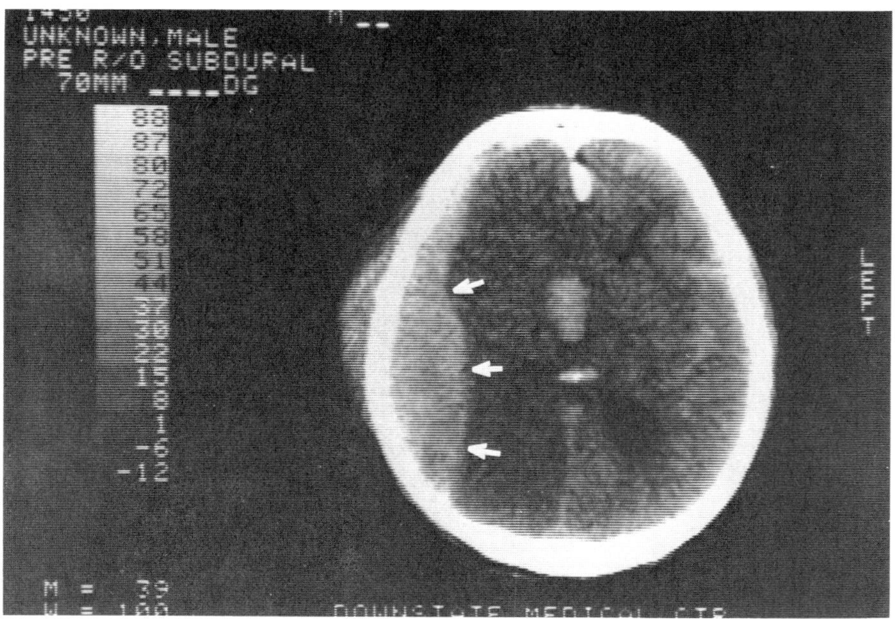

Figure 2.9. This computed tomogram of the head reveals a massive subdural hematoma (arrows), as well as a large hematoma in the scalp and blood in the third ventricle (center of the photo). Fresh blood is denser than brain tissue and, consequently, appears white in comparison with the brain and cerebrospinal fluid.

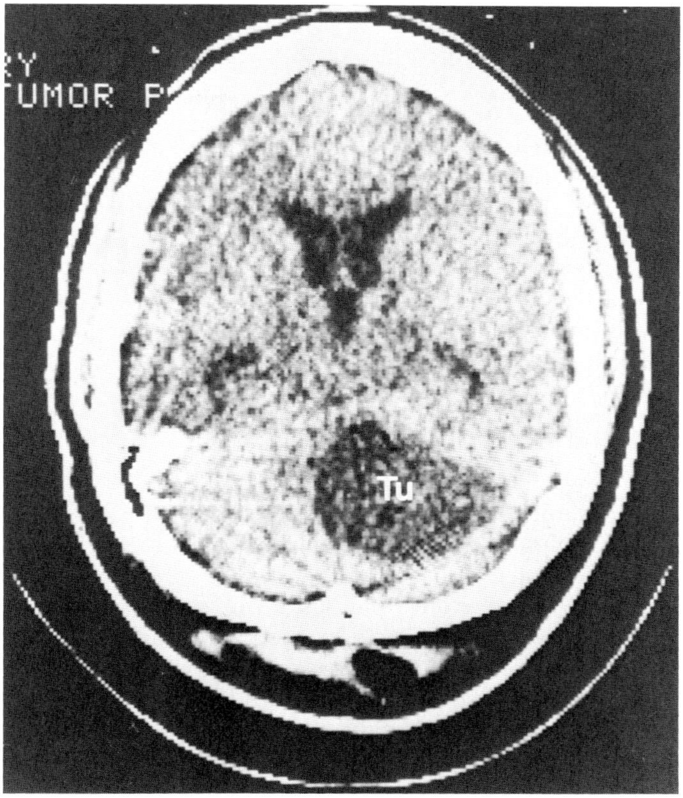

Figure 2.10. The large area of decreased density in the cerebellar hemisphere is a tumor (Tu). Surgical intervention revealed a cerebellar hemangioblastoma.

to the cerebrospinal fluid will help define subtle abnormalities in the subarachnoid space.

The computed tomogram obtained without the administration of intravenous contrast materials is called the precontrast scan. An intracerebral or cerebellar hemorrhage will appear as a dense mass in the brain on the precontrast scan. Tumors with calcifications, such as meningiomas and some gliomas, will appear even denser than blood. If the mass has been growing slowly over the course of several years, the surrounding intracranial structures will be displaced relatively little. An abruptly appearing mass will cause dramatic shifts of the intracranial contents. The postcontrast scan often helps to define the nature of a lesion apparent on the precontrast scan. A brain abscess will appear as an area of decreased density on the precontrast scan; after the injection of contrast material, a ring of enhanced density is likely to appear around the necrotic core of the lesion (21). This may be difficult to distinguish from a cystic tumor (Figure 2.10). A highly vascular tumor may be enhanced over much or all of its area after contrast is given. Areas of infarction are likely to show no enhancement on the postcontrast scan, at least when the lesion is less than 1 week old.

Instillation of metrizamide, a water-soluble, radiopaque material, into the subarachnoid space is useful in assessing lesions about the sella turcica. A common diagnostic problem is the "empty sella," a syndrome in which the patient has an enlarged sella turcica without an intrasellar mass. The excess space in the sella turcica is filled with cerebrospinal fluid, but the resolution of this small area by the computed tomogram is often inadequate. A low density pituitary tumor may be indistinguishable from cerebrospinal fluid. Using the contrast material in the subarachnoid space, one can establish whether the sella turcica is filled with a mass or "empty."

ANGIOGRAPHY

Contrast material injected into blood vessels supplying various parts of the nervous system helps define abnormalities near or involving the blood vessels. If the vessel injected is an artery, the study is called an arteriogram; if it is a vein, a venogram. Abnormalities of the vascular system itself likely to cause nervous system signs include aneurysms, arteriovenous malformations, arterial and venous thromboses, and vascular tumors. Disorders in the nervous system most easily diagnosed with angiography include tumors, infarctions, and hemorrhages.

The technique used to perform the angiogram is dictated by the lesion sought and the special problems of the patient to be studied. The internal carotid arteries and their distal branches could be studied by introducing a needle directly into the neck on either side, but the dangers of dislodging atherosclerotic plaques with puncture of the vessel and of hemorrhage into the neck after removal of the needle prompted development of other techniques (Figure 2.11). Because the right common carotid artery originates with the right subclavian artery off the innominate artery, the internal carotid on the right can be reached by threading a catheter retrograde in the subclavian artery up to the origin of the common carotid artery. The left internal carotid cannot be reached in an analogous fashion because the left common carotid and the left subclavian both arise off the aortic arch, and a catheter threaded into the left subclavian artery would have to make a U-turn to enter the left common carotid after it reached the aortic arch. The vertebral arteries are not accessible by direct puncture because they course through bony channels in the transverse processes of the cervical spine, but they can be reached by catheters threaded retrograde in the subclavian arteries. Both vertebral arteries arise off the subclavian arteries, and so catheters inserted in the brachial arteries can be used to study these vessels supplying the brainstem and posterior fossa. Obviously, any investigation requiring study of all four of these major vessels to the

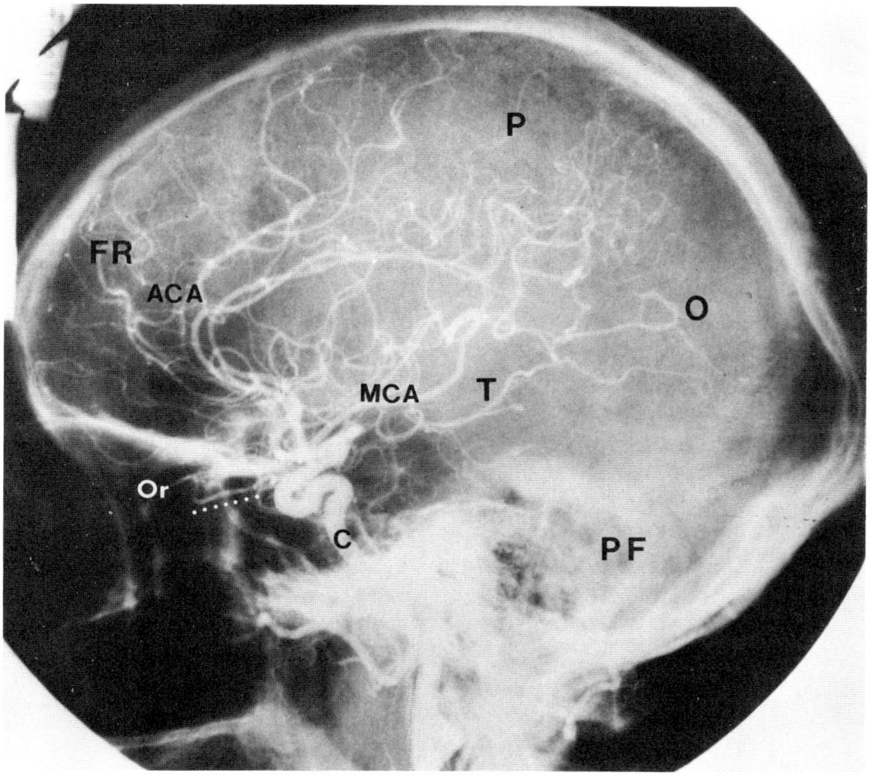

Figure 2.11. Normal carotid arteriogram. MCA, middle cerebral artery; ACA, anterior cerebral artery; C, internal carotid artery; FR, frontal lobe; P, parietal lobe; O, occipital lobe; T, temporal lobe; PF, posterior fossa; Or, orbit; the ophthalmic artery is above the row of white dots (courtesy of Dr. M. Tenner).

head would involve several arterial punctures if the methods described were the only feasible ones. Fortunately, a simpler and safer approach is available through the femoral artery. This artery is punctured just below the inguinal ligament in the thigh and a catheter is threaded retrograde up the aorta and into the aortic arch. The major vessels arising from the aortic arch are selectively catheterized; and, when a test dose of contrast material indicates the catheter is at the origin of the desired vessel, a full set of films is shot while a large bolus of dye is forced through the vessel. As the study of each vessel is completed, the catheter is withdrawn slightly and repositioned in the next vessel to be studied. In experienced hands, this transfemoral approach allows the four major vessels supplying the brain to be studied with only one arterial puncture and no penetration of the carotid artery wall.

Contrast material in the blood vessels will reliably indicate pathology of the blood vessels themselves (Figure 2.12). The radiopaque material will fill and outline aneurysms that may have bled or caused focal deficits by pressing on adjacent nerves. The plexus of abnormal vessels in an arteriovenous malformation will be grossly delineated. Where vessels are obstructed by emboli or thrombi, there will be no filling of vessels distal to the occlusion. An infarction may be indicated by vascular occlusion and displacement of surrounding blood vessels by the swelling of tissue accompanying the brain damage. An intracerebral hemorrhage will appear as an avascular mass producing considerable displacement of surrounding

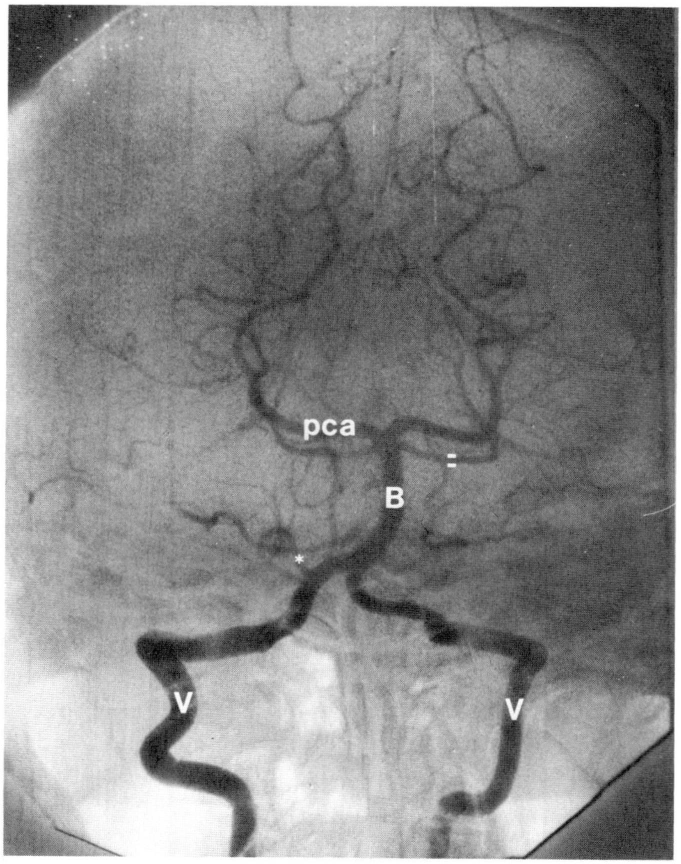

Figure 2.12. This normal arteriogram is an anteroposterior view of the vertebrobasilar system. A special photographic technique, called subtraction, has been used to eliminate structural features outside the blood vessels. The vertebral arteries are labeled V, the basilar artery is B, the posterior cerebral artery is pca, the posterior inferior cerebellar artery origin is marked with an asterisk (*), and the superior cerebellar artery runs through the double lines (=) (courtesy of Dr. M. Tenner).

vessels; most patients with this problem will have an associated hydrocephalus. The cortical plexus of vessels that normally abuts against the inner table of the skull will be displaced away from the bone when there is an overlying subdural or epidural hematoma. In all cases of intracranial hemorrhage, the arteriogram defines the size and location of the clot, but does not establish that the mass delineated is a blood clot. Parasitic cysts and largely avascular tumors are easily confused with clots when arteriography alone is used to study the patient. A brain abscess may have some abnormal perfusion about its margins, but it too will be difficult to differentiate from any other vascular mass on the basis of arteriography alone. The situation is quite different for tumors. Arteriography may be more helpful than computed tomography in establishing precisely the tumor type. Early draining veins are often seen with high grade gliomas of the brain; tumor blushes may appear with meningiomas, as well as astrocytomas. Meningiomas will usually be supplied by vessels from both the internal carotid or vertebrobasilar system and the external carotid systems.

PNEUMOENCEPHALOGRAPHY

Air introduced into the subarachnoid space or the ventricles was useful in studying periventricular pathology before the development of computed tomography. Hydrocephalus, intraventricular tumors, ventricular displacement by masses, and cerebral cortical atrophy could all be assessed by pneumoencephalography, but all of these are now more easily assessed and followed with computed tomography. The limited resolution of computed tomography at the base of the brain, especially about the region of the sella turcica, required continued use of pneumoencephalography until water soluble radiopaque dyes were found for introduction into the cerebrospinal fluid. Using this readily excretable dye, small cisterns about the base of the brain could be discriminated from nervous tissue in the same region. Pneumoencephalography is rarely used in modern medical centers now, and further advances in the application of computed tomography will probably eliminate this highly invasive radiologic technique from the investigation of neurologically impaired patients in the near future.

RADIONUCLIDE STUDIES OF THE CENTRAL NERVOUS SYSTEM

Radionuclide studies were extremely valuable in studying the evolution of central nervous system lesions before the development of computed tomography. The structural lesions most dramatically outlined by radionuclide studies are now more unequivocally demonstrated on computed tomography (Figure 2.13). The main advantages of radionuclide techniques at the present time are their wider accessibility and their dynamic, as well as static, character. Because these techniques are still widely used and are often mentioned in the past histories of patients subjected to new neurologic evaluations, they are worth understanding.

Injection of radionuclide material into the venous blood will not lead to accumulation of the material in or about the brain unless there is a disturbance of the blood–brain barrier. The materials used for radionuclide scanning are chosen specifically because they will not cross a normal

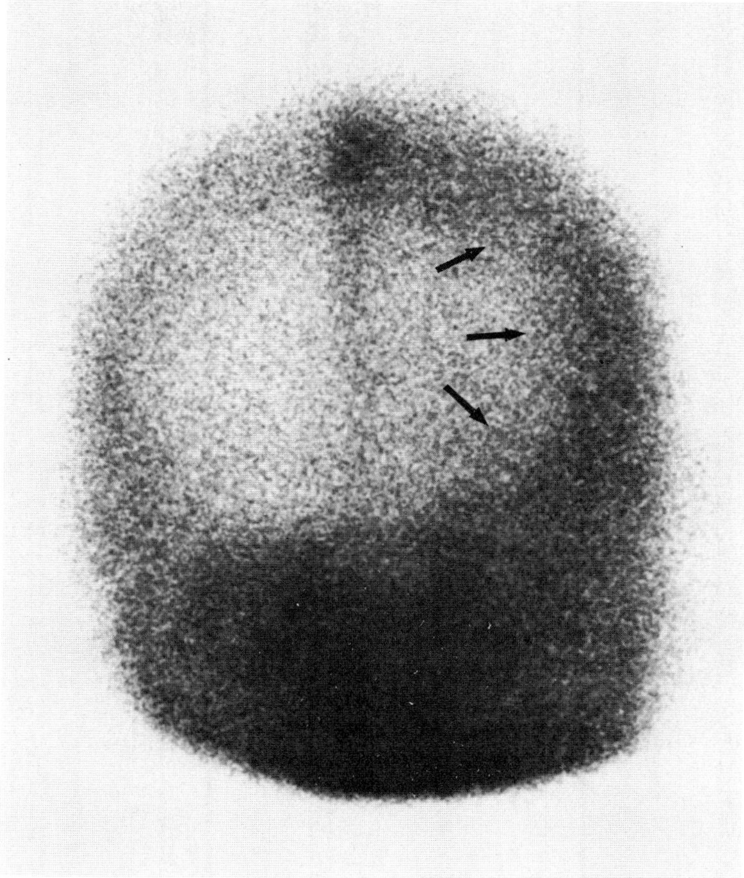

Figure 2.13. The large dark crescent (arrows) along the periphery of this radionuclide brain scan represents radionuclide accumulation in a chronic subdural hematoma. The radioactive material gains access to the intracranial compartment because the traumatic lesion disturbs the blood–brain barrier that would normally exclude this material from all areas outside blood vessels.

blood–brain barrier, and so any focal accumulation of isotope in the head necessarily indicates a disruption of the blood–brain barrier. Superficial injuries in the scalp or lesions in the skull can also produce focal collections of isotope, and so these must be discounted before the radionuclide study can be interpreted. Many brain tumors adequately disturb the blood–brain barrier to induce focal isotope uptakes in the affected area, but the lesions most consistently indicated by radionuclide scanning are subdural hematomas, epidural hematomas, and brain abscesses. Subdural hematomas will collect isotope throughout much of the blood clot, and so the photographic image of the radiation emission from the head will often appear as a crescent of activity overlying the brain on one or both sides. With chronic subdural hematomas the clot may be the same density as the adjacent brain tissue; this occasionally leads to a failure to clearly define the lesions with computed tomography (22). If the lesion is unilateral, the computed tomogram will usually show a shift of the ventricles away from the isodense mass. If the chronic subdural hematoma is bilateral, pressure from both sides of the brain may nullify the shift, and the chronic lesion may be "invisible" as a result. With radionuclide scanning, the isodense clots will be apparent, and confirmation of the subdurals will be provided by an arteriogram. The arteriogram should reveal a space between the outer margin of the cerebral cortex and the overlying skull. This space will coincide with the area of radionuclide collection revealed on the isotope scan.

Brain abscesses are invariably visualized on radionuclide scans, the usual pattern of isotope collection being a ring of radioactive material around the abscess cavity. This pattern also develops with some tumors, but it is most suggestive of brain abscess or focal encephalitis. Computed tomography with contrast enhancement will provide similar images in patients with brain abscesses.

Before computed tomography, infarction was often confirmed by obtaining a pair or a series of radionuclide scans at set intervals from the onset of symptoms. This was helpful because with cerebral infarction there was no focal uptake of isotope acutely, but after 7 to 10 days an area of uptake corresponding to the area of infarction would be apparent. After several weeks or months the isotope studies would no longer outline the area of infarction, a change presumably reflecting the restoration of a fairly normal blood–brain barrier. Computed tomography with contrast enhancement provides a more graphic delineation of cerebral and cerebellar changes with infarction than was ever achieved with radionuclide scanning.

Isotope Flow Studies

Studies of changing patterns of isotope concentrations in the brain early after the injection of the material suggested that this technique might be valuable in evaluating focal changes in cerebral blood flow, but the equipment routinely used for such "flow" studies is generally not sensitive enough to provide useful information (Figure 2.14). If impaired perfusion of a hemisphere is suggested by the radionuclide flow study, then an arteriogram should be done to confirm this impression before any surgery is performed to correct the defect. An asymptomatic patient, that is, one without recurrent neurologic signs, who has evidence of poor perfusion on a radionuclide flow study would not be studied with an arteriogram anyway. Without symptoms, he is not a candidate for surgery, and, if surgery is not contemplated, there is no point in subjecting the patient to the dangers of arteriography.

Intrathecal Studies

A radionuclide technique still widely used is the intrathecal isotope study for evaluating normal pressure hydrocephalus. Normal pressure hydro-

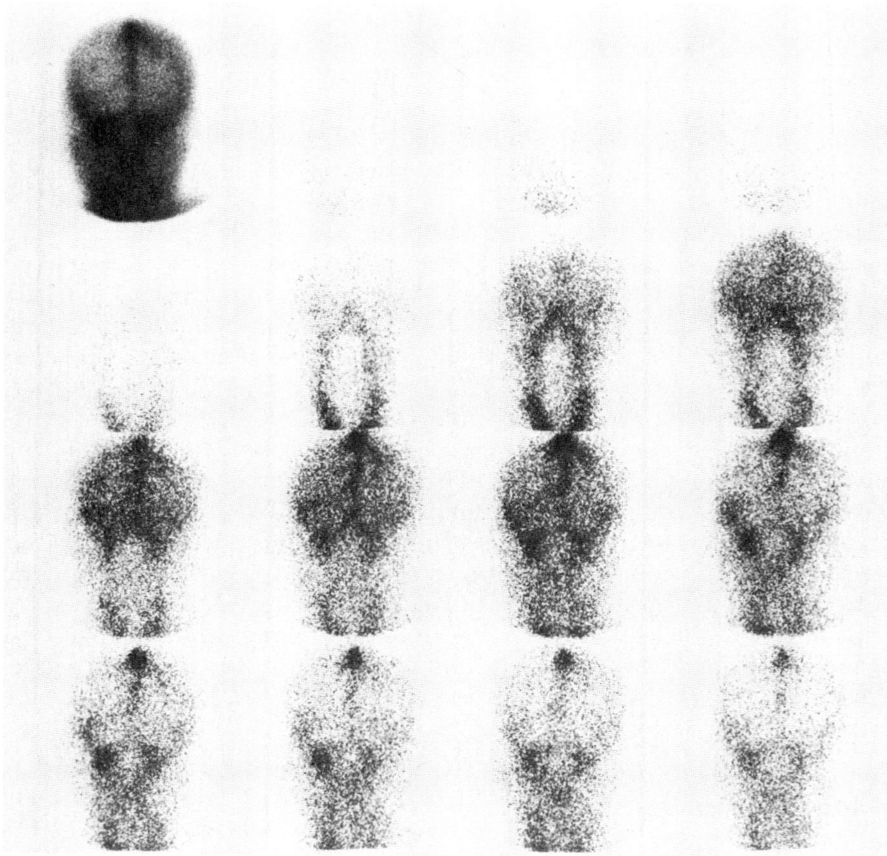

Figure 2.14. These sequential films, obtained during a radionuclide brain scan, show slightly asymmetric filling of blood vessels on the two sides of the head.

cephalus is a theoretic cause of intellectual impairment, gait difficulty, and urinary incontinence in individuals with normal cerebrospinal fluid pressure who have improved neurologic functions after a ventricular shunt instillation (23). Radionuclide iodinated serum albumen (RISA) or another radionuclide bound to a protein is placed in the cerebrospinal fluid in the lumbosacral sac to study flow patterns in patients with this syndrome. Instead of showing rapid clearance of the radioactively-tagged protein from the cerebrospinal fluid, sequential scans over the course of a few days show a relative stagnation of the material in the ventricles. Normally, the radionuclide is distributed over the convexities of the cerebral hemispheres within a few hours and is absorbed into the blood within 24 hours. Patients with hydrocephalus for any reason do not have a normal pattern of cerebrospinal fluid flow. The radioactive material introduced into the subarachnoid space of such individuals "backs up" into the ventricles and is still obvious on scans done 48 or 72 hours after instillation of the isotope intrathecally. Although the true nature of the normal pressure hydrocephalus syndrome is controversial, intrathecal radioisotope studies are still widely employed in the evaluation of patients being considered for shunting.

Perfusion Studies

Experimental perfusion studies using numerous highly collimated probes to follow blood flow in the brain in a variety of pathologic states have provided considerable information on intracranial hemodynamics, but they are still not widely used in clinical practice. Changes in cerebral blood flow patterns with specific cognitive, motor, or sensory activities have been documented and integrated with current concepts of neurophysiology. Little of this information has yet been helpful in clinical diagnosis.

ELECTROMYOGRAPHY AND NERVE CONDUCTION STUDIES

Electrical studies of nerve and muscle activity are routinely performed in cases of suspected muscle disease, peripheral nerve injury, or spinal cord disease. Study of the electrical activity in the muscle is called electromyography (Figure 2.15). Examining the transmission of signals along the nerve to a particular muscle or set of muscles is called the nerve conduction study. These two techniques are combined in a variety of ways to assess the integrity of neuromuscular activity from the level of the anterior horn cell in the spinal cord to the level of the individual muscle fiber.

The speed with which an impulse is conducted along the nerve is well defined for many nerves in the limbs. If an electric shock is applied to the nerve proximally and the time interval to the appearance of the action potential in the innervated muscle is measured, problems in nerve conduction can be detected. Slowing of the nerve conduction time indicates a problem affecting virtually all the motor fibers in the nerve tested. If any of the motor fibers were intact, the impulse would be carried along them to the muscle and arrive without delay. Diabetes mellitus, amyloidosis, and periarteritis nodosa are among the systemic diseases that may cause peripheral nerve disease. Rare metabolic diseases, such as metachromatic leukodystrophy, cause peripheral neuropathies in association with changes in intellectual function. Systemic lupus erythematosus commonly causes psychotic behavior and occasionally produces a peripheral neuropathy. The nerve conduction study provides an objective way of assessing peripheral nerve function in patients who may be unable to cooperate for more subjective tests.

Repetitive stimulation of a nerve can reveal disturbances at the point of contact between the nerve and the muscle, the neuromuscular junction. Myasthenia gravis, a neuromuscular junction disorder characterized by generalized weakness and easy fatigability, will produce a typical decrementing pattern of muscle action potentials when the nerve innervating the muscle is stimulated several times a second. A clinically similar cause of weakness, the Eaton-Lambert syndrome, will produce a typical incrementing response with the same repetitive stimulation. The size of the muscle action potential appearing with this myasthenia-like disease may increase by as much as fourfold when the nerve is stimulated several times per second.

Disease in the muscle itself will change the appearance of the action potentials in ways distinct from the changes developing with peripheral nerve or spinal cord disease. An acute or chronic inflammation of the muscle produces action potentials with an excessive number of components, so-called polyphasic potentials, or action potentials that are lower in amplitude and shorter in duration than normal potentials. Anterior horn cell disease will evoke low amplitude, high frequency potentials called fibrillations that indicate abnormal spontaneous activity in individual muscle fibers. The clinical impression that the patient has fasciculations, an early sign of lower motor neuron disease, can be documented with electrical studies of the abnormal muscles (Figure 2.16). Abnormal electrical activity, such as large positive deflections recorded from the muscle, will also appear with spinal cord diseases. Injury to a peripheral nerve may decrease the size and uniformity of voluntary action potentials recorded within a few weeks of the injury, but the potentials will be

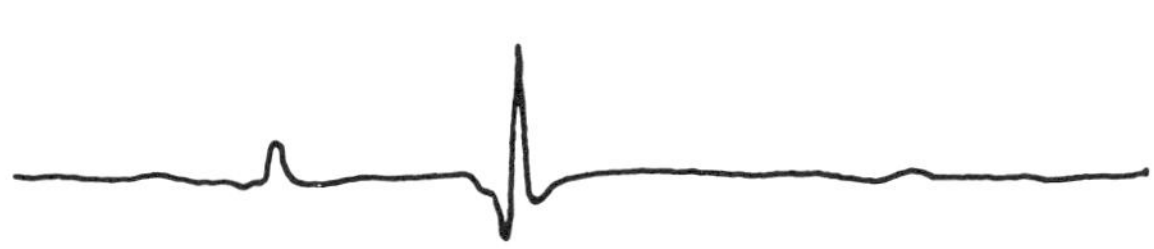

Figure 2.15. Electromyographic recording of a normal voluntary motor unit potential.

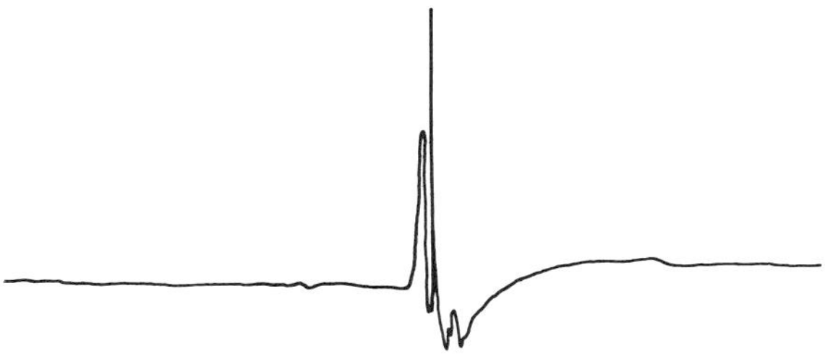

Figure 2.16. Fasciculations are single motor unit contractions that can be seen on physical examination as twitches or writhing movements in the resting muscle. This is an electromyographic recording of the electrical changes occurring during the involuntary muscle activity. Fasciculations usually indicate degenerative disease of the spinal motor neurons.

complex and of prolonged duration if the condition is more chronic with recurrent damage interfering with full recovery. The usefulness of electromyography and nerve conduction techniques in assessing the objectivity of weakness or sensory loss is obvious, but this technique can also help clarify the basis for disorders that are not strictly motor or sensory in character. Patients with labile affect may have amyotrophic lateral sclerosis, a degenerative disease of the central nervous system that causes anterior horn cell damage that will be apparent on electromyography before the patient has substantial weakness. Peripheral nerve damage appears with some diseases responsible for progressive dementias, such as pernicious anemia, and so evaluation of nerve function can narrow the diagnostic options.

BIOPSY

Histologic examination of brain, nerve, or muscle tissue is informative but necessarily destructive. A biopsy of the brain is always a last resort, unless the procedure is performed as part of a treatment protocol. Progressive intellectual impairment in a young person that remains unexplained despite numerous invasive studies may prompt a brain biopsy. The procedure is intended to reveal treatable lesions before irreversible damage is done. Unexpected findings on brain biopsy include tuberculous granulomas, fungal infections, and viral encephalitides.

A peripheral nerve biopsy is done routinely in the investigation of peripheral nerve disease because the sural nerve, a nerve in the lower leg providing sensory innervation to the heel of the foot, is easily reached and causes little functional loss when damaged. Histologic examination of this nerve and its associated vasculature may ultimately spare the patient many painful and fruitless therapeutic trials. Hereditary neuropathies, periarteritis nodosa, and other causes of peripheral nerve damage can be confidently diagnosed with the nerve specimen available for study.

Muscle biopsy is even simpler than nerve biopsy and is often more informative. Characteristic changes in the muscle may indicate peripheral nerve or spinal cord damage, as well as primary muscle disease. Hereditary myopathy, acute myositis, collagen vascular disease, sarcoidosis, parasitic infestation, and other disorders of muscle will be established with routine and special stains of the muscle tissue. The biopsy produces no functional deficits. The amount of muscle required for a thorough evaluation of any myopathic disorder is relatively small.

A biopsy of any part of the nervous system or musculoskeletal system is stressful for both the patient and his family. A brain biopsy is usually only performed as part of an unavoidable neurosurgical procedure, such as for the evaluation of a brain tumor, or in the course of a dementia investigation. The demented patient would generally not appreciate what was being done, but his family would not only be aware of what was being done but would also be responsible for agreeing to the procedure. This is an extraordinary responsibility that must be assumed by some family member. Although the risk that the patient will die or deteriorate as a consequence of the procedure is small, patients undergoing brain biopsy routinely develop seizure disorders after the procedure and are at risk for infections and hemorrhages at the site of the biopsy. Psychiatric assistance in dealing with the family of the patient scheduled for brain biopsy is often as helpful as psychiatric assistance in evaluating the cause of the patient's unexplained cognitive disorder. Nerve and muscle biopsies are less traumatic than brain biopsies, but the patient often has lingering concerns about the damage done by such invasive procedures. Chronic complaints of pain at the biopsy site or weakness in the muscle on which the biopsy was performed may originate in fears that unrevealed disease was discovered or unmentioned damage was done during the procedure. Ascertaining precisely what the patient fears most may allow the physician to review the questionable information with the patient and thereby relieve his fears and associated symptoms.

OTHER NONINVASIVE TECHNIQUES

Evoked Potential Studies

Potential changes occur in the brain when a patient hears a click, sees a flash of light, or is shocked with electricity. The potentials evoked by these stimuli are generally too small to discriminate from the background noise of nonspecific electrical activity in the brain unless special techniques are used to amplify the stimulus-evoked potential (Figure 2.17). Such techniques are available and have been applied to studying the brain wave and

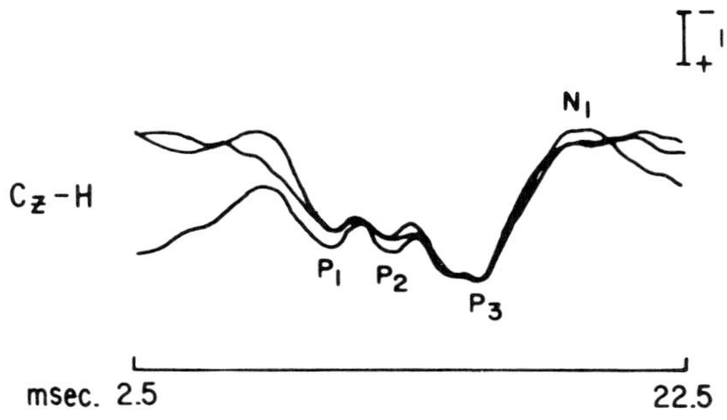

Figure 2.17. Stimulating the median nerve and recording from the scalp produced recurrent potential changes that were enhanced by repetitive stimulation and voltage-averaging techniques. The various components of this somatosensory evoked potential arise at different levels in the nervous system as the sensory information is transmitted to the cerebral cortex (courtesy of Dr. R. Q. Cracco).

in some cases spinal wave patterns elicited by a variety of stimuli (24). Their clinical applications are still extremely limited, but visual evoked potentials are now commonly used to help in the diagnosis of multiple sclerosis and auditory evoked potentials have shown some value in the diagnosis of brainstem disorders. The evoked potentials are altered in these diseases because the structures along the path of the evoked potentials are damaged and consequently interfere with the propagation of a normal evoked potential.

Electronystagmography

Nystagmus can be objectively studied with the same kind of equipment used for recording brain waves. The back of the eye carries a negative electrical charge relative to the front of the eye, and so the globe of the eye acts as a dipole, generating changes in electrical potentials around the eye as the globe moves. By monitoring these changes in potential around the eye, the movement of the eye can be reconstructed. In electronystagmography, nystagmus is induced by caloric stimulation of the semicircular canals in the ears, by having the patient stare at a set of moving stripes, or by rotating the patient on a chair. The patterns of nystagmus elicited are stereotyped in normal individuals and exhibit characteristic patterns of change with disease in different parts of the nervous system. Damage to the inner ear may decrease the amplitude of the nystagmus when that ear is stimulated, whereas damage to the cerebellum may produce an exaggerated nystagmus (15). The principal discomfort associated with this test is nausea. The information that it can provide in the evaluation of balance problems and vertigo is substantial.

Doppler Studies

Attempts to study blood flow in arteries to the brain have included the application of high frequency sound. Noninvasive sonar probes can map the lumen of the carotid artery with fairly convincing accuracy, but the level of resolution achieved with these techniques and the fundamentally two-dimensional view of the artery they provide have limited their clinical usefulness. A patient with suspected carotid artery disease would not be operated upon without an arteriogram of the vessel, and, if treatable disease of the carotid is suspected, an arteriogram is appropriate. Any symptoms justifying a Doppler study would justify an arteriogram, and so the noninvasive study will not eliminate the need for the more invasive arteriogram.

Proton Emission Tomography

Proton emission tomography is a radionuclide study combining the techniques used in computed tomography of the brain, radionuclide brain scanning, and perfusion studies. Radioactive material that emits protons is introduced into the nervous system as part of a molecule used in energy production or structural revision in brain cells. Where the radioactive material accumulates indicates what materials are used in various parts of the brain and what neural structures are most active in normal and pathologic situations. The neural activity during an epileptic fit or transient ischemic attack can be mapped out with the computerized system that reconstructs the metabolic outline of the brain from the proton emissions it records. This is still a strictly experimental technique that requires a linear accelerator near at hand for its operation.

REFERENCES

1. Denny-Brown D: *Handbook of Neurological Examination and Case Recording.* Cambridge, Harvard University Press, 1967.
2. DeJong RN: *The Neurologic Examination.* New York, Harper & Row, 1979.
3. Adams RD, Victor M: *Principles of Neurology.* New York, McGraw-Hill, 1977.
4. Merritt HH: *A Textbook of Neurology,* ed 5. Philadelphia, Lea & Febiger, 1973.
5. Geschwind N: Aphasia. *N Engl J Med* 284:654, 1971.
6. Task force on nomenclature and statistics, American Psychiatric Association: *Diagnostic and Statistical Manual of Mental Disorders (Third Edition).* Washington, DC, American Psychiatric Association, 1980.
7. Brodal A: *The Cranial Nerves,* ed 2. Oxford, Blackwell, 1965.
8. Blumer D: Temporal lobe epilepsy and its psychiatric significance, in Benson DF, Blumer D (eds): *Psychiatric Aspects of Neurologic Disease.* New York, Grune & Stratton, 1975, p 171.
9. Lessell S: Optic neuropathies. *N Engl J Med* 299:533, 1978.

10. Heilman KM, Valenstein E: Mechanisms underlying hemispatial neglect. *Ann Neurol* 5:166, 1979.

11. Blackwood W, Dix MR, Rudge P: The cerebral pathways of optokinetic nystagmus: A neuroanatomical study. *Brain* 98:297, 1975.

12. Plum F, Posner JB: *The Diagnosis of Stupor and Coma*, ed 3. Philadelphia, FA Davis, 1980.

13. Lance JW: Headache. *Neurology (NY)* 10:1, 1981.

14. Shallop JK: The measurement of middle ear function, in Singh S (ed): *Measurement Procedures in Speech, Hearing, and Language*. Baltimore, University Park Press, 1975, p 279.

15. Gilman S, Bloedel JR, Lechtenberg R: *Disorders of the Cerebellum*. Philadelphia, FA Davis, 1981.

16. Harner RN: EEG evaluation of the patient with dementia, in Benson DF, Blumer D (eds): *Psychiatric Aspects of Neurologic Disease*. New York, Grune & Stratton, 1975, p 63.

17. Babb RR, Eckman PB: Abdominal epilepsy. *J Am Med Assoc* 222:65, 1972.

18. Goldensohn ES, Koehle R: *EEG Interpretation*. Mount Kisco, NY, Futura Publishing, 1975.

19. DeVaul RA, Hall RCW: Hallucinations, in Hall RCW (ed): *Psychiatric Presentations of Medical Illness*. New York, SP Medical and Scientific Books, 1980, p 91.

20. Korein J, Cravioto H, Leicach M: Reevaluation of lumbar puncture. *Neurology (NY)* 9:290, 1959.

21. Parker SW: Case records of the Massachusetts General Hospital. Case 2-1981. *N Engl J Med* 304:100, 1981.

22. Jacobson RL, Farmer TW: The "hypernormal" CT scan in dementia: Bilateral isodense subdural hematomas. *Neurology (NY)* 29:1522, 1979.

23. Hakim S, Adams RD: The special clinical problem of symptomatic hydrocephalus with normal cerebrospinal fluid pressure: Observations on cerebrospinal fluid hydrodynamics. *J Neurol Sci* 2:307, 1965.

24. Anziska B, Cracco RQ: Short latency somatosensory evoked potentials: Studies in patients with focal neurological disease. *Electroencephalogr Clin Neurophysiol* 49:227, 1980.

3
The Unresponsive Patient

The unresponsive patient may be unconscious, paralyzed, psychotic, or uncooperative. A careful neurologic examination will clarify whether the altered response to the environment is from an altered level of consciousness, a defective neuromuscular system, a thought or affective disorder, or a contrived neurologic problem. Differentiating between these disorders is usually complicated and occasionally hazardous. Sophisticated patients can feign comatose states convincing enough to prompt intervention with life support measures, such as intubation, and investigation with highly invasive procedures, such as emergency arteriography. The motivations for feigning comatose states are as diverse as the forms the contrived unconsciousness may assume. Even when physicians and family members can offer no reason for the patient's feigning coma, factitious unresponsiveness still must be considered as a possible explanation for the patient's apparently altered consciousness. Of course, skepticism is also appropriate when the patient with a long psychiatric history or clear basis for secondary gain is found unresponsive. Careful neurologic evaluation of such a patient may demonstrate signs of structural brain damage or of acute drug overdose. Every patient with altered consciousness, regardless of the psychiatric history, must be examined and observed without prejudice. Both the psychiatrist and the neurologist are obliged to see that all appropriate and only appropriate measures are taken to investigate and support the patient.

COMA AND PSEUDOCOMA

To be considered unresponsive a patient need only remain unreactive and inattentive to stimuli directed toward him. Unresponsiveness may be from impaired consciousness, but there are several other possible causes including simple refusal to respond. Attempts to arouse an unresponsive patient routinely include calling his name, using a threatening visual stimulus, or applying pain to some part of his body. The type of response the patient exhibits to these different maneuvers determines the severity of his unresponsiveness. If all the evidence suggests that the patient has impaired consciousness (obtundation), it is important to establish the severity of the impaired consciousness at the time of the initial examination. Whether the level of consciousness is progressively deteriorating or improving has diagnostic and therapeutic implications in most conditions that can cause obtundation. There are several degrees of impaired consciousness, the most severe being coma and the mildest being stupor. If noxious stimuli elicit only reflex or semipurposeful activity, the patient is considered comatose. Such patients do not open their eyes when they are stimulated. They produce no comprehensible verbal response to questions and fail to move their limbs on command (1). If the patient can be aroused temporarily to a nearly normal level of consciousness with verbal or noxious stimuli, he is considered stuporous. Stuporous patients quickly revert to their inattentive, obtunded state when the stimulus is removed. Most comatose patients do not have alert facial expressions or purposeful eye movements, but some patients with structural damage deep in the cerebral gray matter may appear paradoxically alert despite their being mute, immobile, and unresponsive to noxious stimuli. These are the patients with so-called coma vigile. In sharp contrast to these profoundly impaired neurologic patients are the psychiatric patients with no brain disease who attempt to appear unconscious. The factitiously comatose patient may be so intent upon appearing obtunded that he will be inappropriately unreactive to noxious stimuli. Patients with intact or only mildly impaired cognitive function who fail to respond purposefully or appropriately to a variety of stimuli are said to be in pseudocoma (2). Such patients include the factitiously comatose individuals, who are willfully unresponsive to noxious stimuli, and the fully conscious victims of brainstem disease, who are unresponsive only because nervous system damage has blocked conventional pathways for responding.

Evaluation of the Unresponsive Patient

The evaluation of any unresponsive patient must determine whether or not the patient is unresponsive because of structural or physiologic damage to the brain and whether or not the patient is awake but simply unable to communicate his awareness of events around him. Obviously, considerable attention must be paid to metabolic status and drug history in the acutely comatose patient. Serum levels of electrolytes, hepatic enzymes, glucose, urea nitrogen, and creatinine should be checked as soon after the patient is seen by the physician as possible. Even if no respiratory problem is apparent, arterial blood gases must be examined for an unsuspected acidosis or alkalosis. A complete blood count may suggest a profound anemia or overwhelming infection is part of the patient's problem. Blood pressure, pulse, and temperature, as well as a hasty assessment of the patient's overall physical status, may point to the origin of the coma before any systematic attention is paid to the patient's neurologic signs. In special cases a little history is more valuable than an exhaustive physical examination. A known diabetic with an irregular diet and regular insulin injections is likely to have hypoglycemia as the basis for an abruptly appearing coma. A patient with several years of epileptic attacks is likely to be in a postictal state when he is found unconscious moments after being observed alert and talkative. The administration of glucose to the diabetic and patient observation of the epileptic will clarify the basis for unresponsiveness in these commonly encountered situations. More difficult to assess is the previously well patient who is found unreactive but without evident trauma, drug ingestion, or intravenous injection sites. The initial step in the evaluation is determining whether or not the patient is, in fact, in coma.

Clinical Signs in the Comatose Patient

Attention to breathing patterns, eye signs, spontaneous movements, and reflexes in all unresponsive patients is especially informative (3–5). An abnormal breathing pattern can be feigned, but certain breathing patterns are too complex or strenuous to be encountered ordinarily in patients voluntarily unresponsive. Rapid breathing at rates greater than 30 breaths per minute, varying respiratory rates and volumes, and prolonged cessation of breathing are fairly reliable indicators of a primarily metabolic or central nervous system disorder. Prolonged apnea, that is, an interruption in breathing lasting 20 to 30 seconds, typically occurs during the first few minutes of a grand mal seizure. Cheyne-Stokes cyclical breathing may signal a cardiac or brainstem problem. Hyperventilation in the patient with no metabolic reason to breathe rapidly and deeply may reflect extensive damage to brainstem structures. Of course, normal breathing patterns persist with most structural and metabolic central nervous system disorders, and a normal breathing pattern alone cannot be construed as evidence of hysteria, malingering, or psychosis.

Any initial examination must look for trauma, even when there is no history of an accident or injury. A young child may be the victim of a beating by a parent who denies any knowledge of trauma to the child. Evidence of a beating may be extremely subtle. A small hematoma in the scalp may be the only superficial change associated with a skull fracture. Burn marks on a child's skin should raise the physician's level of suspicion that child abuse is involved in the current case of unresponsiveness. Slash marks on the wrist or "track marks" along the limbs of an unresponsive adolescent or young adult increase the probability that a drug overdose is responsible for the patient's coma. The patient with fresh urine or feces on his clothes probably had incontinence during an epileptic fit and is unresponsive because he has not yet recovered from the seizure activity. Bite marks on the tongue will reinforce this suspicion. A very superficial examination of the patient may provide important clues to the cause of the patient's unresponsiveness.

Neurologic Signs Associated with Coma

Most patients with structural brain disease causing coma have signs of focal central nervous system damage. Flaccid limbs and absent reflexes restricted to one side of the body are likely with a deep intracerebral hemorrhage or extensive cerebral infarction. In many cases the impaired consciousness is the most obvious sign of an extensive brain lesion. There may be little more than obtundation and swelling of the optic nerve (papilledema) in a patient with a massive brain tumor. The optic nerve appears swollen because the tumor interferes with the flow of cerebrospinal fluid and precipitates an abrupt rise in intracranial pressure. A blood clot forming over the dural lining of the brain (epidural) or between dural and arachnoid layers of the meninges (subdural) will induce a progressive impairment of consciousness in patients with head trauma or other predisposing factors, such as chronic hemodialysis for kidney failure. Fortunately, most patients with space-occupying lesions inside the head will have asymmetric neurologic deficits that indicate the site, if not the nature, of the lesion.

Blood clots overlying the brain beneath the dural lining of the brain (subdural hematomas) are a common cause of coma, and are especially important because they require immediate surgical intervention (Figure 3.1). About 11 percent of all patients admitted for coma will have subdural hematomas, and fully one-third of those admitted in coma after documented head trauma will have a subdural, epidural, or intracerebral hematoma (6). Most of the patients developing this problem of intracranial bleeding with clot formation are young to middle-aged men involved in vehicular accidents (6). Increased intracranial pressure is always associated with subdural hematomas, but the pressure may increase so abruptly that the patient will not have papilledema until after the coma has been evident for several hours. The brain is often diffusely damaged from the head injury, and although there is a focal mass in the head that is life threatening, the signs of the head injury may be so diffuse that a focal lesion is not suggested by the physical findings. An acute alteration in consciousness may develop with intracranial bleeding without head trauma if the patient has a vascular abnormality in the brain, such as an arteriovenous malformation (Figure 3.2).

More systemic evidence of disease can also help to narrow the probable causes of an apparently rapidly evolving coma (4). A stiff neck, fever, and petechial skin rash in a young man is meningococcal meningitis until proven otherwise. The abrupt onset of ocular deviation, facial weakness,

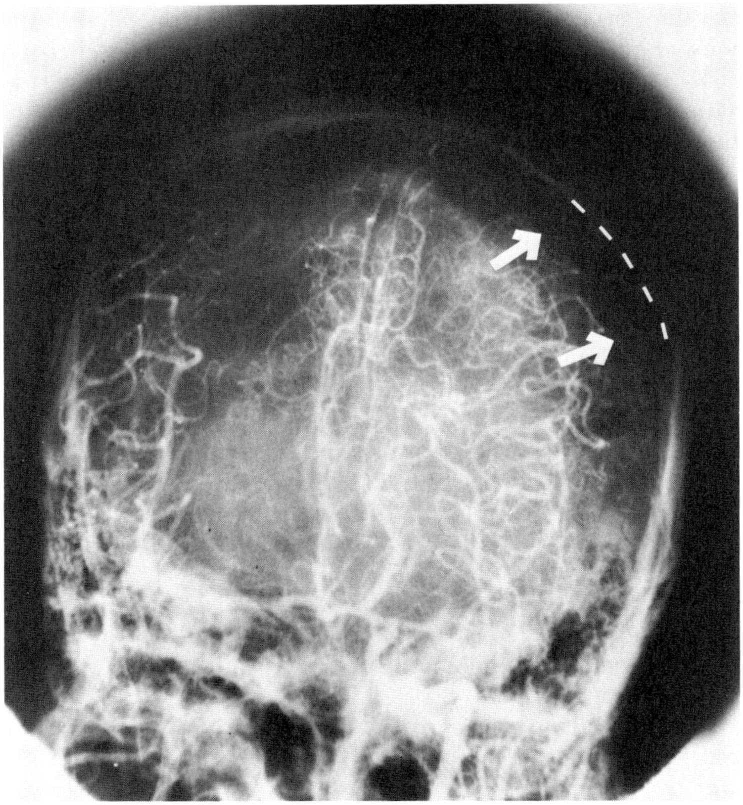

Figure 3.1. This arteriogram was performed on a 40-year-old man who was brought to the hospital unconscious. There was no history available. Neurologic examination revealed a dilated left pupil and bilaterally upgoing toes. The patient had a right focal seizure after admission. The arteriogram revealed a massive subdural hematoma (arrows). The broken white line marks the inner table of the skull. The subdural appears black because it is an avascular mass.

altered breathing rate, and decreased muscle tone on one side of the body in an elderly hypertensive woman suggests a massive intracerebellar hemorrhage. Yellowish discoloration of the whites of the eyes (scleral icterus) incriminates the liver or kidney as the causes of a metabolic encephalopathy leading to obtundation. In any patient, the preserved neurologic functions are just as important in arriving at a diagnosis as those lost or disordered. This is especially true when factitious coma is responsible for the obtundation.

Eye Movements in Coma and Pseudocoma

The normal awake person has two forms of eye movements, saccadic and pursuit. Saccadic eye movements are used to look from one point to another. These are the movements used in reading, glancing to-and-fro, and abruptly shifting gaze. Pursuit movements are used to follow steadily moving targets. The saccadic eye movements are steplike movements characterized by their abrupt onset and arrest. Pursuit movements are fluid changes in eye position, characterized by the continuity of their movement. For either of these movements to accurately keep the eyes on a target, one must have some vision, that is, some conscious registration of the image by the patient. If a person can follow or fix his vision on a target, he must be conscious and able to see. Indeed, true saccadic eye movements and pursuit eye movements are typically present only in the

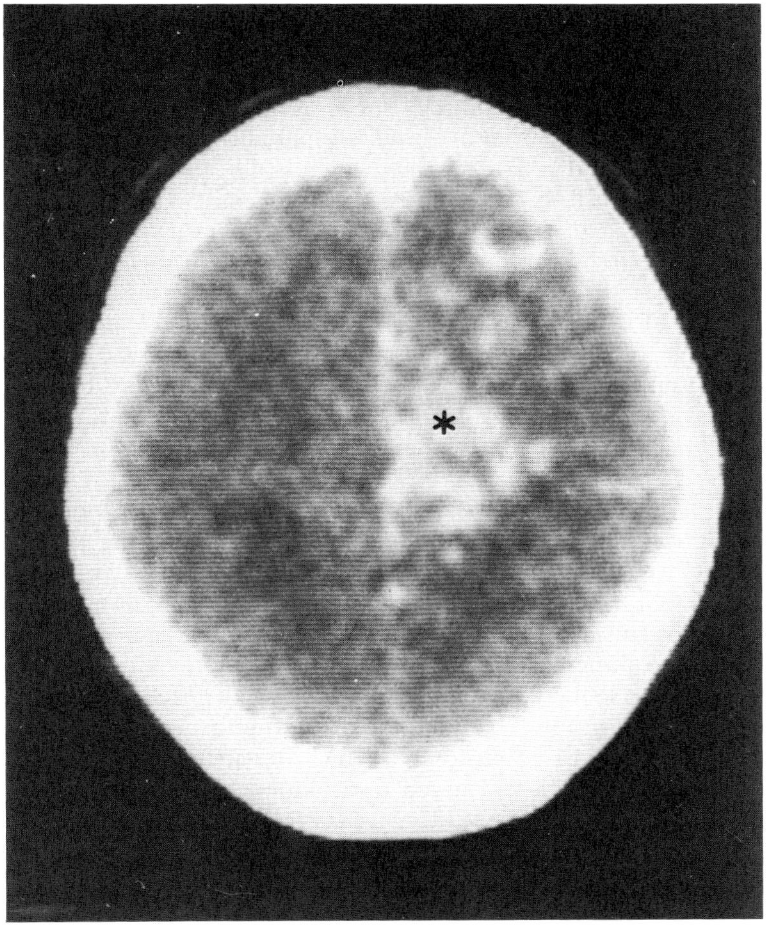

Figure 3.2. This computed tomogram of the head with contrast enhancement reveals a large arteriovenous malformation (*) in the parietal lobe that was responsible for a subarachnoid hemorrage. The 29-year-old patient with this lesion suffered an abrupt alteration in consciousness at the time of the hemorrhage.

conscious patient. A patient can be paralyzed by damage to the brainstem and be left mute and immobile, but maintain fully normal eye movements (Table 3.1).

Locked-in Syndrome. One clinical situation known to produce this combination of deficits is the "locked-in" syndrome (2,4). This results from damage to the ventral pons of the brainstem with sparing of the ocular motor nuclei and reticular activating systems but with loss of the corticospinal tract fibers. The patient maintains voluntary control over his eye movements but loses control of face and limb movements. Facial paralysis may eliminate grimacing or smiling, but allow eye blinking. Damage to fiber tracts from the cerebral cortex to the medulla oblongata of the brainstem will leave the patient mute. Speech is lost because of the resulting laryngeal paralysis, and breathing is occasionally impaired or completely lost. There is no loss of consciousness although the patient appears unresponsive. The best evidence that the patient is awake is the preservation of saccadic and pursuit eye movements. On instructions to look to the right, the eyes will move in one step to the right. When instructed to follow a moving light, the eyes will sweep smoothly along the same trajectory as the light. Patterned blinks may be used for communication. This locked-in syndrome is often only a transient state in the progressive deterioration of a terminally ill patient. The responsible brainstem lesion, whether it be infarction or neoplasia, is likely to progress, destroy vital respiratory centers, and result in respiratory failure. Even if the patient is supported on a respirator, blood pressure and pulse irregularities often cause death.

Eye Movements in Factitious Coma. Eye movements will be preserved in the patient feigning coma, but they may be abnormal (7). The patient may resist efforts to open his eyes or may roll his eyes about when the lids are retracted. A blink response to visual threat indicates intact vision, but in the absence of this conscious response, certain ocular motor reflexes will be intact if the patient is neurologically intact. Opticokinetic nystagmus appears when a striped cloth is drawn across the field of vision. The patient with intact vision has nystagmus with the fast component, or jerk, in the direction opposite that toward which the stripes are moving. If an unresponsive patient has preserved opticokinetic nystagmus, he is awake

Table 3.1. Causes of Pseudocoma

Factitious coma
Catatonia
Locked-in syndrome
Neuromuscular junction disease

and able to see. Doll's eye movements are ordinarily not found in the awake patient, but these are an unreliable indicator of obtundation (4). Simply stated, doll's eye movements are reflex eye movements in response to rapid changes in head position. In the stuporous patient, rotation of the head to the right will produce conjugate deviation of the eyes to the left. It is as if the patient were fixing his gaze on an imaginary point in space and staring at that point despite the involuntary head movements. With a deepening level of coma, this oculocephalic reflex may be entirely absent (8). The loss of this reflex also may occur with some drug overdoses, such as phenytoin overdose. Ophthalmoplegia, that is absent eye movements, is not typical of authentic stupor.

Eye movements similar to those seen with the oculocephalic (doll's eye) reflex can also be feigned. An awake patient may simply stare at a remote point in the examining room and thereby appear to have a prominent doll's eye response. Staring at such a point would also suppress the random saccadic eye movements that would suggest the patient is awake. This voluntary fixation can be broken by filling the patient's central field of vision with a mirror and rapidly moving the mirror. With no stable point in the environment to fixate on, the patient with vision will have eye movements in concert with the movements of the mirror. Such maneuvers are usually unnecessary. A patient in authentic coma usually has disordered eye movements, and a patient unresponsive but awake usually has saccadic and pursuit eye movements.

Roving Eye Movements. With depressed consciousness, eye movements may become roving and dysconjugate. Roving eye movements are slow, fluid, apparently purposeless, changes in eye position. The eyes may move synchronously in the same direction and so remain conjugate, or they may drift separately, more or less independently, and so become dysconjugate. Dysconjugate roving eye movements are a reliable indicator of stupor or coma. The patient with a long depressive history appearing acutely unresponsive with these eye signs would be suspected of a depressant overdose (9). A common combination is coma, mildly dilated pupils, and dysconjugate roving eye movements with glutethimide overdose (2). Barbiturate excess in the epileptic patient treated with phenobarbital as an anticonvulsant may produce a similar picture, but this causes smaller pupils. Atropinic drugs, such as those used in many over-the-counter sleep medications, will produce a similar pattern of unresponsiveness but with widely dilated pupils.

Nystagmus and Ocular Bobbing. Considerably more ominous than roving or dysconjugate gaze are the various forms of jerking eye movements called nystagmus. A spontaneous down-beating nystagmus affecting both eyes synchronously is strong evidence for a brainstem lesion at the junction of the cervical spinal cord and the medulla oblongata of the brainstem.

Spontaneous lateral nystagmus with both eyes deviated in the direction of the fast component may reflect a massive cerebellar hemorrhage. Less rapid, less frequent, conjugate downward deviation of the eyes with a slow phase returning the eyes to the primary position may represent ocular bobbing, a sign often associated with massive brainstem damage at the level of the pons. Ocular bobbing is especially common with basilar artery occlusion, a lesion producing brainstem infarction likely to be fatal. Nystagmus or ophthalmoplegia, that is, paralysis of eye movements, may appear with gait problems and impaired mentation just before the onset of coma in patients with Wernicke's encephalopathy, a progressive disease affecting the hypothalamus and periventricular brainstem structures in thiamine-deficient alcoholic patients.

All these disorders emphasize the clinical significance of eye movements. Careful observation of eye signs is invaluable in correctly reconstructing the events surrounding the patient's lapse into stupor or coma. Not only do they help in determining the presence of coma rather than pseudocoma, but they also help define the basis for the coma when it is authentic.

Inconsistent Signs in Pseudocoma

A more casual examination of the unresponsive patient is appropriate when a systematic examination of neurologic signs has failed to establish whether the physician is treating a truly unresponsive patient or one who is feigning coma. Random movements when not under overt scrutiny should be consistent with deficits found on formal examination. A paralyzed arm should not reach for an irritating strap or intravenous line. Alternatively, reflex positioning of the arms and legs, called "posturing," may be more apparent when the patient is left undisturbed for a few moments. This posturing is an ominous sign; it often reflects increased intracranial pressure and warrants emergency computed tomography of the head and cerebral angiography to search for an intracranial mass. When such signs are not immediately apparent, the physician is obliged to periodically reevaluate the patient's neurologic status. He will not only be able to assess the consistency of the deficits, but he will also be able to observe the evolution of signs. A patient with progressive decrease in the tone on one side of his body may have an enlarging intracranial blood clot, whereas a patient with confused movements after a period of apparent paralysis may be recovering from an epileptic fit. The evolution of signs is often much more informative than the signs themselves.

CATATONIA: PSYCHIATRIC AND NEUROLOGIC

In practice, hysterical coma or a contrived state of unresponsiveness, consciously directed toward secondary gain, is easily distinguished from a metabolic coma or coma arising with structural central nervous system disease. The signs already discussed are usually an adequate basis for deciding between these psychogenic and neurogenic "comas." Such a distinction is not so easily made with psychotic disorders producing various catatonic states. Psychogenic catatonia may be identical in symptomatology to neurogenic stupor or coma; and, alternatively, catatonic states associated with a clear history of psychosis may prove to arise from metabolic or toxic causes (10–13). All the classic signs of catatonia, such as waxy flexibility (catalepsy), negativism, mutism, posturing, and rigidity, appear with some focal brain lesions and during the postictal period of some seizure disorders (Table 3.2) (10).

Parkinsonism and Catatonia

The strictly motor phenomena associated with a psychogenic catatonia are reminiscent of motor signs in neurologic disorders characterized by decreased movement, such as Parkinson disease. Abnormal postures persist in the catatonic and parkinsonian patient. The catatonic patient may hold his head slightly off the bed when he is lying down or he may hold his legs in remarkably flexed postures for long periods of time (14). Maintenance of such awkward postures is also typical of the parkinsonian individual. Also exhibited by the catatonic patient is a susceptibility to 'magnetic' movements. In this, a limb will move toward light pressure exerted by the examiner or it may spring mechanically back to its original position when released by the examiner (14). Paralleling the "on-off response" exhibited by Parkinson disease victims on levodopa, the psychotic

Table 3.2. Causes of Catatonia

Psychogenic catatonia
Lethal catatonia
Hyperpathic akinetic matism
Postictal confusion
Subarachnoid hemorrhage
Viral encephalitis
Postconcussion syndrome
Parkinsonism
Hyperparathyroidism
Hypothyroidism
Medial temporal lobe lesions
Midbrain lesions
Neurotoxin or hallucinogen ingestion
Tumors of the fornix
Medial frontal lobe damage
Carbon monoxide poisoning
Methioninemia with homocystinuria

catatonic patient may precipitately, but transiently, become akinetic in the midst of excessively brisk speech or motor activity (14).

Metabolic and Structural Causes of Catatonia

Some metabolic diseases cause similar symptoms. Occasional patients, initially diagnosed as schizophrenic with catatonia, actually have hyperparathydroidism with abnormally high serum calcium levels. The psychotic disturbance in hyperparathyroid patients abates with treatment of the disordered calcium metabolism (11,13). Clearly, this misdiagnosis is fostered by the high probability that an apparently catatonic patient will have schizophrenia (15). Five percent of schizophrenics have catatonic symptomatology at some time during the course of their disease, and only rare individuals with hyperparathyroidism or other metabolic disorders ever exhibit catatonic signs (10). Distinguishing between the psychiatric and metabolic conditions is further complicated by the psychiatric signs that develop in patients with metabolic diseases. Some patients with catatonia and metabolic disorders have episodes of typical schizophrenic behavior. Homocystinuria with hypermethioninemia, a congenital disorder of metabolism of the amino acid homocystine, can produce the signs of a paranoid schizophrenia with catatonic episodes (12). Rare patients with this disorder have a folate-responsive "schizophrenia." The diagnosis is worth considering if the patient's urine reacts positively with cyanide nitroprusside. This reaction indicates elevated homocystine levels in the urine (12). Treating the patient with folate abolishes many of the psychiatric phenomena.

Structural lesions of the nervous system also may produce transient catatonic states (16). After a severe concussion or with subarachnoid hemorrhage the patient may pass through a catatonic phase, which may even have the hyperthermia and excitement seen with psychogenic catatonia (10,16–18). Medial temporal lobe damage and even midbrain lesions have been associated with catatonic states (16). Twelve percent of patients with catatonia have some evidence of focal temporal lobe dysfunction, whether the catatonia is associated with schizophrenia or not (10,17). Neurotoxins and hallucinogens, such as mescaline, ethyl alcohol, amphetamines, and phencyclidine, may all precipitate catatonic states (10). Tumors of the fornix impinging upon the septum pellucidum, the membrane dividing the lateral ventricles from each other, also produce such unresponsiveness. Even degenerative diseases, such as Pick disease, may produce discrete episodes of recurrent catatonia (19). Mood fluctuations, impaired judgment, restlessness, indecisiveness, and other signs suggestive of strictly psychiatric disease may evolve before the appearance of catatonia in focal degenerative disease (19). Neurosyphilis, cerebral cysts, systemic lupus erythematosus, and tuberous sclerosis all have been associated with catatonic stupors (15,20).

Objective neurologic investigations are occasionally misleading in distinguishing catatonia on a psychiatric basis from that on a neurologic basis. The electroencephalogram in catatonic states associated with typical schizophrenia is often abnormal despite the absence of structural brain damage in these patients (21). Brain wave activity may, in fact, reflect physiologic dysfunction secondary to attempts at treatment. For example, before the diagnosis of schizophrenia is reached, some patients are treated with electroconculsive therapy for their withdrawn behavior. As late as 10 months after this electroconvulsive treatment, the electroencephalogram will show persistent abnormalities.

Lethal Catatonia

Straddling the line between patients with psychogenic and neurogenic catatonia are those with lethal catatonia (Table 3.3). This disorder is characterized by protracted episodes of unresponsiveness, preceded or interrupted by periods of profound agitation, aimless combativeness, confusion, and delirium (18,27). These patients have fevers that may be extremely high. They become dehydrated and die from cardiovascular collapse (27). The entire disease lasts days to weeks. Autopsy examination of the brain rarely shows any abnormalities; and, when pathology is present, it is not adequate to explain why the patient died (18). There is some focal loss of nerve cells in the second to fifth cortical layers of the frontal lobes, but this probably develops secondary to the hyperthermia and dehydration that develop in these severely catatonic patients (17). Symptoms indistinguishable from those appearing in lethal catatonia occur with general paresis, viral encephalitis, and brainstem strokes; but a substantial number of patients are left with the diagnosis of idiopathic lethal catatonia when these possible causes of brain damage are excluded (26,28).

This is a rare disorder, appearing in only 0.23 percent of psychiatric admissions (27). It develops in men three times as often as in women and is fatal in about one-third of cases (27). Fifty-two to 84 percent of the patients who do not die during the catatonic episode have signs of schizophrenia when they have fully recovered from the lethal catatonia (18). Autopsies have been performed on patients dying with lethal catatonia

Table 3.3. Diagnostic Considerations in Lethal Catatonia

Acute schizophrenia
Viral encephalitis
Neuroleptic malignant syndrome
Malignant hyperthermia

very rarely, but the autopsies obtained suggest that in at least some of these patients a low-grade viral encephalitis played a role in their disease (18,28).

Although some patients have a history of schizophrenia before the development of a lethal catatonia, others have a prodrome of abnormal behavior or a thought disorder that spans a few hours to a few weeks. Prodromal symptoms include delusions, anxiety, insomnia, apathy, behavior disorder, and anorexia. Electroconvulsive therapy is viewed as lifesaving by some, but there is no structured study of the advantages of electroconvulsive therapy in this disorder (18). Treating schizophrenic patients with neuroleptics does not prevent or reverse lethal catatonia and, in fact, may induce a syndrome identical to lethal catatonia (29). Patients on haloperidol or a phenothiazine, especially fluphenazine, may abruptly develop fever, rigidity, and stupor evolving into death (30). This neuroleptic malignant syndrome is an idiosyncratic reaction to the drugs and cannot be used to explain the origin of lethal catatonia since the lethal catatonia syndrome was described before phenothiazines and butyrophenones were introduced into psychotherapy (29). A neuromuscular disorder that also resembles lethal catatonia is malignant hyperthermia, a hereditary muscle disease that causes high fevers, progressive obtundation, and death after exposure to various anesthetic agents (30). This is a hereditary disorder, and typical muscle changes will be apparent at autopsy. It is worth considering as the explanation for the patient's abrupt deterioration if that occurs after general anesthesia.

VEGETATIVE STATES

The chronically unresponsive patients with brain damage who do not appear to be in coma and who clearly do not have a metabolic, endocrine, or infectious basis for their condition fall into various types of vegetative states (22). These patients are said to be in a vegetative state because their neurologic functioning is reduced to automatic or vegetative activities (Figure 3.3). There is no behavioral evidence of a functional cerebral cortex. The patient makes no adaptive responses to the environment, but he does appear to have long periods of wakefulness (23). This is also called the apallic syndrome when it is presumed that the cortical gray matter mantle over the cerebral hemispheres, the so-called pallium, is lost (24). This is not brain death, but it may represent cerebral cortical death (3,22,24).

The Apallic Syndrome

The apallic syndrome is not likely to be confused with factitious coma, if only because of the circumstances usually surrounding its appearance.

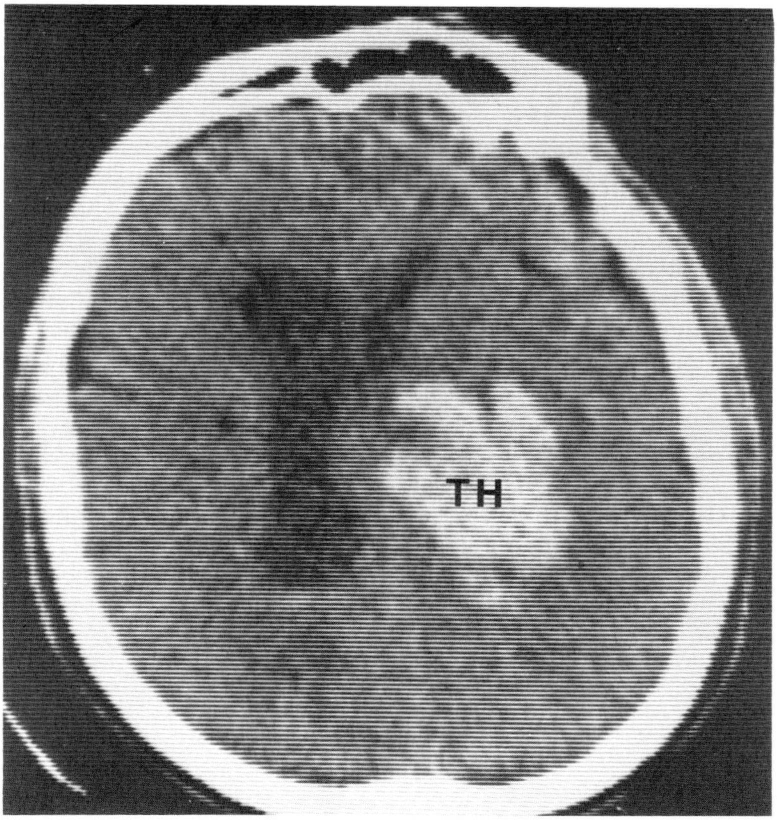

Figure 3.3. A 63-year-old man with a long history of hypertension developed right-sided weakness and severe obtundation over the course of a few hours. This computed tomogram of his brain without contrast enhancement shows a large collection of fresh blood (TH) extending from the left thalamic area. Although this patient survived the stroke, he remained in a vegetative state for more than 1 year after the acute hemorrhage. He required a nasogastric tube for feeding, but breathing was regular and adequate without any assistance (courtesy of Drs. J. Loh and W. Hotson).

This vegetative state appears most commonly after cardiopulmonary arrest, head trauma, and occasionally brainstem stroke (3,22,25). What gives these patients a deceptively alert appearance is their tendency to open their eyes a few weeks after the insult and to blink in response to threat. Teeth grinding (bruxism), chewing, and swallowing may occur spontaneously or with placement of food in the mouth. Eye movements may be roving, but smooth; and the mute patient may appear to follow the examiner about the room. Primitive avoidance reactions, such as withdrawal of a limb from painful stimuli, often develop (24).

Those patients with vegetative states resulting from strictly cerebral cortical destruction will have an electroencephalogram with low voltage waves. In the most severe cases, the electroencephalogram will be diffusely flat-line, a record termed isoelectric (24). Applying noxious stimuli to patients in stupor with preserved cortical mantles will produce changes on the electroencephalogram typical of arousal. With the apallic state, there is no registration of noxious stimuli at the cortical level, and so there is no arousal pattern on the electroencephalogram (24). That an isoelectric electroencephalogram does not invariably indicate brain death is apparent in those vegetative patients whose electroencephalographic rhythms may vary from isoelectric to slow, low voltage activity over the course of months (22). Any patient who has suffered profound hypothermia, massive head trauma, or barbiturate intoxication may have a transiently isoelectric electroencephalogram.

The impression that the patients in vegetative states are actually conscious is reinforced by the appearance of reflexes that seem purposeful. Within a few weeks of the onset of the unresponsiveness, the patient may grasp objects placed in his hand (22). This is a reflex elicited by any stimulus drawn across the palm. Hopeful relatives misconstrue this grasp reflex as an attempt by the patient to acknowledge their presence. Mild tactile stimuli may trigger flexion reflexes in one or several limbs, again prompting speculation that the patient has become more alert and restless. The appearance of alertness in these patients has prompted the title coma vigile in some descriptions of this condition (22,24).

Akinetic Mutism

The patient in a vegetative state because of destruction of his cerebral cortex has no real prospect of intellectual recovery, but there are transient vegetative states. Akinetic mutism was a term first applied to describe a young girl in a vegetative state who had remissions of her unresponsiveness (22). She had a craniopharyngioma, a cystic growth in the anterior part of the brain, which produced episodes of unresponsiveness as it enlarged. Each time the cyst was drained the patient awoke and remained alert and responsive for months at a time. Similar patients have been described with lesions of the brainstem, basal ganglia, and cingulate gyri (22,26).

Although akinetic mutism is a fairly accurate descriptive term, there is a spectrum of unresponsiveness in these patients (Table 3.4). At one end is the "hyperpathic" akinetic mutism in which the immobile, mute, inattentive patient intermittently becomes restless, excited, and even combative (26). When adequately stimulated, this ordinarily mute patient may respond with one or two words. In fact, the first patient designated akinetic mute occasionally spoke in whispered tones. These hyperpathic akinetic mute patients have no impairment of eye movements and appear so awake

Table 3.4. Signs of Catatonia and Akinetic Mutism

Catatonia	*Akinetic Mutism*
COMMON FEATURES	COMMON FEATURES
Mutism	Mutism
Posturing	Intact reflex response to noxious stimuli
Waxy flexibility	No retention of imposed postures
Rigidity	Spastic or flaccid limbs
Intact eye movements	Intact eye movements
Apparent vigilance	Apparent vigilance
Recall of events during catatonia	Amnesia for events during unresponsiveness
Negativism	
OCCASIONAL FEATURES	OCCASIONAL FEATURES
Episodic excitement	Episodic excitement and combativeness (hyperpathic form)
Hyperthermia	Hypersomnia or disturbed sleep-wake cycle (apathetic form)
	Paralysis of vertical gaze

that they are often described as in a vigilant coma or coma vigile (26). The patient appears unwilling to speak or move.

The alternative to coma vigile or hyperpathic akinetic mutism is the apathetic akinetic mutism. Victims of this disorder have hypersomnia and may have disturbances of sleep-wake cycles (26). These patients also have paralysis of vertical gaze and other forms of ophthalmoplegia. The pupillary light reflex, which is preserved in hyperpathic akinetic mutism, may be lost in the apathetic mutism. The episodic excitement and combativeness characteristic of the hyperpathic form does not occur in the apathetic form. The basic feature of akinetic mutism, that is, an apparently awake but unresponsive patient, occurs in both the hyperpathic and apathetic forms of akinetic mutism. The electroencephalogram with apathetic mutism may show diffuse slowing (26). The lesions in the apathetic form are similar to those in the midbrain, hypothalmus, and thalamus seen with the hyperpathic mutism, but there is more extensive damage. The syndrome of apathetic akinetic mutism from brainstem damage probably represents disconnection of the thalamus from its reticular system inputs.

Episodes of catatonia alternating with agitation, screaming, and combativeness can develop with structural damage to the mesial aspect of the frontal lobe, as well as with damage in the midbrain (mesencephalon) (26). The cortical areas usually involved with this frontal lobe disorder are the cingulate gyri, areas of cortex implicated in the "limbic system" of the brain. Because the frontal lobe lesions are rarely limited to this anterior mesial aspect of the cortex, the patients with this form of vigilant coma routinely also demonstrate seizures, hemiplegias, or at least, extensor plantar responses. Other causes of akinetic mutism include damage to the basal ganglia bilaterally. Carbon monoxide poisoning may selectively destroy these deep gray matter structures (26). Patients so affected may remain in coma vigile for years before dying.

Unlike the catatonic patient who may recall vividly events occurring around him during the period of unresponsiveness, the rare patient with akinetic mutism or coma vigile who recovers from his unresponsiveness will have no recall of events during the paradoxical coma (2). Obviously, the amylobarbitone injection test helpful in interviewing the catatonic patient will yield no information from the vegetative or akinetic patient.

FAINTING (SYNCOPE)

Fainting spells, "blackouts," and "drop-attacks" elicit considerable anxiety in those subject to them, but the etiology of this syncope is relatively benign in most individuals. To be a true syncopal episode, the patient must have had a transient loss of consciousness. If the period of unresponsiveness is observed to be longer than 2 to 3 minutes, then epilepsy, metabolic encephalopathy, or psychogenic unresponsiveness should be suspected (Table 3.5). True syncope involves an apparent loss of consciousness, rather than just altered consciousness, with no tonic or clonic muscular contractions. The patient will fall if he is standing, but there is rarely any vertigo preceding the attack. Characteristically, the individual feels unsteady or weak and his vision grays as he loses postural tone. The interval from unsteadiness to falling and loss of consciousness is generally less than 30 seconds. Immediately after syncope, there is no confusion or focal weakness to suggest a seizure disorder. Syncopal episodes may occur several times a day or several times a decade. Their frequency will be determined by their etiology.

The basic event inducing syncope is a brief alteration in the blood supply to the brain. Either the amount of blood is inadequate or the

Table 3.5. Causes of Syncope

Hysterical unresponsiveness
Hyperventilation syncope
Cardiac arrhythmias
Postural hypotension
Epilepsy
Subclavian steal syndrome
Transient ischemic attacks
Hypersensitive carotid sinus
Basilar impression

content of the blood is inappropriate for maintaining consciousness. A precipitate drop in intracranial perfusion will develop with cardiac arrhythmias and postural hypotension. These cardiovascular problems should be considered leading possibilities in elderly individuals and any individual with a history of heart disease. Postural hypotension is especially likely in patients treated for hypertension with antihypertensive medications. When the patient stands or sits up quickly, his blood pressure falls abruptly and syncope occurs. This is most easily dealt with by decreasing the dose of antihypertensive medications used. Unfortunately, postural hypotension also develops in diseases affecting the autonomic nervous system. Diabetic patients and victims of Parkinson disease are prone to problems with maintaining a normal blood pressure and are largely untreatable (32,33). Cardiac arrhythmias may be associated with an abnormal resting electrocardiogram; but, more frequently, the arrhythmia is reflected in electrocardiographic changes only during the episode. By attaching a recording device to the patient for a day or more, transient arrhythmias can be detected, identified, and treated with the appropriate antiarrhythmic drugs. Stokes-Adams attacks are transient cardiac arrhythmias that produce syncope because there is inadequate cerebral perfusion. Some individuals with unusually sensitive carotid sinuses will faint when slight pressure is applied over this part of the carotid artery. The syncope results from excessive slowing of the heart rate, an exaggeration of a normal reflex.

Hyperventilation Syncope

Most patients with syncope do not have cardiovascular problems as the basis for syncope. If the individual is young or middle-aged and on no medications that could cause episodic falls in blood pressure, the most likely explanation for the syncope is hyperventilation. This inadvertant overbreathing usually appears in a setting of acute stress or chronic depression. Syncope results from a metabolic problem induced by the hyperventilation. Excessive carbon dioxide is lost from the blood during overbreathing and an acute respiratory alkalosis develops. This alkalosis leads to syncope, which stops the hyperventilation and allows blood carbon dioxide levels to return to normal. The syncope can be aborted by halting air exchange either by breathing into a largely airtight container or by not breathing at all. The victim of hyperventilation syncope is unaware of the deep breathing that leads to the fainting spells. Most will comment that they make a conscious effort to breathe deeply when they start to feel unsteady or their vision begins to gray. The physiology involved in this syncope is not at all abnormal. The patient is having a normal response to an abnormal breathing pattern. This might justly be called a type of conversion reaction since a disability is self-imposed in the absence of organic pathology, but the syncope is not factitious. Explaining the mechanism for the syncope will allow the patient to minimize its occurrence, but other symptoms will appear if the underlying stress or maladjustment is not eliminated.

Basilar Impression

Syncope occasionally develops with basilar skull abnormalities, but associated signs, such as unilateral weakness and lingering memory difficulty, help distinguish this structural problem from hyperventilation syncope. The patient may complain of dizziness, tinnitus, altered vision, altered hearing, and syncope developing on extension of the neck (34). Presumably, posterior fossa blood flow supplied by the vertebrobasilar system of arteries is compromised where it enters the skull because of the basilar skull malformation (34). A skull x-ray will identify the problem and relatively minor surgery may correct it.

Orthostatic Hypotension

Orthostatic hypotension is a fall in blood pressure associated with assuming an upright position. If the fall in blood pressure is substantial enough, the patient will faint (Table 3.6). Orthostatic hypotension occurs with a decrease in the total blood volume, such as that which occurs after substantial bleeding and with Addison's disease, with diminished cardiac output and with impaired reflex increase in peripheral resistance (35). Fortunately, this is rarely a chronic problem, but there are disorders of the central or peripheral sympathetic nervous system that will produce intractable orthostatic hypotension and, consequently, recurrent syncope (31). This is a disorder of the sympathetic nervous system because it is this part of the autonomic nervous system that regulates arteriolar vasoconstriction, venomotor tone, myocardial contractility, and cardiac rate in response to gravity (31)

Table 3.6. Nervous System Diseases Causing Fainting from Orthostatic Hypotension

Diabetes mellitis
Amyloidosis
Thiamine deficiency
Parkinson disease
Shy-Drager syndrome
Tabes dorsalis (neurosyphilis)
Combined system disease (vitamin B_{12} deficiency)
Antihypertensive medication
Primary orthostatic hypotension

Diabetes mellitus, amyloidosis, and thiamine deficiency can cause autonomic damage substantial enough to produce orthostatic hypotension, but patients so severely affected by their metabolic disease invariably have disturbed bowel function, abnormal sweating, and impotence as other signs of the dysautonomia (35,36). Orthostatic hypotension secondary to disease in the central nervous system is seen most often in the rare degenerative disorder called the Shy-Drager syndrome (32,33,35). This is discussed in detail in the section on impotence because the initial sign of the dysautonomia in this syndrome usually is impaired sexual function. Spinal cord disease alone can cause orthostatic hypotension, and this occasionally develops with tabes dorsalis and combined system disease (33). Sympathetic blocking agents used in the treatment of hypertension, such as guanethidine, can produce orthostatic hypotension (33).

If there is no iatrogenic basis or discrete nervous system disorder to explain the orthostatic hypotension, it is called primary orthostatic hypotension (33,35). The affected individual may have an intact peripheral autonomic system but a defective central autonomic system. Neurotransmitters of both major types usually involved in autonomic nervous system function, specifically, cholinergic and adrenergic neurotransmitters are involved in this postural problem. Because both of these elements of the autonomic system are affected, the patient has none of the cholinergic signs typically developing in most conditions before a faint. With an intact cholinergic response to impending syncope, the patient would notice perspiration and would develop bradycardia. With this system inactive along with the adrenergic system, the patient has no warning that syncope is imminent and simply faints on standing (33). Ordinarily, the adrenergic system prevents the pooling of blood in dependent elements of the body when the normal individual stands up. Failure of this system to increase vascular tone deprives the brain of adequate perfusion. After prolonged bedrest, elderly patients will have transient problems with this reflex adrenergic activity, and fainting may occur if an upright posture is not reassumed gradually (33).

Primary orthostatic hypotension is difficult to treat. Approaches have included transvenous coronary sinus atrial-demand pacemakers, elastic stockings, antigravity suits, mineralocorticoids, and sympathomimetic amines (31). No treatment has had much lasting success. This is usually a progressive disorder.

REFERENCES

1. Brooks DN, Aughton ME, Bond MR, et al: Cognitive sequelae in relationship to early indices of severity of brain damage after severe blunt head injury. *J. Neurol Neurosurg Psychiatry* 43:529, 1980.

2. Posner, JB: Coma and other states of consciousness: The differential diagnosis of brain death. *Ann NY Acad Sci* 315:215, 1978.
3. Snyder, BD, Ramirez-Lassepas M, Lippert DM: Neurologic status and prognosis after cardiopulmonary arrest: I. A retrospective study. *Neurology (NY)* 27:807,1977.
4. Plum F, Posner JB: *The Diagnosis of Stupor and Coma,* ed 3. Philadelphia, FA Davis, 1980.
5. Williams M: Memory disorders associated with electroconvulsive therapy, in Whitty CWM, Zangwill OL (eds): *Amnesia. Clinical, Psychological and Medicolegal Aspects,* ed 2. London, Butterworths, 1977, p. 183.
6. Grossman RG: Treatment of patients with intracranial hematomas. *N Engl J Med* 304:1540, 1981.
7. Rodin EA: Psychosocial management of patients with complex partial seizures, in Penry JK, Daly DD (eds): *Advances in Neurology.* New York, Raven Press, 1975, vol 11, p. 383.
8. Mladinich EK, Carlow TJ: Total gaze garesis in amitriptyline overdose. *Neurology (NY)* 27:695, 1977.
9. Bird TD, Plum F: Recovery from barbiturate overdose coma with a prolonged isoelectric electroencephalogram. *Neurology (NY)* 18:456, 1968.
10. Gelenberg AJ: The catatonic syndrome. *Lancet* 1:1339, 1976.
11. Gatewood JW, Organ CH, Mead BT: Mental changes associated with hyperparathyroidism. *Am J Psychiatry* 132:129, 1975.
12. Freeman JM, Finkelstein JD, Mudd SH: Folate-responsive homocystinuria and "schizophrenia." *N Engl J Med* 292:491, 1975.
13. Karpati G, Frame B: Neuropsychiatric disorders in primary hyperparathyroidism. *Arch Neurol* 10:387, 1964.
14. Marsden CB, Tarsy D, Baldessarini RJ: Spontaneous and drug-induced movement disorders in psychotic patients, in Benson DF, Blumer D (eds): *Psychiatric Aspects of Neurologic Disease.* New York, Grune & Stratton, 1975, p 219.
15. Raskin DE, Frank SW: Herpes encephalitis with catatonic stupor. *Arch Gen Psychiatry* 31:544, 1974.
16. Teuber HL: Prospects for research on schizophrenia: Effects of focal brain lesions. *Neurosci Res Program Bull* 10:381, 1972.
17. Plum F: Prospects for research on schizophrenia: Neuropathological findings. *Neurosci Res Program Bull* 10:384, 1972.
18. Penn H, Racy J, Lapham L, et al: Catatonic behavior, viral encephalopathy, and death. *Arch Gen Psychiatry* 27:758, 1972.
19. Ruff RL, Russakoff LM: Catatonia with frontal lobe atrophy. *J Neurol Neurosurg Psychiatry* 43:185, 1980.
20. Bennett R, Hughes GRV, Bywaters EGL, et al: Neuropsychiatric problems in systemic lupus erythematosus. *Br Med J* 4:342, 1972.
21. Abenson MH: EEG's in chronic schizophrenia. *Br J Psychiatry* 116:421, 1970.
22. Jennett B, Plum F: Persistent vegetative state after brain damage. *Lancet* 1:734, 1972.
23. Sisler GC: Psychiatric disorder associated with head injury, in Hendrie HC (ed): *The Psychiatric Clinics of North America.* Philadelphia, WB Saunders, 1978, vol 1, p 137.
24. Ingvar DH, Brun A, Johansson L, et al: Survival after severe cerebral anoxia with destruction of the cerebral cortex. The apallic syndrome. *Ann NY Acad Sci* 315:184, 1978.
25. Ingvar DH, Sourander P: Destruction of the reticular core of the brainstem. *Arch Neurol* 23:1, 1970.
26. Segarra JM: Cerebral vascular disease and behavior I. *Arch Neurol* 22:408, 1970.
27. Laskowska D, Urbaniak K, Jus A: The relationship between catatonic-delirious states

and schizophrenia, in the light of a follow-up study (Stauder's lethal catatonia). *Br J Psychiatry* 111:254, 1965.

28. Glaser GH, Pincus JH: Limbic encephalitis. *J Nerv Ment Dis* 149:59, 1969.
29. Morris HH, McCormick WF, Reinarz JA: Neuroleptic malignant syndrome. *Arch Neurol* 37:462, 1980.
30. Henderson VW, Wooten GF: Neuroleptic malignant syndrome: A pathogenic role for dopamine receptor blockade. *Neurology (NY)* 31:132, 1981.
31. Moss AJ, Glaser W, Topol E: Atrial tachypacing in the treatment of a patient with primary orthostatic hypotension. *N Engl J Med* 302:1456, 1980.
32. Shy GM, Drager GA: A neurological syndrome associated with orthostatic hypotension: A clinical-pathologic study. *Arch Neurol* 2:511, 1960.
33. Hickler RG: Orthostatic hypotension and syncope. *N Engl J Med* 296:336, 1977.
34. Taylor AR, Chakravorty BC: Clinical syndromes associated with basilar impression. *Arch Neurol* 10:475, 1964.
35. Ziegler MG, Lake CR, Kopin IJ: The sympathetic-nervous-system defect in primary orthostatic hypotension. *N Engl J Med* 296:293, 1977.
36. Low PA, Walsh JC, Huang CY, et al: The sympathetic nervous system in diabetic neuropathy. *Brain* 98:341, 1975.

4
Seizure Disorders

Disorganized electrical activity in the brain that appears paroxysmally and produces impaired intellectual function, altered perceptions, or stereotyped motor phenomena is called epileptic or seizure activity. If seizure activity occurs independently of a stimulus that would produce this type of disorganized electrical activity even in a perfectly normal individual, such as an electrical shock or massive head trauma, the affected individual is said to have epilepsy. This disorder occurs in 0.4 to 0.5 percent of the general population (1). The neurophysiologic abnormality is presumed to involve inappropriate discharges by a massive number of neurons in the cerebral cortex. Structural and metabolic lesions in the brain increase an individual's susceptibility to seizures, but many people without brain lesions have epilepsy. What makes some individuals free of apparent brain disease more susceptible to seizure activity than others is unknown.

Seizure activity and altered consciousness often occur together. Loss of consciousness is routine in certain types of seizures, and, because of this, epilepsy is often suspected when a patient claims he has had a brief loss of consciousness. Unfortunately, altered consciousness and even loss of consciousness are impossible to establish by history alone. This is important only because some patients claim impaired consciousness when it never occurred. Factitious seizures are a common cause of pseudocoma, a voluntary lack of response to the environment. Determining whether a seizure is an authentic epileptic disorder or simply a contrived fit may be difficult, if not impossible, on clinical grounds alone. The more sophisticated the patient, the more difficult that determination will be. Distinguishing between real and contrived seizures is the first step in treating a seizure disorder, because the medications used to control authentic seizures all have unwanted side effects. Not only is the patient with factitious seizures unnecessarily exposed to the hematologic and neurologic effects of anticonvulsants when these medications are needlessly administered, but they may also develop further psychiatric problems as an adverse effect of the drugs.

Patients with true seizure disorders often have psychiatric problems associated with their epilepsy, and it is not at all unusual for a patient with authentic seizures to have contrived seizures as well. Factitious seizures occur in patients with all types of epileptic disorders and even occur in patients without apparent psychologic problems. Any secondary gain provided by the contrived fits is usually fairly obvious to the physician familiar with the patient. The increased incidence of personality disorders and frank psychosis in special forms of epilepsy, such as psychomotor epilepsy, is recognized by most physicians dealing with epileptics, but less appreciated is the risk of depressive illnesses and attempted suicide in patients with seizure disorders. Patients with epilepsy account for 3 to 10 percent of mental hospital admissions in the United States each year (1). The specific psychiatric effect of the seizure disorder depends on many factors, including the type of seizure experienced, the premorbid personality of the patient, and the behavior of people interacting with the epileptic individual. Focal sensory and focal motor epilepsy are notably free of psychiatric complications.

The psychiatrist dealing with a patient with suspected or established epilepsy must deal with both the patient's reasonable concerns about the neurologic disorder and with the complex psychiatric problems that develop in association with the neurologic disorder. Identifying the type of epilepsy affecting the patient helps limit the types of psychologic problems that must be anticipated. The character of the seizure disorder is often confusing early in the course of the epilepsy, and the burden of deciding precisely what type of epilepsy the patient has usually falls on the physician most closely supervising the patient. In the patient with psychologic problems, this is often the psychiatrist.

ETIOLOGY OF SEIZURES

Seizure disorders may be idiopathic or secondary to central nervous system disease. The older the patient at the onset of seizures, the more likely that he has a progressive pathologic process in the brain. Seizures appearing for the first time in a patient over 30 years of age are often secondary to a brain tumor. Seizures at any age that are initially well controlled and later recur despite effective anticonvulsant drug levels may be from structural brain damage, such as that caused by an arteriovenous malformation (2). Structural damage late in life from stroke or transient hypoxia often leads to a seizure focus within weeks or months of the initial insult. A viral or bacterial encephalitis may produce a confusing picture of altered behavior and seizures initially but within days or weeks of these symptoms, the more malignant character of the disease will be apparent (3). Systemic lupus erythematosus, a collagen vascular disease of unknown etiology, will commonly produce seizures and altered behavior as its initial neurologic manifestations (4). Seventeen percent to 50 percent of patients with central nervous system lupus erythematosus have seizure disorders. In more tropical areas, such as Mexico and Central America, parasites, including cysticercosis from pork, may produce foci for seizure propagation. In the Orient, schistosomiasis of the brain is another parasitic infestation producing seizures. Head trauma often produces an amnestic state in which the patient does not recall the trauma, but seizures may be the first indication of cerebral contusion. A wide range of metabolic disorders, including uremia, anoxia, hepatic encephalopathy, and disorders of calcium metabolism, are associated with seizures, but additional signs of dementia or movement disorders are likely to be present (5). Congenital abnormalities producing seizures include hereditary malformations of the nervous system, such as tuberous sclerosis, and prenatal infections, such as toxoplasmosis of the brain. Obviously, very diverse lesions can produce seizures. The character of the seizure generally does not give any clue to the nature of the responsible lesion.

EVALUATION OF SEIZURE TYPE

Seizures produce symptoms ranging from involuntary movements in a limb to complex delusions in a patient with altered consciousness. Different types of seizures respond to different types of medication and have different natural histories. To help in the treatment and monitoring of epileptic disorders, these disorders have been classified according to features that they share (Table 4.1). Specific features involved in this grouping of epilepsies include the symptoms and signs before, during, and after the epileptic fit; the electroencephalographic changes associated with the seizure; the age of the patient affected; the area of the brain that seems to be most involved by the abnormal electrical activity; and the clinical or electroencephalographic progression of the disorder.

Generalized Seizures

Based upon both clinical and electroencephalographic characteristics, seizure disorders fall into two major categories, generalized and partial (6). With generalized seizures, both cerebral hemispheres seem to be involved by abnormal electrical activity at the same time. The most common types of generalized seizures are the major motor, or grand mal, and absence, or petit mal, forms. The pathology underlying the generalized seizure disorder occasionally is familial, resulting in an incidence of some type of epilepsy in 5.4 percent of the relatives of patients with grand mal or petit mal epilepsy (1). Generalized seizures as an entity are not inherited. Some diseases that cause grand mal or petit mal epilepsy can be inherited.

Grand mal seizures are manifest in both children and adults by an abrupt loss of consciousness followed by convulsive movements of the

Table 4.1. Common Types of Epilepsy

Current Terminology	*Alternative Names*
Generalized convulsive	Grand mal Tonic-clonic
Generalized nonconvulsive	Petit mal Absence attacks
Partial with elementary symptomatology	Elementary partial Focal (sensory or motor)
Partial with complex symptomatology	Complex partial Psychomotor Temporal lobe

body. These convulsive movements are usually called tonic-clonic because there are two phases of muscle activity, one in which the patient has persistent contraction of several muscle groups and one in which the contraction alternates with abrupt relaxation. In the tonic phase the patient will arch his back or extend his legs and arms. In the clonic phase the limbs and trunk thrash about as contractions become more rhythmic and interrupted. This type of seizure is often accompanied by tongue biting and urinary incontinence. After these acute epileptic or ictal phenomena, which last a few minutes, the patient is poorly responsive to all stimuli for minutes or hours, an interval designated the postictal period.

The patient with petit mal epilepsy is usually a child, does not lose postural tone, and is unresponsive for seconds with little, if any, associated motor phenomena. The electroencephalogram during the attack has a characteristic 3 cycles per second, spike-and-slow-wave pattern, and this electroencephalographic abnormality can often be induced by flashing lights or hyperventilation (Figure 4.1) (7). There is no substantial confusion following the seizure. The patient may not even realize that he had an episode of altered consciousness. At one time these were called centrencephalic seizures, a term meant to convey the deep brain or upper brainstem origin of the abnormal electrical activity, but this origin for the seizure has never been established and is probably inaccurate (7). This type of seizure is a disorder invariably appearing in affected individuals while they are still children. Adults developing absence attacks for the first time do not have petit mal epilepsy. Absence attacks in children usually evolve into more complex seizure phenomena, such as psychomotor or grand mal epilepsy, or simply become associated with other types of seizures.

Partial Seizures

Partial seizures include epileptic phenomena with complex or simple symptomatology. Partial seizures with simple symptomatology include focal

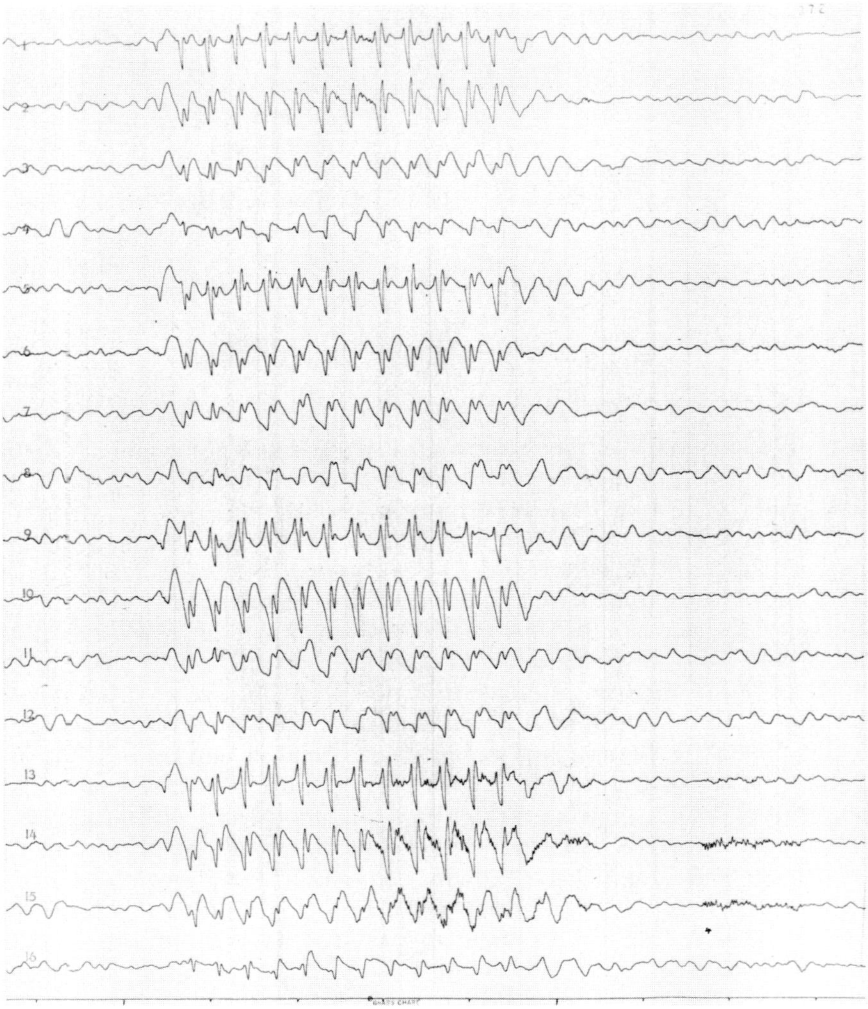

Figure 4.1. This electroencephalogram exhibits the typical 3 per second spike and slow-wave pattern characteristic of generalized nonconvulsive (petit mal) seizures. The patient was a 9-year-old girl with a history of recurrent staring spells.

motor and focal sensory epileptic fits. During these simple partial seizures, the patient may remain entirely alert and responsive while part of a limb or an entire limb has rhythmic involuntary contractions. There is also a group of seizure disorders that start out as partial phenomena and become generalized. The Jacksonian march is a focal motor seizure that progresses to become a generalized motor seizure. Some authorities consider these sequential seizures in a category completely separate from the generalized and partial seizures (7).

The most interesting seizure disorder from a psychiatric viewpoint is the partial seizure with complex symptomatology. The complex symptomatology may be peculiar behavior or unusual movements. The combination of psychiatric and motor phenomena as symptoms of this type of epilepsy inspired the classical name, psychomotor epilepsy. Most brain lesions producing this type of seizure disorder involve the temporal lobe. Even when there is no obvious structural lesion responsible for the seizures, the focus of epileptic activity defined by electroencephalographic studies is usually in the temporal lobe. Because of the importance of the temporal lobe in the development of complex partial seizures, these fits are also called temporal lobe seizures.

Factitious Seizures

The two most difficult diagnostic situations likely to be encountered by a psychiatrist while dealing with seizure patients are the contrived seizure in the true epileptic and the initial seizure in a previously nonepileptic individual. Patients with seizures learn from those who care for them what their seizures look like. They feign seizures to manipulate those obliged to deal with them or for more subtle secondary gain. Motivation for the true epileptic feigning seizures is much the same as that for the nonepileptic who has contrived fits. A common feature of most contrived or hysterical fits is that the contrived seizure solves a conflict (8). Whether this behavior appears to be prompted by an anxiety attack, acting out, or simple malingering, it should extricate the patient from some difficulty or place him in an advantageous position (8). On purely clinical grounds, a contrived seizure by a well-informed patient will be indistinguishable from a true seizure. Fortunately most patients with psychologic problems severe enough to induce them to feign seizures are not adequately careful in contriving the features of their factitious seizure to mislead an informed and critical observer.

Overlooking authentic seizures is also a hazard of dealing with unfamiliar patients. A patient brought to the emergency room immediately after his first epileptic fit may be misconstrued as psychotic or psychologically disturbed because of his aphonia, incoherent speech, or disorganized behavior. If his relatives and friends have never seen an epileptic fit before, they may only report that the patient blacked out. Quite often the family will suspect that the patient is insane because the abrupt alteration in consciousness is followed by a more or less protracted period of confusion or frank dementia. During this period immediately following the seizure, especially when the seizure is a generalized motor seizure (grand mal seizure) or partial seizure with complex symptomatology (psychomotor seizure), the patient is said to be in a postictal state. The postictal period, that is the interval between the acute seizure activity, which ordinarily lasts only a few minutes, and the return to normal mental and motor function, is usually 10 to 20 minutes, but it may be as long as 24 hours. It is common for the patient to appear awake but remain confused and inactive during much of this postictal period. Efforts to examine the patient during the postictal period are usually frustrated by the patient's poor cooperation. Signs elicited during the postictal period are often misleading even when they can be consistently observed. Asymmetric reflexes, unequal limb tones, extensor plantar responses, and even unilateral pupillary dilatation may all be unequivocal but transient neurologic signs during the postictal period. Urinary or fecal incontinence and lacerations of the tongue or cheek reinforce suspicions that the patient had an authentic seizure disorder with postictal unresponsiveness or altered responsiveness confusing the picture. The unsophisticated patient may be unresponsive during the "tonic-clonic" phase of a lengthy hysterical seizure but abruptly return to normal mentation with cessation of the motor activity (8). He will often open his eyes abruptly and volunteer, "I had a fit" or simply look about with mock surprise and ask, "What was that?" Thrashing about of the arms and legs, pelvic thrusting movements, and rolling of the eyes are common manifestations of a hysterical seizure. The patient rarely injures himself during a contrived fit, and only the most sophisticated patient will have urinary "incontinence." Most will resist any efforts to interfere with their breathing during the ictal phase of their seizure, a reaction not seen with authentic epileptic fits (8). Women have hysterical seizures several times more frequently than men (9), but both men and women disposed to hysterical seizures have a much higher than average incidence of psychiatric disease in their families. Most have well-established histories of personal psychiatric problems, commonly depressive in character and often punctuated by suicide attempts (9). Sexual problems are a frequent element in the psychiatric history (10). The mean age of patients exhibiting hysterical seizures is about 32 years old (9). Electroencephalographic activity during the acute attack will be normal, except for movement artifacts, or unchanged from preseizure recordings.

Rare disorders predisposing the patient to have psychiatric problems will also induce authentic seizures. The most striking case of this is systemic lupus erythematosus, a collagen vascular disorder. Central nervous system involvement occurs in 59 percent of patients with systemic lupus erythematosus, and the most common sign of this central nervous system involvement is altered mentation. Severe depression is usually prominent (4). Such an affective disorder may precede other signs of the collagen vascular disease by years, but quite often a progressive dementia will appear at the same time as the seizure disorder. Because of the common appearance of an unexplained depression, the patient's seizure disorder may be misconstrued as factitious when it first develops. Seventeen to 50 percent of patients with systemic lupus erythematosus and central nervous system involvement will have seizures. Although these patients may be puzzling early in their course, their neuropsychiatric problems should be attributed to their organic disease when the collagen vascular disease is recognized. The seizures and dementia attending the collagen vascular disease will become more prominent with every exacerbation of the systemic lupus erythematosus (4). Treatment of this disease with antimalarial drugs or corticosteroids may cause further confusion because the treatments themselves often have psychiatric effects. Antimalarials may produce personality changes and psychotic episodes. Corticosteroids may produce euphoria or frank psychosis (4).

A transient loss of consciousness with an authentic neurologic basis may also be labeled hysteria or seizure activity and, in fact, be neither. There are many causes of fainting or syncope, some of which are discussed in the chapter on altered consciousness. In the elderly, cardiac problems will be responsible for many cases of transient unconsciousness. Subtle cardiac arrhythmias may profoundly affect cerebral perfusion. A Holter monitor recording of cardiac activity over the course of 24 hours may be needed to detect the arrhythmia. Younger people may have metabolic or structural problems leading to syncope. Coughing or urinating will trigger an exagerrated vascular (vasovagal) reflex in some individuals and induce fainting. With the skeletal deformity known as basilar impression, an abnormally formed junction between the skull and the spine may be associated with recurrent attacks of unconsciousness spanning an interval of years (11). Compounding the confusion between the syncopal episodes caused by basilar impression and the loss of consciousness induced by seizure activity is the common association of vertigo, tinnitus, visual alterations, and prolonged amnesia with the loss of consciousness caused by basilar impression. This syncope is presumed to result from ischemia to the brainstem developing with impaired arterial blood flow secondary to the skeletal anomaly (11). Hyperventilation, a response to stress often occurring in women, may also produce syncope and may be confused with a seizure disorder (2). Transient hypoglycemia is a frequently diagnosed, but rarely occurring, basis for syncope. A largely normal electroencephalogram or diffuse changes on the electroencephalogram not typical of epilepsy occurring during one of these misdiagnosed "seizures" will help clarify the etiology of the loss of consciousness.

If an electroencephalogram can be obtained during the seizure, its authenticity can be readily established. A normal electroencephalogram during a generalized convulsion indicates an hysterical seizure disorder. Even when the electroencephalogram cannot be obtained during the fit, the electrical study will usually help establish the authenticity of the seizure. For several hours after the generalized seizure, the brain waves will be abnormal with diffuse or focal slowing likely. During the interval when the patient is free of seizures, the so-called interictal period, the electroencephalogram will be abnormal in about 90 percent of truly epileptic individuals if repeated records are obtained on the patient (8).

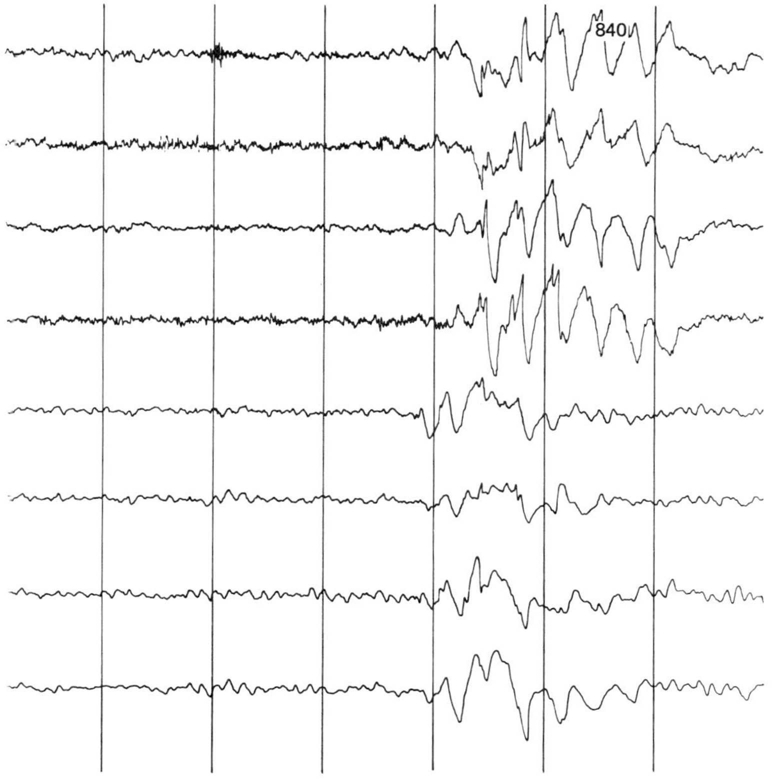

Figure 4.2. This electroencephalogram shows a generalized spike and slow-wave discharge that lasted 2 seconds and occurred only during photic stimulation. The patient was a 9-year-old girl who had only one seizure in her life, at the age of 6 years. She had no deficits on neurologic examination.

Inducing sleep or hyperventilation in the patient will increase the yield of abnormalities. Photic stimulation and special electrode placement can further increase the likelihood of detecting abnormal brain wave activity in the epileptic patient during the interictal period (Figure 4.2). Normal records on several occasions despite these provocative measures are highly suggestive of an hysterical seizure disorder. Anticonvulsants should not be given to these suspect patients, but vigorous efforts should be made to obtain an electroencephalogram during or immediately after a typical seizure.

EPILEPSY AND SUICIDE

Attempted suicide is common among patients with all types of convulsive disorders (12). The prevalence rate of suicidal individuals in the epileptic populations is 32.5/1,000 (12). This is five times the prevalence rate of individuals attempting suicide in the general population. Two factors place patients with epilepsy at special risk: (*1*) they have an inordinately high incidence of depressive illness, and (*2*) they have easy access to nonviolent instruments of suicide, specifically anticonvulsants. Despite dramatic advances in the control of seizure disorders over the past few decades, 17 to 25 percent of ambulatory patients with epilepsy have significant psychiatric problems, which require hospitalization in many cases (1). About 10 percent of all patients with any form of epilepsy require hospitalization in a psychiatric setting at some time during their lives (1). Attempted suicide is often the reason for the psychiatric hospitalization. Eighty-four percent of the epileptics attempting suicide use self-poisoning, and in 65 percent of these instances anticonvulants are used (12). Phenobarbital has always been especially popular with this group attempting suicide. The respiratory depressant action of this drug is often purposely enhanced by alcohol abuse coinciding with the drug overdose. Men with epilepsy are more likely to attempt suicide than women with epilepsy, but both men and women are more inclined to make a serious suicide gesture when they are unemployed. Sixty percent of the epileptics attempting suicide are under 30 years of age and a disproportionate fraction of the suicidal individuals have psychomotor epilepsy. Repeated attempts at suicide are twice as common in epileptics as in nonepileptics. Seventy-four percent of patients with seizures who attempt suicide and fail will try again.

Effective seizure control provides no protection against this behavior. In fact, the patient's psychiatric problems may frustrate all efforts to effectively control seizure phenomena. Poor compliance with the recommended medication regimen is the most common cause of recurrent seizures in a previously well-controlled patient. The patient's decision to stop all anticonvulsants may precipitate the often lethal convulsive disorder called status epilepticus. Although this behavior is generally not included in statistics on suicidal gestures, it probably accounts for as much morbidity and mortality as frank suicide attempts. The epileptic individual can inflict considerable self-injury with minimal effort and planning.

PSYCHOMOTOR (COMPLEX PARTIAL) SEIZURES

Complex partial seizures (psychomotor or temporal lobe seizures) are the most common type of partial seizure. Twenty to 30 percent of all epileptics have this form of partial epilepsy. Most of those developing complex partial seizures have their first epileptic fit about the time of puberty (1). "Temporal lobe epilepsy" is an inaccurate but widely used term that emphasizes the probable site of origin of the epileptic activity that leads to this type of partial seizure with complex symptomatology. It is misleading because epileptogenic activity arising in the temporal lobe does not necessarily produce just psychomotor seizures, and psychomotor seizures do not necessarily occur only with a temporal lobe lesion (7). Despite these reasons for discarding the term temporal lobe epilepsy it has survived several decades of use simply because the epileptogenic activity on the electroencephalograms of patients with psychomotor seizures usually arises in one or both of the temporal lobes. Discrete damage in the temporal lobe can be found in some patients with complex partial seizures, but most patients have no apparent structural basis for the seizure disorder (1). Although most of the known causes of complex partial seizures are not hereditary, 2.6 percent of the relatives of these epileptic patients will themselves have some form of epilepsy, though not necessarily complex partial epilepsy (1).

Complex partial seizures are often difficult to recognize because the signs and symptoms associated with these epileptic fits are remarkably diverse. One-third of the patients developing psychomotor seizures have typical fits only after years of generalized epilepsy (grand mal or petit mal) (1). Sixty-four percent of temporal lobe epileptics have generalized seizures, as well as complex partial seizures, and so it is not surprising that an individual may be told he has different types of epilepsy by different physicians. The variability in seizure phenomena associated with psychomotor epilepsy often leads the physician involved to suspect a psychologic basis for much, if not all, of the abnormal behavior observed. Conversely, patients with personality disorders and episodic psychoses may be inaccurately diagnosed as temporal lobe epileptics. Many patients with psychomotor epilepsy have psychiatric problems distinct from their seizure disorders, but deciding which symptoms arise from the epilepsy and which arise from the psychiatric disorder may be impossible.

Seizure Elements

Every seizure has several discrete stages. This is most obvious with complex partial seizures. The stage with the most obvious electrical disorganization is the ictus of the seizure. This is often preceded by some type of warning, called the aura, and followed by a period of abnormal consciousness, called the postictal period. The interval between obvious epileptic fits is the interictal period (Figure 4.3).

Aura

Patients with complex partial seizures report auditory, olfactory, and visual hallucinations preceding their seizures or independent of any apparent seizure activity. Automatic or stereotyped behavior of some sort may also precede the seizure and is likely to occur despite the patient's being relatively alert and communicative (13,14). The epileptic patient will often realize that he is going through a familiar ritual just before his seizure and announce that he is going to have a seizure. This perception or behavior preceding the seizure is called the aura (15). The distinction between the

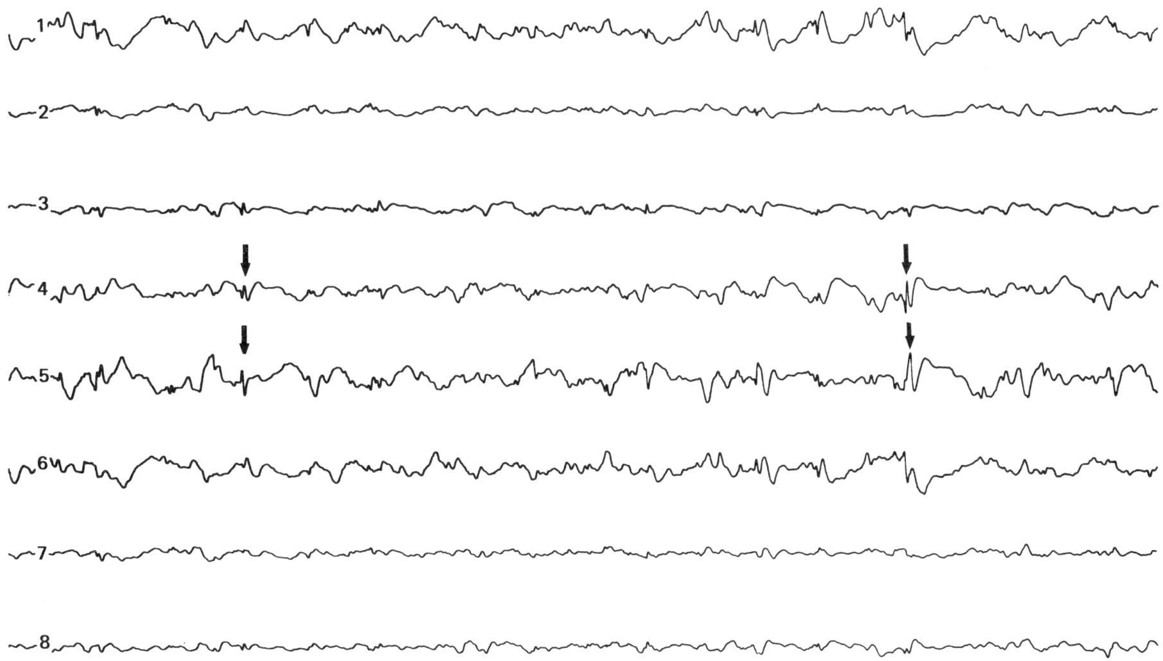

Figure 4.3. A 22-year-old man developed generalized seizures after head trauma. He was poorly controlled on anticonvulsant medication when this electroencephalogram was obtained. Focal spike activity is apparent on the record (arrows); it was most prominent over the right anterior temporal lobe.

ictus, that is, the seizure proper, and the aura is arbitrary, since abnormal electrical discharges are usually quite prominent on the electroencephalogram while the patient is having the aura. What makes the aura truly distinct from the remainder of the epileptic fit is the way the patient perceives it. After the attack is over, he will usually recall the aura. Auras may occur with other partial or generalized seizures, but they are remarkably complex and occasionally protracted with psychomotor (complex partial) seizures.

The aura often involves stereotyped behavior. The patient may feel compelled to make some type of movement. He is obliged to turn his head to the right or left, or he feels he must to sit down. Quite frequently, he will have an irrepressible urge to demand, pour, or drink water (16). This obsession with water and other compulsive activities seen during the aura may also be prominent during the seizure proper. If the obsession is part of the seizure proper, the patient usually does not remember it. Chewing movements, lip-smacking, spitting, or grimacing all occur as part of the aura in some individuals, although these automatic movements also may appear during the seizure proper. With the "uncinate form" of psychomotor seizures, the patient senses and often complains of a disagreeable smell or taste (13). The name refers to the uncus of the temporal lobe, which was presumed to play a prominent role in the perception of olfactory stimuli. Complaints of nausea or abdominal cramps are also fairly common in uncinate fits. These olfactory and gustatory auras have a slightly more serious meaning than other auras because they are often associated with brain tumors (16). Auditory hallucinations are usually of music or of a buzzing sound, but occasionally they are more menacing and involve voices threatening great harm or predicting inevitable tragedy. Visual hallucinations occur less frequently than auditory hallucinations, but, when they do occur, they are usually more complex than auditory hallucinations (17,18). The frequent appearance of hallucinations in this disorder that develop at puberty or during adolescence in most affected individuals arouses concern that the patient may actually be schizophrenic rather than epileptic.

Thought disorders routinely occur during the aura. The patient may recall having feelings of depersonalization or paranoid ideas. Complaints of bizarre delusions and ideas of reference contribute to these patients occasionally being diagnosed as schizophrenic (15,19). Characteristic of psychomotor auras are the feelings of intense familiarity with events just occurring or total unfamiliarity with events that have occurred many times before (1). These feelings are called déjà vu and jamais vu. They are not true hallucinations in the same way that the auditory and visual phenomena are hallucinations, but the feeling of familiarity with the déjà vu may be exaggerated to the point where the patient actually perceives himself back in an old, often unpleasant, situation. This is often referred to by the patient as a flashback, because the features of the delusional experience are so vivid that he seems to relive the old experience.

Other phenomena occurring during the aura include disturbances of emotions or mood and embarrassing automatisms (17). Attacks of intense, groundless fear are occasionally associated with complex partial seizures. This is presumably mediated by the amygdala of the temporal lobe acting alone or in coordination with other temporal lobe structures (20). Stimulation of the amygdala experimentally will induce these same feelings of intense fear (20). The fear may last minutes to hours and is occasionally the only symptom of the seizure disorder (20). In most cases, the fear is accompanied by visceral symptoms and is limited to the aura (20).

Before the patient loses consciousness, he may urinate or defecate (17). Vomiting, sweating, and pallor accompany many of these more visceral phenomena in both psychomotor auras and other epileptic auras. Visceral phenomena of this sort are not compelling evidence that the seizure disorder is in fact complex partial epilepsy, because 20 percent of the patients with convulsive disorders of any sort may have visceral auras that include epigastric pain and borborygmi, as well as nausea and vomiting (21).

Although many of these phenomena appearing during the aura are suggestive of psychiatric difficulty and some of the patients with complex partial seizures have psychiatric problems, there is no connection between the type of aura the patient will exhibit and the psychopathy to which he will be subject. In fact, patients with auras that involve complex delusions and automatisms need not exhibit any psychopathology at other times. All of these different types of auras occur in patients without thought disorders as well as in those with persistent psychiatric problems.

Ictus

The seizure proper or ictus may be little more than a prolonged staring spell or it may evolve into a generalized tonic-clonic (grand mal) seizure. Fairly complex but pointless behavior such as undressing, running, laughing, or crying may occur (1,18,22). Rare patients have sexual climax during the seizure, a phenomenon more likely in patients with seizures triggered by sexual excitement (1). These sexual seizures affect both men and women, but patients reporting such unusual ictal phenomena should be viewed suspiciously.

During the ictus, the patient loses consciousness or has a profoundly altered state of consciousness for which he is amnestic later. The seizure lasts seconds to minutes and is usually not associated with fecal or urinary incontinence. During this period of altered consciousness the patient may drink water, go to the bathroom to urinate or defecate, or simply hide (16). The patient does not bite his tongue or exhibit clonic muscle activity unless the seizure generalizes and becomes grand mal in type.

Postictal Period

Unlike patients with petit mal epilepsy, victims of psychomotor seizures invariably pass through a postictal period after the seizure proper. The postictal state lasts 2 to 10 minutes in most cases and is characterized by marked confusion and poor responsiveness (14,19,23). Initially, the patient will be unable to answer questions regarding events just occurring, and, as his level of consciousness improves, it will be evident that he is amnestic for events occurring just before the seizure. Within a few minutes, this retrograde amnesia will shrink, and the patient will be able to report on events up to the point of the seizure onset. Occasionally he will be unaware of any alteration in his consciousness and the only indication that something actually happened will be the memory gap left for the time of impaired consciousness (1). In patients with generalized seizures, postictal irritability is not uncommon and occasionally patients will injure others about them during this confused period. In psychomotor epilepsy, postictal violence is uncommon, and a sudden burst of anger during this period by these patients is unlikely (1). If the patient is at all violent during the postictal period he will be amnestic for the events. Sexual motives are occasionally ascribed to these patients during the postictal period because they may undress during this confusion. Fostering the notion that these patients are exhibitionists is the occasional phenomenon of sexual arousal as the confusion clears (1). The postictal period may in fact be the most obvious clinical manifestation of the seizure initially. Because of this, both the patient and those observing his confused behavior may assume that he is suffering from a psychiatric disturbance and seek psychiatric, rather than neurologic, assistance. With repeated epileptic fits, the convulsive nature of the disorder will usually be evident.

The Interictal Period

Over the past few decades, considerable controvery has arisen over the nature and significance of interictal behavior in patients with complex partial seizures (2,24). The fundamental issue has been whether or not patients with complex partial seizures exhibit more psychopathology between discrete seizures than other epileptics. Studies 2 decades ago alleged that psychiatric problems were prominent during seizure-free intervals in 63 percent of patients with psychomotor epilepsy, whereas only 30 percent of patients with grand mal seizures had similar problems (15). Various reports more recently have indicated special problems experienced by patients with psychomotor seizures in areas ranging from hyperkinetic behavior and aggression to sexual function and hypochondriasis (1,12,18,25). Schizophrenia and psychotic depression have been more frequently linked to patients with complex partial seizures than with any other type of seizure, an observation that reinforces the general impression that these patients with seizures originating in temporal lobe foci have a special vulnerability to psychiatric disorders (18,25–27).

Truly psychotic thought disorders with features characteristic of schizophrenia are not very common in patients with temporal lobe epilepsy, but they do occur. Affected patients use neologisms, condensed words, loose associations, inconsequential sentences, and considerable verbiage in their speech and reflect delusions of persecution or special privilege in their remarks (18,26). Occasionally, these patients will exhibit hebephrenic, catatonic, or paranoid elements in their thought disorders, but this occurs less commonly, at least for the hebephrenic and catatonic traits, than in the conventional schizophrenic population (15,18). Obsessive and paranoid traits are especially characteristic of the temporal lobe epileptics who develop their seizures before puberty; this paranoid ideation has a distinctly religious coloring (18). Some of these patients report religious conversions after mystical experiences (18). They often ascribe great significance to commonplace occurrences, insisting that an everyday event has religious significance or universal implications (28). Inconsequential events will be recorded in minute detail as part of a compulsion to write down everything that happens on a daily basis (28). Problems with abstraction are common. Traits routinely present in the psychomotor epileptic that are inconsistent with schizophrenia are a generally warm and appropriate affect and a higher incidence of dementia rather than hebephrenic deterioration after years of cognitive difficulty (1,18).

Psychomotor Fugue States

Occasionally, patients with psychomotor seizures have prolonged episodes of aimless wandering followed by retrograde amnesia (29). These episodes have a superficial resemblance to schizophrenic fugue states, but the basic defect in these epileptic patients appears to be disordered memory, rather than a dissociative state (29). These confused wandering episodes are most likely to occur when the patient has poorly controlled seizures, and one seizure is occurring within a short interval of another. The patient has relatively short interictal periods, and the return to normal intellectual functioning may be incomplete even when the patient is behaving in a somewhat organized and unobtrusive manner. When seizure control improves, the patient may be unable to recall any of the events that transpired during the period of high seizure frequency. Amnesia for these events is usually permanent. Most prolonged confusional states bearing any resemblance to psychotic fugues are generally not of epileptic origin, even if the patient denies all recall of events preceding the episode of wandering (1).

Epileptic Twilight State

Prolonged seizure activity can produce abnormal behavior, whether the seizure has a temporal lobe focus or not, but such protracted ictal periods are exceedingly rare in complex partial epilepsy (29,30). These bouts of closely spaced seizures, which have no real interictal periods, are called complex partial status epilepticus. During this status epilepticus, the patient may continue his routine activities in a slow, confused, somewhat stuporous manner for hours (14). This is often called an epileptic twilight state, and throughout the entire period of semiautomatic activity the patient's electroencephalogram will have continuously or nearly continuous abnormal wave forms (14,18). Paradoxically, elderly patients in this epileptic twilight state may have the typical 3 cycles per second, spike-and-slow-wave pattern on the electroencephalogram that is characteristic of petit mal or absence status epilepticus (30).

The clinical differences between patients with absence status and complex partial status are minimal. Both types of status epilepticus are equally rare. The patient may be somewhat communicative, and he may complain that his surroundings are remote. More rarely, this confused behavior will be associated with screaming and destructive behavior. Additional indications that an epileptic twilight state is the basis for the altered behavior is cyclical vomiting in infants and very young children and shocklike (myoclonic) limb jerks in adults (14,30). Distinguishing these twilight states from schizophrenic fugues or factitious amnesia is generally impossible unless the patient can be monitored with an electroencephalogram during the episode (18).

Psychosis and Temporal Lobe Epilepsy

The initial reports that temporal lobe epileptics had schizophreniform and affective disorders prompted several studies of psychotic patients with the specific aim of looking for a connection between their psychoses and evidence of temporal lobe dysfunction (15,31). Sporadic reports of psychotic patients with focal temporal lobe lesions have strengthened the notion that temporal lobe seizure foci can dispose a patient to schizophreniform disorders (31). Temporal lobe epilepsy was found more commonly in mentally ill patients than any other seizure disorder. Sixty-five percent of patients with epilepsy of some sort and schizophreniform symptoms independent of a family history of schizophrenia had psychomotor epilepsy (15). The similarity of symptoms with temporal lobe damage and schizophrenia raised the possibility that the seizure activity per se was not essential for the development of psychopathology. Experience supports this notion. Lateral temporal lobe lesions may produce the visual and auditory hallucinations characteristic of both schizophrenia and temporal lobe epilepsy (17,31). The seizure disorder is less significant in the development of psychotic signs than is the temporal lobe lesion.

Schizophreniform Disorders

Eleven percent of temporal lobe epileptics have overt psychoses and 36 percent have psychologic problems unrelated to adjusting to their disease

(32). Psychotic episodes in these temporal lobe epileptics last days or weeks, a duration atypical for a simple postictal state, and the psychosis occasionally will terminate with an epileptic fit (15). Indeed, the schizophreniform psychosis appears most often in temporal lobe epileptics when the seizure frequency is low and the seizure focus is on the dominant side (15,27). Psychopathology is most typical of temporal lobe epileptics with clear-cut epileptogenic foci on electroencephalographic recordings from the left temporal lobe (32). Although the seizure disorder appears before the psychiatric problems in most of these patients, psychiatric problems are apparent by adolescence in 85 percent of the epileptics who develop psychiatric problems (32). To have seizures appearing before the psychopathology, these disturbed patients must develop psychomotor fits at a fairly young age, and, in fact, 67 percent have their first seizure between 5 and 10 years of age (32). There is an apparent latency of several years between the first seizure and the first signs of psychologic problems (18). A study of patients treated with temporal lobe resections for poorly controlled seizures concluded that temporal lobe epileptics were more often psychotic if they were women, if they developed epilepsy after 10 years of age, and if they had neoplastic or retained "embryonic" (hamartomatous) tissue in the temporal lobe (33).

Affective Disorders

Schizophreniform psychoses are the most common clearly psychotic phenomena developing in temporal lobe epileptics, but affective disorders also occur with significant frequency. These affective disorders at their worst result in psychotic depressions leading to suicide attempts and rage attacks that prompt psychiatric admissions (12,32). In children with temporal lobe epilepsy, episodes of minimally provoked rage and hyperkinetic behavior may develop when the seizures first begin (1). Although this hyperkinetic behavior and rage occur less frequently as the epileptic individual gets older, depressive affective disorders become more prominent (1). The adult with psychomotor epilepsy is often quite irritable and may have excessive mood swings. These patients are easily manipulated. By changing the topic of conversation, an interviewer can shift the patient's affective display from friendly and even infantile to angry and aggressive (22).

Electroencephalographic Changes in Schizophrenia

Electroencephalographic studies also link temporal lobe lesions and schizophrenic behavior. Early reports claimed a 10 percent incidence of electroencephalographic abnormalities in the temporal lobes of patients diagnosed schizophrenic (34). More recent studies on schizophrenics have shown no consistent pattern of abnormality, but temporal lobe abnormalities still occur in at least 11 percent of the patients (34). An association between psychoses and temporal lobe electroencephalographic abnormalities is not well established, but it is generally accepted that there is a higher than expected incidence of nonpsychotic sociopathy in patients with temporal lobe abnormalities, whether or not the patient has a seizure disorder (35). Obviously, a temporal lobe electroencephalographic abnormality is not proof of temporal lobe epilepsy. Even fugue states, visual and auditory hallucinations, déjà vu, and sexual disorders associated with abnormal electroencephalograms are not evidence of a clear connection between the seizure disorder and the psychiatric symptoms (19). Truly psychotic symptoms may, in fact, be inversely related to seizure activity in the temporal lobes. Twenty-five percent of the patients with psychiatric disorders and temporal lobe epilepsy in one study had more normal electroencephalograms during periods of increased psychotic activity (15).

Aberrant Behavior in Psychomotor Epileptics

There is no consensus on the validity of a link between psychomotor or temporal lobe epilepsy and psychoses or behavior disorders. One study found psychiatric disturbances in about 30 percent of all epileptics with no difference between the incidence of psychiatric disturbances in psychomotor and nonpsychomotor epileptics (36). Much of what is interpreted in epileptic patients as psychopathology may be fairly routine postictal signs of a neurologic disturbance. Patients with temporal lobe seizures may have problems with word-finding during the interictal period as a protracted sign of disturbed temporal lobe function (37). Circumlocution and circumstantiality are often used to compensate for this subtle language difficulty, and these adaptive techniques may provide part of the impression that the patient has a psychogenic cognitive disorder (37). Character changes unequivocally do occur with partial resection of the temporal lobe cortex, but this gross maneuver need not reflect changes developing with a seizure focus in this same cortex (35). Psychologic test data and psychiatric interviews on temporal lobe epileptics and nontemporal lobe epileptics show no significant differences in psychopathology in some studies (35). Patients with psychomotor epilepsy who do ultimately require psychiatric hospitalization have a slightly higher incidence of schizoid character traits (35).

Despite all the controversy generated by the debate over the association between psychomotor epilepsy and psychosis, what has emerged from the study of these patients that is well documented and widely accepted is that there is a remarkably high incidence of certain personality disorders and maladaptive traits. Studies of patients with psychomotor seizures and psychiatric problems initially pointed to an unexpectedly high incidence of aggressive tendencies in these patients, especially in those with seizure phenomena appearing before they were 10 years old (18,27). Most of these aggressive epileptics were not, in fact, psychotic, but rather demonstrated substantial character disorders. Advocates of surgical control of these seizure disorders showed evidence of increased postoperative control of aggression when the diseased temporal lobe was resected early after the onset of the seizure disorder (27). The relationship between aggression and psychomotor seizures is discussed at length in the chapter on affective disorders.

Sexual Dysfunction

More common, but less dramatic, than the aggressive behavior exhibited by these epileptic individuals is the abnormal sexual behavior developing in these individuals. Sexual dysfunction is often very prominent, hyposexuality appearing much more commonly than hypersexuality (19,24). "Impotence" and frigidity occur in as many as 50 percent of the patients with temporal lobe epilepsy; these sexual disorders appear in only 30 percent of patients with grand mal epilepsy and other chronic medical illnesses (1). The hyposexuality exhibited by these patients is a problem with interest rather than with ability (38). The men are not physiologically impotent and the women do not have pain with intercourse; they simply lack interest in initiating any kind of sexual activity, heterosexual or homosexual. If the temporal lobe epilepsy starts before puberty or at puberty, these individuals are likely to remain without sexual experience or partners (1). If the temporal lobe epilepsy starts later in life, the patient and often the patient's spouse will complain of a profound deterioration in sexual interest. Effective anticonvulsant control of the seizures may improve libido and performance in some of these patients, another indication that the seizure disorder itself underlies the change in behavior (1).

Personality Traits

Anecdotal accounts report eccentric traits that include compulsive writing and idiosyncratic writing (24). These patients show meticulous attention to definitions, produce volumes of detailed information largely devoid of content, and may even reverse their writing direction so that their script can only be deciphered in a mirror. These hypergraphic patients also speak in a strikingly pedantic and circumstantial manner (24). Hyperreligiosity is common in these patients. They have remarkably inflexible views of right and wrong, good and evil, and often exhibit fanatical commitments to their personal moral opinions (1). They characteristically lack any sense of humor.

Formal assessments of personality profiles in these patients support the anecdotal reports of peculiar personality traits. Efforts to correlate characteristic thinking styles with the side of the temporal lobe focus initially suggested that a reflective cognitive style was typical of patients with left temporal lobe foci and an impulsive cognitive style was more typical of patients with right temporal foci (22). One of the most revealing studies on these character traits compared results obtained by objective tests and interviewer opinions with the epileptic's opinions of himself (25). Patients with right temporal lobe foci were more obsessive and emotional than patients with left temporal foci, and they often exhibited an extraordinary moralistic fervor. They denied being depressed although they appeared to be somewhat depressed and had a high incidence of suicide attempts. Whenever the suggestion was made to the patient that there might be negative features to his behavior, he violently denied the possibility and argued that he never participated in behavior that was improper. This affective coloring to all events, regardless of how minor, was not apparent in the patients with left temporal lobe foci. The patients with left temporal foci were remarkably self-critical and paranoid. They exhibited considerable anger but were clearly quite dependent in their behavior. These patients also expressed a strong sense of destiny, and they frequently expended considerable energy looking for the meaning behind remarks and the implications of events. The patients with left temporal lobe foci were generally quite self-conscious.

Psychiatric hospitalizations were high for patients with both right and left temporal lobe epileptic foci, with more than 30 percent reporting hospitalizations at some time in the past (25). Despite this high incidence of psychiatric hospitalizations, most of these patients were never psychotic by any measure. Their personality traits were unusual, but they rarely led to schizophrenic or manic-depressive disorders. The principal features seen in the patients with right temporal lobe foci were a tendency toward excessive emotionalism and obstinate denial of any deficiencies. The patients with left temporal foci exhibited a tendency to intellectualize and to react to all deficiencies with a typically catastrophic response (25). The "right-sided" patient denied that he had any problems and made his denials with inappropriate vehemence; the "left-sided" patient examined the smallest of problems with extraordinary thoroughness and proclaimed himself overwhelmed by the problem (25). Patients with foci on either side are notably circumstantial in their speech and dependent in their behavior. These behavioral abnormalities show no correlation with seizure frequency although they do correlate with the duration of the epileptic disorder. The longer the patient has suffered from psychomotor seizures, the more likely he is to have a personality disorder more unequivocally developed (25).

Temporal Lobe Lesions and Personality Disorders

Despite this evidence of a statistical connection between psychomotor seizures and various types of psychopathology, it is possible, as already mentioned, that the seizures are not directly responsible for the abnormal psychosocial profiles and the higher than expected incidence of schizophrenic traits. The pathology causing the seizures may be directly responsible for the cognitive and affective disorders seen in these patients. Seizure control clearly has no bearing on the development of psychotic features or of personality disorders. Lesions in the temporal lobes that may lead to the appearance of schizophreniform psychoses quite often produce generalized tonic-clonic seizures rather than complex partial seizures (23). Mental symptoms appear in 75 percent of patients with temporal lobe tumors regardless of whether or not any form of seizure disorder develops (23). Lesions on the inner or mesial aspects of the temporal lobes are associated with the déjà vu, jamais vu, fear, and despair typically seen in patients with psychomotor seizures (31). About 12 percent of patients with catatonia have focal lesions in a temporal lobe; the patient may exhibit catatonia in association with or independent of a seizure disorder (39). Even the remarkably long interval between the onset of psychomotor seizures and the appearance of psychotic features in those patients who eventually develop them suggests that the psychiatric disorder is an uncommon effect of pathology that may induce seizures. The mean interval between the onset of seizures and the appearance of a psychosis is 14 years, clearly enough time for a slowly evolving lesion to produce considerable neural change (25). This latency is independent of the effectiveness of seizure control during the intervening years. The psychopathology and the seizures appear to be more coincidental than causally related.

Treatment of Psychomotor Epilepsy

Complex partial seizures can usually be controlled with anticonvulsant drugs. The drug of choice is carbamazepine. It is usually effective in 200 milligram doses given three to five times daily. Some patients are not seizure-free on this medication alone, even when the serum level of the drug is at the therapeutic level. These patients may do better on primidone, 250 milligrams three to five times daily, but many require a combination of primidone and carbamazepine. Other anticonvulsants, such as phenytoin, may be added to the regimen if these two drugs in combination are not effective in eliminating all seizures. In rare cases, the seizures cannot be controlled with medications. This may be because there is a progressive lesion in the brain that must be removed or because the epileptic activity in the temporal lobe is so severe that it cannot be suppressed. Because speech has vital centers in the dominant temporal lobe, surgery to control the seizures is often hazardous, unless there is a circumscribed lesion very far anterior in the temporal lobe. When there is no obvious structural lesion in the temporal lobe, an electroencephalographic recording obtained directly from the surface of the brain (electrocorticogram) at the time of surgery will help identify precisely which part of the cortex has the most epileptogenic activity. This limited resection of temporal lobe tissue often decreases the frequency of seizures in patients uncontrolled on medication and may allow anticonvulsant medication to control the previously uncontrolled epilepsy.

STATUS EPILEPTICUS

Status epilepticus is a frequently lethal seizure phenomenon producing unresponsiveness. In status epilepticus, one seizure follows another without the patient's returning to normal consciousness. This is easily and often feigned. The hysterical or psychotic patient appears to have a major motor seizure every few minutes and remains unresponsive between motor episodes. Conversely, true status epilepticus may be overlooked. The episodic seizure activity may be manifested in a comatose patient by little more than conjugate deviation of the eyes to one side. Once suspected, status epilepticus may be confirmed with an electroencephalogram which will show the episodic changes in brain wave patterns typical of this convulsive disorder. Such confirmation should generally be reserved for those patients strongly suspected of factitious seizures. Any patient with well-documented seizures who presents in status epilepticus must be treated immediately to avoid brain damage or death.

Intravenous anticonvulsants at the doses appropriate for treating status epilepticus will stop the factitious seizure activity of the hysterical or psychotic patient by abruptly sedating him. The danger of treating factitious status epilepticus is that the patient is subject to the same drug effects regardless of whether the seizures are real or feigned. Phenobarbital, phenytoin, diazepam, and paraldehyde are most commonly used to treat this disorder. Respiratory arrest, hypotension, and even occasional cardiac arrhythmias are acceptable complications of these drugs if the patient truly is the victim of a life-threatening condition.

There are rare forms of status epilepticus that are not as lethal as the commonly encountered generalized convulsive status epilepticus. These include epilepsia partialis continua, a condition in which the patient has constant partial seizures with elementary motor symptoms (focal motor seizures) (2). Despite constant limb or facial movements, these patients may have normal or only mildly altered consciousness. In petit mal status, abnormal movements will not be apparent, but altered consciousness will be obvious (30). A confused, dreamy state will develop rather than coma, but the altered mentation may not stop the patient from carrying out fairly routine activities. In both of these situations, an electroencephalogram is usually essential for diagnosis. Intravenous anticonvulsants may be very effective in petit mal status, but are generally ineffective against epilepsia partialis continua (2). When the status epilepticus is factitious, efforts to control it may prove lethal despite the patient's good physical health.

Status epilepticus is caused by several disturbances. The most common cause is discontinuation of anticonvulsant medications. Patients free of seizures for several months or years often stop taking pills to see if the epilepsy is still a problem. Unfortunately, withdrawal from some anticonvulsants, including phenobarbital and primidone, increases the risk of seizures and may precipitate status epilepticus. Sleep deprivation plays a role in causing status epilepticus in about ten per cent of cases (40). Any type of extreme physical stress will lower the patient's seizure threshold, but sleep deprivation is much more effective at lowering the threshold than are other deprivation states, such as starvation.

PSYCHIATRIC AND OTHER SIDE EFFECTS OF ANTICONVULSANT DRUGS

All of the currently used anticonvulsant drugs have numerous adverse effects, some of which are manifest as thought disorders or affective disorders. The risk of exposing the patient to unwanted side effects is minimized by using the anticonvulsants most likely to be effective against the type of seizure observed in the patient (Table 4.2). Unfortunately some patients are not seizure-free on only one anticonvulsant. Two or three drugs in combination will be used in these refractory cases and the likelihood of adverse side effects is correspondingly increased. Either toxic serum levels of specific anticonvulsant drugs or an idiosyncratic reaction to the drug may produce psychiatric signs in vulnerable patients (41). The most common psychologic signs of anticonvulsant toxocity are acute confusion, mood changes, lethargy, and schizophreniform reactions (Table 4.3) (41).

Phenytoin

Phenytoin (Dilantin, Epanutin) is an effective anticonvulsant in generalized and partial seizure disorders and is the drug of choice for generalized tonic-clonic (grand mal) seizures. Although it occasionally produces blood

Table 4.2. Anticonvulsant Drugs of Choice

Seizure Type	*Preferred Anticonvulsant Drugs*	*Common Brand Names*
Generalized convulsive (tonic-clonic, grand mal)	Phenytoin Primidone	Dilantin Epanutin Mysoline
Generalized nonconvulsive (absence, petit mal)	Valproic acid Ethosuximide Methsuximide	Depakene Zarontin Celontin
Complex partial (psychomotor, temporal lobe)	Carbamazepine Primidone Phenytoin	Tegretol Mysoline Dilantin Epanutin
Elementary partial (focal)	Phenytoin	Dilantin Epanutin
Myoclonic	Clonazepam	Clonopin

Table 4.3. Anticonvulsant Drug Side Effects

Drug	*Common Nonpsychiatric Phenomena*	*Common Psychiatric Phenomena*
Phenytoin	Sedation, nystagmus, blurred vision, gait ataxia, dysarthria, coarsening of facial features, hypertrichosis, gingival hyperplasia, pseudolymphoma	Poor concentration, intellectual slowing, logorrhea, hallucinations, schizophreniform reactions, personality change
Phenobarbital	Sedation, nystagmus, gait ataxia	Depression in the elderly, hyperactivity in children, visual hallucinations
Primidone	Sedation, nystagmus, gait ataxia, impaired memory	Acute confusion, persecutory delusions
Carbamazepine	Nausea, vertigo, diplopia, paresthesias, thrombocytopenia	Confusion
Ethosuximide	Lethargy	Acute confusion, affective disorders, night terrors
Valproic acid	Lethargy, gastrointestinal disturbances, tremors, anorexia, headache, enuresis, insomnia, thrombocytopenia	Confusion
Clonazepam	Choreoathetoid movements, lethargy	Stereotypy, autism, paranoid delusions, labile affect, auditory hallucinations, hostility

disorders, the commonly encountered adverse reactions are neurologic and psychiatric. A staggering gait, slurred speech, blurred vision, and mild sedation are the most common complaints. On examination, the toxic patient will have a staggering gait, nystagmus, and mildly slurred speech as the serum level exceeds 20 micrograms per milliliter. Years of phenytoin use often cause persistent but mild gait problems and sensory loss. These result from cerebellar degeneration and peripheral neuropathy induced by the drug (42,43). Young patients routinely complain of coarsening of facial features, darkening of limb and facial hair, and overgrowth of the gums.

Psychiatric problems are rarely a manifestation of an adverse reaction to phenytoin, but the range of psychiatric reactions that do occur is broad. Many patients complain of intellectual slowing and impaired concentration, but rare patients will actually develop tactile or visual hallucinations (41). Even more rarely an acute psychosis will appear that is indistinguishable from schizophrenia (41,42). The patient may have uncoordinated movements, garbled speech, urinary and fecal incontinence, and acute withdrawal (42). Acute conversion reactions may appear in patients, with no prior history of psychiatric problems (2). Occasional patients have stereotyped movements, autistic thinking, loose associations, and infantile affects (44). Patients with mild organic brain disease seem to be especially vulnerable to cognitive disorders as an early sign of phenytoin toxicity (44). Fortunately, this toxic effect of phenytoin is seen much less often than minor intellectual and personality changes. Problems with memory or calculations may be reported by the patient and impatience or irascibility may be reported by those around him (42).

These cognitive and affective changes will resolve when the serum phenytoin level falls below the toxic range. Depending upon the serum level of the drug, this may take 5 to 10 days in the severely toxic patient (43). The time required to drop the serum level to half its initial level (half-life) is also affected by several drugs often used in patients with psychiatric problems. Diazepam, chlorpromazine, prochlorperazine, methylphenidate, and chlordiazepoxide all increase the half-life of phenytoin, thereby slowing its clearance from the blood (43).

The simplest way to check for phenytoin toxicity is to obtain a serum level. The serum level should reach a plateau after the patient has been on the drug for about 5 days. This plateau is ideally between 10 and 20 micrograms per milliliter (43). With higher anticonvulsant levels, toxic signs and even increased seizure frequency may appear. Toxic effects aside from an acute allergic or gastrointestinal reaction should not arise for several hours after oral administration of the drug, because absorption is so slow that peak serum levels are not reached until about 4 to 8 hours after an oral dose (43). Suicide attempts with this drug are not usually successful, because gastric irritation will trigger vomiting of a massive oral dose. Most patients find it difficult to take more than 500 milligrams (five capsules) at one time. If more than 10 or 15 pills are swallowed and retained, the principal danger of the drug is in its cardiac action. Fatal arrhythmias with phenytoin overdose rarely occur even after massive oral doses. Although a rapid intravenous infusion of phenytoin carries substantial danger, most patients do not have the means to inject the medication, and phenytoin injected into muscle is very poorly absorbed (43).

Phenobarbital

Phenobarbital is one of the oldest anticonvulsants in use, and it is currently not the drug of choice for any seizure type. It is used as a second drug in patients with generalized seizure disorders if the patient has persistent seizures after a therapeutic trial of the drug of choice alone has failed. The high incidence of side effects has increasingly curtailed its use as alternative drugs have been developed. Children given the drug often become hyperactive, irritable, aggressive, and tearful (41). These hyperactive children have reduced attention spans, easy distractibility, and marked destructiveness. Most adults have no adverse reactions to phenobarbital except for mild sedation until toxic levels are reached, and then the patient usually develops a staggering gait, slurred speech, and nystagmus (41). Toxic confusional states may develop in adults with serum phenobarbital levels of over 60 micrograms per milliliter, but this is so much in excess of the therapeutic range of 15 to 40 micrograms per milliliter that the patient will usually develop other signs first (41,43).

Elderly adults are more vulnerable to the side effects of phenobarbital than are young adults, and they may have restlessness, confusion, and severe depression at relatively low levels. Rare patients develop visual hallucinations or a delirium-tremems type psychosis. Paradoxically, some patients develop psychotic reactions when the phenobarbital is stopped (41). More commonly, abrupt phenobarbital withdrawal causes seizures even in patients not previously known to have seizures.

An additional disadvantage of the drug is its abuse potential. Patients may use the drug for its mood altering effects or take a large number of pills in a suicide attempt. The drug is well tolerated orally and the peak serum level will not be reached until 12 to 18 hours after an oral dose (43). A high enough dose will suppress breathing and result in death. Phenobarbital has a half-life of 3 days. Toxic effects may take several weeks to clear after an overdose (2,41). The high level of toxic reactions with phenobarbital also leads to a high level of noncompliance. About 20 percent of the patients advised to take phenobarbital do not comply with their physician's instructions (2).

Primidone

Primidone is related to phenobarbital structurally, and it is converted in part to phenobarbital during its breakdown. Both primidone and its metabolic products, phenobarbital and phenylethylmalonamide (PEMA), are effective anticonvulsants. Generalized tonic-clonic (grand mal) and complex partial seizures are suppressed by primidone (43). Adverse reactions include those developing with phenobarbital, but they are less likely to occur because the serum phenobarbital level is less significant in controlling seizures in patients on this medication than the serum primidone level. A therapeutic level of primidone is 4 to 15 micrograms per milliliter (41). Toxic and idiosyncratic reactions to this drug include sedation, staggering gait, memory disturbances, acute confusional states, and persecutory delusions (2,41). Toxic manifestations of a primidone dose may appear much sooner after an oral dose than those of phenobarbital, because peak serum levels of primidone are reached within 3 hours (43). Many of the toxic effects of primidone, especially the sedation, can be minimized by starting the patient on a low dose and increasing it over the course of 2 to 3 weeks.

Carbamazepine
Carbamazepine is chemically related to the tricyclic antidepressants, but has no antidepressant effects (43). It is the drug of choice for complex partial (psychomotor) seizures but is also effective against elementary partial and generalized tonic-clonic seizures (2,43). Although there was considerable concern when the drug was first introduced that platelet disorders would be a common problem, the most frequently observed toxic reactions are neurologic. Vertigo, dizziness, and diplopia develop as the serum level of the drug increases above the therapeutic range of 4 to 12 micrograms per milliliter (41,43). Pins-and-needles sensations and excessive fatigue develop in some patients taking the drug, and they may persist for several days after the drug is stopped. The half-life of carbamazepine is 15 to 30 hours (41).

Ethosuximide
Ethosuximide and related substances, like methsuximide, are the drugs of choice in petit mal epilepsy (2). Signs of toxicity occur at serum levels greater than 40 to 80 micrograms per milliliter (41). Toxic and idiosyncratic reactions to the drug include acute confusional states and affective disorders (41). The abnormal affect may range from extreme lethargy and lack of initiative to unfounded euphoria. Patients with long-standing cognitive disorders may develop extreme paranoia and aggressiveness. Night terrors may become a substantial problem for children taking this drug (41).

Valproic Acid
Dipropylacetic (valproic) acid is unrelated structurally to any other anticonvulsant. It is very effective against several different types of generalized seizure disorders and it is probably the drug of choice for myoclonic seizures. Toxic effects occurring above the therapeutic range of 23 to 43 micrograms per milliliter include fatigue, nausea, thrombocytopenia, and elevated hepatic enzyme levels (45). Neurologic reactions include fine resting and postural tremors, headache, enuresis, insomnia, and anorexia. These toxic effects will clear rapidly when the drug is stopped because the drug's half-life is only 7 to 10 hours.

Benzodiazepines
Benzodiazepines have limited usefulness as anticonvulsants, but there are some notable exceptions. Diazepam is extremely effective for short periods when administered intravenously to treat status epilepticus. Clonazepam is effective against myoclonic seizures. Unfortunately, this group of drugs has a high level of adverse psychologic effects. Both clonazepam and flurazepam may induce aggressive behavior and marked hostility (41). Overmedication with clonazepam has produced stereotyped behavior with compulsive cleaning, forceful eye rubbing, and choreoathetoid limb and

body movements (44). The patient may have autistic thinking, paranoid delusions, labile affect, and auditory hallucinations (44). These psychotic signs will disappear as the dose of medication is decreased. This is not necessarily true for all benzodiazepines. Patients on chronically high doses of diazepam, a drug which is ineffective as an anticonvulsant when given orally, may have psychosis with delirium 3 to 5 days after the drug is abruptly stopped (41).

REFERENCES

1. Blumer D: Temporal lobe epilepsy and its psychiatric significance, in Benson DF, Blumer D (eds): *Psychiatric Aspects of Neurologic Disease.* New York, Grune & Stratton, 1975, p 171.
2. Booker HE: Management of the difficult patient with complex partial seizures. *Adv Neurol* 11:369, 1975.
3. Corsellis JAN, Goldberg GJ, Norton AR: "Limbic encephalitis" and its association with carcinoma. *Brain* 91:481, 1968.
4. Bennett R, Hughes GRV, Bywaters EGL, et al: Neuropsychiatric problems in systemic lupus erythematosus. *Br Med J* 4:342, 1972.
5. Karpati G, Frame B: Neuropsychiatric disorders in primary hyperparathyroidism. *Arch Neurol* 10:387, 1964.
6. Gastaut H: Clinical and electroencephalographical classification of epileptic seizures. *Epilepsia* 11:102, 1970.
7. Goldensohn ES: The classification of epileptic seizures, in Tower DB (ed): *The Nervous System.* New York, Raven Press, 1975, vol 2, p 261.
8. Massey EW, Riley TL: Pseudoseizures: Recognition and treatment. *Psychosomatics* 21:987, 1980.
9. Roy A: Hysterical seizures. *Arch Neurol* 36:447, 1979.
10. La Barbera JD, Dozier JE: Hysterical seizures: The role of exploitation. *Psychosomatics* 21:897, 1980.
11. Taylor AR, Chakravorty BC: Clinical syndromes associated with basilar impression. *Arch Neurol* 10:475, 1964.
12. Hawton K, Fagg J, Marsack P: Association between epilepsy and attempted suicide. *J Neurol Neurosurg Psychiatry* 43:168, 1980.
13. Hecker A, Andermann F, Rodin EA: Spitting automatism in temporal lobe seizures. *Epilepsia* 13:767, 1972.
14. Goldensohn ES, Gold AP: Prolonged behavioral disturbances as ictal phenomena. *Neurology (NY)* 10:1, 1959.
15. Flor-Henry P: Ictal and interictal psychiatric manifestations in epilepsy: Specific or non-specific. *Epilepsia* 13:773, 1972.
16. Rémillard GM, Andermann F, Gloor P, et al: Water-drinking as ictal behavior in complex partial seizures. *Neurology (NY)* 31:117, 1981.
17. Mulder DW, Daly D: Psychiatric symptoms associated with lesions of temporal lobe. *J Am Med Assoc* 150:173, 1952.
18. Slater E, Beard AW: The schizophrenia-like psychoses of epilepsy. i. Psychiatric aspects. *Br J Psychiatry* 109:95, 1963.

19. Mohan KJ, Salo MW, Nagaswami S: A case of limbic system dysfunction with hypersexuality and fugue state. *Dis Nerv Syst* 36:621, 1975.
20. McLachlan RS, Blume WT: Isolated fear in complex partial status epilepticus. *Ann Neurol* 8:639, 1980.
21. Babb RR, Eckman PB: Abdominal epilepsy. *J Am Med Assoc* 222:65, 1972.
22. Rodin EA: Psychosocial management of patients with complex partial seizures. *Adv Neurol* 11:383, 1975.
23. Malamud N: Psychiatric disorder with intracranial tumors of limbic system. *Arch Neurol* 17:113, 1967.
24. Waxman SG, Geschwind N: Hypergraphia in temporal lobe epilepsy. *Neurology (NY)* 24:629, 1974.
25. Bear DM, Fedio P: Quantitative analysis of interictal behavior in temporal lobe epilepsy. *Arch Neurol* 32:454, 1977.
26. Slater E, Beard AW: The schizophrenia-like psychoses of epilepsy. Psychiatric aspects. *Br J Psychiatry* 109:95, 1963.
27. Serafetinides EA: Aggressiveness in temporal lobe epileptics and its relation to cerebral dysfunction and environmental factors. *Epilepsia* 6:33, 1965.
28. Valenstein E, Heilman KM: Emotional disorders resulting from lesions of the central nervous system, in Heilman KM, Valenstein E (eds): *Clinical Neuropsychology*. New York, Oxford University Press, 1979, p 413.
29. Mayeux R, Alexander MP, Benson DF, et al: Poriomania. *Neurology (NY)* 29:1616, 1979.
30. Niedermeyer E, Fineyre F, Riley T, et al: Absence status (petit mal status) with focal characteristics. *Arch Neurol* 36:417, 1979.
31. Teuber HL: Prospects for research on schizophrenia: Effects of focal brain lesions. *Neurosci Res Program Bull* 10:381, 1972.
32. Pritchard PB, Lombroso CT, McIntyre M: Psychological complications of temporal lobe epilepsy. *Neurology (NY)* 30:227, 1980.
33. Taylor DC: Aggression and epilepsy. *J Psychosom Res* 13:229, 1969.
34. Abenson MH: EEG's in chronic schizophrenia. *Br J Psychiatry* 116:421, 1970.
35. Stevens JR: Interictal clinical manifestations of complex partial seizures. *Adv Neurol* 11:85, 1975.
36. Mignone RJ, Donnelly EF, Sadowsky D: Psychological and neurological comparisons of psychomotor and non-psychomotor epileptic patients. *Epilepsia* 11:345, 1970.
37. Mayeux R, Brandt J, Rosen J, et al: Interictal memory and language impairment in temporal lobe epilepsy. *Neurology (NY)* 30:120, 1980.
38. Taylor DC: Sexual behavior and temporal lobe epilepsy. *Arch Neurol* 21:510, 1969.
39. Plum F: Prospects for research on schizophrenia: Neuropathological findings. *Neurosci Res Program Bull* 10:384, 1972.
40. Roth N: Sleep and motility. *Dis Nerv Syst* 38:778, 1977.
41. Tollefson G: Psychiatric implications of anticonvulsant drugs. *J Clin Psychiatry* 41:295, 1980.
42. McLain LW, Martin JT, Allen JH: Cerebellar degeneration due to chronic phenytoin therapy. *Ann Neurol* 7:18, 1980.
43. Penry JK, Newmark ME: The use of antiepileptic drugs. *Ann Intern Med* 90:207, 1979.
44. Franks RD, Richter AJ: Schizophrenia-like psychosis associated with anticonvulsant toxicity. *Am J Psychiatry* 136:973, 1979.
45. Bruni J, Wilder BJ: Valproic acid. *Arch Neurol* 36:393, 1979.

5
Speech Disorders

Speech abnormalities often provide evidence of a psychiatric problem, but structural lesions in the brain can also produce changes in speech. Identifying the speech disorders that have strictly psychiatric or strictly neurologic bases is difficult and often frustrating. If the patient has a long psychiatric history, the appearance of a peculiar speech pattern is often ascribed to the antecedent mental illness, but this reliance upon the patient's history occasionally allows a new problem to be overlooked. Altered speech develops with a variety of psychiatric and neurologic disorders. The changes in speech appearing with profoundly different diseases are often remarkably similar, these changes ranging from the permanent loss of all communication skills to transient disturbances in accent or intonation. Determining whether the language problem represents a thought disorder, an emotional conflict, or a structural lesion in the brain is the most important, if not the most difficult, distinction made in the evaluation and treatment of speech-impaired patients.

Most speech disturbances can be categorized as either aphonia, aphasia, or dysarthria. There is no significant overlap between these three forms of language disturbance, although there are rare speech problems that do not fit clearly into one class or another. Aphonia is a loss of verbal production, such as that occurring in the catatonic schizophrenic and the akinetic mute individual. These patients do not speak, and their understanding of spoken or written language is often difficult to assess. The dysarthric patient speaks but with specific defects in the sound of the language produced. He has intact word-finding abilities, excellent speech comprehension, and normal grammatical skills; but, articulation, the production of appropriate sounds, is impaired. The rate, rhythm, clarity, volume, or even continuity of words and sentences may be defective. With aphasia, the content or comprehension of speech is defective. The aphasic patient has difficulty following instructions or producing meaningful replies, problems in language handling that are not explained by any deficits the individual may manifest in hearing or articulating. An aphasia may involve both the comprehension and production of speech, or it may be limited to language comprehension or meaningful speech production alone. The speech defect in aphasia may be so restricted that only a particular element of language function is lost, such as the ability to name objects.

Aphonia usually has a psychologic basis, whereas dysarthria usually indicates underlying structural disease. Aphasia causes the most difficulty for clinicians trying to distinguish organic from psychogenic language disorders. This speech disorder is occasionally interpreted as evidence that the affected individual has some form of schizophrenia (1). If the patient has focal neurologic signs other than impaired language, this error is less likely; but the patient with disordered language alone may be referred for psychiatric evaluation by very well informed clinicians. Complicating the recognition of specific types of aphasia are the aphasic disorders characterized by a disturbance in a single aspect of language. A patient may follow written instructions, appear deaf to verbal instructions, and simultaneously show intact recognition of nonverbal stimuli (2). The patient's abilities do not fit sensibly with his deficits, even though the language problem typically has an organic basis. Attention over recent years to patients with reading problems has made restricted problems in this area much less suspect (3–6). It is now generally recognized that individuals with no psychologic difficulty may have virtually intact language function with selective deficits in reading or even in reading certain forms of written language (3,4). These rare syndromes of pure word deafness and pure word blindness (dyslexia) do not fit well into any established scheme of language function.

APHONIA: THE MUTE PATIENT

The awake adult who interacts with his environment nonverbally, but persistently refuses to produce any vocal sounds usually has no destructive or metabolic lesion in the central nervous system. Akinetic mutism, as discussed in the section on the unresponsive patient, certainly can occur with both psychiatric and neurologic disorders, but patients with this syndrome exhibit little or no interaction with their surroundings (7). The patient with a seizure disorder may be mute, but relatively active, during the period of confusion that follows most epileptic fits; but this aphonia is transient (7). Postictal mutism, as it is called, usually lasts minutes, rather than hours. The persistently mute patient who can walk and hold objects and follow examiners is generally the victim of a psychiatric disorder or the perpetrator of a factitious symptom. The obvious exception to this is the patient with structural damage to the organs of speech. A patient with a damaged larynx or severed laryngeal nerves will be mute, but awake, just like the mentally ill patient and the malingerer, but the cause of the aphonia in the patient with laryngeal disease will usually be evident. Direct examination of the larynx by an otolaryngologist will establish whether or not the vocal cords can move normally. If structural disease is not present and a psychiatric disorder is apparent, the patient's aphonia still cannot be automatically ascribed to a strictly psychologic basis. The psychiatric problem itself may be secondary to an organic lesion, such as hyperparathyroidism. The victim of this endocrine problem may have aphonia as part of a depressive reaction that appears as serum calcium levels rise (8).

At the acute onset of an aphasia, the patient is rarely ever mute. Mutism does occur in children with a lesion producing an aphasia, but even in childhood, an abrupt loss of speech must be viewed suspiciously (4,9). Just as aphasia in childhood more frequently produces aphonia than in adult life, so too does stress in childhood evoke an acute mutism as a psychogenic disorder more often than in adult life (4). Indeed a mute patient cannot be considered aphasic until some speech function has been demonstrated (10). Aphasia is disordered language, not absent language.

Transient Mutism

Transient mutism does occur with some circumscribed lesions in the brain. When the patient cannot combine sounds to form anything resembling words, he is described as aphemic (Figure 5.1). This is a rare language disorder appearing with strokes that damage the left frontal lobe (11). Patients with this language problem are usually mute when they are first seen by a physician, but there is little question of a psychiatric problem because right-sided weakness invariably accompanies the aphonia (11). Speech returns within days of the onset of the problem, but it has an abnormal rhythm and poor clarity. The patient has good grammar, vocabulary, and writing if these were present before the development of the aphemia. These patients are not truly aphonic. Even while the patient is mute, he will make vocal noises usually by humming or grunting. In those patients without obvious right arm weakness, there may be some question of an underlying psychiatric problem. An amobarbital interview will establish the organic character of the mutism: psychogenic aphonia will abate as the patient receives the depressant drug.

Patients with aphemia will follow a stereotyped pattern of speech recovery. Initially, singing and repetitive speech will be much better than spontaneous speech (11). More extensive frontal lobe damage produces the more complex language disturbance of Broca's expressive aphasia. Aphemia is most easily distinguished from a Broca's expressive aphasia by the preservation of written language in aphemia, but not in an expressive aphasia. The aphemic patient writes clearly even when he is unable to express himself at all in spoken language. The lesion responsible for aphemia probably lies between Broca's area in the prefrontal cortex and the motor cortex controlling the muscles involved in speech.

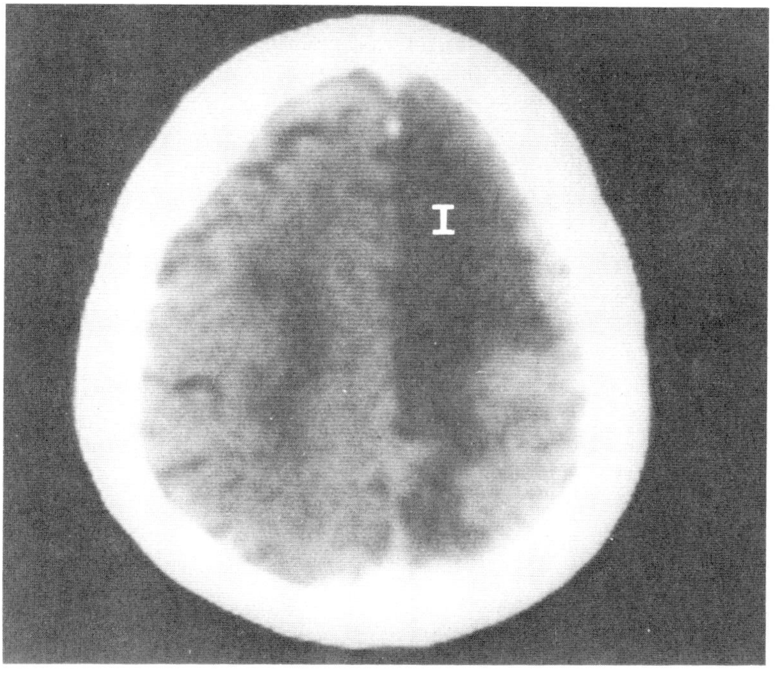

Figure 5.1. An 80-year-old man developed weakness in his right leg that progressed over the course of a few days. As the weakness increased, the patient became less vocal. With complete paralysis of the leg, he became mute but entirely alert and otherwise cooperative. A computed tomogram revealed infarction (I) in the distribution of the left anterior cerebral artery. The patient was presumed to have an aphemia secondary to left frontal lobe damage.

Bilateral thalamic lesions will produce transient loss of all speech in rare individuals (12). With recovery from the acute insult, which may be a stroke, the patient will exhibit persistent defects in speech. This thalamic mutism occurs occasionally in patients treated for Parkinson disease by placing small lesions in the thalamus. Obviously, an adverse psychologic reaction to the surgery is not usually considered as the cause of aphonia in these patients, but the preoperative depression manifest by many parkinsonian patients may cause some initial concern that the mutism does not have a purely structural basis. Characteristic of these mute patients is preserved writing ability (10). Although most of the patients selected for this type of thalamic surgery are under treatment for Parkinson disease and have slow, compressed writing, given enough time they will write meaningful words and sentences. Thalamic lesions that produce aphonia are invariably bilateral (12). Hesitancy in speech and loss of fluency routinely last 6 to 9 months, and the patient is invariably aware of his speech problem.

The intracranial events producing transient mutism usually cause numerous other signs of brain damage. The loss of speech may be just an early deficit in a long chain of problems terminating with death within a few days or weeks of this initial problem. If the patient survives the neurologic catastrophe, speech impairment may remain as permanent evidence of the brain damage suffered. Mutism occasionally follows hemorrhage into the gray matter about the aqueduct of Sylvius in the midbrain and into the pons, but these patients are usually akinetic, as well as mute, during the first few days after the bleeding (12). The akinetic mutism gradually resolves and leaves a mute, but active, patient. The multiple cranial nerve deficits occurring with the brainstem hemorrhage simplify recognition of patients with this structural lesion in the brainstem. Abnormal eye movements, complaints of double vision, and facial weakness appear along with the aphonia when midbrain and pontine structures are damaged. Confusion rarely develops over what caused the loss of speech in these patients.

Speech Hesitation

Cerebral lesions produce a reluctance to talk that is easily misconstrued as aphonia (11). The rare aphasia in which repetition is remarkably intact while spontaneous verbal expression is poor, the so-called transcortical motor aphasia, often leaves the patient apparently mute initially, but, with considerable coaxing, the patient will repeat short phrases (13). Transcortical aphasias, as discussed in the following section, recover spontaneously at a relatively rapid rate with language function passing through phases of more common aphasias, so that a psychogenic basis for the patient's mutism is rejected at least in retrospect (13).

Less likely to show resolution is the disorder of speech recognition called pure word deafness or auditory verbal agnosia. The specific unresponsiveness to words, rather than sounds, in a largely mute patient frequently prompts a psychiatric hospitalization for these patients (2). If the patient with pure word deafness can be coaxed into speaking by way of written commands, his speech will sound clearly abnormal. The intonation and rhythm of normal speech will be absent and the word-deaf patient will seem to wail as much as speak (2). The schizophrenic patient who acutely loses all speech may be coaxed into verbalizing by similar maneuvers, but the resulting speech will sound fairly normal, though flat and reluctant. Patients with bilateral thalamic tumors also show a profound reluctance to talk, but with adequate manipulation they will exhibit relatively normal speech (12). Neurologic deficits associated with the speech abnormality help distinguish speech hesitancy caused by structural lesions from that caused by schizophrenia.

APHASIA

Aphasia is a group of speech disorders that share the one feature that they are all language dysfunctions (12). The dysfunction may be in the comprehension, production, repetition, structuring, or application of language, but it is language, not sound, that is mishandled. If a severely dysarthric patient's garbled speech proves to be accurately structured, meaningful speech when it is transcribed into a comprehensible form, then the patient is not aphasic (10). Distinguishing between different types of aphasias is simplified by recognizing traits, such as the fluency of the patient's speech, which correlate with damage to specific areas of the brain. Fluency is an especially important aspect of every patient's speech, since no matter what else can be established for an individual's language abilities, his speech can at least be defined as fluent or nonfluent (Table 5.1). Fluent speech has the normal sound and flow of the patient's native tongue even if the content is an endless string of meaningless sounds. Nonfluent aphasia is usually an expressive problem, that is, a problem with producing words and sentences despite intact language comprehension (14). Fluent aphasia is usually a "receptive" problem, that is, a disorder characterized by facile vocal output with limited comprehension of spoken and written language (10). Of course, there is much more to language than the fluent production of a string of words and the facile comprehension of spoken and written phrases. Syntax, interpretation of word order, naming, repetition, and inflection of verbs and nouns all have roles in language, and all may be defective in aphasic patients (17).

The side of the brain associated with most language disturbances when it is damaged is called the speech dominant side. Less than 1 percent of right-handed people are right hemisphere dominant for speech, and at least 60 percent of left-handed people are left hemisphere dominant for speech (10,18,19). About 93 percent of adults are right-handed (4). This means that most language functions are disturbed with left cerebral hemisphere disease, and the right cerebral hemisphere has limited, though real, importance in speech (20). Aphasia of any kind indicates a left-sided cerebral lesion in 95 percent of the individuals affected regardless of the patient's handedness (19). The precise location of various speech functions

Table 5.1. Aphasia Types

Fluent	*Nonfluent*
Wernicke's (sensory, receptive)	Broca's (motor, expressive)
Conduction	Isolation of speech area
Transcortical sensory	Transcortical motor
Anomic	Global

in the left hemisphere is much more controversial than the thesis that the left hemisphere is almost always dominant for speech.

Any structural lesion may produce an aphasia, but the type of lesion and site of damage influence the course of recovery followed, if in fact language does recover. The most common cause of aphasia is stroke. The amount and location of the brain damage suffered in the stroke both affect the outlook for recovery of language abilities. Patients with small areas of damaged cerebral cortex because of infarction or hemorrhage generally do better than patients with extensive areas of damage, but lesions centering directly on vital speech areas may produce dense, persistent aphasias, even when the extent of the lesion is small. Aphasias appearing with head trauma usually have a better recovery than aphasias developing with stroke (13). Thirty percent of posttraumatic aphasias remit over the course of a few weeks (13). The remaining patients with posttraumatic aphasia generally recover within 3 months. Younger patients recover from aphasia more quickly than older patients, regardless of the insult producing the language disorder.

Impaired Language Production: Expressive Aphasias

Patients who understand language, but struggle to produce words, despite adequately functional mouth and laryngeal structures, often have an expressive or Broca's aphasia. Broca's aphasia is a speech impairment long recognized as a problem in language production (14–16). The third frontal convolution of the speech dominant hemisphere is the most common site for lesions producing this type of aphasia (17). Because the left cerebral hemisphere is almost always the speech dominant hemisphere, patients with this nonfluent aphasia usually have disease of the left frontal lobe. The exact site that must be damaged to produce a Broca's aphasia is still disputed. A few pathologic studies suggest that Broca's area for expressive language functions is in the precentral gyrus of the frontal lobe, a site distinctly posterior to the classically defined area (18).

With Broca's aphasia, speech is halting and labored. The patient makes errors in producing words and displays exasperation as he recognizes his mistakes. "Book" may come out "B . . . b . . . b . . . bog." Speech becomes telegraphic as the patient omits less important words (14). A simple statement like "I put the book on the table" is reduced to "I . . . put . . . book . . . table." In addition to the lost fluency, there is considerable lost flexibility in speech. Verbs and nouns are not inflected, and syntax is largely eliminated (17). The patient seems to be speaking a language with which he is only slightly familiar; yet, when he listens to someone else speak the same language, he has almost flawless comprehension. Broca's area is apparently involved in setting the rules for coordinating the simultaneous and sequential motor activities of speech (4). The patient with a Broca's aphasia seems to have limited skills in articulating or, rather, in programming motor systems for the articulation necessary for the production of accurate speech (17). This phonetic problem is compounded by a limited capacity to deal with grammar. Comprehension of speech deteriorates for these nonfluent aphasic patients when syntax is essential to the understanding of a statement. Producing grammatically accurate statements is much more of a problem for the patient with an expressive aphasia than is interpreting statements with complex syntax. Faulty interpretation of some instructions with complex grammatical structure does, however, occasionally give the impression that the patient has a significant problem with language comprehension. The ability to name objects is sometimes preserved out of proportion to other facets of speech.

Written speech is generally affected in much the same way as spoken language (14). The patient with a Broca's aphasia writes in the uninflected telegraphic manner characteristic of his speech. The patient can repeat phrases or words, but usually only after many preliminary attempts to initiate the test phrase. Reading is impaired in these nonfluent patients, but some reading competency will remain, regardless of the severity of the expressive aphasia (5). It may be that problems develop with reading because the lesion in the frontal lobe that produces the expressive aphasia damages systems important in interpreting syntax and maintaining the appropriate sequence in verbal information (5). Whether the reading problems seen in Broca's aphasia develop because of disturbed language center function or more concrete neurologic dysfunctions, such as impaired eye coordination from damaged lateral gaze centers, it is worth noting that reading ability in this language disorder is generally better than in other forms of aphasia.

Neurologic signs associated with a Broca's aphasia may be quite subtle, but most patients have substantial right-sided weakness accompanying the language disorder. Because of the frontal lobe site most often involved in Broca's aphasia, these patients usually have weakness or paralysis in the right arm and the right side of the face (10). The lower half of the face is characteristically more impaired than the forehead. Innervation from both cerebral hemispheres controls movements on both sides of the forehead. Visual field problems are notably absent. Right leg strength may be entirely intact. When weakness is not at all obvious, the organic nature of the speech problem is suggested by both the pattern of the language disorder and by the patient's apparent anxiety and frustration.

This language disorder is rarely confused with psychiatric disease, but psychiatric problems do appear in patients with an unequivocal Broca's aphasia. The psychiatric problem may be a reaction to the neurologic deficits or a further complication of the structural lesion that produced the aphasia. Whatever the cause of the psychiatric problem, the most common form it assumes is as an affective disorder. Depression complicates the recovery of some patients with expressive aphasias, but if an affective disorder does appear in these patients, it is usually apathy or loss of initiative, a complication of the frontal lobe damage rather than of the aphasia (19).

Receptive Aphasias

The most common fluent aphasia is Wernicke's aphasia, a language disorder usually arising with damage to the left posterior temporal gyrus (10,21). Comprehension of spoken and written language is disproportionately affected in this language disorder (14,17). Unlike the Broca's or expressive aphasic, the patient with a receptive aphasia is unaware of the errors in his speech (Table 5.2). He seems to understand his own language to the same extent he understands that directed toward him by others. Individual sounds, called phonemes, may be in error, resulting in "sut" for "cut." These substitutions, whether they involve parts of words or entire words, are called paraphasias. Substituted phonemes are called literal paraphasias (10); entire words erroneously substituted are called

Table 5.2. Signs of Aphasia

Aphasia Type	*Characteristics*
Broca's aphasia	Nonfluent speech
	Intact comprehension
	Poor repetition
	Poor reading
	Poor writing
	Errors in syntax
	Associated right arm and face weakness
Wernicke's aphasia	Fluent speech
	No comprehension
	No repetition
	Poor naming
	No reading
	No writing
	Frequent paraphasias
	Associated right visual field cut
Global aphasia	Nonfluent speech
	No comprehension
	No repetition
	No naming
	No reading
	No writing
	Frequent paraphasias
	Associated right hemiparesis
	Associated right visual field cut

verbal or semantic paraphasias. With verbal paraphasias a legitimate word replaces a similar noun or verb, such as "transigent" for "transient," or an entirely new word, a neologism, is placed in the stream of words. Paraphasias, neologisms, and inappropriate responses to instructions are all characteristic of the fluent Wernicke's aphasia. With a very mild aphasia, the errors made by the patient are often overlooked by listeners, and a significant speech problem may go undetected for weeks or months. Substitution of "t" for "d" is an especially common phonemic error, and this usually goes unnoticed even if it develops abruptly (17).

The patient does not write as fluently as he speaks, but he demonstrates all the errors characteristic of his speech in his writing (10). Logorrhea or excessive verbal production develops in some patients with Wernicke's aphasia, but it is never paralleled by an associated graphorrhea (4). This trait is useful in distinguishing aphasic patients from schizophrenic patients. The latter may fill pages with written jargon similar to the disconnected paraphasic speech they produce when they have logorrhea (4). To explain this discrepancy between speech fluency and writing, Norman Geschwind proposed that speech is overlearned through practice much more than is likely with writing (4). Most people talk several hours every day, using similar words and phrases repeatedly, but the same is not true of writing. Broca's area is overtrained for verbal output, but not for written output, and so when it is released from regulation by other cortical areas, such as Wernicke's area, it can produce an acoustically fairly normal speech output; however, it does not have enough ingraining of writing to allow fluent written output. Supporting this notion is the rarity of fluent aphasias in children under 10 years of age (9). Presumably, the child's Broca's area has not developed enough independent activity before that age to function without constant instruction from other cortical areas (4). Despite the observed lack of fluency in writing with Wernicke's aphasia, penmanship is better preserved than with Broca's aphasia (4).

Repetition is severely impaired in Wernicke's aphasia because the patient does not understand what is being said. He is unable to follow simple instructions whether written or spoken. Reading comprehension is impaired in this fluent aphasia presumably because of the verbal association techniques used by most people learning to read (4). Printed matter would normally evoke auditory association as a person reads, but in Wernicke's aphasia, the normal pathway is disrupted. With more severe language disturbances the patient often omits nouns and inappropriately arranges items of speech (17). As the aphasia resolves, it is likely to change considerably in character. Neologisms and phonemic paraphasias are replaced by verbal paraphasias, and, with further resolution, the patient will exhibit difficulty in naming objects rather than in avoiding paraphasias (13). This does not mean that patients with Wernicke's aphasia invariably get better. Those with the worst aphasic disorders are least likely to show improvement (13).

Schizophrenic Jargon and Receptive Aphasia

The fluent aphasic is easily mistaken for a patient with a thought disorder. If the lesion develops from a small embolus to the middle cerebral artery, the principal blood supply to the superior temporal gyrus, there may be little evidence of additional neurologic disease. A small visual field cut in the right superior quadrant of the visual field may be the only evidence of a structural brain lesion other than the aphasia. Apparently tangential and irrelevant speech with numerous neologisms and widely varying content appropriately suggests an acute schizophrenic reaction to the examining physician (4). The verbigeration of psychogenic catatonia, in which the patient produces repeated, meaningless words and sentences is easily confused with a Wernicke's aphasia, unless a psychiatric history or signs of catatonia point to the psychiatric basis for the language disorder (7). Both the schizophrenic patient and the patient with a receptive aphasia are vague, have loose associations, use circumlocution, and produce a vast amount of meaningless verbiage (1). Both patients also often show no appropriate response to an examiner's instructions or questions. Although the aphasic patient is more likely to stutter, both the schizophrenic patient and the fluent aphasic will exhibit blocking of specific words and phrases (1).

That paraphasias are not characteristic of schizophrenic speech may help in distinguishing the two types of patients from each other, just as the aphasic's tendency to perseverate is likely to set him apart (Table 5.3). Other characteristic differences between the thought disordered and language disordered patients are their modes of interacting with an interviewer. The aphasic patient will pause to get the listener's aid in finding the word that eludes him, a maneuver never used by the schizophrenic. Syntax is often preserved in schizophrenic language but is invariably disturbed in aphasic disorders (1). Patients with a receptive aphasia occasionally appear depressed, but they are much more commonly euphoric and apparently undisturbed by their communication problem (19). Unfortunately, when all criteria for discriminating between the schizophrenic patient and the aphasic patient are considered, the most useful item is the patient's history and the context of the current speech disorder.

Recovery from a Receptive Aphasia

Recovery of speech in the patient with a receptive aphasia does occur with nonprogressive lesions. A receptive aphasia developing with cerebral infarction will usually improve over the course of days or weeks. The recovery follows a fairly consistent pattern: neologisms subside and phonemic paraphasias are replaced by semantic paraphasias (13). As the aphasia becomes more subtle, the only apparent deficit may be a problem with naming. The patient with the least jargon early in the course of his aphasia will have the best recovery from the aphasia. Progressive lesions,

Table 5.3. Distinctions Between Receptive Aphasia and Schizophrenic Jargon

Receptive Aphasias	*Schizophrenic Jargon*
Interaction with examiner	Little reaction to examiner
Paraphasic speech	Blocking
Difficulty reading	Altered intonation
Difficulty writing	Fluent writing
More likely to stutter	Inexact word usage
Likely to perseverate	Does not perseverate
Enlists examiner's help in word-finding	Overly concrete or overly abstract
Usually 40- to 70-year-old patients	Usually 20- to 30-year-old patients
Speech defect evolves to anomia	Pedantic speech
Logorrhea without graphorrhea	Logorrhea with graphorrhea
	Reiteration of bizarre themes
	Verbigeration
	Inappropriate affect
	Condensation of words
SHARED FEATURES	
Neologisms	
Reiteration	
Pauses	
Circumlocation	
Verbal substitution	
No echolalia	

such as Alzheimer disease, which produce a receptive aphasia in some patients, will obviously not be associated with remission of the aphasia regardless of how slowly the central nervous system disease progresses.

Conduction Aphasia

Normal language relies upon interaction between speech comprehension centers and speech production centers (Figure 5.2). Although there are several sites important in various aspects of both functions, the connections between the superior temporal gyrus and the third frontal convolution of the left cerebral hemisphere are of special significance in normal language production (14). This connection, which probably includes a fiber tract known as the arcuate fasciculus, necessarily runs through the parietal lobe as it courses from the temporal lobe to the frontal lobe (4,14). Damage deep in the left parietal lobe consequently produces a fluent aphasia called a conduction aphasia.

Phonemic paraphasias occur with this aphasia, but to a lesser extent than that seen with Wernicke's aphasia (13). Fluency is only fair in conduction aphasia, but comprehension of written and spoken language is excellent (22). Repetition, especially of short syntactical words, such as

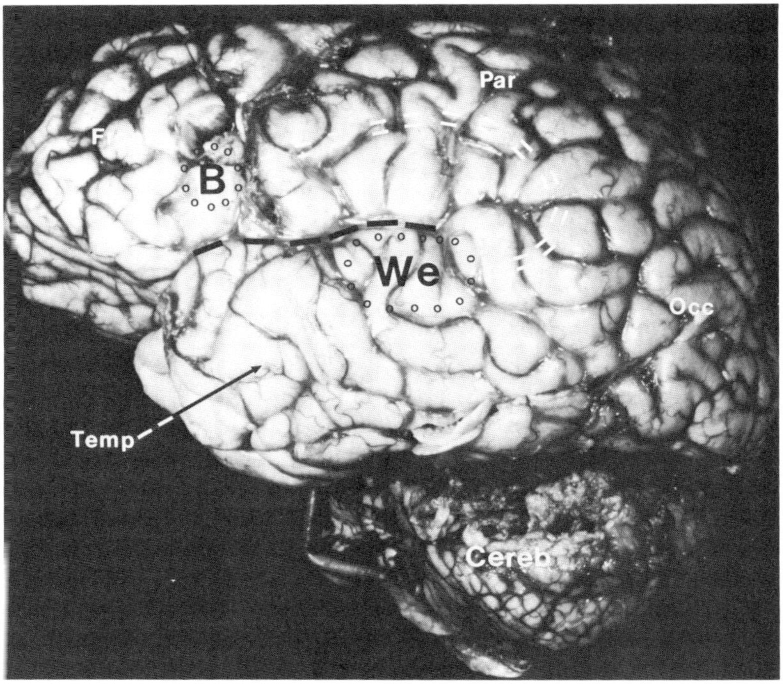

Figure 5.2. The approximate locations of Broca's area (B) and Wernicke's area (We) are indicated on this lateral view of a formalin-fixed brain. The broken black line above Wernicke's area lies in the Sylvian fissure, and the broken white lines extending from Wernicke's area to Broca's area represent the subcortical connection between the two speech centers. Interruption of this connection, which is probably the arcuate fasciculus, presumably causes a conduction aphasia. Other landmarks indicated are the cerebellum (Cereb), the frontal lobe (Front), the parietal lobe (Par), the occipital lobe (Occ), and the temporal lobe (Temp).

"no ifs, ands, or buts" is impaired out of proportion to all other deficits, although naming of objects is also quite poor (6,10). Reading comprehension is variably affected, but it too is usually impaired (6). A distinctive paraphasic disorder in this form of aphasia is the repetition of related paraphasias as the patient seems to focus in on the desired word. The resulting sentence may be interrupted by a paraphasic sequence of "dock . . . clock . . . clerk . . . work" (22).

Conduction aphasia rarely occurs as an isolated neurologic finding. A right-sided visual field defect and right-sided sensory deficit often occur with this aphasia (4). Patients may have lesions extending deep into the motor fibers that course through the internal capsule, in which case they will also have right-sided weakness or paralysis. The prognosis for recovery of language with this type of aphasia is relatively good. The other neurologic problems appearing with the aphasia more commonly cause long-term disability than does the aphasia.

Global Aphasia

All of the structures discussed with Broca's aphasia, Wernicke's aphasia, and conduction aphasia are relatively close to each other, and all are supplied by the same internal carotid artery branch, the middle cerebral artery. It is not at all unusual for the inferior frontal lobe, superior temporal lobe, and inferior parietal lobe to be simultaneously damaged with a middle cerebral artery occlusion. The resulting language disorder involves speech production, comprehension, and repetition (10). This is a global language dysfunction and is, accordingly, called a global aphasia. These patients understand little or no spoken or written language, and their speech is limited to fairly banal phrases (13). They also have the other neurologic signs of a left middle cerebral artery occlusion, which include right arm and face weakness, right-sided sensory deficits, and right visual field cuts. Recovery from global aphasia is usually protracted and incomplete.

Naming Difficulty: Anomic Aphasia

Despite the predictability of language dysfunctions with focal lesions in the left frontal and temporal areas, there is a wide range of language dysfunctions that have no currently established anatomic bases. Anomic aphasia is the most common of these nonlocalized language disorders. The principal defect is in naming objects or recalling words (14). Comprehension and repetition are preserved (10). This is a fluent aphasia because the patient usually avoids the words he cannot recall, although this may result in considerable circumlocution. A typical manuever used by such aphasic patients is to indicate items by their function, rather than by their name. A "watch" is "the time teller" and a "pen" is "that thing you write with." Syntax is generally preserved, but the store of words, that is, the lexicon, seems to be deficient (17).

Anomic aphasias occasionally develop with lesions limited to the dominant angular gyrus, an area of cerebral cortex in the parietal lobe at the junction of parietal, occipital, and temporal lobes (4). This is, however, not the only site of injury that can cause anomic aphasias. Alzheimer disease, metabolic encephalopathy, and structural lesions in the basal temporal region of the dominant hemisphere can all cause anomic aphasias (23). Because the language defect is so elementary, even hysterical patients can exhibit a clinical anomia that is convincing (23). Epileptic patients may have transient anomic aphasias during the postictal state, the recovery stage after a seizure; and patients with temporal lobe epilepsy may even exhibit some anomia during seizure-free periods, a defect probably reflecting the importance of a normal temporal lobe in word recall (23,24).

As other aphasic disorders resolve, they most often leave the patient with an anomic aphasia, if any aphasia persists at all (13). The site of the initial lesion producing the aphasia does not affect this tendency to pass through an anomic aphasia as the initial aphasia resolves. Metabolic disorders, head trauma, and presenile dementia producing an aphasia usually produce an anomic aphasia (10). These are nonfocal disorders, and that they preferentially affect word-finding ability supports the notion that long-term memory for words is a diffuse cortical function (17). Anomic aphasias are occasionally associated with an inability to read or write (13).

Isolation of the Speech Area

A rare fluent aphasia, which supports the schema of language organization outlined above, is the isolation aphasia. This is rare because the lesion responsible effectively isolates the frontal cortex and the temporal cortex with their intervening connections from the cortex around them (10). This can occur with a watershed infarct of the cerebral hemisphere, a stroke affecting areas supplied by the most terminal branches of the cerebral arteries. Watershed infarcts develop with profound hypotension. Isolation of the speech area is manifest by a largely mute patient whose principal language ability is repetition (10). Comprehension is lost and spontaneous speech is virtually absent. Echolalia occurs when the patient is asked a question or given an instruction. Rather than responding to the inquiry or following the order, the patient repeats the examiner's statement. Occasionally the patient will complete extremely familiar phrases in an almost reflex manner (19). Provided the stock greeting "Merry Christmas and a Happy . . ." the patient may respond with "New Year."

Patients with this type of aphasia are severely impaired and generally do not recover much speech or intellectual function. The common setting for the hypotension producing the responsible stroke is a cardiac arrest. Isolation of the speech area may be evident only after the patient passes through a vegetative state lasting weeks or months. Multiple infarcts occurring over the course of years may also produce this type of aphasia, but the affected individual will invariably have a profound multi-infarct dementia. This speech disorder will prompt concern that the patient has a psychogenic catatonia only if the setting for the onset of the deficit is unknown.

Transcortical Aphasia

More complex aphasic disorders are called transcortical. The signs in transcortical aphasias do not conform to the simple notion of a few association areas of significance in limited speech functions interconnected by anatomically obvious fiber bundles. To explain these kinds of aphasias with the theories used in explaining more conventional fluent and non-fluent aphasias, hypothetical centers in the brain must be presumed to be disconnected from established speech centers. Transcortical aphasias assume two major forms, fluent and nonfluent.

The nonfluent transcortical aphasia is also known as transcortical motor aphasia (13). In this language disorder, the patient is often mute for tasks requiring spontaneous speech, but repetition of complicated sentences is flawless (13,25). Comprehension is good. Reading and writing are frequently normal (19). The characteristics of transcortical motor aphasia suggest that an area responsible for semantic concepts is disconnected from Broca's area (25). The patient appears to have lost access to verbal concepts not originating in the auditory area.

Transcortical sensory aphasia is the fluent alternative to transcortical motor aphasia. As in the motor aphasia, repetition is remarkably good. Paraphasias, limited comprehension, and poor naming establish it as a sensory or receptive language disorder (13). Writing and reading are severely impaired (19). Again the patient seems to have suffered a disconnection between an area for semantic concepts and the cortical speech center, in this case, Wernicke's area (25).

Just as receptive and expressive aphasias have intermediate forms sharing features of both, the transcortical aphasias have a mixed form in which repetition is excellent, comprehension is poor, naming is fair, and speech is not fluent (25). All of these transcortical aphasias most often occur after head trauma, and all usually resolve spontaneously within a few weeks after their appearance (13).

Pure Word Deafness

Pure word deafness is a language disturbance selectively involving the understanding of spoken words (4). This is also called verbal auditory agnosia (2). Patients affected by this disorder can recognize and respond to nonverbal sounds, but they respond to spoken language as if they were listening to a language they had never before heard (6). Reading, writing, and comprehension of written instructions are intact (4). This selective unresponsiveness to words causes difficulty in distinguishing between patients with this language disorder and victims of psychogenic deafness (2). These patients reinforce the impression of a psychogenic thought disorder by infrequently speaking spontaneously, while maintaining an awake and attentive appearance. Their spontaneous writing may show some impairment, but communication by written messages is usually feasible (2). The patient is aware of his deficit, and he realizes that he cannot understand his own speech when he tries to speak. Oral responses to written questions reveal that the patient's speech has become sonorous, often wailing, with the development of pure word deafness (2).

Although several different lesions have been described with this language disorder, the site probably most important in its production is the hypothetical connection between the primary cortical auditory areas and Wernicke's area (2,19,25). Auditory pathways, as well as corpus callosum connections from the right hemisphere auditory cortex, may be involved (4). The first temporal convolution of both hemispheres would presumably be damaged in a patient exhibiting pure word deafness but such a symmetrical pair of widely separated lesions is unlikely (2). Whatever its anatomic basis, pure word deafness is usually a permanent deficit once it appears (2).

Impaired Reading: Dyslexia

Disturbances in the understanding of written language appear independently of deficits in comprehension of verbal language. This is called dyslexia or alexia, and it occurs with discrete cerebral lesions or idiopathically. Both adults and children are affected by the disorder. The problem with reading may appear when efforts are first made to teach the affected child to read. Reading problems are apparent at this early age in most cases with no apparent antecedent injuries to the brain. The child will have normal speech and writing despite a pronounced reading disability. Dyslexia appearing in an adult is invariably an indication of a structural lesion in the brain. Reading and writing are also more likely to be impaired together in an adult, and the lesion responsible for the dyslexia also will produce a visual field cut. Dyslexia developing in the adult with a stroke may be transient, but dyslexia apparent in a child first learning to read is usually a more permanent problem.

A right-handed patient who abruptly loses his abilities to read and write usually has damage to the angular gyrus of the left parietal lobe (4,6). Presumably the pathways from the visual association areas in the occipital lobe to Wernicke's area in the temporal lobe are destroyed. Comprehension of written language is at least partly dependent upon translating visual symbols into auditory associations which are interpreted in Wernicke's area (6). With damage to areas connecting visual and auditory association cortex, written language cannot be deciphered although it can be perceived. In some patients, the nondominant right hemisphere may participate in reading to a slight extent by extracting semantic meaning from the overall appearance of the word, using the arrangement of lines and curves as if they were actually nonverbal symbols (6). Some patients can use this recognition technique to partly circumvent their reading disability. Its application is usually limited to reading traffic signals and street signs.

That alexia may be just a problem with phoneme recognition or auditory associations in some patients is graphically demonstrated in languages with both ideograms and phonemes as part of the written language. Japanese is one such language. Japanese patients with alexia have been described with intact reading of ideograms and dyslexic reading of phonemic writing (3). In other words, symbols with meaning apart from auditory associations can still be understood even when the comprehension of symbols encoded into letters or phonemes is lost.

Impaired Reading With and Without Impaired Writing

Complete loss of reading ability classically appears in two situations: (*1*) a structural lesion in the dominant parietal lobe, and (*2*) damage to the inferior and medial aspects of the dominant occipital lobe with involvement of the posterior part of the corpus callosum, the fiber bundle connecting the two hemispheres (5). For reading as well as speech, the dominant hemisphere is the left hemisphere in most patients. With the left parietal lobe lesion, the patient will usually have a mild right-sided visual field cut, a mild right hemiparesis, normal speech comprehension, and agraphia, a complete loss of writing ability. This is called alexia with agraphia. With a left occipital lobe lesion, the patient will have a dense right visual field loss, but intact copying and writing (4,5). This is called alexia without agraphia.

Loss of writing, or agraphia, develops with damage to the parietal cortex in the region of the angular gyrus presumably because of damage to pathways from Wernicke's area that pass to writing (graphomotor) areas in the frontal lobe. These patients can copy even though they cannot write script, and their reading difficulty extends to the recognition of individual letters (3). Problems with calculations, finger naming, right-left orientation, and recognizing parts of the body as self often accompany alexia with agraphia (3). Disturbed color naming is also common in this disorder (26). The defect is not in recalling the name of the color but, rather, in associating the name of the color with the color (26).

Pure Word Blindness

Alexia or dyslexia occurs without agraphia with a lesion in the left occipital cortex extending into the posterior part of the corpus callosum because fibers from both the left and the right occipital cortex are destroyed. This usually develops with a left posterior cerebral artery occlusion (27). Another term for this disorder is pure word blindness, the implication being that the patient cannot see the meaning in written speech, although he is certainly not blind (28). Any visual problem coincident with alexia without agraphia will generally be limited to loss of vision in the right visual field of both eyes, a so-called right homonymous hemianopia (28). Written language is perceived in the intact left visual field, but this information cannot reach the dominant hemisphere because the right occipital cortex, where it is received, is cut off from the left hemisphere by the damage to the corpus callosum. Apparently, visual responses in the right occipital lobe must be transmitted to the left hemisphere for interpretation when the visual task is reading words.

The patient can circumvent this deficit by reading the letters of each word aloud and reconstructing the word from his auditory perception of the spelling. What allows the patient to recognize and name the letter but not the word is unknown (29). It may be that the letter is a less complex stimulus for the visual association center to handle than is the full word. An even more likely explanation is that there is a defect in a visual system specifically responsible for recognizing collections of written letters as words. Other conditions in which parts of an entity can be recognized but the whole not perceived are well documented. This defect in the recognition of an aggregate of parts is called simultanagnosia, and it occurs with damage to the occipitotemporal region of the left hemisphere (29). It may be the basic problem in pure word blindness, but other phenomena associated with this alexia cannot be explained by simultanagnosia alone. Patients with pure word blindness usually have problems naming colors, reading musical notations, and reading numbers (28). Writing is preserved in these patients, presumably because there is no parietotemporal lobe damage.

Treatment of Aphasia

Aphasias do not respond to conventional speech therapy. Whether treated by retraining or not, most patients will show some recovery of normal speech. They will make the most significant gains in the language they are exposed to during the recovery phase even if that language is not the one they learned initially as a child. Setting words to music has helped some aphasic patients improve their speech recovery, but this "melodic intonation" technique has not been widely used (30).

Patients with global aphasias do the most poorly in terms of recovery of normal speech; those with anomic, conduction, and transcortical aphasias do the best (13). The severity of the aphasia when it first develops in acute conditions is fairly well correlated with the prognosis for recovery (13). Patients with severe aphasias recover poorly. The rate of recovery, though not necessarily the degree of recovery, is the fastest in expressive aphasias and conduction aphasias; the rate is slowest in global and anomic aphasias (13). Although the rate of recovery from an anomic aphasia is often very slow, the extent of recovery is usually quite substantial. Patients with anomic aphasias improve slowly, but continue to improve for many months before their deficits approach a plateau. Speech therapy does not directly affect the rate or extent of recovery, but it is still of value in the severely aphasic patient (13). The attention to the patient's speech difficulty and the reassurance that is provided by a therapist who can focus on speech assets rather than disabilities usually provide a substantial psychologic boost that can help in the recovery of other functions.

DYSARTHRIA

Dysarthria is a disorder of the clarity, speed, or rhythm of speech. Language content, grammar, and relevance are intact. Despite the varied ways in which speech can be distorted, dysarthria resulting from disease in the nervous system conforms to a few discrete patterns (31). Discounting an anatomic disorder of the larynx, pharynx, mouth, or nose, the sites of damage in the nervous system capable of producing dysarthria are myriad (12). Structural lesions are less often the basis for speech distortions than are metabolic or toxic disorders. The most familiar dysarthria is the slurred speech of alcohol intoxication (32). This is so familiar to nonmedical individuals that patients with slurred speech from any cause are routinely dismissed as drunk when they ask for help. Individuals with multiple sclerosis and lithium intoxication are at a special disadvantage because of the inebriated sound of their dysarthrias.

Recognition of the basic features of a dysarthria often suggests the site or the cause of the speech disorder. A commonly overlooked speech alteration is the decrementing speech volume associated with parkinsonism (12). The typical staccato or scanning speech of cerebellar disease is diagnostic of the site of central nervous system damage responsible for the dysarthria, and, in a specific context, it may be virtually diagnostic of the disease responsible for the cerebellar damage (32). A 20-year-old woman abruptly developing scanning speech after an earlier episode of visual loss must be presumed to have multiple sclerosis until proven otherwise (33). A 10-year-old boy with progressive gait problems and slowly evolving scanning speech is most likely to have a cerebellar tumor (32). A 60-year-old man with a long history of smoking, a pulmonary mass on chest radiogram, and abrupt onset of hoarseness may have laryngeal disease or laryngeal nerve compression by a carcinoma. The form and the setting of dysarthria provide considerable information on the possible causes of the speech disorder.

Speech characteristics rely upon interaction between several different nervous system networks (12,32,34). The frontal lobe cortex damaged in the patient with a nonfluent aphasia is near, if not in fact overlapping, cortical areas important in the programming of pharyngeal and oral movements. Consequently, a left cerebral hemisphere stroke may leave a patient with dysarthria rather than aphasia. Indeed, any stroke affecting motor pathways to the face, mouth, and pharynx is capable of producing distorted speech. The pure motor stroke so characteristic of hypertensive patients is often associated with slurred, labored speech when facial weakness is apparent. Nerve fibers from frontal motor systems are presumably interrupted in their course to the brainstem nuclei controlling articulatory muscles. Basal ganglia disease apparently interferes with speech modulation (34). With Huntington disease voice pitch may become variable (34). In parkinsonism, speech is characteristically halting, monotonous, and quiet (34). Damage to the ventrolateral nucleus of the thalamus occasionally produces a defect in the initiation of speech (12).

Dysarthria occurring with cerebellar disease is more a disorder of intonation and rhythm than articulation (35). Certainly many patients with cerebellar damage have slurred, slowed speech, but the speech alterations characteristic of cerebellar damage are disturbances of rhythm or modulation (31,32). The patient may speak in a sing-song manner, as if reading a passage of poetry while trying to decipher the rhythm in the passage. This scanning pattern of speech may appear in combination with explosive, poorly modulated speech. These disorders of speech rhythm are often referred to as ataxic dysarthrias or dysprosodic speech (32,35). Since much of the cerebellum is important in regulating muscle tone and coordinating muscle activity, it is possible that dysarthria occurs with cerebellar damage because of a delay in the generation of muscular forces (35). Although the left cerebral cortex connects primarily with the right cerebellar hemisphere, it is the left cerebellar hemisphere that is usually damaged in dysarthric patients (22,32). This implicates the right cerebral cortex in the dysarthrias occurring with cerebellar disease, if indeed any cerebral mechanisms play a role in this dysprosodic speech. Changes in intonation and rhythm of speech with right cerebral cortical lesions do occur, a finding not unexpected in a hemisphere long recognized as important in the appreciation of melodies and other musical functions (20,32,36). The right cerebral hemisphere and the left cerebellar hemisphere play discrete roles in the regulation of speech rhythm, intonation, and variability (20,32).

Metabolic causes of dysarthria produce fairly consistent speech disturbances, but the type of disordered speech may have several possible causes. A patient with monotonous, low volume speech may be on phenothiazines or have Parkinson disease or both. Slurred speech will develop with overdose of the anticonvulsant medication phenytoin, but it will also appear with alcohol intoxication, barbiturate abuse, or even uremia. Recurrent episodes of scanning speech may appear with metabolic disorders, but are more likely to be caused by multiple sclerosis (33).

With the information provided by careful examination of the character of the dysarthria, the physician can investigate the probable causes of the abnormal speech. Systemic problems, throat injuries, and brain damage are the three principal categories into which lesions causing dysarthria will fall. Psychiatric patients exhibiting the type of dysarthria appropriate for their antipsychotic medications need not be investigated unless additional neurologic signs appear along with the dysarthria. As already mentioned, patients taking lithium for several months or years or on toxic doses of the drug may develop slurred speech. Phenothiazines and butyrophenones routinely give speech a monotonous or decrementing quality. Of course a careful neurologic evaluation would be appropriate if the patient on antipsychotics developed scanning or explosive speech. This change would suggest a structural lesion in the cerebellum. Treatment of the underlying disorder will usually eliminate the dysarthria.

APRAXIA

Individuals who cannot perform a task, even though they adequately understand what task is requested, have no focal neurologic deficits interfering with the performance of the task, and may even exhibit all the movements required for performing the task, have an apraxia. Apraxias usually appear in association with expressive aphasias and may affect only one side of the body (37). The left side is more often affected than the right side when only one arm is affected by the apraxia. A typical example of an apraxia is the patient who cannot pretend to hammer a nail into a piece of wood when instructed to, but can readily perform the action when given the actual items to use. Orofacial apraxia is the most common kind of apraxia. The patient will make bizarre noises when asked to blow out an imaginary match, but the task will be accurately and effortlessly performed with the real object. Some patients cannot perform the desired action upon command even when the real objects are available, but they will exhibit their ability to perform the required action when they are not trying to follow the instruction. The patient cannot decide what to do with a key and lock when asked to open the lock with the key, but when uninstructed the patient may simply insert the key in the lock and turn it as part of an effort to gain access to a room. This type of behavior disorder is rarely confused with a psychiatric problem only because of the other neurologic deficits routinely associated with the apraxia. Most patients with this disorder are recovering from frontal lobe strokes with prominent Broca's aphasias as part of the symptomatology. A receptive aphasia cannot be present as part of the patient's problem, simply because of the way an apraxia is defined.

Most neurologists suspect that apraxias develop when Broca's area is disconnected from a motor association area responsible for organizing the intended action. The patient hears and understands the instruction in Wernicke's area and the intent to carry out the instruction is transferred to Broca's area along the arcuate fasciculus, but the patient fails to perform the action because the intended behavior cannot be relayed from Broca's area to the motor cortex. This simple view of apraxia as a disconnection of one area of the cortex from another is supported by the observed development of apraxias affecting only the left side with lesions in the corpus callosum, the thick fiber bundle connecting the two hemispheres

(37). Presumably, the intended action can be relayed from Broca's area in the left frontal lobe to the left motor cortex, but it cannot be relayed to the right motor cortex because of the lesion in the corpus callosum. The right frontal cortex, which controls movements on the left side of the body, is disconnected from language regulation systems, but is still intact. Patients with apraxias can imitate tasks if they can see them done, and some even use this technique to induce their left side to do what their right side has already done. Despite the apraxia from a corpus callosum lesion, the patient can accurately perform an action with the left hand after it has been demonstrated by the right hand.

Most apraxias are transient, but with extensive cerebral cortical damage much of the impairment may persist. Patients usually develop techniques for circumventing their apraxias if they do not have other major intellectual deficits. There is no specific treatment for an apraxia.

REFERENCES

1. Gerson SN, Benson DF, Frazier SH: Diagnosis: Schizophrenia versus posterior aphasia. *Am J Psychiatry* 134:966, 1977.
2. Shoumaker RD, Ajax ET, Schenkenberg T: Pure word deafness. *Dis Nerv Syst* 38:293, 1977.
3. Yamodori A: Ideogram reading in alexia. *Brain* 98:231, 1975.
4. Geschwind N: Neurological foundations of language, in Myklebust HR (ed): *Progress in Learning Disabilities.* New York, Grune & Stratton, 1968, vol I, p 182.
5. Benson DF: The third alexia. *Arch Neurol* 34:327, 1977.
6. Heilman KM, Roth L. Campanella D, et al: Wernicke's and global aphasia without alexia. *Arch Neurol* 36:129, 1979.
7. Gelenberg AJ: The catatonic syndrome. *Lancet* 1:1339, 1976.
8. Karpati G, Frame B: Neuropsychiatric disorders in primary hyperparathyroidism. *Arch Neurol* 10:387, 1964.
9. Woods BT, Carey S: Language deficits after apparent clinical recovery from childhood aphasia. *Ann Neurol* 6:405, 1979.
10. Geschwind N: Aphasia. *N Engl J Med* 284:654, 1971.
11. Ruff RL, Arbit E: Aphemia resulting from a left frontal hematoma. *Neurology (NY)* 31:353, 1981.
12. Botez MI, Barbeau A: Role of subcortical structures and particularly of the thalamus in the mechanisms of speech and language. *Int J Neurol* 8:300, 1971.
13. Kertesz A, McCabe P: Recovery patterns and prognosis in aphasia. *Brain* 100:1, 1977.
14. Geschwind N: Disconnexion syndrome in animals and man. *Brain* 88:237,585, 1965.
15. Broca P: Remarques sur le siège de la faculté du langage articulé, suives d'une observation d'aphemie. *Bull Soc Anat* 36:330, 1861.
16. Broca P: Deux cas d'aphemie tramatique, produite par des lésions de la troisième circonvolution frontale gauche. *Bull Soc Chir* 5:51, 1864.

17. LeDoux JE, Barclay L, Premack A: The brain and cognitive sciences. *Ann Neurol* 4:391, 1978.

18. Trojanowski JQ, Green RC, Levine ON: Crossed aphasia in a dextral. A clinicopathological study. *Neurology (NY)* 30:709, 1980.

19. Sherwin I, Geschwind N: Neural substrates of behavior, in Nicholi AM (ed): *The Harvard Guide to Modern Psychiatry*. Cambridge, Mass, Kelknap Press, 1978, p 59.

20. Ross ED, Mesulam M: Dominant language functions of the right hemisphere? Prosody and emotional gesturing. *Arch Neurol* 36:144, 1979.

21. Wernicke C: *Der Aphasiche Symptomencomplex*. Breslau, Cohn and Weigart, 1874.

22. Allen GI, Tsukahara N: Cerebrocerebellar communication systems. *Physiol Rev* 54:957, 1974.

23. Mayeux R, Brandt J, Rosen J, et al: Interictal memory and language impairment in temporal lobe epilepsy. *Neurology (NY)* 30:120, 1980.

24. Niedermeyer E, Fineyre F, Riley T, et al: Absence status (petit mal status) with focal characteristics. *Arch Neurol* 36:417, 1979.

25. Heilman KM, Tucker DM, Valenstein E: A case of mixed transcortical aphasia with intact naming. *Brain* 99:415, 1976.

26. Geschwind N, Fusillo M: Color-naming defects in association with alexia. *Arch Neurol* 15:137, 1966.

27. Benson DF, Segarra J, Albert ML: Visual agnosia-prosopagnosia. *Arch Neurol* 30:307, 1974.

28. Rubens AB, Benson DF: Associative visual agnosia. *Arch Neurol* 24:305, 1971.

29. Warrington EK, Shallice T: Word-form dyslexia. *Brain* 103:99, 1980.

30. Albert ML, Sparks RW, Helm NA: Melodic intonation therapy for aphasia. *Arch Neurol* 29:130, 1973.

31. Brown JR, Darley FL, Aronson AE: Ataxic dysarthria. *Int J Neurol* 7:302, 1970.

32. Lechtenberg R, Gilman S: Speech disorders in cerebellar disease. *Ann Neurol* 3:285, 1978.

33. McAlpine D, Lumsden CE, Acheson ED: *Multiple sclerosis. A Reappraisal*. Baltimore, Williams & Wilkins, 1972.

34. Zentay PJ: Motor disorders of the nervous system and their significance for speech. Part I. Cerebral and cerebellar dysarthrias. *Laryngoscope* 47:147, 1937.

35. Kent R, Nestell R: A case study of an ataxic dysarthria: Cineradiographic and spectrographic observations. *J Speech Hear Disord* 40:115, 1975.

36. Shankweiler D: Effects of temporal lobe lesions on recognition of dichotically presented melodies. *J Comp Physiol Psychol* 62:115, 1966.

37. Heilman KM, Coyle JM, Gonyea EF, et al: Apraxia and agraphia in a left-hander. *Brain* 96:21, 1973.

6
Cognitive Disorders

Cognitive disorders occur in a wide variety of neurologic diseases and a narrower range of psychiatric disorders. Distinguishing between intellectual disturbances resulting from organic brain disease and those caused by psychiatric disturbances is relatively simple in most cases, but subtle cases do occur with complex neurologic disorders (1). The thought disorder of acute schizophrenia may be easily distinguished from the dementia of Wernicke's encephalopathy, but the cognitive disorder associated with systemic lupus erythematosus is easily mistaken for an acute nonneurologic psychosis. Of course, the diagnostic problems are not limited to neurologic diseases imitating psychiatric disorders. Psychiatric diseases occasionally present with the signs and symptoms typical of organic brain disease. Patients with severe depression occasionally develop profound intellectual impairment (2). This usually leads to considerable delay in the treatment of the psychiatric disturbance, because a structural or physiologic basis for the cognitive disorder is sought before a psychologic etiology is considered. The affective disorder is unsuspected while the patient is investigated for the intellectual disorder simply because this cause of dementia is so unusual and more organic causes, such as Alzheimer disease and chronic subdural hematomas, are so common.

Complicating the assessment of patients with intellectual disturbances is the absence of consistent traits to identify the dementia of organic brain disease and distinguish it from the cognitive disorders of psychiatric illness. Dementia is nothing more than a deterioration in intellectual functions. The functions affected include abstraction, memory, judgment, calculations, constructional skills, and language (3). A single intellectual function or several at once may be disturbed with either a dementing process or a psychiatric illness (3). Occasionally, there are indications that the intellectual problem has a primarily psychiatric basis. For instance, patients with "dementia" secondary to a depressive psychosis have problems with abstract interpretations, but have normal scores on vocabulary tests (4). The problems with abstraction are less severe in the depressed patient than they are in schizophrenic patients, but they may be just as severe as the conceptual difficulties appearing in patients with an organic brain syndrome. An additional clue that the apparent dementia in the depressed patient is from a psychiatric problem is the paradoxical observation that as the psychotic depression deepens the patient shows improved abstract thinking (4).

Neurologic and systemic diseases that produce cognitive disorders also may produce unequivocal signs of psychosis and, therefore, be overlooked when the patient's abnormal mentation is being assessed. Systemic lupus erythematosus, a collagen vascular disease that can cause a cerebral arteritis, routinely causes acute psychotic episodes. Obviously, patients known to have systemic diseases that can cause central nervous system damage usually have their underlying problem recognized early in the course of the psychosis. This is not true in diseases which present with little more than cognitive disorders for years. A victim of a slowly progressive degenerative disease of the brain with prominent intellectual and affective problems, such as Wilson disease, may be confined to institutions and die without the organic basis for the cognitive disorder being recognized. Two to five percent of individuals with Huntington disease are admitted to psychiatric facilities with the diagnosis of schizophrenia several years before other signs of the degenerative disease appear (5). After severe head injuries, as many as 14 percent of patients will have symptoms typical of schizophrenia; this can produce considerable confusion if the patient does not recall the injury and no one else witnessed it (5). Even patients with multiple sclerosis, a disturbance of the myelin coating of nerve fibers, may develop a thought disorder associated with a flat affect.

Unequivocal signs of psychosis in the patient with no focal neurologic deficits do not guarantee that the patient is free of central nervous system damage. Typically schizophrenic individuals occasionally have structural brain diseases, such as infarction, subdural hematoma, or intracranial tumor, that may be responsible for at least part of their cognitive disorders (1). Unsuspected structural lesions are found in the brains of 5 to 10 percent of chronic psychiatric patients (1). Meningiomas, for example, occur twice as often in psychiatric patients as they do in the general population (1). In some situations these brain lesions are simply incidental findings with no relevance to the individual's mental disorder, but the real test of the importance of a brain lesion is treatment of the lesion. If the patient improves when the meningioma is removed, it is reasonable to assume that the tumor was important in the development of the psychiatric problem.

Time often limits the physician's opportunity to respond effectively to nonpsychiatric cognitive disorders. A chronic subdural hematoma may produce subtle changes in the patient until herniation and death ensue. Unrecognized drug-related dementias may lead to inappropriate evaluation and treatment of patients. Benzodiazepenes, such as diazepam (Valium), may cause confusion, forgetfulness, and gait difficulty, especially in the elderly (6). Amphetamine abuse produces a psychosis with paranoid delusions and repetitive, compulsive movements, which is easily misdiagnosed as schizophrenia when no drug history is available (7). The early recognition of the structural or physiologic basis for a thought disorder is vital if the deficits that may develop are to be limited or reversed. Because there is no simple formula for distinguishing between functional psychoses and organic cerebral disease, both must be considered in any patient with an acute or chronic cognitive disorder (8).

A potentially reversible basis for the cognitive disorder can be found in at least 15 percent of the patients with organic dementias, and therapeutic intervention of some sort is feasible in over 25 percent of these patients (8). In elderly patients an organic basis for an acute psychosis is more likely to be suspected and sought than in younger people. "Delirium" is the organic psychosis most often found in the elderly (8). This old and somewhat vague term is generally used to denote a reversible thought disorder that produces agitated behavior and hallucinations or withdrawn behavior with inattention and little response to the environment (Table 6.1). Twenty to 30 percent of hospitalized patients experience delirium to some extent at some time during their hospitalization (9). The affected individual is disoriented and has markedly impaired judgment (10). He often appears stuporous and has problems focusing his attention on environmental stimuli. Speech is often incoherent or rambling (10). There is a fairly global, but markedly variable, disturbance of intellectual function (9). Although the patient often has no recall of the period during which he was delirious, the entire episode is occasionally recalled as a chaotic dream or nightmare (11). An electroencephalogram obtained during the delirium will be abnormal even though no structural or infectious brain disease is usually found (12).

Delirium is usually caused by a transient metabolic encephalopathy (10). The variability in the appearance of this disorder is related to the variety

Table 6.1. Characteristics of Delirium

Transient cognitive disorder
Impaired consciousness
Fluctuating signs and symptoms
Inattention
Disorientation
Impaired memory
Delusions or hallucinations
Incoherent speech
Excessive or reduced psychomotor activity
Disturbed sleep-wake cycle

of problems that can cause this transient alteration in cognitive function. Impaired renal function, abnormal liver function, and insufficient pulmonary function can all precipitate delirium in a vulnerable individual. Underlying structural brain disease, such as damage from an old stroke, makes the patient more susceptible to episodes of delirium. Whatever form this altered cognition assumes, a toxic reaction to medication, a mass lesion in the skull, or an occult infection in the central nervous system must be considered. Elderly patients may develop delirium as a response to dramatic changes in their environment coinciding with the acute stress of a systemic illness. Whenever delirium occurs, it interferes with efforts to determine whether or not the patient has an irreversible dementia.

Dementia may appear together with movement disorders, sensory abnormalities, gait problems, auditory hallucinations, or other signs and symptoms of nervous system damage. The progressive dementias of Huntington disease and Parkinson disease are usually overshadowed by the movement disorders appearing in these syndromes. Multi-infarct dementia rarely appears as an isolated problem; there are usually significant motor or sensory deficits associated with the intellectual deficits. Patients with epilepsy may have transient cognitive disorders at or immediately after an epileptic fit. The seizure preceding the postictal confusion generally clarifies the basis for the cognitive disorder even when the postictal signs persist for more than one day. These disorders, which produce dementia as an incidental or minor phenomenon, will be discussed in the chapters that deal with their most prominent signs and symptoms.

LIMITED COGNITIVE DISORDERS

MEMORY DISTURBANCES: AMNESIA

Memory may be fairly selectively disturbed in patients with well-circumscribed neurologic dysfunctions. The memory deficit may be transient or permanent, and the type of memory disturbed may be immediate, recent, or remote. Immediate memory involves little more than the registration and repetition of information, such as the recall of a list of numbers within a few seconds of hearing the list. Remote memory deals with information more or less permanently stored from past experience. Recent or short-term memory involves registering and retaining information for hours, days, or weeks. Short-term memory generally requires a minimum of distracting material between the presentation of the information and its recall (13). This type of memory deteriorates rapidly and has a small capacity. For immediate recall, the capacity of the system is usually limited to seven or eight unrelated items (13). There is no apparent limit to the capacity of long-term memory and the items held in long-term memory are less vulnerable to decay (13). Obviously, the boundaries between these types of memory are not distinct, and the patterns of memory disturbances in a number of disorders reflect the arbitrary character of these functional distinctions. Amnesia is a disturbance of some type of memory; and, because there are different types of memory, there are necessarily different types of amnesia. Whether long-term or short-term memory is impaired, the amnesia may be transient or permanent. Even the distinction between transient and permanent amnesia is arbitrary. What appears to be a permanent memory loss after 1 week of impairment may prove to be a transient loss after 1 month of observation.

Problems with immediate recall are often related to inattention, rather than defective memory. To recall an item, the individual must register the information, an activity which is little more than attention. Inattention often appears with metabolic encephalopathy, but if structural brain damage is responsible, the lesion will most often be found in the right parietal lobe.

Systemic diseases, as well as focal brain disease, can cause transient amnesia (Table 6.2). With infectious diseases, including bacterial pneumonia, typhoid fever, and other conditions causing sepsis, the patient may have a well-defined period of memory loss coincident with a period of altered consciousness induced by the overwhelming infection (14). Problems with memory commonly wax and wane in concert with the metabolic disturbances in hepatic and renal failure. Hypoglycemia can induce a transient memory disturbance, which is often associated with abnormal behavior (14). More local disturbances, such as complicated migraine, will

Table 6.2. Causes of Transient Memory Loss

Fugue states
Epilepsy
Head trauma
Alcoholic blackouts
Transient ischemic attacks
Complicated migraine
Metabolic encephalopathy
Sepsis
Meningoencephalitis
Hypoglycemia
Electroconvulsive Therapy
Cerebral arteritis
Meningeal Carcinomatosis
Basilar impression
Neurosyphillis

occasionally disturb memory function for 1 to 4 hours (14). Presumably ischemia produces these well-defined episodes of amnesia in complicated migraine as well as in other diseases of cerebral blood vessels, such as systemic lupus erythematosus and thromboangiitis obliterans (14).

Posttraumatic Amnesia

Transient amnesia is likely after head trauma or seizure activity. With head trauma, immediate recall is least affected and recent or remote memory is variably affected (15). This memory disturbance involves more than just the transient disorientation that typically occurs with even relatively mild head trauma (11). With substantial head trauma, the victim is usually amnesic for the trauma, some minutes or hours immediately following the trauma, and some minutes or hours immediately preceding the trauma (16). The retrograde amnesia, that is, the loss of information acquired before the trauma, usually clears as the patient recovers from the head injury over the course of days or weeks. The recovery of memory and other intellectual functions is, of course, dependent upon the site of the injury, the severity of the injury, the age of the patient, and the complexity of the functions tested (15).

Posttraumatic amnesia occurs because the patient fails to continuously record events happening about the time of the head injury. The duration of the posttraumatic amnesia is defined as the interval between the injury and the reappearance of consistent recall of day-to-day events (16). Because it is closely tied to many other cognitive functions, the duration of the posttraumatic amnesia is a useful indicator of the severity of the damage incurred by the brain during the injury. The duration of the amnesia is inversely related to the prognosis (17). Patients with protracted posttraumatic amnesia have more problems with intellectual function when their condition has stabilized, whether that requires several weeks or several months (16). Even the age of the patient at the time of severe head trauma is less important in predicting the long-term intellectual recovery than is the duration of the posttraumatic amnesia (16).

Selected areas of damage in the brain will produce specific memory defects. Bilateral temporal lobe lesions usually produce defects in short-term memory (18). The age of the patient plays an especially important role in the severity of the memory problem exhibited by patients with these focal lesions. Severe temporal lobe contusions will produce more apparent memory defects in an elderly patient than in a child. The course of recovery may be deceptive, especially in older individuals. Intellectual functions showing initial improvements may later deteriorate (15). The decline may not be apparent for months or years after the injury. Of course, with any dementia appearing weeks or months after the injury, chronic subdural hematomas must be suspected (19).

Seizures occasionally occur at the time of a severe head injury or within hours of the injury. These posttraumatic seizures complicate the memory disturbance ordinarily suffered with head trauma. After a seizure, patients are generally amnesic for activities performed during the seizure, even if fairly complex automatic behavior occurred (14). The patient is also likely to deny recall of coherent purposeful activity he was engaged in immediately before the seizure. Prolonged seizure activity associated with ambulatory behavior for which the patient has no recall is exceedingly rare (20). This is discussed in greater detail in the section on postictal confusion. Postictal confusion and memory disturbances are often difficult to distinguish from transient global amnesia, a temporary disturbance of recent memory ascribed to poor blood flow to temporal lobe structures.

Metabolic, Degenerative, and Structural Causes of Amnesia

More complex memory disturbances appear with metabolic, degenerative, and other nontraumatic lesions of the brain (21). A profoundly low serum sodium or calcium concentration impairs recent memory, but concentration and orientation are usually affected along with memory (22). Affective changes are usually more prominent in such electrolyte disorders. As discussed in detail below, thiamine deficiency disturbs recent memory more than remote memory, but remote memory may also be impaired, the deficits being less apparent as the patient is questioned on more remote items. Events occurring before the thiamine deficiency produces a memory disorder are recalled more accurately than those occurring after the patient develops an amnesic syndrome (13). Immediate recall may be fairly good if the patient with thiamine deficiency is attentive, but the patient has obvious problems with organization and more long-term recall of material (13).

Defects of remote memory are also likely to develop in association with other cognitive disorders. In Alzheimer disease, patients characteristically have their major problems with recall when the information requested involves remote memory (18). Patients with postencephalitic dementias may have a problem with retention of new information that is profound in comparison to that exhibited by the more strictly amnesic victims of Korsakoff syndrome (13). Tumors producing memory disorders as a major feature are usually in the deep gray matter of the diencephalon or the frontal lobe (14). Strokes do not usually disturb memory selectively, but vascular accidents involving the vessels supplying the hippocampal structures of the temporal lobes may produce permanent memory deficits (14). The defects with these vascular lesions usually appear in the patient's immediate recall and his ability to acquire new information and skills (14). Surgical or traumatic damage to structures on the inner face of the temporal lobe will impair retention of new information and generally induces some retrograde amnesia (14). Surgical destruction of the anterior thalamic nuclei, a stereotactic procedure commonly used in the past to treat Parkinson disease, also occasionally produces severe memory disorders (14).

Psychogenic Amnesia

Some individuals without apparent neurologic disease suffer profound memory disorders. When there is considerable gain for the patient in forgetting what he has done or even who he is, a psychiatric problem or attempted deception must be considered. Distinguishing between a psychotic memory disorder and a contrived amnesia may be extremely difficult.

In those amnesic states seen with the psychiatric confusional states called fugues, the patient wanders away from his customary environment, at all times exhibiting behavior rational enough upon cursory inspection to limit suspicion in casual observers. Clouding of consciousness is slight, if at all present, during the hours or days involved in the fugue (23). If the wandering individual is asked for a statement of who he is, he is likely to give a false identity, and all sense of true personal identity seems to be lost (23). Most characteristic of the fugue is that the patient seems unaware of this loss of identity (23). At the end of the fugue, the patient usually denies recall of any events occurring during the period of apparently altered consciousness and resumes his prior identity. That identity is exactly the same as the identity exhibited by the patient before the fugue (23). Even more dramatic is the patient who resumes normal mentation at the end of the fugue but denies recall of all prior life events. This patient is aware of his loss of personal identity, but exhibits no other cognitive disorders and no problems with acquiring and retaining new information. This type of fugue provides the victim with an opportunity to start his life afresh with no recall of or responsibility for prior events.

Individuals most likely to profit from fugues are precisely those who most often have them: patients chronically depressed over what they see as unalterable situations develop fugues with inordinate frequency (23). The fugue allows an escape from the intolerable situation. An exacerbation of the chronic depression is often the acute setting for the fugue. The forgotten material is usually painful, shameful, or guilt-provoking; and, even though the patient claims no recall of the unpleasant material, his behavior and dreams are affected by the unacknowledged events (24).

A history of suicide attempts is common in these fugue victims, but the suicide attempts never occur during the fugue (23). Although half of the patients develop the amnesic fugue state after head trauma, the trauma itself only serves as a catalyst. An acute profound amnesia, with or without an accompanying fugue, is likely to appear in the chronically depressed patient when an especially traumatic event heightens his chronic anxiety level (23). Multiple personalities is a somewhat more complex functional amnesic system that patients adopt as an alternative to suicidal gestures (24). The shallowness of the amnesia is apparent with amobarbital narcosis, during which the patient recalls events before the fugue without difficulty. Hypnosis may help the patient recall many of the items that were forgotten or repressed (23).

Psychomotor epilepsy (complex partial seizures) is often suspected by both psychiatrists and neurologists when a patient is found wandering aimlessly and denies recall of recent events. These fugue-like states actually occur quite rarely in patients with psychomotor seizures, but they certainly do occur. Whether they are prolonged postictal automatisms or dissociative phenomena associated with depression is controversial (20). The rarity of this fugue-like state in epileptic patients and the high incidence of depression in those exhibiting the behavior suggests that this wandering state is, in fact, a fugue with the same psychiatric basis as the fugue exhibited by nonepileptic individuals. The rare fugue-like wandering that does occur as an authentic manifestation of an epileptic condition need not be secondary to psychomotor (complex partial) seizures alone. Other types of epilepsy exhibit fugues, but with subtle features usually simplifying the recognition of the confusional episode as an epileptic phenomenon. Epileptic individuals with aimless wandering during a nonconvulsive generalized status epilepticus (petit mal status) will be able to recall their purposeless behavior when the seizure ends; this feature alone is enough to distinguish them from patients with true fugues (20). The important element appearing in the patient with wandering and complex partial seizures is the amnesia, but the amnesia is not necessarily from the seizure activity. Patients with well-documented psychomotor (complex partial) status epilepticus as a rule do not exhibit aimless wandering (20).

Transient Global Amnesia

The acute onset of a selective impairment in the ability to form new memories develops in very few neurologic disorders. When that acute memory disturbance resolves in a matter of hours, it is called transient global amnesia, and it is usually from cerebrovascular disease. Memory impairment is difficult to assess in a patient feigning forgetfulness or refusing to cooperate, but the setting of the transient memory disorder may be helpful in assessing its authenticity. Most affected individuals are elderly, that is, over 60 years of age, and most have only one or two episodes of transient amnesia ever (25,26).

Men are affected more often than women. The attack will last hours, and memory will return intact after resolution of the transient global amnesia. The memory impairment is characteristically limited to short-term memory, with old memories left unimpaired and immediate recall retained (27). Digit span is normal during the attack, but retention of new information is reduced to minutes. The patient characteristically asks the same questions repeatedly. There are usually no other signs of neurologic disease, and, during the attack, the patient will be able to function in routine activities, such as driving a car, copying figures, and dressing himself. The patient will not be aware of any problem with his memory; and, when the attack subsides, he will not recall events occurring during the transient amnesia. In fact, he may be amnesic, at least transiently, for the few hours preceding the attack (26). Transient global amnesia may last up to 24 hours, but it rarely persists more than 3 or 4 hours (26). Once the memory disorder starts to clear, it generally resolves completely within minutes. Objective tests of verbal performance involving long-term memory may show some permanent deficiencies, but memory function will otherwise be as good as before the episode once the amnesia resolves (28).

There is little that can be done during the attack to objectively assess it. An electroencephalogram may show bilateral slow wave and sharp wave activity over the temporal lobes (25). This paroxysmal activity suggests an epileptic basis for the global amnesia, but most investigators believe that ischemia of the hippocampal areas of the temporal lobe or of the mammillary bodies in the hypothalamus is responsible for the transient cognitive disorder (25). Obviously, transient global amnesia can occur with seizure activity, but in that context the memory disorder is likely to be associated with other signs or symptoms of an epileptic problem, such as incontinence, tonic-clonic movements, or an aura preceding the amnesia. Usually there is no antecedent illness to point to as responsible for the transient amnesia although essential hypertension is fairly common in affected individuals (26).

Patients experiencing this dysfunction exhibit no psychiatric abnormalities except for an appropriate level of apprehension and anxiety (26). A history of psychiatric illness is a distinctly uncommon feature in transient global amnesia. Factitious transient global amnesia is difficult to distinguish from the neurologic disorder simply because there are so few objective features characterizing the authentic memory disorder. Any obvious advantages for the patient in claiming amnesia should call the diagnosis of transient global amnesia into question. An isolated defect in memory should be viewed skeptically, especially in a young person with no prior history of typical seizure activity or essential hypertension.

More enduring memory impairment will result from encephalitis of viral and other origins, as well as from meningeal carcinomatosis, the dissemination of cancer cells in the subarachnoid space (29,30). If inflammatory changes in the brain are largely limited to the structures classically included in the limbic lobe, the encephalitis is called limbic encephalitis. Memory impairment routinely occurs in limbic encephalitis, the memory disorder resembling that occurring with transient global amnesia. Specifically, short-term memory will be defective with good remote memory and occasionally intact immediate recall (29). Unlike the amnesia in transient global amnesia, the memory problem developing with this limbic encephalitis is likely to last months or years if the patient survives (29). Consistent with the presumed site of vascular disease in transient global amnesia, the brain areas damaged in patients with limbic encephalitis include the hippocampus and mammillary bodies (29). The electroencephalogram in these patients also shows paroxysmal temporal abnormalities.

Patients with extensive bilateral hippocampal damage, an extremely unlikely lesion, do have selective deficits in recent memory, another observation supporting the importance of these temporal lobe structures in short-term memory problems. The hippocampus seems to be primarily implicated in short-term memory storage (31). Bilateral hippocampal damage will be associated with permanent short-term memory impairment.

Transient global amnesia is necessarily a retrospective diagnosis. A variety of permanent memory disorders may appear acutely and only their duration distinguishes them from transient amnesia. The permanent amnesic disorder of Korsakoff syndrome usually produces the same kind of memory dysfunction as transient global amnesia (30). Short-term or recent memory is also the facet of memory most sensitive to electroconvulsive treatment (25), and so transient amnesia may confuse the treatment of a patient with an affective disorder. The appearance of the memory defect may arouse concern that the affective problem is actually developing from a progressive neurologic disease, but the course of the patient's signs and symptoms will clarify the basis for the memory disturbance. As already noted in the section on syncope, the skeletal malformation at the base of the skull called basilar impression may produce transient episodes of amnesia associated with syncope which last as along as a week (32). Other neurologic signs, such as blindness or hemiparesis, make confusing basilar impression with transient global amnesia unlikely. There is no treatment for transient global amnesia; but, as with any disorder presumed to reflect transient ischemia to the brain, predisposing conditions, such as valvular heart disease and hypercoagulable states, must be sought.

Confabulation

Confabulation is a sign of neurologic disease rather than a syndrome by itself. Interpreting a patient's false statements as confabulation presumes he is not willfully lying or feigning confusion. The authentic confabulator cannot restrain himself from answering a question even if he does not know the answer (33). He does not monitor his answer and fails to correct himself, even when he has made an obvious mistake. Confabulation is not necessarily related to suggestibility, disorientation, or even the degree of memory disorder, but memory impairment and confabulation are in some ways related (33). Severe confabulators have grossly impaired recent memory, but they generally have good long-term memory (33). These patients seem to be aware of when an answer to a question is not required, and they will not answer when asked such rhetorical questions. They confabulate when they are obliged to provide some information, and they characteristically do not hesitate in answering the questions and make no effort to correct their totally false answers. Patients with mild degrees of confabulation will usually confabulate only on questions involving recent memory, and even then they are likely to hesitate before supplying the contrived answer and may correct themselves. The mild confabulators seem more able to draw on environmental cues in composing their answers. Whether the degree of confabulation is mild or severe, the confabulators use entrenched memory items, facts and issues of longstanding importance (33). These items seem more important than conflicting information provided by the examiner and the environment.

What induces some patients to confabulate is unknown. It is not strictly a result of a memory disorder, since many patients with severe amnesia never confabulate (34). Patients with extensive frontal lobe damage are more likely to have "fantastic" confabulation than "momentary" confabulation (34). Fantastic confabulation involves the elaboration of false memories which direct the patient's remarks and behavior as if they were accurate (34). With momentary or "embarrassment" confabulation, the patient fabricates past events by expanding upon fragmentary memories. The events reported in this type of confabulation may be accurate but misplaced in time or location (34). Immediate recall may be quite good in these patients. Recent memory is the function that is usually most defective (34). What role the frontal lobe plays in inducing confabulation when it is defective is unknown.

The line between confabulation and delusion is a fine one. Patients with posttraumatic confusion occasionally exhibit complex delusions in which they will reconstruct a detailed history of their lives over the course of several years that is totally fictitious. One especially provocative form of this delusion-centered confabulation is the situation in which the patient has an unshakable belief that the people closest to him are impostors (11). The paranoid delusion and the history the patient provides to defend his conviction are called Capgras syndrome, and it most often appears in paranoid schizophrenics (11). This is not a problem with recognition; the patient readily identifies the faces associated with relatives and friends, but he insists that those posing as relatives and friends have switched places with the real individuals. Assertions that he witnessed the massacre or kidnapping of his family will be offered by the patient to bolster his claim that the people he is dealing with cannot be the people they claim to be even though they are identical in every detail with the individuals they claim to be. This delusional system can appear after head trauma. It is presumed to reflect frontal and parietotemporal damage (11). Gradual resolution of the cognitive disorder may occur.

The most common setting for confabulation is the Korsakoff psychosis of Wernicke-Korsakoff syndrome. Neither frontal lobe nor parietotemporal lobe damage are responsible for the confabulation in this disorder.

Presumably, this means that confabulation can appear with damage to at least two different areas in the brain. Confabulated perceptions, such as those in Anton syndrome of cortical blindness, indicate that confabulation may occur even with restricted deficits in nonverbal systems (25). Again the separation between delusions and confabulations becomes very imprecise when patients with sensory problems are considered.

Wernicke-Korsakoff Syndrome

Memory may be fairly selectively impaired in alcoholism-related thiamine deficiency (25). When impaired recent memory is the most prominent or only apparent neurologic problem, the patient is said to have a Korsakoff psychosis or syndrome. These are misleading names since the memory disturbance is in no sense a psychosis and is more a symptom than a syndrome. Actually, Korsakoff psychosis is just a limited expression of the more diffuse and often lethal encephalopathy called Wernicke disease, which is generally caused by thiamine deficiency. Patients surviving Wernicke encephalopathy have memory impairment in about 60 percent of cases. Those with memory disorders have persistent confabulation in three out of four cases (14). The combination of focal neurologic signs, such as gait difficulty and eye movement abnormalities, with a confabulatory memory disorder is called the Wernicke-Korsakoff syndrome. Alcoholism is the usual setting for the signs and symptoms of Wernicke-Korsakoff syndrome, but they occasionally develop with vascular disease and may even appear transiently after head trauma (25).

This amnesic syndrome is distinct from acute alcoholic "blackouts" in which the intoxicated patient does not register events occurring while he is inebriated. The amnesia reported by the individual who has had a blackout will include the entire period of acute intoxication and may even extend to just before this. This type of transient amnesia is reported by 64 percent of alcoholics and is not associated with any persistent neurologic or psychiatric defects (14). It occurs more often after drinking spirits than after wine. Wernicke-Korsakoff syndrome may develop in patients with alcoholic blackouts, but the blackouts are not an indication that the patient is at high risk of developing Wernicke disease.

In its most uncomplicated form, Korsakoff psychosis is characterized by defective recent memory with relatively good immediate recall and remote memory (Table 6.3). Intact immediate recall in these patients is helpful in distinguishing them from hysterics; patients with hysterical amnesia occasionally recall recent and remote events but fail to register new information (35). The patient with Korsakoff psychosis cannot retain new information for more than a few minutes, and, although remote memory is generally good, there is invariably a gap in memory for events extending back months or years before the appearance of the amnesic syndrome (36). With cues to help with recall, the victim of Korsakoff syndrome will

Table 6.3. Causes of Korsakoff Psychosis

Wernicke disease (thiamine deficiency)
Third ventricle tumors
Herpes simplex encephalitis
Anoxic encephalopathy
Alzheimer disease
Temporal lobe contusion, infarction, or resection

perform better on memory tasks (36). The patient often confabulates to fill gaps in his memory, and he exhibits no insight into his deficit (14). New tasks cannot be learned but there is good retention of tasks learned early in life (37). There is invariably some loss of memory for events and skills acquired before the onset of the syndrome; this retrograde amnesia is more substantial than that likely with head trauma or a seizure disorder (35). Although other cognitive functions are largely intact, there may be some impairment of concentration, spatial organization, and visual abstraction (35). Problem solving is usually intact, and aphasia is never an aspect of this disorder in the adult. Naming and vocabulary are generally not affected. Children developing Korsakoff syndrome are often aphasic, as well as amnesic. Presumably, speech in this age group is a recently learned skill (37).

More extensive damage with thiamine deficiency results in classical Wernicke disease or encephalopathy. The three major features of this nutritional disorder are dementia, usually in the form of Korsakoff psychosis, ocular motor abnormalities, usually manifest as nystagmus, and gait difficulty, usually limited to a staggering gait (36). An internuclear ophthalmoplegia (median longitudinal fasciculus syndrome), a complex abnormality of eye coordination, is common, and disturbed conjugate gaze may appear (35). These patients rarely have tremors or slurred speech, but they usually have signs of peripheral nerve disease. Other signs of cognitive dysfunction besides the Korsakoff psychosis include agitation and hallucinations, especially when a steady intake of alcohol is stopped. Global confusion, apathy, inattention, and drowsiness are also common features of Wernicke encephalopathy (35,36).

Attention and the appropriateness of answers and remarks usually improve dramatically when the patient is given intravenous thiamine. Without thiamine, the course of the illness is rapid. Neurologic signs evolve over the course of hours, and the patient may die within a few days. Mortality is 17 percent in the acute phase of the disorder. If the patient survives, he usually has persistent gait difficulty. The ocular motor difficulty will improve much more rapidly than any limb incoordination that has evolved. Recovery from the Korsakoff psychosis is seen in only 20 percent of patients (35,36). When this recovery does occur, it is slow and usually only after a delay of months.

Lesions found in patients with Wernicke encephalopathy include hemorrhagic necrosis of the periaqueductal gray matter, the mammillary bodies, and other hypothalamic structures. The Korsakoff psychosis is probably from damage to subcortical gray matter structures in the diencephalon, specifically the medial dorsal nuclei of the thalamus and the mammillary bodies of the hypothalamus (13,35). The thalamic changes associated with Korsakoff psychosis are actually less constant than the mammillary body damage, and the mammillary body changes alone may be responsible for the memory disorder (36). Presumably, the mammillary bodies provide structures, classically considered part of the limbic lobe, access to the cerebral cortex (36). In the fully developed Wernicke-Korsakoff syndrome, cerebellar damage is likely, and all of the neuronal elements in the superior vermis are especially vulnerable (35). With more diffuse intellectual deterioration, there is widespread evidence of degeneration in the cerebral hemispheres (36). An increase in the number of astrocytes in the cerebrum will be an early sign of this degeneration.

GERSTMANN SYNDROME

Patients with cerebral lesions damaging the dominant parietal hemisphere may have a collection of selected cognitive problems referred to as the Gerstmann syndrome. The principal features include right-left confusion, problems with finger identification (finger agnosia), impaired arithmetic abilities (dyscalculia), and impaired writing ability (agraphia) (25,38). Patients may also have difficulty with their ability to construct or draw, but this is less specific for a dominant hemisphere lesion. These deficits most often develop with infarction of the left parietal lobe. The optic radiation responsible for vision in the right visual field courses through the white matter of this lobe on its way to the occipital lobe. Unless the parietal cortex alone is damaged, a right visual field cut will occur along with the cognitive disorders. With such a field cut, the structural basis for the cognitive disorder is obvious. The optic radiation for the right inferior visual quadrant is most often affected.

Speech may be normal in patients with the Gerstmann syndrome, but they, in fact, usually have a conduction or receptive aphasia (39). That the four main features of the Gerstmann syndrome preferentially cluster together with lesions in the dominant parietal lobe is an oversimplification. Each of the cognitive defects may occur alone or together with a field cut, language disturbance, reading impairment, constructional apraxia, impaired visual recognition, or a pervasive dementia (39). In fact, the problem with right-left confusion, one of the major features of the syndrome, may be just part of a receptive aphasia and not represent a distinctive intellectual deficit (39). The finger agnosia is part of a defect in recognition of body parts or of their relation to each other (39). With specialized tests, a defect in word finding or maze learning may be detected with limited parietal lobe lesions, whether they be dominant or nondominant. This limited cognitive defect is called topographagnosia (25).

Selected cognitive defects of the sort that occur with parietal lobe damage arouse suspicion that the patient has a strictly psychologic problem. The family and physician dealing with the patient ascribe this neurologic disorder to a psychiatric basis simply because the patient appears so intact. The defects are severe for restricted functions and intact for other functions. Despite the family's insistence that this problem appeared in the setting of severe emotional stress, the physician responsible for the patient must look for structural lesions in the parietal area. The deficits may be reversible if the cause of the damage is reversible. A low grade encephalitis can cause these signs transiently in individuals without structural brain disease. Slow evolution of these limited cognitive defects occurs with expanding brain tumors and arteriovenous malformations. Most patients developing the Gerstmann syndrome abruptly have suffered a stroke. Occasionally, head trauma will produce a cerebral contusion in the dominant parietal lobe and precipitate these signs. Treatment of the syndrome is dictated by the kind of lesion responsible for the syndrome.

DENIAL OF ILLNESS

Some patients with structural brain damage deny that they have any disabilities even when the most cursory examination will reveal profound deficits in strength, sensation, or coordination. This denial of illness or handicap occasionally develops on a purely psychiatric basis, but an exaggerated version of this denial occurs with nondominant (right) hemisphere damage. When the denial has a strictly neurologic basis, it is called anosognosia. Parietal lobe damage most commonly produces anosognosia (11). What compels the patient to deny that he has a problem or even to acknowledge that a disabled limb belongs to him is unknown.

Anosognosia is usually associated with paralysis of the left side of the body simply because the lesions responsible for the denial syndrome are usually large. A massive nondominant hemisphere stroke is the most common setting for the disorder. Intracerebral hemorrhages and extensive parietal lobe tumors can also produce anosognosia. Regardless of how profound the paralysis or sensory deficit accompanying the anosognosia, the patient will refuse to recognize any changes in his ability to function normally. Elaborate explanations may be developed to explain the failure of a limb to perform a routine action. The patient may even dismiss the examiner's requests by claiming that he performed the desired movement in the recent past and was simply refusing to repeat it. The denial of motor and sensory disability is often associated with a disturbed perception of the self. On asking a patient if his left arm is the paralyzed one held by the physician, the examiner is likely to be told that it is not. Alternatively, the patient may complain that one arm or leg is shorter than the other or even that an extra limb has been added to his body (40). Paranoid delusions occasionally accompany the disturbance of self-image (11).

At least part of this denial syndrome involves neglect of all elements in the half of the environment contralateral to the injured hemisphere (41). Even if the intact limbs are used, movements are more slowed and awkward when the patient attempts to do something in the neglected half of the environment. Clothes will be carelessly draped over the left side, or the arm and leg will be simply omitted from garments. The patient does not react to stimuli in the neglected space as quickly as he will to stimuli in the normal space even if the stimulus is as nonspecific as a loud noise (41).

Denial of illness causes special problems, whether the underlying lesion is a stroke, tumor, vascular malformation, or brain abscess. Rehabilitation is difficult because the patient is not attentive enough to his deficits to compensate for them. Other cognitive functions may remain relatively intact, but, more commonly, the patient also exhibits problems with constructions (25). These right-handed individuals develop substantial deficits in drawing and figure completion while exhibiting no difficulty with writing or calculation. Recovery of these cognitive functions will depend upon the nature of the lesion causing the right parietal lobe damage. A stroke will usually produce permanent, disabling deficits. A brain abscess may cause transient deficits that clear with evacuation of the pus.

ACUTE DIFFUSE COGNITIVE DISORDERS

POSTTRAUMATIC DEMENTIA

Cerebral Concussion and Contusion

Head trauma often produces transient or persistent cognitive disorders. Amnesia for the head injury and even retrograde amnesia for the minutes or hours preceding the head trauma are common and upsetting for the patient, but they do not indicate significant brain damage. When the patient has no persistent signs of cerebral damage, he is said to have had a concussion. This assumes that no structural damage was done to the brain, and so there should be no late effects of the head trauma. In a contusion, the brain is damaged, often with apparent bleeding into the cerebrum or subarachnoid space. Contusions generally produce more lasting deficits and may cause seizures as late sequelae of the head injury.

Motor vehicle accidents account for most of the head injuries in the United States; and, consequently, the sites of contusion most often encountered are the frontal and temporal lobes. These suffer preferentially with the abrupt deceleration on impact when the head hits the windshield or other unyielding element of the car. The resulting hemorrhage and edema may be so massive that only resection of these injured lobes will prevent fatal herniation of the brain.

The type of cognitive disorder that will appear with a concussion or contusion will depend upon the part of the brain most traumatized. A receptive aphasia will develop with damage to the dominant temporal lobe. A blunted affect with loss of initiative might appear with frontal lobe damage (42). Cognitive deficits will usually resolve in minutes or hours with a concussion, but they routinely progress for hours or resolve slowly over the course of weeks or months with a contusion. A rapidly progressing cognitive disorder after a severe contusion is a worrisome sign and necessitates aggressive investigation and management. This may mean resection of the damaged lobes. If the head trauma involves a penetrating injury to the brain, cognitive or affective disorders usually develop even if no brain tissue is resected. Aggressive and criminal behavior is seen with an unexpectedly high frequency after penetrating injury of the frontal lobes (43). Intellectual disturbances are most likely with lesions in the left parietal and temporal lobes (43). As expected, the severity of the injury and the cognitive dysfunction are closely related (16).

Transient changes in behavior and intellectual function are so common after relatively minor head trauma that they are often considered a syndrome, aptly called the postconcussion syndrome. This syndrome is characterized by poor concentration, easy intellectual and physical fatigue, irritability, pervasive anxiety, hypersensitivity to noise, intractable headache, and dizziness (42). These signs often last weeks or months after the accident and occasionally worsen during the first few weeks after the concussion. The prolonged disability associated with these relatively minor neurologic signs prompted some psychiatrists to call this a traumatic neurosis (42). Implicit in this term is the assumption that organic brain disease is not a factor in the patient's behavior, and that is probably an unfair assumption. It is true that the duration of disability related to the concussion is often shortest in those patients suffering the most severe concussions, but this does not prove that patients with mild concussions are malingering (42). What it does suggest is that victims of concussions exhibit behavior after the injury not typically found in patients suffering minor injuries to other parts of the body. Obviously, social factors may be playing a role in this curious pattern of increased disability with minor head trauma, but it is also possible that a protracted convalescence is a nervous system reflex to relatively minor trauma. More serious trauma may activate other reflexes that increase the rate of recovery.

Acute Subdural and Epidural Hematomas

A rapidly progressive dementia following head trauma is invariably a serious sign and often indicates that there is a blood clot overlying the brain. If the clot forms between the dura mater and the arachnoid layers of the meninges, it is called subdural. If it develops outside the dura mater, between that fibrous tissue and the skull, it is called epidural. Epidural hematomas usually progress rapidly and develop only after severe head trauma. Mild confusion and disorientation may be followed by coma within minutes or hours. This is an especially common lesion when a fracture of the parietal bone crosses the groove of the middle meningeal artery. The rapidly enlarging clot overlying the frontal lobe may initially induce misleading changes in personality, such as irritability or combativeness. The subsequent impairment in consciousness may be misconstrued as bizarre behavior, rather than coma. Epidural hematomas always require emergency surgical removal. The diagnosis is readily made with computed tomography or arteriography.

Subdural hematomas may develop more slowly than epidural hematomas, but they are often just as lethal. Eleven percent of all patients admitted in coma after severe head injuries have subdural hematomas, and mortality with this lesion when the patient is already comatose when first seen is 60 to 90 percent (44,45). All subdural hematomas are not necessarily caused by head trauma. Patients on hemodialysis may develop subdurals with no head trauma and the elderly may develop them with remarkably minor head trauma. Fluid shifts and anticoagulant treatment for dialysis probably cause the subdurals seen in hemodialysis patients. A fragile vascular system and increased occurrence of accidents probably contribute to the development of these hematomas in the elderly. These atraumatic subdurals often cause no deficits early in their evolution but cause slowly progressive dementia, gait problems, or personality changes as they enlarge. Acutely, they may be too small and too continuous within the cranium to be apparent on computed tomography. Where there is reason to suspect a subdural hematoma, repeated computed tomograms are indicated to allow identification of the subdurals. This is discussed further in the section on chronic subdural hematomas.

Temporal Lobe Damage

Lesions in the temporal lobe often produce visual or auditory hallucinations, especially if the patient has a concurrent seizure disorder (40). With severe head trauma causing primarily temporal lobe damage some patients develop an acute psychosis that is largely indistinguishable from an acute schizophrenia (11). Specific symptoms are characteristic of damage to specific parts of the temporal lobe. Imagined recall and inappropriate unfamiliarity, so-called déjà vu and jamais vu phenomena, usually appear with medial temporal lobe damage. Selective deficits in verbal memory develop with damage to the hippocampus in the left temporal lobe (46). Most of the changes apparent in individuals with temporal lobe damage are changes in affect, rather than in intellectual function. Affective paroxysms, such as intense fear, baseless anxiety, or profound despair, occur more often than any cognitive disturbances when the patient suffers temporal lobe damage, but both are often seen to varying extents in the affected patient.

Frontal Lobe Damage

Frontal lobe damage characteristically blunts affect and cognition. Affective changes are characterized by a general lack of concern and an apparent shallowness of response. Socially inappropriate actions, such as random defecation and urination, will arouse concern in family members long before any cognitive difficulty is appreciated. The most common cognitive defects are problems with abstraction, attention, and memory (47). Memory may be impaired, and, when it is, recent memory is usually most affected. This defect in recent memory leaves the patient disoriented (47). Forced thinking and hallucinations also develop in some patients with frontal lobe damage. The most prominent psychologic changes with damage to the frontal lobes are invariably disturbances of affect, rather than cognition. These are discussed in the chapter on affective disorders.

Subarachnoid Hemorrhage

Bleeding into the cerebrospinal fluid commonly occurs with significant head trauma, but a subarachnoid hemorrhage may develop without any associated trauma. Clinically, the patient usually exhibits a dramatic change in cognition, affect, consciousness, or all of these faculties. If there has been substantial head trauma, a subdural or epidural hematoma must be considered and sought. Often the subarachnoid blood will extend from a cerebral contusion. Some patients complain of severe headache and subsequently act inappropriately or become stuporous even when there has been no antecedent head trauma. Misdiagnosis is more likely in this situation than when a head injury is reported. The patient's family may complain that the patient suddenly became confused, argumentative, or assaultive. A psychiatric basis is reasonably suspected if this abrupt change in personality developed during a heated argument or, alternatively, during sexual activity. These are common settings for spontaneous subarachnoid hemorrhages.

If the source of bleeding has allowed extension of the hemorrhage into the brain, then focal neurologic deficits in association with cognitive or affective disorders simplify the diagnosis. Unfortunately, bleeding is often from defects in very superficial vascular structures, and the irritating blood may bathe the entire central nervous system. Focal signs may develop with strictly subarachnoid blood, but more often than not they are not found when intracerebral bleeding does not occur. Because subarachnoid blood irritates the meninges, the patient almost always has a stiff neck. Seizures and coma develop in the most severe cases. Little more than impaired speech volume and substantial confusion may develop in the most benign cases. Unfortunately, what starts as little more than a cognitive disorder can evolve into a more serious problem, especially if a subarachnoid hemorrhage is not suspected and appropriate measures are not taken.

Spontaneous subarachnoid hemorrhages are caused by aneurysms, arteriovenous malformations, occult tumors, and blood clotting disorders. Bleeding from a mycotic aneurysm may be the first indication that the patient has subacute bacterial endocarditis. Metastatic tumors, especially malignant melanoma and choriocarcinoma, may have intracranial bleeding as the first sign of neoplastic disease, but these tumors are usually in the brain itself and, consequently, cause intracerebral bleeding with prominent signs of brain damage. This is also true of hypertensive bleeds. The patient with longstanding hypertension is at high risk for intracranial hemorrhage, but the bleeding usually starts in the basal ganglia, thalamus, pons, or cerebellum. An arteriovenous malformation at the surface of the brain or abutting one of the ventricles may bleed with little destruction of surrounding brain tissue, but this is less likely with the complex system of abnormal vessels in an arteriovenous malformation than with the focal blood vessel defect of the saccular aneurysm. This outpouching on an artery may cause neurologic signs as it enlarges, but more commonly it is silent until it bursts. A sudden increase in intracranial blood pressure plays a role in many cases. This would explain the observed frequency of bleeds with fornication, defecation, and agitation.

Although examination of the cerebrospinal fluid will quickly establish whether or not a subarachnoid hemorrhage has occurred, concern for subdural or massive intracerebral hematomas usually demands that a computed tomogram be the initial investigation. Even when there is no focal accumulation of blood, the relative density of fresh blood when compared to normal brain tissue often allows recognition of intraventricular blood on a computed tomogram. If the computed tomogram is negative and a lumbar puncture is performed, the cerebrospinal fluid obtained will usually have red blood cells with few white blood cells in the fluid.

Red blood cells do not form clots in the cerebrospinal fluid unless bleeding occurred at the time of the lumbar puncture. This is useful in distinguishing between a traumatic spinal tap and a subarachnoid hemorrhage. Also helpful is the elevated cerebrospinal fluid protein that will develop within hours of the subarachnoid bleeding. The normal cerebrospinal fluid protein will be elevated about 1 milligram per deciliter for every 700 red blood cells per cubic millimeter of fluid. If the cerebrospinal fluid protein is elevated in excess of this ratio, the blood in the fluid was almost certainly there for a few hours before the tap. The pigments contributed to the cerebrospinal fluid as the blood cells break down will produce a yellow color in the supernatant when the fluid is centrifuged. This yellow color, or xanthochromia, is also a reliable indicator that the blood in the fluid was not introduced inadvertently at the time of the lumbar puncture.

Having established that the patient has had a subarachnoid hemorrhage, the physician is obliged to look for the source. Arteriography of the four major arteries to the brain is indicated whether a saccular aneurysm, mycotic aneurysm, or arteriovenous malformation is suspected. Aneurysms are often multiple. All of them must be identified to allow effective treatment of the disorder. A blood coagulation profile will uncover clotting abnormalities in most cases. Transient clotting disorders develop with the ingestion of warfarin (rat poison, Coumadin) and with platelet dysfunction (idiopathic thrombocytopenic purpura).

The treatment of subarachnoid hemorrhage is determined by the cause of the hemorrhage. If an aneurysm is responsible, surgical clipping will be attempted when the patient is stable enough to survive the surgery. This ordinarily means an interval of at least 2 weeks between onset of symptoms and corrective surgery. If a mycotic aneurysm is responsible, treatment of the underlying cardiac disease will be vital. Mycotic aneurysms usually develop over the surface of the cerebral convexity and so are relatively accessible for clipping, a trait not shared with saccular aneurysms, which are most often found on the undersurface of the brain about the circle of Willis. Arteriovenous malformations may be excised if they are superficial, but they often lie deep in the brain, making them inaccessible to surgery. Embolization with small spheres or glue is currently used to decrease flow through these anomalous vascular systems. If a clotting defect underlies the subarachnoid hemorrhage, hematologic investigations will be needed to determine the reversibility of the defect.

POSTICTAL CONFUSION

After a partial or generalized seizure, most patients are confused for minutes to hours. This is not true for generalized nonconvulsive (petit mal) seizures, but it is consistently so with generalized tonic-clonic (grand mal) and complex partial (psychomotor) seizures. The duration of this postictal confusion is usually no more than 20 minutes, but some patients will have cognitive disorders lasting as long as 24 hours after the seizure. Some investigators believe that the disturbance in cognitive function occurring after psychomotor seizures may last much longer; this is discussed in detail in the section on complex partial seizures. Postictal confusion may involve a fairly selective impairment of attention or memory or it may appear as a dramatic personality change with inappropriate hostility, denial of illness, and combativeness. Regardless of what affective or cognitive defects appear during the postictal period, the patient's intellectual functioning will return to normal when all seizure activity has ceased for a few hours. No cognitive defects remain as a permanent consequence of the seizure.

The two special situations in which the necessarily transient nature of the postictal thought disorders may not apply are patients recovering from days of continuous seizure activity (status epilepticus) and some patients with temporal lobe foci. The patient in status epilepticus probably suffers structural damage to the brain in the form of neuronal loss. Abnormal patterns of blood flow and excessive neuronal metabolic activity are probably responsible for this seizure-related brain damage. Even in status epilepticus, a condition in which one seizure may follow another in rapid succession for days or until death occurs, the damage suffered by the brain does not become appreciable until the condition has persisted for many hours.

Patients with temporal lobe foci for their complex partial seizures occasionally have a schizophrenia-like psychosis associated with their epilepsy, but the relationship between the epilepsy and the thought disorder is still controversial. With temporal lobe damage, patients commonly have persistent thought disorders, whether or not they have epilepsy. Although some neurologists have described problems with naming in patients with temporal lobe epilepsy, standard testing of intellectual abilities, including memory, in these patients during interictal periods reveals no consistent impairment (48). Patients with complex partial seizures are occasionally misdiagnosed as schizophrenic because of the similarity in the cognitive disorders developing in these two problems, but even those epileptic patients with prominent cognitive disorders are distinct from most schizophrenics in several respects. There is a religious character to many of the epileptic's delusions and preoccupations. Despite his paranoia and complaints of menacing auditory hallucinations, he maintains a warmth unlikely in a truly schizophrenic individual (49). Inconsequential sentences, neologisms, ideas of influence, and hallucinations are all evident in some of these epileptic individuals, but the affect they display is generally appropriate (49). It is quite likely that the cognitive disorder appearing in some patients with temporal lobe epilepsy is a distinct entity unrelated to schizophrenia and more closely tied to the temporal damage than the paroxysmal seizure activity.

INFECTIOUS DISEASES

Bacterial Meningoencephalitis

Bacterial meningitis or meningoencephalitis usually produces rapid deterioration of consciousness, rather than mild signs of dementia, but altered cognition or affect may be the initial or residual signs of a bacterial infection in the central nervous system. The cognitive disorder with bacterial infection ranges from disorientation to florid hallucinations. Transient amnesia may develop in the initial stages of tuberculous meningitis, but cranial nerve signs or altered consciousness are much more typical of this infection. Syphilis is most often responsible for a chronic, rather than acute, dementia, but neither is commonly seen in the United States because of the rarity of all forms of neurosyphilis. Acute cognitive disorders develop with meningococcal and pneumococcal meningitis, but these thought disorders rapidly progress to stupor and coma if the infections are not treated within hours of their initial symptoms. The disorientation, hallucinations, paranoid delusions, and memory disturbances appearing in patients with such virulent bacterial infections are rarely confused with an acute nonneurologic psychosis unless the patient has a long history of psychiatric disturbances. Even in these psychiatric patients, the appearance of a fever and neck stiffness usually dispels any doubts that the cognitive disorder has a neurologic basis.

Viral Encephalitis

Viral infections of the central nervous system can produce intellectual changes that evolve over the course of weeks, months, or years. The kind of cognitive or affective disorder developing with the infection is usually fairly specific for the type of virus causing the encephalitis. Encephalitis lethargica, a common antecedent to postencephalitic parkinsonism in the 1920s, often presented with an acute memory disorder and confabulation that was rapidly overshadowed by obtundation (14). Congenital rubella is clearly associated with a higher incidence of autistic behavior in affected children than is found in the general population (50). Minor behavioral or cognitive disturbances commonly occur after infections with relatively benign causes of meningoencephalitis, such as mumps virus and enterovirus. The full extent of the disability produced by a viral agent may not be apparent for years after an acute illness. Mental retardation and speech difficulty developing in western and eastern equine encephalitis of childhood may prove more substantial as the child matures (50). The agent producing St. Louis encephalitis will cause intellectual and motor deficits in 20 to 60 percent of the elderly patients infected up to 1 year after the acute illness (50). A delay of years between viral encephalitis and intellectual decline is most characteristic of subacute sclerosing panencephalitis. This disease affects individuals from 2 to 21 years old, but children about 7 years old are most commonly affected. Behavior problems, declining school performance, and progressive dementia occur over the course of months. The patients develop myoclonic jerks and die within 1 to 3 years. The disease is attributed to a congenital measles infection or mumps infection.

How viruses cause the often lethal damage they are responsible for is still largely unknown. This is especially true for the so-called slow viruses, which are likely to kill the victim without inciting any apparent immune response. Access to the central nervous system is usually by way of the bloodstream, but some viruses probably travel along nerve fibers to reach the brain and spinal cord (50). However they gain access to the nervous system, these viral agents can produce central nervous system damage that is ineffectively dealt with by the nervous system's own immune mechanisms and by the antiviral agents yet developed.

Herpes Simplex Encephalitis

Psychiatric symptoms commonly appear early in the course of herpes simplex encephalitis. Disordered memory, profound personality changes, marked irritability, and complaints of intractable headache are the initial problems in most victims of this disease. These nonspecific signs and symptoms may appear days or weeks before more substantial signs, such as seizures or obtundation (25,14). An acute psychosis occasionally develops after the early confusion and personality change, and this usually prompts psychiatric observation or treatment of the patient. Visual and auditory hallucinations or delusions develop as features of this psychosis and suggest an acute schizophrenia. Bilateral hippocampal involvement may be manifest as a transient memory deficit or even as a permanent Korsakoff-type amnesic syndrome if the patient survives this viral encephalitis (50). Global dementia and focal motor deficits usually develop as the disease progresses. Bitemporal headaches, back pain, fever, and neck stiffness appear days or weeks after the cognitive and affective disorders.

The responsible virus is *Herpes simplex* type 1, the same virus that causes herpetic gingivostomatitis and recurrent herpes labialis (30). There is no seasonal pattern to the disease. Herpes simplex encephalitis occurs sporadically throughout the year in all age groups and in all communities. There is no apparent patient to patient spread.

Diagnosing herpes encephalitis is usually difficult before the patient is severely impaired. An early check of the herpes antibody titers in the blood and in the cerebrospinal fluid does not usually show any rise in the titers until the infection has been active for weeks. Other clinical tests may provide substantial indirect evidence of the infection. The electroencephalogram is diffusely slow and often has repetitive sharp waves, most prominent in the temporal leads. A computed tomogram may show edema in the temporal lobes, but a lumbar puncture usually reveals normal cerebrospinal fluid opening pressure, sugar, and protein (30). There may be some mononuclear blood cells, some red blood cells, and slight elevation of protein content in the cerebrospinal fluid. Radionuclide brain scan generally indicates radionuclide uptake in the temporal and parietal lobes.

Definitive diagnosis requires brain biopsy. The disease produces widespread hemorrhagic necrosis of cerebral cortex and subcortical white matter and tends to affect the orbital surfaces of the frontal lobes and the bulk of the temporal lobes preferentially (30). Grossly, these lobes appear swollen. Microscopically there is an extensive inflammatory cell infiltrate in the perivascular spaces, and, occasionally, there are eosinophilic intranuclear inclusions in some of the cells (30). Much of the cortex will be necrotic. Biopsy is especially important since many of the patients with what appears to be herpes simplex encephalitis have unexpected, often treatable, brain diseases. These include tuberculosis, cryptococcal meningitis, parasitic infections, lymphocytic choriomeningitis, and cerebral tumors (51). Other diseases that mimic herpes encephalitis, but are not treatable, include subacute sclerosing panencephalitis, Reye's syndrome, toxic encephalopathy, and other viral encephalitides (51).

There is still no clearly effective treatment. Trials with the antiviral agent adenine arabinoside (vidarabine) have been promising, but limited. In some studies, mortality with the drug is about 40 percent, whereas that for patients left untreated or given other drugs is 70 to 90 percent (51). The extent of functional recovery is marginally better in those patients surviving after treatment with adenine arabinoside. Patients do best if they are under 30 years of age and are not obtunded at the time the antiviral agent is started (51). Psychiatric problems developing with the disease may persist to some extent after the patient recovers from the acute illness. Intellectual and psychiatric problems in survivors occasionally demand permanent institutionalization.

Rabies

Psychiatric symptoms are often the most prominent early manifestation of rabies. After months of incubation, the virus produces a profound change in the patient's behavior with rage attacks often alternating with periods of apparent terror (25). Affective changes overshadow cognitive changes. The course of the illness is too fulminant to allow confusion with strictly psychiatric disorders. Brain damage is obvious if a biopsy is performed to help in diagnosis. This virus, like that causing herpes simplex encephalitis, shows an affinity for the temporal lobes. The patient develops seizures as the disease progresses and commonly dies in convulsions (25).

Progressive Multifocal Leukoencephalopathy

Dementia and weakness progressing over the course of weeks or months in a patient with an impaired immune system is often from progressive multifocal leukoencephalopathy. This is a demyelinating disease of the brain that usually develops in patients with chronic lymphocytic leukemia, Hodgkin disease, or sarcoidosis (52). The common factor in all of the adults affected is a longstanding defect in the reticuloendothelial system. Patients on immunosuppressive therapy are also at risk (53). The initial signs of progressive multifocal leukoencephalopathy include confusion, emotional lability, gait difficulty, and speech problems (50). The patient is usually apathetic, slightly paranoid, and inattentive (52). This intellectual and affective change is usually associated with aphasia, seizures, blindness, hemiparesis, and clumsiness as the disease progresses (50). Death is likely within 10 weeks to 1 year of the onset of the symptoms (52).

Multiple areas of demyelination with considerable sparing of nerve cell bodies and axons are the most apparent pathologic changes. This is presumed to involve a virus, because a papovavirus appears in the oligodendrocytes damaged in the disease. These are myelin producing cells, and the myelin they elaborate is disrupted (50). There is little or no inflammatory response to the viral injury, and, accordingly, the cerebrospinal fluid is normal (53).

Any patient susceptible to this disease is also especially susceptible to bacterial and fungal meningitis. The real danger in these chronically ill patients is that their initial personality changes will be misconstrued as a depressive reaction to their systemic disease, and this psychiatric disturbance will be treated. Progressive multifocal leukoencephalopathy is not a treatable disorder, but a bacterial or fungal meningitis mistaken for progressive multifocal leukoencephalopathy is treatable if it is detected early in the disease.

Subacute Sclerosing Panencephalitis

Subacute sclerosing panencephalitis causes progressive intellectual and motor deterioration over the course of a few months (54). This is an invariably fatal disease of children and young adults that is apparently caused by a viral infection. Children affected by this disease become irritable, inattentive, destructive, and disobedient. Jerking movements of the limbs develop as the disease progresses, but these are easily confused with habit spasms (tics). The initial signs may be misconstrued as a behavior problem, but the lethal nature of the problem becomes evident within a few weeks as the child deteriorates. A persistent measles virus infection is responsible for the central nervous system destruction in most, if not all, cases (54). Mumps virus has been implicated in some cases. There is no treatment for this disease.

VASCULAR DISEASES

Impaired blood flow to the brain can cause acute or chronic changes in cognitive function, but other signs of brain damage, such as weakness and impaired sensation, usually occur with the cognitive changes. If blood flow to the brain is severely restricted for more than a few minutes, the tissue deprived of its blood supply will be irreversibly damaged. Nerve cells are much more sensitive to this ischemia than are glial cells, the nonneural elements in the brain, and once the nerve cells are lost there is no chance of regeneration in the damaged tissue. Inflammatory lesions of the cerebral blood vessels may cause protracted periods of ischemia without producing permanent brain damage, but in any situation where blood flow to part of the brain is decreased there is the risk of infarction. This is obvious in the usually benign ischemia that develops with migraine headaches. Patients with this type of vascular disorder often develop transient neurologic signs that recur for years without becoming permanent deficits. For no apparent reason, this uncomplicated headache may progress to a more serious disorder with cerebral infarction developing during an ischemic episode. Profound affective changes often occur with vascular headaches, but the other symptoms of the disorder clarify the cause of the psychiatric changes. Vascular disease of any kind causing strictly psychiatric symptoms is unusual, but this does occur with collagen vascular disease and, much more rarely, with stroke.

Systemic Lupus Erythematosus

Cognitive and affective disorders frequently occur in systemic lupus erythematosus. This is because 59 percent of the patients with systemic lupus erythematosus have central nervous system involvement (55). Disordered mentation in systemic lupus erythematosus may develop years before other signs of the collagen vascular disease (55). Memory may be disturbed transiently and repeatedly. Other signs of intellectual impairment occasionally occur, but an endogenous depression is more common. Movement disorders, especially chorea, develop along with the cognitive and affective changes in some patients, but they are often misconstrued as reactions to antipsychotic drugs if the patient is being treated for his psychiatric symptoms. Fortunately, from a diagnostic viewpoint, 17 to 50 percent of patients with central nervous system lupus erythematosus develop seizures, and as many as one-third have cranial nerve dysfunctions. Unfortunately, neuropsychiatric symptoms appearing with one episode of systemic lupus erythematosus often recur with each exacerbation of the disease (55).

The fundamental lesion in the central nervous system with symptomatic systemic lupus erythematosus is presumed to be a vasculitis. Inflammatory changes in the blood vessels may be so extensive that fixed neurologic deficits, such as a hemiplegia, develop. Because vascular changes in lupus are often transient, neuropsychiatric deficits are usually transient.

The treatments frequently employed in systemic lupus erythematosus may cause as much psychologic dysfunction as the disease itself. Antimalarial drugs used during exacerbations of the systemic lupus erythematosus may precipitate psychotic episodes, personality changes, or convulsions. Corticosteroids may produce a euphoria or even frank psychosis (55). Defining whether the disease or the treatment is causing the cognitive and affective disorders can usually be accomplished by increasing the dose of the drug being used and assessing its impact on the psychiatric symptoms.

Stroke

There is no correlation between atherosclerotic changes in cerebral vessels and the dementia exhibited by patients with the atherosclerotic changes (56). Vascular disease causes dementia in most patients through multiple small strokes or one major stroke. This destruction of brain tissue by infarction or hemorrhage will usually appear as discrete episodes of intellectual disturbance with limited recovery after the catastrophic event. Substantial intellection deterioration is caused by vascular disease in less than 10 to 15 percent of all demented patients over 65 years of age, even though the elderly are most at risk for complications of cerebrovascular disease (8,57–59). Sensory and motor deficits usually appear coincidentally with the intellectual disturbances, but these "elementary" signs of brain disease may largely resolve despite persistence of the dementia (3).

A progressive dementia from vascular disease is unusual. It will occur with cerebral infarctions or hemorrhages over the course of years, but even then it generally does not have a smooth course (3). Typical stroke episodes will punctuate the progressive decline in intellectual function. An acute dementia that completely resolves after a few weeks or months is much more common than progressive dementias with atherosclerotic disease. There is pathologic evidence of cerebral infarction in more than 50 percent of apparently normal individuals over 65 years of age (57). The volume of brain infarcted in these relatively normal individuals is less than 50 cubic centimeters, but it is probably the location of the infarction, rather than its size, that determines whether or not dementia develops (57).

If a multi-infarct dementia is responsible for the patient's cognitive dysfunction, diagnostic tests should readily document this. Multiple areas of damage will be evident on the electroencephalogram, even if the lesions are too small to be apparent on a computed tomogram of the brain. The electroencephalogram will reveal several areas of focal slowing, and sharp waves or spikes may originate about the area of structural damage. Cerebrospinal fluid examination will not usually reveal any abnormalities. An arteriogram will confirm the vascular etiology for the intellectual disturbance by demonstrating multiple branch occlusions.

Recovery of intellectual function between stroke episodes may be fairly impressive. If the patient continues to have recurrent nonfatal strokes, he will generally deteriorate to a vegetative state. Survival in this condition can extend for months or years. Death usually results from massive infarction, systemic infection, or severe dehydration. There is no treatment for multi-infarct dementia or for the intellectual deficits that may appear with a single stroke.

METABOLIC DISEASES

Confusion, disorientation, and subsequent amnesia for the period of altered cognition occurs with several metabolic and endocrine disorders (Table 6.4). Patients with hepatic failure or renal failure may hallucinate and react violently to paranoid delusions as toxic metabolites accumulate in their blood. Adrenal insufficiency (Addison disease), Cushing disease, thyrotoxicosis, hypothyroidism, hyperparathyroidism, and hypoparathyroidism may all lead to impaired cognition because of inappropriate hormonal activity (14,60). More strictly metabolic than hormonal bases for dementia include acute intermittent porphyria, severe hypoxia, hypoglycemia, hypocalcemia, and hypercalcemia (14,61). Serum glucose levels of about 30 to 40 milligrams per deciliter often produce mild disorientation, inattention, and poor concentration; lower levels produce more global impairment of cognitive function and lead to coma (61). Hypercalcemia at levels in excess of 16 milligrams per deciliter will induce paranoid ideas, hallucinations, and disorientation. Profoundly low calcium levels produce an acute confusional syndrome similar to the thought disorder developing in delirium tremens with acute alcohol withdrawal (61). Hallucinations, disorientation, paranoid ideation, and inattention also develop with severe hypoxia, an acute metabolic problem in patients with pulmonary emboli

Table 6.4. Treatable Causes of Dementia

Depression
Frequent epileptic fits
Drug intoxication
Poisoning
Benign brain tumor
Chronic subdural hematoma
Brain abscess
Hyponatremia
Hypercalcemia
Uremia
Pulmonary insufficiency
Hepatic encephalopathy
Hyperthyroidism
Hypothyroidism
Hyperadrenalism
Hypoadrenalism
Hydrocephalus
Bacterial or fungal meningoencephalitis
Pernicious anemia
Pellagra
Systemic lupus erythematosus

or collapse of a lung. All of these acute cognitive disorders appear much earlier in the deterioration of normal serum levels when the change in the serum glucose, oxygen, or electrolyte content is precipitate. A very gradual change in the serum level of any of these essential elements may be tolerated fairly well until the deviation from normal is extreme.

Poisoning with arsenic, lead, manganese, mercury, or thallium affects memory function fairly selectively early in the course of exposure, but other neurologic and systemic signs appear as the degree of poisoning becomes more severe. Affective disturbances and cerebellar tremor were especially characteristic of the hatters using mercury to cure their pelts when beaver fur was a major raw material for hat making. The psychomotor retardation evident in children eating lead-based paint is familiar to any pediatrician working in city slums. Vitamin deficiencies also lead to metabolic problems producing dementia as a major feature in several instances. Nicotinic acid deficiency is manifest as pellagra, a disorder occasionally causing memory impairment as well as other disturbances of cognition (14). The anoxic cerebral damage developing with carbon monoxide poisoning will be manifest as persistent problems with memorization in mild cases and profound dementia and affective dysfunction in more severe cases. Both of these cognitive changes may be delayed until 2 to 3 weeks after the acute poisoning (14).

Thallium Poisoning

Psychiatric reactions and dementia are common manifestations of thallium poisoning (62). Fortunately, most patients who have inadvertently ingested this substance have numerous systemic signs suggesting the diagnosis. Gastrointestinal disorders are especially common; some patients develop a paralytic ileus (62). Vomiting and diarrhea regularly occur. The patient usually has hair loss and often develops a peripheral neuropathy or a parkinsonian-type tremor. Sleep disturbances are prominent, and the patient is often apathetic and stuporous during the day. Seizures occasionally occur.

The confusing patients are those with primarily psychiatric symptoms. Affective disorders are likely, but paranoid delusions may be a prominent part of the syndrome (62). Hallucinations often occur. If psychiatric symptoms develop before the other signs of the disease, the patient may be misdiagnosed as a paranoid schizophrenic or victim of a schizoaffective disorder.

Patients will die of heart failure if the poisoning is severe (62). Treatment of the disorder involves eliminating as much of the toxin as possible. Magnesium sulphate and diuretics may expedite clearance of the poison. If kidney damage is substantial, hemodialysis may be necessary (62).

CHRONIC DIFFUSE COGNITIVE DISORDERS

Chronic intellectual impairment and perceptual problems develop with depressive psychoses, degenerative brain disease, metabolic disorders, and other illnesses affecting the central nervous system. Determining the cause of a diffuse cognitive disorder is useful because many of the diseases producing intellectual and perceptual problems are treatable (Table 6.4). Even when the underlying problem cannot be treated, identifying the cause of the mental deterioration will help predict the course of the illness. This prognosis is important for those caring for the demented individual. With realistic predictions of the patient's rate of deterioration and duration of survival, the family or friends can make the necessary practical and emotional adjustments to the chronic disease.

DEPRESSION AND DEMENTIA

Elderly patients with a depressive psychosis may develop all the characteristics of an "organic" dementia and are commonly misdiagnosed as victims of Alzheimer disease (2,57,63). This type of pseudodementia accounts for only a few percent of all the elderly patients with severe dementia, but it is important because it is a treatable dementia that may lead to fatal complications if it is not dealt with vigorously early in its evolution (57). The pattern that the dementia assumes is not at all distinctive. The patient will be disoriented to time and place; memory, especially for recent events, will be defective; and reasoning may be faulty. Psychometric test scores will be generally low, and a significant discrepancy between verbal and performance scores on the Wechsler Adult Intelligence Scale (WAIS), typical of an organic dementia, will appear (63).

Initially, the patient loses interest in his usual activities and displays a lack of confidence and initiative (2). He fails to perform effectively at work and exhibits progressive difficulty with memory. Abstract thinking is clearly defective (4). To further support the impression of central nervous system disease are the changes in movements that appear in these patients. Bradykinesia, stooped posture, and rigidity of the type developing in Parkinson disease may evolve with the cognitive disorder (63). Changes in psychomotor function appear insidiously or abruptly (2). In the initial stages of this affectively-based thought disorder the patient is often hostile, inaccessible, and panicky.

Even when the intellectual defects seem to have developed quite abruptly, a careful history will usually reveal typical signs of depression preceding the rapid deterioration in intellectual function by weeks or months. The usual story is that of rapidly progressive dementia, appearing over the course of days, in a patient with chronic depression or wide swings in mood each day. The patient usually has delusions of loss, failure, isolation, poverty, or infirmity (63). Before the appearance of the dementia, the depressed patient usually expresses considerable guilt. He will have weight loss and early morning awakening, as well as other vegetative signs of depression. Although the neurologic examination of this patient will reveal unequivocal cognitive dysfunction, the associated signs of anxiety, depression, or even elation should suggest an affective disorder as the basis for the thought disorder (2).

Laboratory tests are not very helpful in reaching the correct diagnosis, except to the extent that they rule out structural and metabolic causes of dementia. The patient may become mute and incontinent of urine, but throughout all this the electroencephalogram will look relatively normal. Objective assessments of brain integrity, such as computed tomography, cerebrospinal fluid examinations, and radionuclide flow studies, will all be normal. Since most patients affected by this depression-triggered dementia are over 60 years of age, the most common misdiagnoses are Alzheimer disease and Parkinson disease (57). Distinguishing which of these disorders is responsible is of considerable importance. Without appropriate treatment, the depressed patient will die from aspiration or starvation (63). With antidepressants and electroconvulsive therapy, the patient may recover fully. The dementia clears as the depression remits.

DEGENERATIVE DISEASES OF THE BRAIN

Cognitive disorders develop when parts of the brain involved in intellectual activity degenerate. The cerebral cortex is usually the principal site of damage in degenerative diseases causing dementia, but damage to other elements in the nervous system can also produce intellectual or perceptual impairment. The neural elements lost are often in systems not routinely considered important in cognitive activity; profound dementia can develop with little apparent damage to the cerebral cortex. Basal ganglia degeneration, such as that associated with Parkinson disease, may be accompanied by profound intellectual deterioration. The causes of central nervous system degeneration are unknown, but several different etiologies are likely simply because there are several different degenerative syndromes. Some follow hereditary patterns and are presumably from metabolic defects, but many are sporadic or too common to link to heredity. Once the degeneration is clinically apparent, it is generally progressive regardless of the specific syndrome developing. No treatment is currently available for any of these degenerative disorders of the central nervous system.

Alzheimer Disease

Much of the dementia in individuals over 60 years of age which is dismissed as "old age" is Alzheimer disease, a progressive degenerative disease of the brain. About 4.4 percent of people more than 65 years old have moderate to severe dementia. The cause of this senile dementia in 65 percent of cases is Alzheimer disease (58). Alzheimer disease can occur in individuals under 65 years of age in which case it is called presenile dementia. There is no basis, other than age, for distinguishing between presenile dementia and senile dementia (56). This cause of intellectual deterioration is the fifth most common cause of death in the United States, but it is an indirect cause of death in most cases, because patients with this degenerative disorder die from complications of the overwhelming central nervous system disease. Systemic infections, dehydration, and starvation will be the immediate causes of death in most cases (8,57). More than three individuals out of every 1,000 in the population have Alzheimer disease (58). More than half of the patients in nursing homes and municipal hospitals over the age of 65 carry the diagnosis of senile dementia. This is an idiopathic disease, but pathologic criteria for establishing the diagnosis are clearly defined.

Presentation

The cognitive disorder initially appears between 45 and 65 years of age in 80 percent of patients with Alzheimer disease (25). Characteristically, there is no early change in personality. The early changes are strictly cognitive; and, in fact, the victim of the disease is often the first to note any change in mental acuity. With an increasing awareness of deficits evolving with the disease, the patient commonly becomes severely depressed. Memory or word-finding are often impaired initially, long-term memory being affected, as well as short-term memory (18). Decreased learning ability, impaired social judgment, labile affect, and loss of familiar skills all appear as the patient deteriorates (59). Deficits in memory, language, and constructional abilities are most prominent. A frank expressive or global aphasia may be prominent 3 to 5 years after the first signs of Alzheimer disease (63). Personality traits change insidiously; the initially withdrawn patient becomes boisterous and assaultive as the dementia becomes profound (56).

Pathology

The pathologic hallmarks of this disease include neuronal loss, neurofibrillary tangles, and senile plaques (58). Neurofibrillary tangles are collections of intraneuronal fibers that stain with silver and appear to be bundles of paired helical filaments when examined with an electron microscope (58). The senile plaque is a collection of degenerating nerve processes surrounding an amyloid core. Neuronal loss is most prominent in cortical association areas, with the precentral and postcentral gyri consistently spared. Parietal and temporal lobes are often altered early in the course of the disease. The concentration of senile plaques and neurofibrillary tangles in the brain corresponds to the degree of intellectual deficit exhibited by the patient (58). The entire brain will be reduced in size and weight in late stages of the disease (Figure 6.1).

Although these pathologic features are most characteristic of Alzheimer disease, they do appear in other conditions. Down syndrome, progressive supranuclear palsy, idiopathic and postencephalitic parkinsonism, post-traumatic dementia, and the amyotrophic lateral sclerosis-Parkinson com-

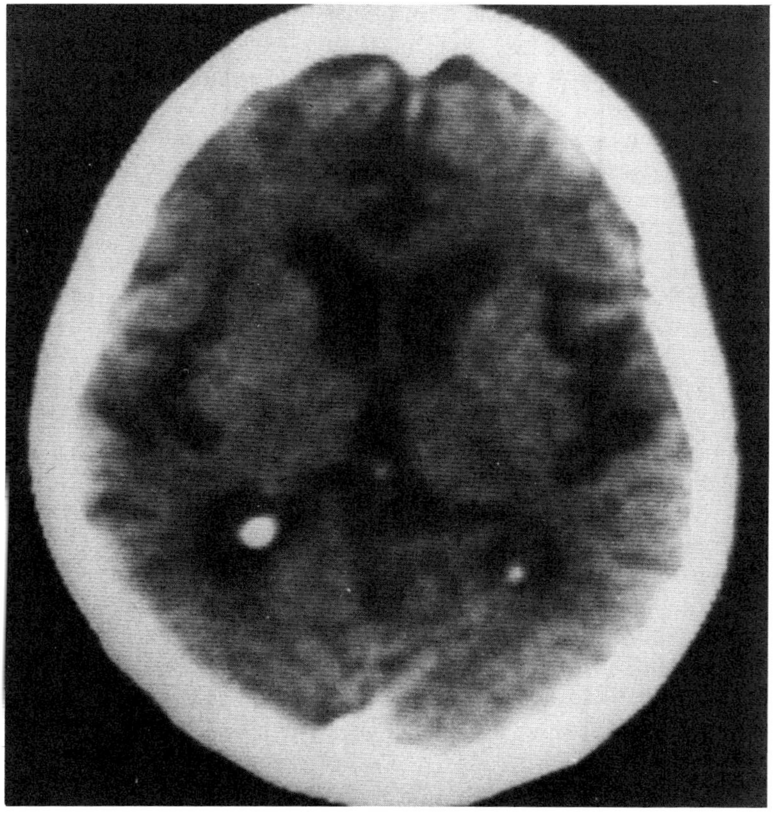

Figure 6.1. Cerebral atrophy and hydrocephalus *ex vacuo* can be seen in this computed tomogram of an 82-year-old man with progressive dementia and gait difficulty. The sulci and gyri of the cerebral cortex are prominent because nerve cells have been lost from superficial and deep gray matter structures. The ventricles have enlarged in response to a decrease in the brain volume, even though there is no increased intraventricular pressure.

plex of Guam all commonly exhibit neurofibrillary tangles and senile plaques (64). How these different dementing diseases are related is unknown.

It is also clear that these pathologic changes alone are not proof that the patient has Alzheimer disease or that he will have a progressive dementing illness. Senile plaques are found in 70 percent of all people over 65 years of age, regardless of their intellectual abilities (57). The first plaques develop in people while they are still in their third or fourth decade of life and increase with age. What affects the rate of increase in the number of plaques and whether these pathologic changes will lead to dementia is unknown.

Premorbid Evidence of Alzheimer Disease

With neuronal loss and other cellular changes, the entire cerebrum atrophies. This gross structural change should be simple to identify on computed tomography of the brain, but this is not true in practice. Although much of the investigation of cerebral atrophy with Alzheimer disease has been done with computed tomography, there is still little evidence that cerebral atrophy can be accurately assessed with this radiographic technique (65). Apparent atrophy on computed tomography may be unaccompanied by histologic changes in the brain when the gross tissue is available for study. In patients thought to have Alzheimer disease there is no significant correlation between atrophy, as estimated by computed tomography, and mortality. Only the most profound changes in brain structure can be assessed with radiographic techniques.

As neuronal structures atrophy, the ventricles enlarge to fill part of the additional space available in the skull. Because the ventricles appear dilated in much the same way they would if there was an obstructive hydrocephalus, this is called hydrocephalus ex vacuo. In patients with severe Alzheimer disease, the cortical mantle thins and the sulci, the spaces between surface folds, become wider. Functional impairment, rather than radiographic evidence of atrophy, is valuable in predicting the course of the disease. Neuropsychologic tests, especially those involving memory and language, are more useful in estimating survival with senile dementia than are radiographic tests (66). Of course, there are fairly consistent changes on other objective measures of cerebral function in patients with Alzheimer disease. The electroencephalogram slows; the dominant rhythm shifts from alpha at 8 to 12 cycles per second to theta at 4 to 7 or delta at 0 to 3 (59). Cerebral oxygen uptake and cerebral blood flow decrease as the intellectual impairment increases. Diagnosing Alzheimer disease while the patient is alive without doing a brain biopsy is still impossible.

Prognosis

This disease has a terrible prognosis. Forty-six percent of affected individuals die within 1 year of diagnosed dementia in some studies (66). Of course, this diagnosis is usually made only after 3 or 4 years of slowly progressive symptoms, and the patient's total survival from first cognitive problems to death may span as much as 8 years. Expressive language impairment in presenile or senile dementia seems to indicate an especially poor outlook for survival beyond 1 year from the appearance of this symptom (143).

Etiology

The etiology of Alzheimer disease is unknown. Theories have ranged from viral infection to aluminum poisoning (67). Complicating the evaluation of any theoretical etiology for this disease is its clinical resemblance to other dementing processes caused by a variety of agents. Clinically, the disease is indistinguishable from Pick disease (25), a degenerative disorder of the brain pathologically distinct from Alzheimer disease on the basis of inclusion bodies in neurons. Both of these are fundamentally "cortical" dementias, that is, the neuropathology is primarily limited to the cerebral cortex. Efforts to establish a hereditary pattern for Alzheimer disease have been unsuccessful. There may be an increased risk of acquiring the disease in certain families, but it is unlikely that genetic factors alone cause Alzheimer disease (56,58).

Treatment

No treatment has produced any consistent improvement in victims of Alzheimer disease. Because the concentration of the enzyme choline acetyltransferase is reduced in the brains of patients with Alzheimer disease, some investigators have tried treating the disease by increasing serum choline levels (68). The assumption is that acetylcholine deficiency is important in this disease, just as dopamine deficiency is important in Parkinson disease. Increasing choline levels should allow the brain to maximize its production of the neurotransmitter acetylcholine. Efforts to force more choline into the brain have involved feeding patients high doses of choline or of lecithin, a more palatable substance that is degraded in the body to choline (69). Results with both of these substances have been unimpressive. Some investigators combined piracetam, a substance that increases metabolic activity and probably increases the rate of membrane revision, with choline (69). Senile patients taking this combination for several months showed little consistent change in their intellectual functioning, although isolated cases of improved verbal memory did occur in some demented individuals (69). Vasodilator treatments are still popular with many physicians, but there is no evidence that these drugs are effective. Giving amphetamines to individuals with Alzheimer disease is dangerous, and improved psychomotor function with this kind of treatment is rare. The current consensus is that there is no effective treatment for Alzheimer disease.

Pick Disease

Pick disease produces a dementia indistinguishable from that developing in Alzheimer disease, but the pattern of brain damage found at death is distinct. Despite its clinical and histologic similarities with Alzheimer disease, Pick disease is only one-fiftieth as common. Clinically, Pick disease should be suspected if the personality structure is relatively poorly preserved as the dementia progresses (3). Patients with this degenerative disease also develop signs of parietal lobe disease, such as constructional difficulty, less often than patients with Alzheimer disease. Early in the evolution of signs, patients with this type of cortical dementia have poor insight and considerable resistance to intellectual testing (70). As in Alzheimer disease, language deficits may develop years after the onset of the disease. Memory is also usually disturbed; mood fluctuations and even frank catatonia appear in some patients (70).

Clinical tests will be abnormal in much the same way as in Alzheimer disease. The electroencephalogram is usually abnormal early in the disease; generalized slowing routinely appears and frontal sharp waves occasionally develop (70). Cortical atrophy largely restricted to the frontal lobes is sometimes evident on computed tomography, but such local atrophy may be inapparent until gross examination of the brain. The histologic changes in the brain are fairly consistent. There is a moderate increase in the number of glial cells in the cortex, and neuronal loss is usually substantial. About 20 percent of the brains affected by this disease will have inclusions in the neurons that stain with silver preparations; these are called Pick bodies. More commonly, numerous neurons will be swollen and will have pale cytoplasm (58). Typically, the cerebral atrophy is most prominent in the frontal and temporal lobes.

There is no cure for Pick disease. If a severe affective disorder accompanies the dementia, the patient may respond to phenothiazines (70). The dementia itself responds to no treatment. A shortened lifespan is the rule with this disease.

Parkinson Disease

James Parkinson observed that patients with the "shaking palsy" subsequently named after him had no intellectual deterioration (64). Unfortunately, he was wrong. Dementia is rarely the presenting symptom in Parkinson disease, but it may be prominent by the time the patient or his family seeks help. It is almost always the movement disorder, rather than the intellectual or mood changes associated with this degenerative disease, that induces the patient or those concerned with his well-being to seek medical attention. Fifty-five percent of patients with Parkinson disease have unquestionable dementia (64). Ironically, it is often the individual with a severe movement disorder, rather than an intellectual problem, who is diagnosed as demented; whereas the patient with significant dementia and no movement disorder goes undetected. The confusion arises because the bradykinesia typical of parkinsonism is routinely misinterpreted as dementia. The patient responds slowly, but accurately, to questions or instructions. This may account for the improved psychomotor performance when parkinsonian patients are started on levodopa or other antiparkinsonian medication (8). Inevitably, this initial improvement is overshadowed by subsequent deterioration in cognitive function despite continued medication. Indeed, some investigators believe that long-term levodopa treatment of Parkinson disease may hasten the appearance of dementia in this disease. One-third of the patients treated with levodopa for 6 years will develop clinically significant dementias (57). Rather than being responsible for a higher incidence of early dementia in patient effectively treated, levodopa may simply allow a greater proportion of patients to survive the common complications of Parkinson disease and consequently produce a larger population of parkinsonian patients available for more chronic effects of the disease.

The kind of dementia developing in Parkinson disease is relatively consistent. Orientation, construction, and memory are particularly involved whereas social behavior, language, and manipulation of old information are less likely to be affected. The aphasia and apraxia typical of Alzheimer disease are notably absent in Parkinson disease (64).

The dementia seen with Parkinson disease may be tied to pathologic changes characteristically seen in Alzheimer disease. Senile plaques and fibrillary tangles of the sort ordinarily seen in Alzheimer disease appear in 33 percent of patients with Parkinson disease (64). Only 5 percent of an age-matched control population have these tangles and plaques (64). Changes in the basal ganglia overshadow the degenerative changes in the cerebral cortex in all patients with Parkinson disease, whether dementia, bradykinesia, rigidity, or tremor is the most prominent sign of the disease. There is no treatment that slows the intellectual deterioration once it starts or that prevents the dementia from developing.

Huntington Disease

Patients with Huntington disease are likely to have cognitive or affective changes before any movement disorder becomes apparent. Sometimes dementia advances to akinetic mutism without the chorea characteristic of the disease ever appearing. The earliest evidence of dementia is usually a subtle change in personality. The patient becomes indecisive, apathetic, and irritable (25). Insight and judgment are often impaired. The pathologic basis for this dementia appears to be neuronal loss. This is prominent in the caudate and other basal ganglia nuclei, the thalamus, the brain stem, the cerebellum, and the cerebral cortex (58). Because many of these patients are treated with neuroleptic drugs for their cognitive disorders, they may be mistaken for chronic schizophrenics with neuroleptic-induced movements when chorea first appears.

Progressive Supranuclear Palsy

Dementia associated with rigidity and opthalmoplegia may develop with the relatively uncommon syndrome of Steele-Richardson-Olszewski, also known as progressive supranuclear palsy. These patients are often mistaken for senile dementia patients suffering from Alzheimer disease or Parkinson disease, because their initial difficulties include deteriorating gait, poor memory, impaired judgment, and more nonspecific personality changes (71). These symptoms usually appear in the fifth and sixth decades of life and progress over the course of months or years (72). Behavior and personality changes precede and overshadow cognitive defects (73). The patient may become irritable, suspicious, and domineering. Attention to personal appearance wavers. The organic basis for the personality change will become more apparent as the patient develops slurred speech and dystonic posturing (71). In this posturing, the patient will be rigid with his head thrust back and his trunk maintained in an abnormal position. Arms and legs will also become rigid, but, unlike in Parkinson disease, tremors usually do not develop.

The first evidence of ocular motor difficulty will be impaired downward gaze (73). Doll's eye movements will be preserved, an indication that this is the result of disease above the level of the ocular motor nuclei. Voluntary lateral eye movements may be slow, but they will be full (73). Caloric stimulation of the semicircular canals will also induce full excursions of the eyes, even in the direction of the apparent gaze palsy. With progression of the disease, the saccadic eye movements will slow, and the patient will have a prominent stare.

Slowing of movements, similar to that developing with Parkinson disease evolves over the course of years (71). Limb movements become more clumsy; swallowing may be defective; and speech is often explosive or absent (73). Further limitation of ocular mobility develops, and convergence is lost. Cerebellar and extrapyramidal signs become prominent as the disease progresses. The patient will develop spasticity in his limbs and a masked appearance to his face (74). The disease progresses slowly over the course of years. Problems with affect may be prominent. The patient routinely develops pseudobulbar affect, a disturbance in the control of emotional displays (71,74).

Half of all affected patients die within 4 to 7 years of their initial symptoms with pneumonia or dehydration (71). There is no effective treatment, but levodopa or anticholinergic drugs will produce temporary improvement in some individuals (71,74). The patients die rigid and bedridden (73).

Pathologically, most of the degenerative changes associated with progressive supranuclear palsy develop in the brainstem (73). Neurofibrillary tangles, gliosis, and neuronal loss are prominent, but demyelination may also occur (74). Demyelination may extend into the basal ganglia, but most of the neuronal loss and neurofibrillary degeneration develops in the brainstem, cerebellum, and diencephalon (72). The dentate nucleus and superior cerebellar peduncle may be so profoundly damaged that frank necrosis occurs (73). Progressive supranuclear palsy is a dramatic instance of a severely dementing illness with primarily subcortical pathology.

INFECTIOUS BASES FOR DEMENTIA

A central nervous system infection can cause slowly progressive cognitive and affective disorders much more suggestive of schizophrenia or of a schizoaffective disorder than of destructive brain disease. Fortunately, relatively few infectious diseases will produce these psychologic changes in the absence of more conventional signs of meningoencephalitis, such as fever, stiff neck, seizures, and focal neurologic deficits. The causes of these atypical infections range from geographically isolated slow-viral illnesses, like kuru, to world-wide bacterial diseases, like tuberculosis. Some of these are treatable diseases, and all are refractory to psychiatric intervention. Recognizing the infectious basis for the cognitive disorder spares the psychiatrist considerable frustration in dealing with the refractory patient.

Kuru

The Fore Islanders of New Guinea believed that kuru, an invariably fatal local disease, was caused by unfriendly sorcery. Early European investigators dismissed witchcraft as the etiology of this dementing disease and ascribed it to hysteria. They apparently believed the native explanation for the tremors developing with kuru; the name "kuru" meant trembling with fear, and the victims of the disease started trembling when they became aware of having been cursed. Victims of the disease usually first became aware of the curse when their gait became unsteady. Profound personality disorders and clumsiness of all limbs soon followed these initial gait problems (75). That this was an invariably fatal disease made some investigators doubt a purely psychiatric basis for this disorder, and some suggested that it might be a hereditary illness (75). No one suspected a viral etiology, simply because the course of the disease was impossibly slow for a viral illness. When the agent was recognized to be a transmissible virus, its unconventional behavior warranted its being called a slow virus.

The initial signs in this progressively dementing illness are not cognitive or affective at all. Most patients developed leg pains, leg tremors, or difficulty walking as their first symtom(75). Profound dementia, impaired emotional control, and depression or euphoria routinely followed this locomotor problem within months. Many victims of the disease were suspicious, angry, aggressive, and even randomly abusive. Death inevitably ensued within 1 year of the cerebellar signs, the patient terminally exhibiting loss of virtually all cognitive functions.

The victims of the disease were usually children or young women, a population determined by exposure to the viral agent during cannibalistic rituals, rather than by special susceptibility. Significant incapacity before death lasted from 3 months to as long as 9 months (76). The actual incubation period for the infecting agent proved to be years.

The central nervous system lesions found with this illness were similar to those found in other slowly dementing illnesses, such as Creutzfeldt-Jakob disease. Dendrites, axons, and neuronal cell bodies developed vacuoles which gave the brain a "spongiform" appearance. Cerebellar damage was often extensive, a finding consistent with the clinical evidence of early cerebellar disease. Unlike other viruses, the slow viral agent did not evoke any inflammatory response in the brain. Although there was no immune response to the infecting agent, patients with the disease had no immune system defects (76).

This disease has been eradicated with the abolition of ritual cannibalism in New Guinea, but it provided considerable insight into a previously unrecognized cause of dementia. This insight led to the identification of other so-called subacute spongiform encephalopathies. Creutzfeldt-Jakob disease is the best understood of these slow-viral diseases producing cognitive disorders in humans.

Creutzfeldt-Jakob Disease

Creutzfeldt-Jakob disease is a sporadically occurring cause of presenile dementia found all over the world. The slow virus responsible for this disease has been transmitted accidentally during corneal transplants, but the conventional mode of transmission is unknown (76). A familial pattern can be found in 10 percent of cases, but this probably reflects common exposure. The prevalence of the disease approaches one case per million individuals in densely populated areas of the United States, and there is a disturbingly high incidence of the disease in patients who have had brain surgery (76). The average age at onset of the disease is 58 years old; men and women are equally affected (77). Signs and symptoms may be obvious for only 2 or 3 months before death, but more than one-third of affected individuals have a prodromal illness lasting months that involves mild, but variable, affective or cognitive disturbances. The kinds of symptoms developing during this prodrome are so inconsistent that they can be recognized as part of the disease only in retrospect.

Intellectual deterioration with Creutzfeldt-Jakob disease is fairly global;

memory, language, constructions, reading, and calculations will all be disturbed as the disease progresses. Forty-nine percent of patients have changes in mentation as the only neurologic abnormalities apparent during much of the early part of the disease (78). Lethargy and chronic fatigue appear months before any intellectual changes in one-fourth of affected individuals; this asthenia progresses to a clinically apparent depression in 15 percent of patients before a slow-viral dementia is suspected (78). Memory loss and inappropriate behavior are often the first unequivocal signs of disease. About 14 percent of patients have hypersomnia or insomnia before cognitive changes; this, in association with weight loss and irritability, allows this progressive dementia to be readily confused with a psychotic affective disorder. As the disease evolves, the patients have involuntary muscle jerks, increased muscle tone, clumsiness, tremors, visual loss, weakness, and a generalized slowing of movements. A fluent, receptive aphasia may develop; many patients have problems with constructions and are inattentive to objects and events in one-half of their environment (unilateral neglect) (63).

Intellectual and perceptual deficits increase steadily over the course of several months. Eighty-one percent of individuals developing this disease survive 4 months from the appearance of unequivocal neurologic signs (78). The disease occasionally has a much more acute onset and rapid course. A stroke-like illness with vertigo, transient blindness, and rapidly progressive aphasia occurs in about 10 percent of affected individuals, and these invariably die within 2 months of the onset of the disease.

Some form of mental deterioration is obvious in all patients with this slow virus, but in 65 percent this is more accurately characterized as a behavior abnormality than as a cognitive disorder (78). Loss of initiative and irritability are commonly reported personality changes. Many patients are paranoid, depressed, and withdrawn (77). A functional psychosis is routinely misdiagnosed during this early stage of the disease (Table 6.5). Many patients with Creutzfeldt-Jakob disease develop involuntary movements as they deteriorate, but these movements are not at all specific for the disease, and so are not helpful in clarifying the diagnosis. These movements range from choreoathetosis to convulsive muscular jerks. Visual hallucinations also frequently develop, providing even more evidence of a basically psychiatric disorder; but, with the appearance of gait difficulty, aphasia, blindness, and seizures, the organic origin of the disease will usually be recognized (79). A receptive or "jargon" aphasia similar to that seen with Alzheimer disease also often evolves, and this is easily confused with a schizophrenic speech disorder (80). Sensory complaints are unusual, except for the common problems with vision. The patient occasionally becomes mute early in the illness and is invariably mute at its termination (77).

Associated neurologic signs as the disease progresses are myriad (77, 81, 82). Problems with recognition, loss of writing skills, and neglect of

Table 6.5. Signs Suggesting a Functional Psychosis in Cruetzfeldt-Jakob Disease

PRODROMAL
Paranoia
Withdrawal
Depression
Sleep disorders
ACUTE OR SUBACUTE
Visual hallucinations
Mutism
Episodic writhing or convulsive limb movements
Dystonic posturing
Jargon aphasia

body parts increase as the patient's cognitive functions deteriorate. Evidence of basal ganglia disease includes abnormal postures, resting tremors, and hypokinesia. Signs of cerebellar disease, such as gait difficulty, nystagmus, vertigo, and hypotonia, develop in most patients. Nine percent of patients develop a seizure disorder (78). Cranial nerve signs appear sporadically. Terminally, the patients are akinetic and mute. Death is from cachexia, infection, or cardiopulmonary collapse (78).

Diagnostic studies may establish the diagnosis even when the virus has not been cultured from infected brain tissue, but definite diagnosis usually requires a brain biopsy or autopsy. Cerebrospinal fluid examination will reveal an elevated protein, and pneumoencephalography or computed tomography will show atrophy (77). Electroencephalographic changes are distinct but variable (Figure 6.2). Focal slowing is occasionally prominent, but most suggestive of the diagnosis is a pattern of periodic spikes or sharp waves (12,77). Electroencephalographic abnormalities usually appear when the disease is well advanced and the characteristic dementia and myoclonus are unequivocal (78). Diffuse irregular bursts of high amplitude slow waves occasionally develop, but more typically there are diffuse, regularly recurring single or multiple sharp waves or spikes occurring at a frequency of one per second (78,83). Whatever form these periodic discharges assume, they are usually imposed upon a generally slow background and their periodicity, that is the interval between each discharge, is extraordinarily regular (83).

Pathologically, there is loss of nerve cells in much of the cerebral cortex and to a lesser extent in subcortical structures. A fine-meshed vacuolation, or spongy state, develops throughout the cortex in both the cerebrum and the cerebellum. This spongy appearance is from the accumulation of fluid in dendritic and astrocytic processes. Plaques that stain with periodic acid-Schiff stain are found in the cerebellum (79). The basal ganglia are also

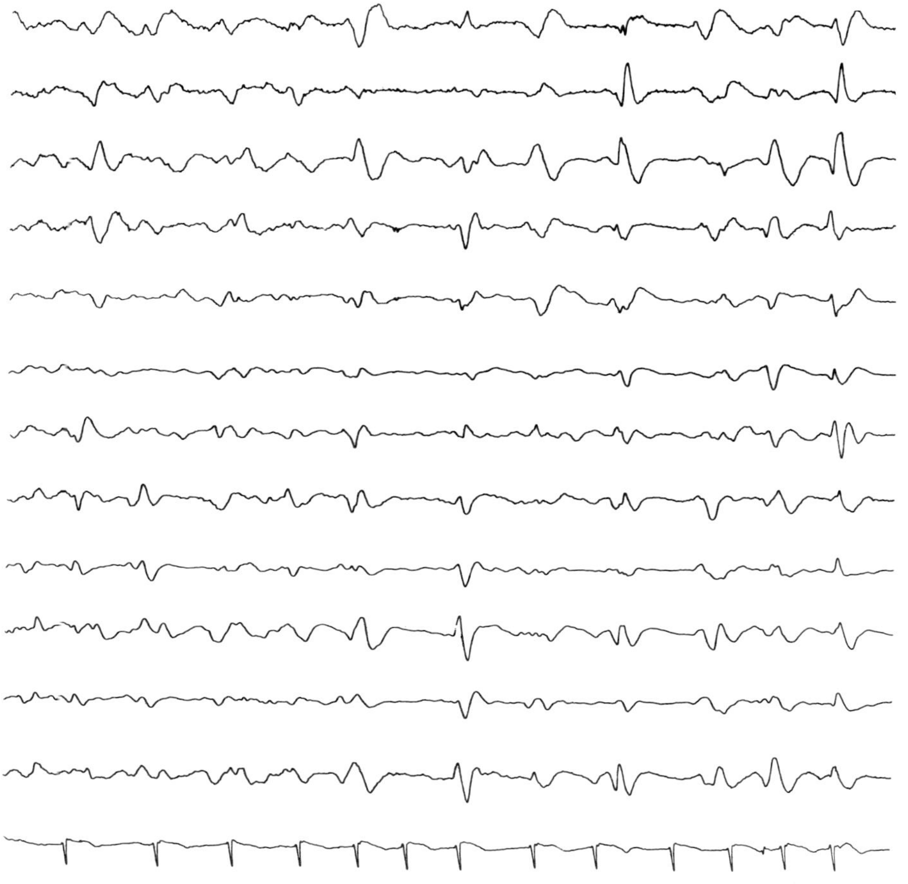

Figure 6.2. This elderly woman had rapidly progressive dementia over the course of 4 months. At the time this electroencephalogram was obtained, she had myoclonic jerks. The recording shows periodic, high-voltage sharp waves and slow waves, a pattern consistent with the diagnosis of Creutzfeldt-Jakob disease. The bottom line of the electroencephalogram was recorded from a muscle in the arm to show the frequency of myoclonic jerks occurring during the recording. The myoclonic jerks and the periodic waves are not strictly in phase, but some of them are synchronous.

involved, a finding consistent with clinical signs of extrapyramidal disease (79). The degree of pathologic change varies greatly from one case to another and the severity of these degenerative changes is unrelated to the duration of the disease (82).

There is no treatment for Creutzfeldt-Jakob disease. The character of the disease causes considerable disruption of the patient's professional and personal life before obvious neurologic signs develop, and consequently a psychiatrist may be involved with the patient himself or with other family members before it is realized that the problem is a progressive brain disease. Most families with an affected member have many concerns about the disease and about the implications of the patient's behavior that are best addressed in family meetings or family therapy. The rarity of the disease arouses fears that the problem might be hereditary, and as with any infectious illness, individuals near to the patient are routinely concerned with spread of the disease to themselves or their children. Allaying these fears will simplify the terminal care of the patient.

Neurosyphilis

The most common cause of presenile dementia only a few decades ago was syphilis. Neurologic disease caused by this infection was usually a late event in the course of the illness. Effective treatment of the infection before it reached the nervous system became feasible with the introduction of penicillin, and this dramatically curtailed the high incidence of neurosyphilis in the United States. When neurosyphilis was a common disease, it presented in several different forms. The most common form was general paresis, a progressive dementia produced by direct invasion of the *Treponema pallidum* organism into the cerebrum. Other forms included meningovascular syphilis, a syndrome similar in character to a typical bacterial meningitis with associated arteritis, and tabes dorsalis, a primarily sensory disorder developing with spinal root and spinal cord damage (39). Affective and cognitive defects were most common in the general paretic form.

General paresis produces dementia with the characteristics of frontal lobe damage (25). Initially, changes in affect and personality are usually prominent (39). The patient complains of headache, insomnia, lethargy, apathy, and poor impulse control. His family reports emotional lability with outbursts of unprovoked rage, as well as a progressive deterioration in the patient's customary social skills. The patient's behavior becomes more vulgar and egocentric (39). The first sign of intellectual deterioration is usually forgetfulness. This is intermittent initially, but it becomes more persistent as the patient deteriorates. The patient's attention span shortens, his interests become more restricted, and his ability to think quickly becomes blunted. Problems with calculations, speech, writing, and abstraction all appear early in the course of general paresis (39). Signs of more focal central nervous system damage include dysarthria, tremor, optic atrophy, lid ptosis, urinary incontinence, and spastic paraparesis; but these need not develop until years after the initial signs of general paresis. Affective changes in these patients are extremely diverse, but most develop a grandiose personality disorder with delusions of wealth and power early in the evolution of the disease (39). The first sign of general paresis appears abruptly in 50 percent of the affected individuals, and that first sign may be an epileptic fit, a suicide attempt, transient amnesia, or delirium (39). A gradual deterioration of intellectual function will occur in all affected individuals.

Serologic tests for syphilis are appropriate in most patients presenting with psychotic behavior or signs of central nervous system damage. If there are signs of focal neurologic damage associated with a progressive dementia in a psychotic patient, a cerebrospinal fluid examination is justifiable. The diagnosis is established by a positive response to flagellated treponemal antigen test of the cerebrospinal fluid, even if all other fluid parameters are normal. The disease may be arrested if it is treated early enough. Penicillin is the treatment of choice, and 80 percent of affected individuals will be cured with this drug alone (25). Although the infection is cured, the brain damage done by the infection will persist, and any cognitive disorders present at the time the therapy is started may be permanent.

POSTTRAUMATIC CHRONIC DEMENTIA

A slowly progressive deterioration in intellectual function after head trauma is relatively uncommon. Patients often complain that their thinking steadily changes after an accident, but this is usually not supported by objective testing. One situation in which the patient's unremitting intellectual decline is authentic is with chronic subdural hematomas (Figure 6.3). These gradually enlarging blood clots will produce personality changes, memory problems, lethargy, gait difficulty, urinary incontinence, and progressive confusion over the course of weeks or months. The head trauma producing a subdural hematoma may be minor, especially if the patient is elderly or on anticoagulants. When the subdural hematoma has increased in size very slowly over the course of several months, a careful examination of the patient will often reveal no focal deficits. The gait is likely to be shuffling; primitive reflexes, such as grasp and suck, may be evident; and plantar responses may be extensor (Babinski sign). Rather than increasing the examiner's level of suspicion, these physical findings are likely to reinforce the physician's prejudice that the patient has a degenerative central nervous system disease. Chronic subdural hematomas may be lethal if they enlarge enough to produce herniation of the brain, but even the insidious dementia they produce is adequately disabling to make their detection and treatment important.

Computed tomography often reveals the lesion since it is usually fairly large when it is symptomatic. If there is a unilateral hematoma, the shift of the brain away from the mass will confirm the presence of the hematoma. Subdural hematomas several months old are less dense than brain tissue and so can usually be readily identified on computed tom-

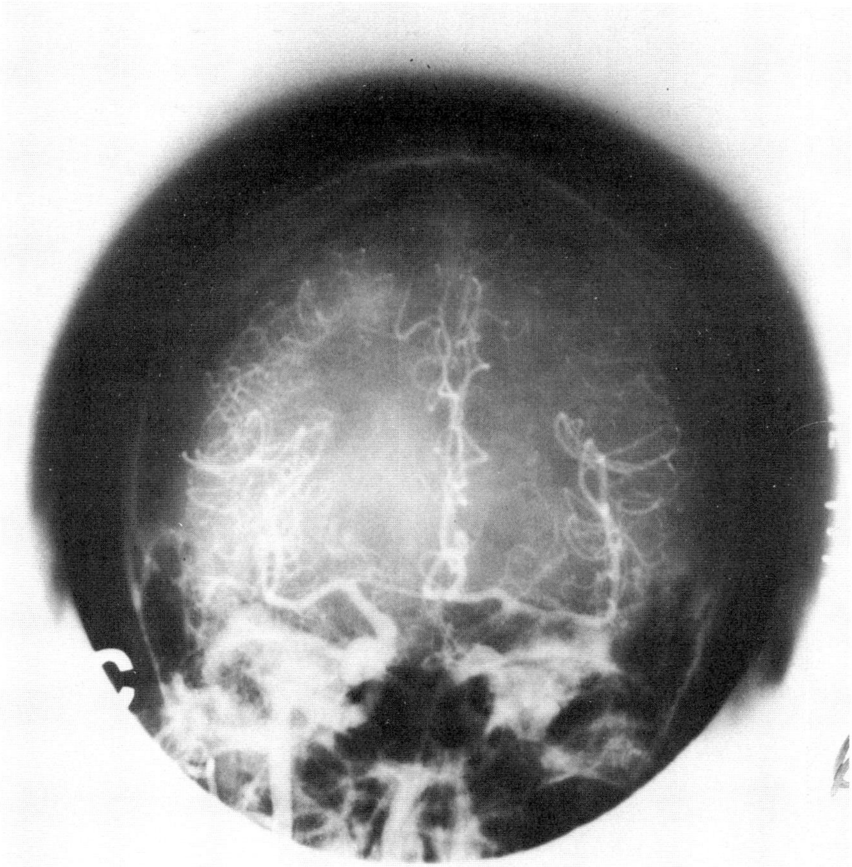

Figure 6.3. This arteriogram was performed on a 56-year-old man who had been under psychiatric treatment for 2 years. He was being treated for an unexplained change in behavior with psychotic features. Neurologic examinations at the time his mentation first changed and at the time of this arteriogram revealed no signs other than the cognitive disorder. The arteriogram was obtained because he had a seizure. The study revealed massive, bilateral subdural hematomas, which appear as dark crescents over both hemispheres between the outermost cortical blood vessels and the inner table of the skull. At surgery, the fluid in the subdural accumulations was found to be typical of chronic subdural hematomas.

ography. Unfortunately, the hematoma may be the same density as brain tissue when the clot is a few weeks or months old (19). A significant shift in the position of the ventricles may be the only indication of an intracranial mass. Even this will be absent if the chronic subdural hematomas are bilateral. With these collections pressing on the brain from both sides, the ventricles may be small, and the cortical sulci, inapparent. When this computed tomographic picture is seen in a demented patient, chronic subdurals should be suspected. Eighty percent of patients with dementia who are over 60 years of age will have enlarged ventricles and prominent sulci (19). Presumably this reflects the generalized atrophy of the brain. When the "isodense" chronic subdural hematomas produce an unexpectedly normal computed tomogram of the brain, a technetium Tc 99m pertechnetate scan of the head will reveal focal collections of isotope bilaterally over the convexities of the cerebral hemispheres. This technique will reveal 91 percent of subdural hematomas more than 10 days old but only 50 percent less than 10 days old (19). Any uncertainty over the nature of the radionuclide uptake can be settled with an arteriogram, which will reveal the extracerebral character of the crescent-shaped masses.

The treatment of chronic subdural hematomas requires surgery. The fluid and clot must be completely removed, and the patient must be closely watched for reaccumulation of the fluid. With evacuation of the subdural hematomas, the chronic dementia may clear dramatically. If the patient subsequently deteriorates, the subdural collection has probably reaccumulated, and reexploration of the patient's head is appropriate.

METABOLIC DISORDERS

Metabolic problems may prove to be the cause of much of what is presently called schizophrenia, but currently there are relatively few thought disorders with established metabolic bases. Problems with electrolytes, metabolic substrates, and blood gases not attributable to a glandular problem routinely produce acute cognitive disorders, but more persistent thought disorders associated with metabolic abnormalities can usually be traced to an abnormal hormone. These hormonal causes of chronic intellectual and perceptual problems are considered under endocrine disorders.

Inborn errors of metabolism usually produce mental retardation while the individual is an infant, but some cause problems later in life. Problems with methionine metabolism producing homocystinuria are well-established bases for disordered thought and behavior (84). The patients develop suspiciousness, religious preoccupations, agoraphobia, ritualistic behavior, and angry outbursts over the course of months or years. They do not have hallucinations or frankly paranoid delusions, but they are distinctly ambivalent and autistic. They have loose associations, concrete thinking, poor judgment, and distorted self-images. Their affect is inappropriate as well as labile. The enzymatic defect underlying this cognitive and affective disorder is cystathione synthetase (84). Homocystinemia and homocystinuria develop with this block in methionine metabolism. Large doses of methionine will exacerbate behavioral disorders in some patients with the more typically schizophrenic symptoms. There is no treatment for this enzyme deficiency.

Acquired metabolic problems causing chronic progressive dementias are usually caused by poisons, but one substance not routinely viewed as a poison that may cause a variety of central nervous system disturbances directly or indirectly is ethanol. Alcohol abuse has been associated with several different dementing disorders in addition to Wernicke-Korsakoff encephalopathy. One that has a less well defined metabolic basis is Marchiafava-Bignami disease. Patients with this disorder develop a dementia characterized by lack of initiative and irritability (25). The personality changes may be gradual, but they are often associated with incontinence and gait difficulty. Lesions evolve at a variable rate, but the patients usually deteriorate over weeks or months and precipitately pass into coma and die. Demyelination of the corpus callosum is the principal defect found at autopsy. The metabolic basis for this is unknown.

HYDROCEPHALUS

Impaired cerebrospinal fluid flow, defective reabsorption, or excessive production usually causes cerebrospinal fluid to accumulate under increasing pressure, a condition generally called hydrocephalus (Table 6.6). As this fluid accumulates, the ventricles become larger, and the cortical mantle is pushed against the skull. Which ventricles become enlarged is determined by the level of obstruction or malfunction in the system. If the aqueduct of Sylvius is blocked, the lateral and third ventricles will enlarge while the fourth ventricle remains small (Figure 6.4). If the problem is at the level of reabsorption, all of the ventricles will enlarge.

Cognitive disorders develop with increased intracranial pressure whether that increased pressure is the result of a mass or of an impairment in cerebrospinal fluid dynamics. The increase in pressure is probably not entirely responsible for the dementia that develops since individuals with pseudotumor cerebri, a condition characterized by very high intracranial pressures, but no hydrocephalus, are not demented. When the increased pressure results from blockage in the flow of cerebrospinal fluid from the ventricles to the subarachnoid space, dementia results despite the absence

Table 6.6. Hydrocephalus

Obstructive		*Nonobstructive*	
Communicating	Noncommunicating	Degenerative (Hydrocephalus ex vacuo)	Destructive
Normal-pressure hydrocephalus	Ventricular mass	Alzheimer disease	Posttraumatic
Posthemorrhagic		Pick disease	

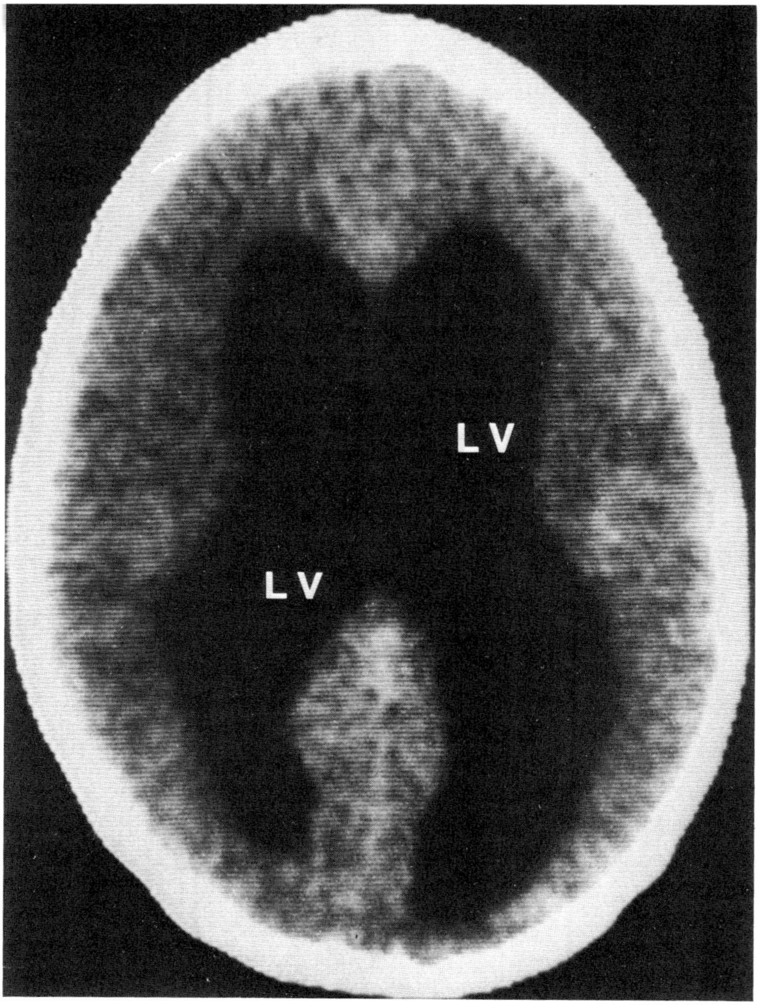

Figure 6.4. The lateral ventricles (LV) are massively distended in this patient with severe hydrocephalus (courtesy of Drs. J. Loh and W. Hotson).

of diffuse cerebrocortical disease; presumably, the distortion of the brain developing as the ventricles enlarge is responsible for the generalized cognitive disorder. Additional signs with acute obstruction of cerebrospinal fluid outflow from the ventricles include nausea, vomiting, obtundation, and ultimately death from transtentorial or tonsillar herniation of the brain (3). It is the patient with a more gradual or partial obstruction of ventricular outflow who has a progressive personality change with impaired judgment, faulty memory, and generally diminished intellect (3).

Enlarged ventricles also develop with chronic degenerative diseases of the cerebrum, such as Alzheimer disease, but the resulting dementia is not because of the ventricular enlargement. Indeed, this change in ventricular size is called hydrocephalus ex vacuo only to stress the apparent tendency of the ventricles to increase in volume as the cortical volume decreases. In most conditions producing increased ventricular size, either with or without increased intracranial pressure, dementia develops apace with the hydrocephalus, and may be relieved by reversing the hydrocephalus.

Normal Pressure Hydrocephalus

Apparent hydrocephalus with no associated increased intracranial pressure has recently been viewed as a distinct cause of dementia associated with urinary incontinence and a gait disorder (72,85). That this is an authentic syndrome or a distinct entity is still being debated, but patients are generally treated to relieve the hydrocephalus if they seem to have this normal pressure hydrocephalus. Clinically, the patient usually has deteriorating cognitive function over the course of months or years with prominent deficits in orientation, memory, attention, and abstraction (63). The severity of the dementia varies from a slight alteration in personality to a vegetative state. Although incontinence is not invariably present when the dementia first appears, problems with urinary incontinence are usually out of proportion to the severity of the dementia present (3,85,86). Unlike patients with Alzheimer disease, patients with normal pressure hydrocephalus do not develop an aphasia (63). Rigidity and bradykinesia, much like that appearing in Parkinson disease, often do develop; and gait deteriorates to small, shuffling steps. Terminally, the patient will be akinetic and mute.

The syndrome appears generally at a younger age than Alzheimer or Parkinson disease, but its peak incidence in the fifth decade of life causes some confusion in distinguishing this from progressive supranuclear palsy (72). Also complicating the recognition of this syndrome is its high probability of occurring as a late effect of subarachnoid hemorrhage, head trauma, or meningitis. Patients surviving these disorders and developing dementia are usually viewed as victims of damage done by the initial process, rather than as patients with a new complication. The distinction is important since dementia resulting from brain damage with meningitis, subarachnoid hemorrhage, or head trauma is usually irreversible, whereas dementia appearing with hydrocephalus often remits when the hydrocephalus is relieved.

Recognition of the syndrome depends on associating the typical clinical triad of dementia, incontinence, and gait difficulty with radiographic evidence of hydrocephalus. With computed tomography, enlarged ventricles can be seen easily, and the lack of deep sulci and prominent gyri to suggest hydrocephalus ex vacuo justifies further investigation of the hydrocephalus (86). On lumbar puncture, the cerebrospinal fluid pressure will be normal; and, if a radionuclide, such as radioactive iodinated serum albumin (RISA) or ytterbium-169-citrate is injected into the subarachnoid space, the disordered cerebrospinal fluid dynamics can be documented. Isotope will appear in the ventricles within 2 hours of isotope instillation in the cerebrospinal fluid, and the isotope will remain in the ventricles 48 hours later, rather than being quickly reabsorbed from the spinal fluid (86). Excessive accumulation of the radionuclide in the ventricles is of itself abnormal, since the flow of cerebrospinal fluid is out of the ventricles. The failure of the radioactive material to rapidly disperse in the subarachnoid space over the cerebral convexities and disappear within 24 to 48 hours suggests that there is a force inside the ventricles pressing the cerebral hemispheres against the inner table of the skull. The electroencephalogram is not diagnostic in this condition; diffuse slowing is evident, but this change occurs with many diseases producing dementia (3).

The accepted treatment for this syndrome is ventriculoperitoneal or ventriculopleural shunting of the cerebrospinal fluid. Unfortunately, the improvement after shunting is variable, and the risk of subdural hematoma as a complication of the surgery is substantial. Even if a subdural hematoma does not develop, the patient is at risk for meningitis introduced by the shunt or recurrent hydrocephalus with shunt obstruction for whatever reason (3). When the syndrome was first described and shunting was introduced to treat it, 66 to 76 percent of the patients treated improved after shunting (86). The patients who did best were those with relatively mild dementia, appearing less than 1 year before the shunt procedure, with incontinence apparent from the start of the dementia (86). Although subsequent experience with shunting in these patients has been much less gratifying than the initial experience, most neurologists still view the procedure as justifiable in patients who have all the classical features and radiologic signs of normal pressure hydrocephalus (63,86,87).

Third Ventricle Masses

Tumors and other masses in the third ventricle can produce cognitive disorders by obstructing cerebrospinal fluid flow and by interfering with subcortical gray matter functioning. Masses at this level can easily obstruct the aqueduct of Sylvius or even the foramina of Monro, as well as press on the thalami or hypothalamus. In one series, 90 percent of third ventricle tumors were associated with symptoms of cognitive dysfunction (88). Lesions in this area occasionally produce cognitive disorders similar to schizophrenia, but the other signs of neurologic disease routinely present limit the frequency of misdiagnosis with these masses. Cases of third ventricle tumors may be dominated by psychiatric symptoms, but eventually with enlargement of the tumor altered consciousness routinely appears (88). Removal of tumors in this region may be difficult or impossible, in which case radiation therapy or cerebrospinal fluid shunting or both may prove effective in reducing the symptoms of the lesion, if not in effecting a cure.

BRAIN TUMORS

Cognitive defects will develop with neoplasms of the brain or of adjacent structures as the cerebral cortex is destroyed or compressed. The type of cognitive defect will depend upon the site of the tumor (Figure 6.5).

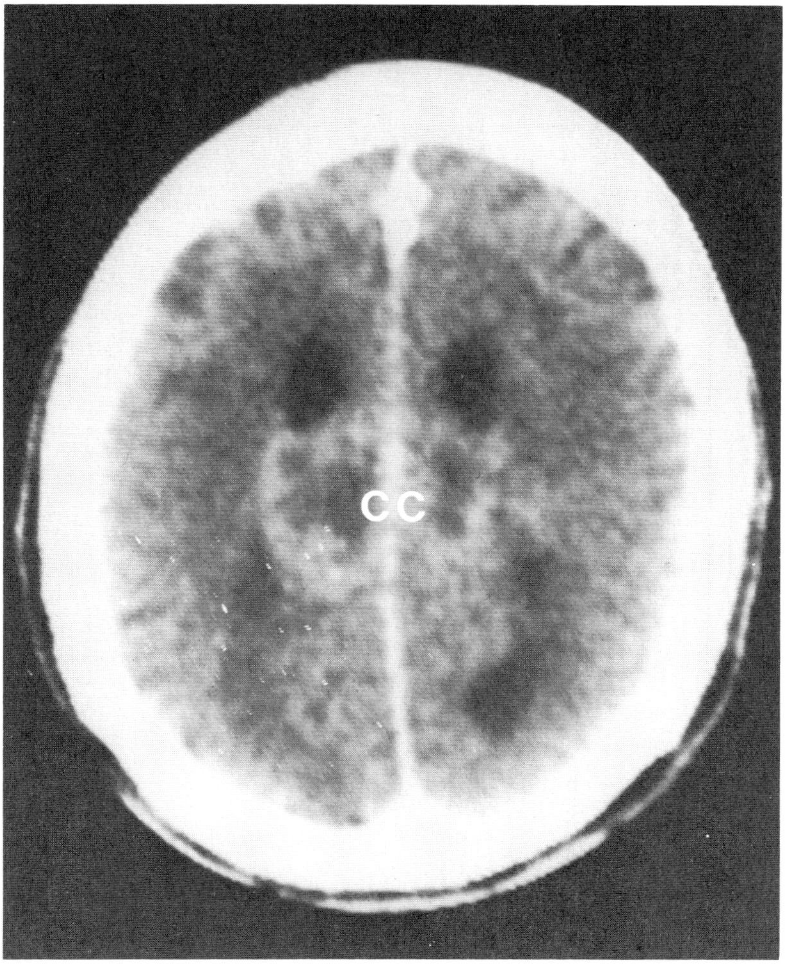

Figure 6.5. A 75-year-old man had a slowly progressive dementia that was complicated by epilepsy. He never had seizures before the development of his intellectual impairment. A computed tomogram of his brain revealed a large tumor (CC) in the corpus callosum (courtesy of Drs. J. Loh and W. Hotson).

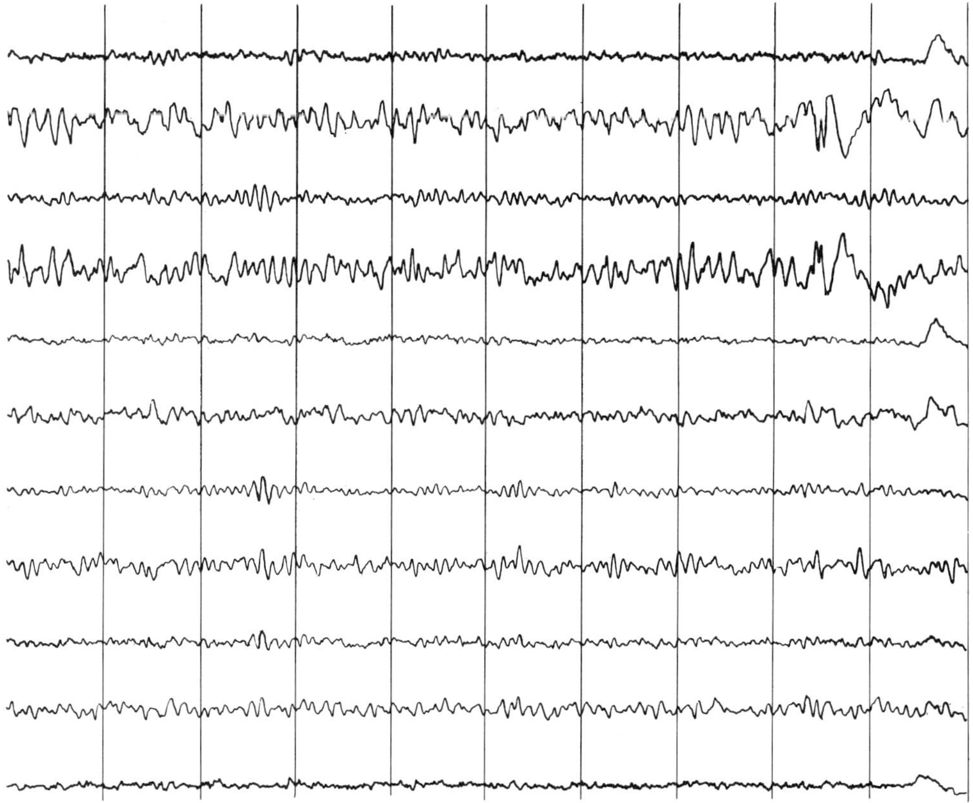

Figure 6.6. An electroencephalogram recorded from an adult with a slowly progressive dementia revealed focal slow-wave activity. The second and fourth lines in this recording have high-voltage, low-frequency waves that indicate a structural lesion in the right anterior temporal area. Further studies revealed a meningioma in this location that was apparently responsible for the patient's progressive intellectual deterioration.

Aphasia may develop with a frontal or temporal lesion. Memory difficulty may appear with temporal or parietal neoplasms, and impaired reading may evolve with a parietal or occipital lesion. Treatment is determined by the type of lesion. Biopsy may be necessary for establishing the precise tumor type.

Cognitive symptoms develop with 80 percent of tumors in the frontal lobe, 75 percent in the temporal lobe, 45 percent in the parietal lobe, 10 percent in the posterior fossa, and 90 percent in the third ventricle (88). That tumors in the structures classically included in the limbic system more commonly cause psychiatric symptoms than tumors elsewhere in the brain is debatable; but limbic tumors certainly can present with signs of schizophrenia or psychotic depression. Obviously, many patients with tumors in these deep brain structures have focal deficits or seizure disorders with no apparent psychosis. A series of over 250 cases of temporal gliomas failed to reveal one case of clearly psychotic behavior (88). Problems with intellectual function are especially common with frontal lobe tumors. Sixty to 90 percent of patients with frontal lobe tumors will have cognitive defects, such as impaired memory, shortened attention span, and disturbed abstraction (47). Blunting of emotional response and loss of spontaneity is more typical than impaired cognition in patients with frontal lobe tumors, but both affective and cognitive dysfunctions can usually be detected in these individuals (Figure 6.6) (47). A rapidly growing frontal lobe tumor is especially likely to be associated with profound confusion.

ENDOCRINE DISORDERS

Hypothyroidism

Abnormal thyroid function will produce several kinds of nervous system dysfunction if it persists long enough. The severely hypothyroid patient will have psychomotor slowing, abnormal ("hung-up") deep tendon reflexes, and a flat affect. Systemic signs will include coarse hair, thickening of the skin, and hypothermia (8). The severe organic mental syndrome that may develop with hypothyroidism is called myxedema madness and involves disorientation, impaired memory, global confusion, and problems with concentration (60,61). Affective disorders also develop with this dementia, the most prominent feature of this mood disturbance usually being depression. Associated neurologic signs include clumsiness from cerebellar dysfunction, hand numbness and weakness from median nerve compression at the wrist (carpal tunnel syndrome), impaired hearing, and generalized weakness associated with peripheral nerve dysfunctions (61). Suspecting abnormal thyroid function in a patient with all of these signs and symptoms is unavoidable.

When hypothyroidism is relatively mild and only slowly progressive, typical systemic signs of myxedema may be inapparent, whereas psychiatric symptoms may be quite prominent. The mildly hypothyroid patient may have a severe depression with prominent paranoid features as the principal neuropsychiatric symptom (89). Systemic signs of hypothyroidism are easily overlooked in these psychotically aggressive individuals. Low serum levels of triiodothyronine (T3) or thyroxine (T4) will establish the diagnosis. Measurements of thyroid stimulating hormone will help determine whether the hypothyroidism is primary or secondary to pituitary insufficiency. Radionuclide studies of thyroid function are helpful in equivocal cases.

The treatment in all cases of hypothyroidism is replacement of the missing hormone. Thyroid replacement must be gradual, regardless of how severe the systemic signs of hypothyroidism are, because an abrupt jump in the serum thyroxine level may exacerbate the psychosis (89). In nonpsychotic patients thyroid replacement may provoke complaints of irritability and anxiety. The patient feels "pushed" if the thyroid replacement is advanced precipitately, and poor compliance may be misconstrued as a psychologic reaction to medication intervention rather than the endocrine response it actually represents. The later in life the hypothyroid cognitive disorders first appear, the more likely they are to be completely reversible.

Other Endocrine Disorders

Hyperthyroidism may produce a severe dementia without the agitation usually seen in overactivity of the thyroid (8). This is called apathetic hyperthyroidism and may be reversed with treatment of the hyperthyroidism. With excessive corticosteroid production, as in Cushing syndrome, the patient may develop a diffuse cognitive disorder, but this is routinely associated with changes in facial and body appearance to suggest the appropriate diagnosis (8). Overactivity of the glands responsible for these two disorders, the thyroid and adrenal glands, is easily assessed by measuring the substances they produce, specifically thyroxine and triiodothyronine for the thyroid and cortisol for the adrenal. A variety of medical and surgical approaches are used to decrease the activity of such hyperactive glands.

An elevated serum calcium will develop with metastatic bone tumors, sarcoidosis, and protracted immobilization, but the cause most amenable to treatment is overactivity of the parathyroid glands. Hyperparathyroidism is commonly associated with depression, constipation, fatigue, and weight loss, but occasional patients will have profound confusion and disorientation as well (90). Forty-two percent of patients with primary hyperparathyroidism have psychiatric and neuromuscular signs and symptoms (91). Headache develops in 50 percent of the patients with neuropsychiatric symptoms, the pain usually being described as a continuous dull ache (91). Psychiatric disorders range from acute depressive reactions to psychotic aggressive behavior. Florid paranoid states with hallucinations and periods of apparent catatonia are well described in primary hyperparathyroidism (91). Amnestic states and generalized dementia may also develop (91). The altered mentation is routinely associated with an elevated serum calcium level, but when the calcium level is not checked the patient may be mistaken for schizophrenic. Skull films will help make the diagnosis of hyperparathyroidism because the cranial vault may have a "salt and pepper" appearance and the dense lamina dura usually outlining the roots of the teeth will be lost (90). Primary hyperparathyroidism is treated by removing some of the parathyroid glands. If the disorder is secondary to kidney disease, management of the renal problem is essential.

MINIMAL BRAIN DYSFUNCTION

Behavior disorders of childhood occasionally develop with cognitive or perceptual problems (92). Presumably, the intellectual handicap interferes with the child's ability to learn social skills and to develop self-restraint. Children with intellectual impairment fostering behavior disorders usually exhibit hyperactivity, impulsivity, short attention spans, destructiveness, and emotional lability (93). The currently popular term for this syndrome is minimal brain dysfunction (10). As this name implies, signs of focal neurologic damage are generally slight, if at all present. Children with severe brain damage often have behavior disorders, but they are generally not included in the diagnostic category of minimal brain dysfunction unless the focal neurologic deficits present can be elicited only on careful neurologic examination. The profound impairment of attention span often suggests that the child has a hearing problem, and, in fact, subtle auditory or visual deficits do play a role in rare children with this behavior disorder (92). Because there are no obvious focal neurologic signs in most affected children, many children with behavior disorders alone are labeled victims of minimal brain dysfunction with the inherent assumption that they have organic brain disease. Despite this potential for misdiagnosis, the concept of minimal brain dysfunction is useful and probably fairly accurate.

The hyperactivity observed in these children is an excessive restlessness or inappropriate, purposeless movement (94). This is not simply an excess of energy that the child can channel into effective exploratory behavior; learning and exploration are effectively blocked by the chaotic nature of the child's behavior. Misconduct is totally refractory to punishment, and the sharp mood swings characteristic of these children are apparent as early as infancy (94). Infants who later exhibit minimal brain dysfunction sleep poorly and cry readily. Even before they can exhibit much independent activity, these individuals are a substantial burden to their parents.

Neurologic Bases

This is a frequently diagnosed disorder, and it clearly occurs more frequently in children with unequivocal central nervous system disease than in those with no disease at all. As many as 3 percent of school age children exhibit features of minimal brain dysfunction. Boys are affected four times as often as girls (92). Thirty-four percent of children with unequivocal central nervous system disease have behavior, personality, or other psychiatric disorders (93). This is not surprising since children with obvious brain damage have long been recognized as being more susceptible to psychiatric disturbances. Psychiatric problems are five times as common in children with epilepsy, cerebral palsy, and other neurologic diseases as in children in the general population (93). This is not just a reaction to being handicapped. Children with nonneurologic handicaps are much less often affected by these behavior and personality disorders (93).

The kind of psychiatric problem that develops in brain-damaged children is sometimes fairly specific for the kind of brain damage suffered. Children who have had viral encephalitis often develop extrapyramidal movement disorders as evidence of the brain injury, and along with this motor problem they will develop hyperkinetic personality disorders and severely limited capacities for abstraction. With anoxic brain damage at birth, the child is at considerable risk of developing at least some features of minimal brain dysfunction (92). Many of the children who contracted encephalitis during the great epidemic of von Economo's encephalitis in 1918 and survived developed restlessness, easy distractibility, destructive behavior, and poor social skills (92). Head injuries, heavy-metal poisonings, and early childhood central nervous system infections can all lead to signs and symptoms of minimal brain dysfunction. Clearly, structural disease in the brain can produce this hyperactive behavior pattern. What remains a problem for both psychiatrists and neurologists is confidently making the diagnosis of minimal brain dysfunction in the children who have hyperactive, destructive behavior with no associated nervous system disease (93).

Psychologic Characteristics

Children diagnosed as having minimal brain dysfunction are typically in constant motion. Their boundless energy is reflected in profound restlessness and short attention spans. Emotional swings are wide and include temper tantrums, unprovoked attacks, and low tolerance levels (93). This destructive, erratic behavior is extremely frustrating for the parents of the child and often provokes exaggerated permissiveness or extreme rejection of the child by the parents (93). Because these children do not integrate into social groups outside the family, they become an even greater burden on the family. They often see themselves as peculiar and act with even more license because of the differences they sense between themselves and their peers (92). In addition to these social and psychologic problems, children with unequivocal brain damage or dysfunction as the basis for their minimal brain dysfunction usually exhibit easily detected deficits in speech and motor performance (93). Perseveration and learning impairments are noticeable even before the child enters school (93). The intellectual level of most children with minimal brain dysfunction is low normal. They have poor auditory and visual memories (92). Growing out of these limitations are problems with reading and spelling. Motor disorders may be substantial enough to interfere with running, jumping, and tasks requiring fine coordination.

As the child matures, the physical hyperactivity abates during the second decade of life (94). Unfortunately, the intellectual hyperactivity often persists. Their persistent emotional lability and inattentiveness continues to interfere with their learning, and sociopathic behavior will often become a prominent feature of the child's activity.

Clinical Evaluation

The evaluation of children with suspected minimal brain dysfunction should include a careful general examination. Head circumference, stature, skin pigmentation, palmar creases, and general appearance should all be evaluated critically to be sure that a congenital problem is not responsible for the central nervous system disorder (92). Chromosomal analysis is appropriate, and a careful family history may be helpful in uncovering hereditary disorders. An electroencephalogram should be done, but it may be normal even if a seizure disorder is associated with the minimal brain dysfunction. A computed tomogram of the head will reveal any significant structural lesions in the brain. Lead and other reasonable heavy-metal poisons should be sought in the blood. Formal psychologic tests will provide an overview of the child's strengths and weaknesses, which will allow a more effective teaching program to be tailored to the potentials of the individual child.

Treatment

Although most conditions causing minimal brain dysfunction cannot be cured, the affected individual can be treated symptomatically. Perinatal brain injuries cause static encephalopathies: the damage done to the brain does not progress, but it does not resolve either. The symptoms associated with the static central nervous system disorder can be ameliorated with a variety of drugs. The hyperactivity may abate considerably when the child is treated with a central nervous system stimulant. Dextroamphetamine sulfate at doses of 5 to 30 milligrams a day or methylphenidate at 10 to 60 milligrams a day are the two most commonly used stimulants (92,93). If stimulants fail, phenothiazines or butyrophenones are reasonable alternatives, but these drugs often interfere with school performance, even if they decrease the level of hyperactivity (93). The social environment also affects the child's behavior. Traditional educational settings usually fail to teach the child basic skills, and the child's disruptiveness in that setting exacerbates his social isolation. A highly structured environment with clearly defined expectations is essential in educating these children (94). They require individual attention throughout the teaching period and a minimum of potentially distracting elements in the teaching environment.

The family will need as much support and encouragement as the child. Dealing with a child with minimal brain dysfunction is extremely frustrating for parents and siblings. Rather than profiting from the families attention, the child may simply learn to manipulate it by using extremes of behavior to elicit the desired responses from the family. Minimal brain dysfunction is a family problem in a very real sense and psychiatric intervention for individuals with minimal brain dysfunction is most often valuable if it involves the entire family. Parents who become deeply involved in the psychiatric treatment of the affected child while ignoring the resentment of the other children in the family provide a destabilizing environment for the "patient." Even when there are no other children in the family, the excessive dedication of one parent to the child's treatment may disrupt the family by alienating the neglected spouse. Any family with an affected child must be aware of the chronicity of minimal brain dysfunction. Although the hyperactivity and distractibility will lessen with age, the adolescent and young adult who exhibited minimal brain dysfunction as a child will commonly have substantial psychiatric problems (92). Social ineptness and sociopathic behavior are characteristic of the individual as he matures (92).

COGNITIVE DISORDERS WITH NEUROLEPTIC AND ANTIDEPRESSANT TREATMENT

Cognitive disorders occasionally develop as a side effect of antipsychotic drugs, but this is relatively uncommon and fairly obvious when it does occur. On initiating neuroleptic treatment, the most common side effect is sedation, but elderly patients may become profoundly disoriented (95).

Phenothiazines, butyrophenones, and monoamine oxidase inhibitors generally do not disturb memory, but tricyclic antidepressants may (14). With tricyclic antidepressants, as with phenothiazines, the elderly are most susceptible, and the principal manifestation of the drug's toxicity is an acute confusional state with hallucinations and amnesia for the period of disorientation (14). Stopping the responsible drug is essential, but other antipsychotic or antidepressant medication can usually be introduced without substantial risk of precipitating more intellectual or perceptual problems.

DIAGNOSTIC APPROACHES TO COGNITIVE DISORDERS

Every patient with a cognitive disorder must have a careful neurologic examination. In many cases this involves little more than a comprehensive history and physical examination with special attention to signs and symptoms of neurologic disease. From the preceding discussion it is apparent that the number of laboratory tests that could be performed as part of the investigation of the cognitive disorder is enormous; which ones should be performed will be dictated by the precise character of the intellectual or perceptual disorder and by the signs and symptoms associated with the cognitive problem. Vitamin B_{12} levels will be almost invariably normal if they are obtained routinely on every patient with impaired insight and attention, but they will provide valuable information if they are checked whenever the patient has impaired position sense and a spastic gait associated with the intellectual disorder. Certain laboratory tests should be routinely used, and some should be reserved for patients with specific signs or symptoms.

Reasonable screening tests for any patient with diffuse cognitive problems include a complete blood count with a differential of the white blood cells, serum electrolyte measurements, and serologic tests for syphilis. The variety of dementias that can be caused by thyroid disease and by collagen vascular diseases justifies the evaluation of serum thyroid factors (T3, T4, thyroid stimulating hormone), erythrocyte sedimentation rate, antinuclear antibody, lupus erythematosus (LE) cell prep, and rheumatoid factor in any patient with intellectual or perceptual problems. An electrocardiogram and chest x-ray will help exclude cardiopulmonary irregularities as factors in the appearance of an intellectual deficit. A bedridden patient who develops an acute psychosis should have arterial blood gas studies because of the high probability that the episode was precipitated by a pulmonary embolus causing severe hypoxia. Investigations of liver function and renal function with venous blood studies are more routinely in order than an arterial blood study. A routine urinalysis may provide the initial evidence of a metabolic disorder and is consequently justifiable for every patient with a cognitive disorder.

If these routine systemic studies reveal no abnormalities, more specific examinations of the brain should be performed. Even when a diffuse dementia is not apparent, an electroencephalogram should be obtained to be sure there is no metabolic encephalopathy or progressive degenerative disease. A routine skull radiogram will uncover very few of the patients with organic brain disease even when a brain tumor is causing the cognitive problem, but it is so innocuous and inexpensive a test that it is as reasonable a study for every patient admitted with a cognitive dysfunction as is a serologic study for syphilis. Computed tomography of the head is an increasingly available method for revealing structural brain lesions, and a precontrast study of the whole brain is an appropriate screening test for any patient with intellectual dysfunction. Cost and availability currently limit the application of this radiographic study.

Most invasive studies require a more discriminating approach. Cerebrospinal fluid examination is informative; but, unless there is reason to suspect a chronic infection or acute hemorrhage, it is not justifiable as a routine test. The patient with a positive serology for syphilis who has no history of treatment for the infection must have a cerebrospinal fluid examination to assess the likelihood of neurosyphilis. Patients on immunosuppression or with diseases, such as lymphomas, that suppress normal body defenses should have lumbar punctures at the first appearance of altered mentation, because they are at high risk for unusual central nervous system infections, such as cryptococcal meningitis.

The investigation of cognitive disorders should focus on treatable causes of intellectual dysfunction, but the diagnosis of untreatable lesions is also valuable. A clear impression of what the patient's disease is enables the family and the physician involved to decide what resources should be used in managing the patient. A patient with Alzheimer disease cannot profit from psychiatric treatment, and confidently establishing that diagnosis will relieve the family and the physician from the responsibility of dealing with that patient's confused behavior in a psychiatric setting. Huntington disease is not a curable disease, but establishing it as the basis for a suicide attempt spares the physician considerable fruitless effort in looking for the motivation behind the self-destructive gesture. Knowing what motivated bizarre or dangerous behavior also relieves the family of considerable anxiety. If an organic brain syndrome provoked an attack on a family member, much of the guilt and fear prompted by such an action can be dissipated by explaining to the family that there was no hidden motivation behind the incident.

FAMILY COUNSELING

One of the more important elements that the physician must deal with when he is responsible for an intellectually impaired individual is the family surrounding that individual. Obviously, the problems faced by the family are different with different kinds of cognitive disorders, and certain types of patients will be a factor in only certain families. Minimal brain dysfunction will disrupt the lives of parents and siblings, whereas Alzheimer disease will have an impact primarily upon a spouse and adult children. The central problem for the family of a disturbed child is often behavior modification and education; the central problem for the family confronted with a demented elderly individual is usually providing supervision and supportive care. The common factor in all families disrupted by an organic brain syndrome affecting one of its members is the patient himself. The victim of the disease assumes a dependent role, which is new to the family even when the victim is a child. Some families choose to deny that there is a problem; some reject all responsibility for the patient; and some become obsessed with the care and comfort of the intellectually disabled member, much to the detriment of other family members.

Individuals unfamiliar with organic brain syndromes usually do not readily comprehend exactly what the patient's impairments are. Parents, siblings, or children of the intellectually impaired individual routinely treat him as if he were still competent and rational. Although they can readily perceive that a paralyzed limb is no longer able to perform coordinated acts, they hesitate or simply fail to perceive that the intellectual impairments obvious in the patient's statements and acts make him incompetent to direct his own affairs or, for that matter, the family's affairs. A delirious patient may refuse an essential examination, such as a spinal tap, and the involved family members will frequently rally in support of the patient's decision. This is a reasonable reaction for a family dealing with an intact relative; but, when the patient is having paranoid delusions and meningitis is a likely cause of these delusions, such an irrational alliance can be lethal. More commonly, the confused or delusional patient accuses family members of wrongdoing or of abandoning him. The truly concerned relatives are especially likely to take these accusations seriously and try fruitlessly to convince the intellectually impaired patient that he is mistaken. The physician can simplify much of his interaction with the family by explaining to the concerned relatives what the intellectual or cognitive impairment will mean in terms of the patient's insight and judgment. The futility of trying to reason with a demented patient is not intuitively obvious to individuals who have spent years dealing with a recently disabled family member as a responsible person. Viewing the disabled relative differently takes time simply because the old individual is still seen and the new disabilities are initially overlooked.

Neurologic problems are often overlooked for months or years because the affected individual faces skepticism from his family when he complains. This skepticism may persist even after neurologic investigations have established that the patient has an organic lesion. In most cases nothing more malicious is involved then denial of a distressing situation. Despite this, this patient is left isolated and feels obliged to be defensive. This occurs most commonly when a spouse is sick. The threat of a serious illness induces the healthy spouse to dismiss the sick individual's complaints as simply neurotic. This situation can occasionally be defused by confronting the skeptical spouse with his or her refusal to view the partner's illness seriously. Recognizing the healthy member's denial of the illness in the family allows all members of the family to discuss the difficulties imposed upon them by one member's being ill. If the physician does not convince the family or the healthy spouse that the patient needs help with a physical illness, the patient and the physician may find that they have no help available to them from the family when it is most needed.

The most difficult situation for the physician to deal with is abandonment of the patient by his family. Recognizing that a serious and, perhaps, untreatable illness is disabling a family member, the remaining family members may choose to simply deny all responsibility for the sick individual's care. If the sick individual is a child with complex partial seizures, the abandonment can effectively block all efforts to control the patient's seizure disorder. Compliance is a major problem in epileptic individuals with family problems, but it becomes an insurmountable problem when the patient's illness alienates him from the important figures in his life. Sometimes family members are unaware of their estrangement from the patient. When the rejection is this subtle, there is some hope that open discussion of the family's reaction to the illness will minimize the patient's isolation. More forthright abandonment is not amenable to intervention by the physician or mental health professional.

Illness usually affects more than one individual, regardless of the type of illness. Recognizing and dealing with the other individuals affected by the illness often increases the feasibility of good medical or psychiatric care of the disabled person. A helpful family is a valuable asset in the evaluation and treatment of any individual with a cognitive disorder.

REFERENCES

1. Owens DGC, Johnstone EC, Bydder GM, et al: Unsuspected organic disease in chronic schizophrenia demonstrated by computed tomography. *J Neurol Neurosurg Psychiatry* 43:1065, 1980.
2. Post F: Dementia, depression, and pseudodementia, in Benson DF, Blumer D (eds): *Psychiatric Aspects of Neurologic Disease.* New York, Grune & Stratton, 1975, p 99.
3. Harlow JM: Recovery from passage of an iron bar through the head. *Publ Mass Med Soc* 2:329, 1868.
4. Braff DL, Beck AT: Thinking disorder in depression. *Arch Gen Psychiatry* 31:456, 1974.
5. Plum F: Prospects for research on schizophrenia: Neuropathological findings. *Neurosci Res Program Bull* 10:384, 1972.
6. Browne TR: Case records of the Massachusetts General Hospital: Case 43-1977. *N Engl J Med* 297:930, 1977.
7. Snyder SH, Aghajanian GK, Matthysse S: Drug induced psychoses. *Neurosci Res Program Bull* 10:430, 1972.
8. Wells CE: Geriatric organic psychoses. *Psychiatr Ann* 8:466, 1978.
9. DeVaul RA, Hall RCW: Hallucinations, in Hall RCW (ed): *Psychiatric Presentations of Medical Illness.* New York, SP Medical and Scientific Books, 1980, p 91.
10. Task force on nomenclature and statistics, American Psychiatric Association: *Diagnostic and Statistical Manual of Mental Disorders (Third Edition).* Washington, DC, American Psychiatric Association, 1980.

11. Weston MJ, Whitlock FA: The Capgras syndrome following head injury. *Br J Psychiatry* 119:25, 1971.
12. Harner RN: EEG evaluation of the patient with dementia, in Benson DF, Blumer D (eds): *Psychiatric Aspects of Neurologic Disease.* New York, Grune & Stratton, 1975, p 63.
13. Piercy MF: Experimental studies of the organic amnesic syndrome, in Whitty CWM, Zangwill OL (eds): *Amnesia. Clinical, Psychological and Medicolegal Aspects,* ed 2. London, Butterworths, 1977, p 1.
14. Whitty CWM, Stores G, Lishman WA: Amnesia in cerebral disease, in Whitty CWM, Zangwill OL (eds): *Amnesia. Clinical, Psychological and Medicolegal Aspects,* ed 2. London, Butterworths, 1977, p 52.
15. Lezak MD: Recovery of memory and learning functions following traumatic brain injury. *Cortex* 15:63, 1979.
16. Brooks DN, Aughton ME, Bond MR, et al: Cognitive sequelae in relationship to early indices of severity of brain damage after severe blunt head injury. *J Neurol Neurosurg Psychiatry* 43:529, 1980.
17. Artiola I, Fortuny L, Briggs M, et al: Measuring the duration of post traumatic amnesia. *J Neurol Neurosurg Psychiatry* 43:377, 1980.
18. LeDoux JE, Barclay L, Premack A: The brain and cognitive sciences. *Ann Neurol* 4:391, 1978.
19. Jacobson RL, Farmer TW: The "hypernormal" CT scan in dementia: Bilateral isodense subdural hematomas. *Neurology (NY)* 29:1522, 1979.
20. Mayeux R, Alexander MP, Benson DF, et al: Poriomania. *Neurology (NY)* 29:1616, 1979.
21. Heilman KM, Van Den Abell T: Right Hemisphere dominance for attention: The mechanism underlying hemispheric asymmetries of inattention (neglect). *Neurology (NY)* 30:327, 1980.
22. Webb WL Jr, Gehi M: Electrolyte and fluid imbalance: Neuropsychiatric manifestations. *Psychosomatics* 22:199, 1981.
23. Pratt RTC: Psychogenic loss of memory, in Whitty CWM, Zangwill OL (eds): *Amnesia. Clinical, Psychological and Medicolegal Aspects,* ed 2. London, Butterworths, 1977, p 224.
24. Blumer D: Temporal lobe epilepsy and its psychiatric significance, in Benson DF, Blumer D (eds): *Psychiatric Aspects of Neurologic Disease.* New York, Grune & Stratton, 1975, p 171.
25. Sherwin I, Geschwind N: Neural substrates of behavior, in Nicholi AM (ed): *The Harvard Guide to Modern Psychiatry.* Cambridge, MA, Belknap Press, 1978, p 59.
26. Whitty CWM: Transient Global Amnesia, in Whitty CWM, Zangwill OL (eds): *Amnesia. Clinical, Psychological and Medicolegal Aspects,* ed 2. London, Butterworths, 1977, p 93.
27. Shuttleworth EC, Morris CE: The transient global amnesia syndrome. *Arch Neurol* 15:515, 1966.
28. Mazzucchi A, Moretti G, Caffarra P, et al: Neuropsychological functions in the follow-up of transient global amnesia. *Brain* 103:161, 1980.
29. Corsellis JAN, Goldberg GJ, Norton AR: "Limbic encephalitis" and its association with carcinoma. *Brain* 91:481, 1968.
30. Lehrich JR: Case records of the Massachusetts General Hospital: Case 44-1979. *N Engl J Med* 301:987, 1979.
31. Mohan KJ, Salo MW, Nagaswami S: A case of limbic system dysfunction with hypersexuality and fugue state. *Dis Nerv Syst* 36:621, 1975.
32. Taylor AR, Chakravorty BC: Clinical syndromes associated with basilar impression. *Arch Neurol* 10:475, 1964.
33. Mercer B, Wapner W, Gardner H, et al: A study of confabulation. *Arch Neurol* 34:429, 1977.

34. Kapur N, Coughlan AK: Confabulation and frontal lobe dysfunction. *J Neurol Neurosurg Psychiatry* 43:461, 1980.
35. Adams RD, Victor M: *Principles of Neurology*. New York, McGraw Hill, 1977.
36. Mair WGP, Warrington EKL, Weiskrantz L: Memory disorder in Korsakoff's psychosis. *Brain* 102:749, 1979.
37. Geschwind N: Neurological foundations of language, in Myklebust HR (ed): *Progress in Learning Disabilities*. New York, Grune & Stratton, 1968, vol I, p 182.
38. Gerstmann J: Psychological and phenomenological aspects of disorders of the body image. *J Nerv Ment Dis* 126:499, 1958.
39. Lishman WA: *Organic Psychiatry*. London, Blackwell, 1980.
40. Teuber HL: Prospects for research on schizophrenia: Effects of focal brain lesions. *Neurosci Res Program Bull* 10:381, 1972.
41. Valenstein E, Heilman KM: Unilateral hypokinesia and motor extinction. *Neurology (NY)* 31:445, 1981.
42. Sisler GC: Psychiatric disorder associated with head injury, in Hendrie HC (ed): *The Psychiatric Clinics of North America*. Philadelphia, WB Saunders, 1978, vol 1, p 137.
43. Stevens JR: Interictal clinical manifestations of complex partial seizures. *Neurol* 11:85, 1975.
44. Grossman RG: Treatment of patients with intracranial hematomas. *N Engl J Med* 304:1540, 1981.
45. Seelig JM, Becker DP, Miller JD, et al: Traumatic acute subdural hematoma: Major mortality reduction in comatose patients treated within four hours. *N Engl J Med* 304:1511, 1981.
46. Benson DF, Segarra J, Albert ML: Visual agnosia-prosopagnosia. *Arch Neurol* 30:307, 1974.
47. Hecaen H, Albert ML: Disorders of mental functioning related to frontal lobe pathology, in Benson DF, Blumer D (eds): *Psychiatric Aspects of Neurologic Disease*. New York, Grune & Stratton, 1975, p 137.
48. Mayeux R, Brandt J, Rosen J, et al: Interictal memory and language impairment in temporal lobe epilepsy. *Neurology (NY)* 30:120, 1980.
49. Slater E, Beard AW: The schizophrenia-like psychoses of epilepsy. i. Psychiatric aspects. *Br J Psychiatry* 109:95, 1963.
50. Johnson RT: Viral etiology in amentia and dementia, in Katzman R (ed): *Congenital and Acquired Cognitive Disorders*. New York, Raven Press, 1979, p 177.
51. Whitley RJ, Soong S-J, Hirsch MS, et al: Herpes simplex encephalitis. *N Engl J Med* 304:313, 1981.
52. Davies JA, Hughes JT, Oppenheimer DR: Richardson's disease (progressive multifocal leukoencephalopathy). *Q J Med* 42:481, 1973.
53. Glew RH: Case presentations of the Massachusetts General Hospital: Case 27-1979. *N Engl J Med* 301:34, 1979.
54. Hall WH, Choppin PW: Measles-virus proteins in the brain tissue of patients with subacute sclerosing panencephalitis. *N Engl J Med* 304:1152, 1981.
55. Bennett R, Hughes GRV, Bywaters EGL, et al: Neuropsychiatric problems in systemic lupus erythematosus. *Br Med J* 4:342, 1972.
56. Sherwin I, Seltzer B: Senile and presenile dementia: A clinical overview, in Nandy K, Sherwin I (eds): *The Aging Brain and Senile Dementia*. New York, Plenum Press, 1977, p 285.
57. Wells CE: Chronic brain disease: An overview. *Am J Psychiatry* 135:1, 1975.
58. Terry RD: Dementia. *Arch Neurol* 33:1, 1976.

59. Kaszniak AW, Garron DC, Fox JH, et al: Cerebral atrophy, EEG slowing, age, education, and cognitive functioning in suspected dementia. *Neurology (NY)* 29:1273, 1979.

60. Sachar EJ: Psychiatric disturbances in endocrine disease: some issues for research, in Plum F (ed): *Brain Dysfunction in Metabolic Disorders*. New York, Raven Press, 1974, p 239.

61. Ettigi PG, Brown GM: Brain disorders associated with endocrine dysfunctions, in Hendrie HC (ed): *The Psychiatric Clinics of North America*. Philadelphia, WB Saunders, 1978, vol 1, p 117.

62. Prick JJG: Thallium poisoning, in Vinken PJ, Bruyn GW (eds): *Handbook of Clinical Neurology*. New York, American Elsevier, 1979, vol 36, p 239.

63. McHugh PR, Folstein MF: Psychopathology of dementia: Implications for neuropathology, in Katzman R (ed): *Congenital and Acquired Cognitive Disorders*. New York, Raven Press, 1979, p 17.

64. Boller F, Mizutani T, Roessmann U, et al: Parkinson disease, dementia, and Alzheimer disease: Clinicopathological correlations. *Ann Neurol* 7:329, 1980.

65. Fox JH, Kazniak AW, Huckman M: Computerized tomographic scanning not very helpful in dementia. *N Engl J Med* 300:437, 1979.

66. Kaszniak AW, Fox J, Gandell DL, et al: Predictors of mortality in presenile and senile dementia. *Ann Neurol* 3:246, 1978.

67. Delaney JF: Spinal fluid aluminum levels in patients with Alzheimer disease. *Ann Neurol* 5:580, 1979.

68. Renvoize EB, Jerram T: Choline in Alzheimer's disease. *N Engl J Med* 301:330, 1979.

69. Friedman E, Sherman KA, Ferris SH, et al: Clinical response to choline plus piracetam in senile dementia: Relation to red-cell choline levels. *N Engl J Med* 304:1490, 1981.

70. Ruff RL, Russakoff LM: Catatonia with frontal lobe atrophy. *J Neurol Neurosurg Psychiatry* 43:185, 1980.

71. Steele JC: Progressive supranuclear palsy. *Brain* 95:693, 1972.

72. Morariu MA: Progressive supranuclear palsy and normal pressure hydrocephalus. *Neurology (NY)* 29:1544, 1979.

73. Steele JC, Richardson JC, Olszewski J: Progressive supranuclear palsy. *Arch Neurol* 10:333, 1964.

74. Haldeman S, Goldman JW, Hyde J, et al: Progressive supranuclear palsy, computed tomography, and response to antiparkinsonian drugs. *Neurology (NY)* 31:442, 1981.

75. Hornabrook RW: Kuru—A subacute cerebellar degeneration. The natural history and clinical features. *Brain* 91:53, 1968.

76. Gajdusek DC: Unconventional viruses and the origin and disappearance of kuru. *Science* 197:943, 1977.

77. Roos R, Gajdusek DC, Gibbs CJ: The clinical characteristics of transmissible Creutzfeldt-Jakob disease. *Brain* 96:1, 1973.

78. Brown P, Cathala F, Sadowsky D, et al: Creutzfeldt-Jakob disease in France: II. Clinical characteristics of 124 consecutive verified cases during the decade 1968–1977. *Ann Neurol* 6:430, 1979.

79. Chou SM, Martin JD: Kuru-plaques in a case of Creutzfeldt-Jakob disease. *Acta Neuropathol (Berl)* 17:150, 1971.

80. McHugh PR, Folstein MF: Psychiatric syndromes of Huntington's chorea: A clinical and phenomenologic study, in Benson DF, Blumer D (eds): *Psychiatric Aspects of Neurologic Disease*. New York, Grune & Stratton, 1975, p 267.

81. Mayer V, Orolin D, Mitrova E, et al: Transmissible virus dementia. I. An unusual space and time clustering of Creutzfeldt-Jakob disease and of other organic presenile dementia cases. *Acta Virol (Praha)* 22:146, 1978.

82. Mitrova E, Mayer V, Orolin D: Transmissible virus dementia II. Neurohistology of three geographically clustered cases of Creutzfeldt-Jakob disease. *Acta Virol (Praha)* 22:154, 1978.

83. Gloor P: EEG characteristics in Creutzfeldt-Jakob disease. *Ann Neurol* 8:341, 1980.

84. Spiro HR, Schimke RN, Welch JP: Schizophrenia in a patient with a defect in methionine metabolism. *J Nerv Ment Dis* 141:285, 1965.

85. Hakim S, Adams RD: The special clinical problem of symptomatic hydrocephalus with normal cerebrospinal fluid pressure: Observations on cerebrospinal fluid hydrodynamics. *J Neurol Sci* 2:307, 1965.

86. Shukla D, Singh BM, Strobos RJ: Hypertensive cerebrovascular disease and normal pressure hydrocephalus. *Neurology (NY)* 30:998, 1980.

87. Wolf JK, Santana HB, Thorpy M: Treatment of "emotional incontinence" with levodopa. *Neurology (NY)* 29:1435, 1979.

88. Malamud N: Psychiatric disorder with intracranial tumors of limbic system. *Arch Neurol* 17:113, 1967.

89. Easson WM: Myxedema psychosis—Insanity defense in homicide. *J Clin Psychiatry* 41:316, 1980.

90. Gatewood JW, Organ CH, Mead BT: Mental changes associated with hyperparathyroidism. *Am J Psychiatry* 132:129, 1975.

91. Karpati G, Frame B: Neuropsychiatric disorders in primary hyperparathyroidism. *Arch Neurol* 10:387, 1964.

92. Hart EJ, Carter S: Minimal brain dysfunction, in Downey JA, Low NL (eds): *The Child with Disabling Illness.* Philadelphia, WB Saunders, 1974, p 255.

93. Lucas AR, Goodlund LS: Clinical management of children with brain disorders, in Hendrie HC (ed): *The Psychiatric Clinics of North America.* Philadelphia, WB Saunders, 1978, vol 1, p 179.

94. Denckla MB, Heilman KM: The syndrome of hyperactivity, in Heilman KM, Valenstein E (eds): *Clinical Neuropsychology.* New York, Oxford University Press, 1979, p 574.

95. Goetz CG, Dysken MW, Klawans HL Jr: Assessment and treatment of drug-induced tremor. *J Clin Psychiatry* 41:310, 1980.

7 Affective Disorders

Affective disorders develop acutely or chronically with diseases disrupting normal brain function. They usually involve only one or two elements of the patient's range of emotions when organic brain disease is responsible. The pattern of functional disturbance with affective disorders contrasts with that developing with cognitive disorders that have an organic basis. Dementing illnesses will compromise memory, language, calculations, constructions, and abstractions simultaneously; but affective disorders will produce depression, euphoria, violence, or anxiety selectively. Individual elements of the patient's affect are disturbed, and, although some patients with organic brain disease do become psychotic, the mood disturbance need not evolve into a psychosis. Structural lesions and physiologic disturbances in the brain alter the emotions and personalities of affected individuals, but they do not necessarily cause pathologic personality traits or affective disorders (1,2). The duration of the affective disorder and the patient's reaction to it are quite variable. Mood disturbances may be transient or persistent. In some cases the patient is aware of the change and is concerned about it; in others, he is unaware or indifferent. The character of the affective change, the duration of the change, and the patient's reaction to it are all helpful in determining the cause of the mood or behavior disturbance.

The anatomic and physiologic bases for abnormal emotional responses are still controversial even though there have been many, highly invasive studies of the brain over the past few decades involving both experimental animals and humans (3–8). From these investigations it did become clear that the notion of an "emotional brain" sequestered from the remainder of the brain was an oversimplification. "Papez circuit" and the "limbic lobe" are now largely of historic interest; these terms referred to restricted segments of the human brain thought to comprise the emotional brain (9–12). Although the concept of an emotional circuit in the brain was brilliant and useful when it was introduced, the anatomic and physiologic information available to Papez and other early investigators was considerably more limited than it is now. Insights accrued since Papez's original suggestions have made it clear that the structural and functional bases for emotion are exceedingly complex. Structures ranging from the brainstem to the cerebral cortex play roles in various emotions and, consequently, in various affective disorders.

STRUCTURAL ELEMENTS IN EMOTIONS

The so-called limbic lobe includes structures skirting the third ventricle and exhibiting extensive connections with the temporal and frontal lobes. That these parts of the brain were structurally related to each other was suggested by Broca in 1878, and that they had a functional relationship was developed by Papez 6 decades later (9,10). Papez suggested that the cingulate gyrus, hippocampus, fornix, mammillary bodies, and anterior thalamus formed a circuit that was completed by projections from the anterior thalamus back to the cingulate gyrus and that this circuit was important in emotions (10).

Structures phylogenetically derived from parts of the brain involved with smell seemed to be especially important in the functioning of this emotional brain. The importance of these olfactory structures was apparently overstated. It is true that anosmia, the loss of the ability to smell, will disrupt sexual, aggressive, territorial, and maternal behavior in experimental animals, but these changes only develop when the olfactory bulbs are removed (3). Anosmia induced by zinc sulphate will not cause these changes (3). Destructive lesions in the septal region, a gray matter structure in front of the third ventricle with close ties to olfactory structures, do produce affective changes in some patients. Tumors in the septal region occasionally produce rage attacks and irritability in humans. Electrical stimulation of this area in several species will cause sexual arousal (13).

The temporal lobes also seemed to be strategic elements in the emotional brain, and, as more insight into affective disorders accrued, the importance of this part of the cerebrum was confirmed. Inappropriate affect, ambivalence, and antisocial behavior can all develop with temporal lobe tumors, whether or not the patient has temporal lobe epilepsy (14). Bilateral temporal lobe destruction produces marked blunting of affect, often called placidity (13). With mesial temporal lesions, that is damage to the inner face of the temporal lobe, the patient may have recurrent episodes of intense fear or despair (14). Anhedonia, the inability to realize satisfaction or enjoyment from ordinarily satisfying events, appears with temporal, as well as frontal and upper brainstem, lesions (14). The inner face of the temporal lobe is an especially common site for lesions producing anhedonia (14).

Emotional Dominance

A factor in the elaboration of emotions given virtually no attention until just 10 years ago is the interaction of the two cerebral hemispheres. One hemisphere may, in fact, exert a dominant influence over the other. Dominance is clearly exerted by one hemisphere over the other in several functions including speech and handedness, the functions for which the idea of dominance was first proposed. Visuospatial manipulations, facial recognition, musical functions, and perhaps several components of emotion are primarily dependent upon the 'nondominant' hemisphere. The right cerebral hemisphere is almost always nondominant for speech and handedness; that is, it exhibits considerably less of a role in the comprehension and production of language and the elaboration of rapid, precise hand and finger movements than does the left hemisphere. If one hemisphere has an especially weighty role to play in the elaboration of emotions, that is, a dominance in affect, it is probably the right hemisphere (16). The cognitive style of the left hemisphere is analytic: one might say dispassionate (17). Environmental features are dealt with methodically, sequentially. The right hemisphere deals with stimuli in a more holistic manner. It is an essentially nonverbal hemisphere that displays affective responses that may be translated into words by the left hemisphere but does not require the left hemisphere for the emotional response (17). There may be a parallel between nondominant hemisphere activity and mental processes that are repressed (17). In a sense, the right hemisphere is part of the "unconscious" because it is responsible for nonsystematic brain activity that does not usually find verbal expression. Attention, arousal, and initiation of responses may all depend upon right hemisphere structures when affective issues are involved (13). The right hemisphere cannot direct behavior by way of logic, but it may still influence behavior considerably by directing preference.

Patients with primarily left hemisphere lesions often respond dramatically to their illness with excessive emotional displays, self doubts, feelings of worthlessness, and profound pessimism (16). Sixty-two percent of patients with strictly left hemisphere lesions react in this way, and only 11 percent appear indifferent to their deficits (17). This catastrophic reaction to the brain damage is seen in only 10 percent of patients with primarily right hemisphere damage, but 33 percent of these patients exhibit indifference to or denial of their impairment (16,17). Extending this to an experimental level, some investigators have reported similar reactions to right or left hemisphere dysfunction when this is transiently induced by the Wada technique of carotid infusion with amobarbital (17). The implication is that the intact right hemisphere faces no modulation from the left hemisphere in the patient with a left-sided lesion, and, as a result, the affective display is unchecked by the more logical left hemisphere.

Observations on the incidental behavior of patients answering different types of questions also suggest a special role in affect for the right hemisphere. The right frontal lobe directs conjugate lateral gaze to the left in normal individuals. That reflex left conjugate gaze will occur with increased activity on the right side of the brain is purely speculative, but it is interesting that patients required to answer emotionally charged or preferential questions tend to look to the left (16). This same shift of gaze is seen when the individual is asked to deal with spatial problems, a demand clearly drawing on the right side of the brain (16). In dealing with affective disorders, some clinicians have observed a better response to unilateral electroconvulsive treatment when the shock is applied to the right hemisphere (17). Many of these observations have not been widely confirmed, but they remain unrefuted. To extrapolate from these tentative observations to the hypothesis that the left cerebral hemisphere inhibits the emotional right cerebral hemisphere and may be the basis for repression is farfetched but provocative (17).

Surgical Manipulation of Mood

Although midbrain, hypothalamic, frontal, temporal, and other widely dispersed areas of the brain play roles in the elaboration of emotional responses, considerable interest has developed in controlling affective or behavior disorders by surgical lesions in circumscribed areas of the brain (12). Stereotactic lesions in the anterior corpus callosum, the broad bundle of fibers connecting the two cerebral hemispheres, allegedly improve phobias, anxiety states, depressions, and affective components of schizophrenia (15). Some neurosurgeons have placed small lesions in the cingulate gyrus, the band of cortex lying just superior to the corpus callosum on the inner face of the cerebral hemispheres, producing alleviation of depression, hypomania, obsessive compulsive neuroses, anorexia nervosa, alcoholic depression, and anxiety neurosis (15). Why lesions in these cerebral structures cause such wide-ranging affective changes has yet to be explained. The anergia and negativism that develops in depressed patients after the placement of cingulate gyrus lesions is also an unexplained, but, fortunately, transient phenomenon (15). The later sequelae of these procedures and other techniques, such as cryosurgery (freezing) in the medial frontal lobes for obsessional neuroses and depression, have yet to face the scrutiny given earlier psychosurgery, such as prefrontal leucotomy (15). It is clear that the incidental or elective destruction of brain tissue can profoundly alter affect, but it is not known how specific the structures now implicated in emotions are for affective functions alone.

AGGRESSION

Destructive behavior may be an initial sign or a late sequela of central nervous system disease. When that behavior is somewhat goal-directed and stimulus-dependent, it is called aggressive. Aggression in this sense is more than striving for a reasonable goal. It is an affective disorder that leads to hostile attitudes and often sociopathic activities. It is distinct from pathologic rage in that the latter is elicited by nonspecific stimuli, is purposeless, and may be interminable (18).

In many situations, distinguishing between unrestrained rage and aggressive behavior is impossible. Patients with hallucinations may react to imagined auditory or visual threats with violent fits of rage directed toward real individuals in their environment. This occasionally occurs in patients with epilepsy as part of the seizure activity or between discrete seizure episodes (18). Totally unprovoked and undirected rage is more characteristic of acute cerebral infections, such as rabies, in which Ammon's horns of the temporal lobes are damaged by the infecting virus (18). Although most violent crimes are not committed by neurologically disabled individuals, profound emotional disorders and associated violent acts certainly do occur in various forms of viral encephalitis (19,20). Violent, destructive behavior was common in children surviving the influenza epidemic of 1918, an epidemic during which thousands of people developed encephalitis (20). The period of stupor, seizures, or other signs of meningoencephalitis usually simplifies the diagnosis. The organic basis for the violent behavior is rarely in doubt (Table 7.1). When the viral encephalitis is more slowly progressive, the patient's gradual deterioration will correct any misdiagnosis prompted by the slow evolution of neurologic deficits.

Focal brain lesions are associated with antisocial or destructive behavior only rarely. Tumors in the anterior midline, centering about the septum pellucidum and the hypothalamus, are associated with increased emotional lability that may develop into violent behavior (18). These patients seem to react to paranoid ideas. Progressive rage can develop with a dermoid cyst of the third ventricle (19). Occasional victims of temporal lobe tumors

Table 7.1. Neurologic Causes of Aggression

Encephalitis (rabies, influenza)
Cerebral contusion
Lead poisoning
Hypothalamic tumor
Temporal lobe tumor
Psychomotor epilepsy

will react to minor stimuli with violent indiscriminate attacks on people and objects about them (18). These rage attacks are presumed to develop with irritation of the adjacent hypothalamus. Degenerative diseases of the brain can also lead to violent behavior, but this unusual development is routinely in the setting of a preexisting neurologic disease. The usually docile patient with Down syndrome (mongolism) may develop violent behavior during the third decade of life as senile plaques, degenerative changes in the cerebrum, form (19).

Mistaking a brain-damaged individual for an organically-sound sociopath is actually much less a problem than ascribing organic brain disease to healthy criminals. Much of the criminal population previously designated neurologically damaged is, in fact, within the range of normal. Electroencephalographic studies on murderers judged insane at one time revealed abnormal patterns in 65 percent of the group, but this was when such patterns as '14 and 6', a sharp wave discharge found in normal individuals, was considered pathologic (19). Concern that aggressive criminal behavior might be rooted in focal brain lesions prompted considerable study of changes in aggression and violence after lesions in selected areas of the brain. The results of these studies, as well as the procedures used, are controversial. One of the notions developing out of the studies of criminal populations is the episodic dyscontrol syndrome (21). Individuals with this syndrome have discrete paroxysms of violent behavior lasting minutes to hours. These episodes are unprovoked and are occasionally preceded by abnormal sensations and followed by headache or drowsiness. Implicit in the grouping of these individuals into a syndrome is that a common nervous system disorder, perhaps an epileptic disorder, underlies the behavior disorder.

Individuals with episodic dyscontrol, in fact, share several characteristics besides their violent behavior. They are usually from lower socioeconomic strata, exhibit sociopathic behavior by their twenties or early thirties, and have little formal education (21). There is a high incidence of chronic alcoholism in and abuse by their fathers. More than three out of four people exhibiting episodic dyscontrol as adults had hyperactivity as children; and about half report staring spells lasting seconds with "altered consciousness" but no violent behavior (21). These are exceedingly remorseful individuals, and about 50 percent report suicide gestures or attempts. Alcohol routinely increases the frequency and severity of their criminal outbursts. The episode of uncontrolled rage may be preceded by visual illusions, hyperacusis, nausea, or paresthesias (21). After the attack, some patients deny recall of their behavior or any ability to control their behavior. Sixty-eight percent of these individual report some improvement in their episodic dyscontrol while on phenytoin; but, regardless of treatment, episodic dyscontrol rarely appears in individuals over 50 years of age (21). Whether or not this is a seizure disorder is one of the issues avoided by using the term episodic dyscontrol syndrome (22). Objective study of this group is complicated by the substantial secondary gain to the patient when he can provide a convincing picture of a seizure disorder.

When violent behavior does occur in the setting of a seizure disorder, it is likely to be largely undirected and disorganized (19). Despite numerous court pleas ascribing violent behavior to psychomotor (complex partial) seizures, most neurologists do not accept the notion that repeated violence and destructive behavior are commonly related to seizure phenomena (22,23). Seventy-two percent of juvenile offenders involved in violent crimes claim memory lapses, blackouts, dizziness, and dreamlike states experienced during the crime and excessive fatigue after the crime (22). These phenomena may simply represent subjective changes associated with excitement.

Studies indicating that the incidence of epilepsy in prison populations is tenfold that seen in the general population are misleading (19). With the wide acceptance of epilepsy as a cause of violent behavior, a plea based upon an organic nervous system disorder is likely to be proffered and energetically documented during the proceedings leading to imprisonment (24). Since the diagnosis of epilepsy in most cases relies heavily on the patient's own testimony, any population with a vested interest in establishing cerebral dysfunction must be evaluated with some skepticism. Many of these patients admit that intoxication with alcohol or other drugs played a role in their aggressive episodes (24). Psychiatric problems other than drug abuse and alcoholism are also common in patients with episodic dyscontrol. More than 30 percent admit to sexual problems, including impotence, transvestitism, and obsessive abstinence (24). Epilepsy can account for no more than 1 percent of all reported violent acts, and that figure is, at best, an overestimate (19).

Brain lesions in experimental animals clearly can increase aggressive behavior. Lesions of the amygdala, posterior hypothalamus, or brainstem enhance hunting and violence in some animals (22). Although rage attacks in brain-damaged individuals are more characteristic of hypothalamic lesions than of lesions elsewhere in the brain, there are numerous central nervous system disorders that preferentially damage the hypothalamus and associated areas without causing personality disorders (19). These include icteric encephalopathy, a sequela to hyperbilirubinemia in the newborn; Wernicke disease, a consequence of thiamine deficiency; and Boeck sarcoid, a disorder characterized by noncaseating granulomas. Herpes simplex encephalitis involves several structures classically considered part of the limbic system (11). There is necrosis and inflammation of the hippocampus, uncus, amygdala, and anterior perforating substance in over 60 percent of affected individuals, yet aggressive behavior is rarely observed in this viral illness (19). Although some neurologists believe that most repeatedly violent offenders are neurologically impaired, aggressive behavior in man cannot be predicted on the basis of anatomic lesions (22).

Aggression and Temporal Lobe Seizures

Violence as a concomitant of temporal lobe (complex partial) epilepsy has been repeatedly studied with distinctly inconsistent results. There clearly is a high incidence of sociopathy and psychopathology in patients followed in seizure disorder clinics for temporal lobe epilepsy, but these clinic patients are highly preselected (25). They are usually indigent, have poor seizure control, and exhibit numerous psychosocial problems. The highly compliant, socially integrated individual with well-controlled epilepsy is less likely to be in the clinic group; he does not require regular supervision. These considerations aside, there is little consistent data to prove that sociopathy occurs more often in victims of complex partial seizures than in patients with generalized (grand mal) seizures (25). Certainly, patients with complex partial seizures have more personality disorders than other patients with epilepsy, but goal-directed, violent behavior is not typical of temporal lobe epileptics.

Studies linking complex partial seizures with aggressive, destructive, or otherwise sociopathic behavior have been primarily preoperative or postoperative evaluations of epileptic patients subjected to surgery for relief of intractable seizures (26). In these patients, definite temporal lobe structural damage could be found in 80 percent of cases, a relatively high rate of pathology for an epileptic population (26). Aggressive behavior was the most common psychiatric abnormality described, but this was manifested by unpredictable outbursts of anger during periods between frank seizures (the interictal period). Although children with temporal lobe epilepsy alone do not have these unprovoked rage attacks, the epileptics most likely to have irrational destructive or abusive behavior as adults are those whose seizures started early in childhood (25,26). With surgical resection of the anterior temporal lobe, the aggressive behavior remits for more than 6 years in 27 percent of the patients so treated (26). Even in these patients with temporal tip resections, the preoperative significance of the aggressive behavior should not be overrated. Only 16 percent of the aggressive epileptic patients could be legitimately characterized as psychotic (26).

In most patients with complex partial seizures, the angry outbursts seem to follow long seizure-free intervals (23). The actual period of abusive behavior lasts hours to days and may be abruptly terminated if a seizure occurs. During this irritable period, the patient resists all efforts to calm him and broods over imagined slights or insults. Serious injury to those in contact with the patient during this angry period is unlikely; and, when the anger abates, the patient is usually remorseful and apologetic (23). He remembers how he behaved and may promise to avoid such behavior in the future. Of course, the promise is forgotten when the next imagined slight provokes another episode of anger. Control of the seizure disorder may increase the frequency of the episodes; and so some clinicians allow their patients to remain incompletely controlled if violent behavior is a prominent interictal problem (23). This tolerance of recurrent seizures is risky because injury or status epilepticus may result, and so treatment of these patients with phenothiazines may be a better approach to their interictal anger.

Some investigators do claim a high incidence of aggressive behavior in patients with mesial temporal sclerosis and temporal lobe seizures, but the current consensus is leaning away from any clear association between temporal lobe damage and sociopathic behavior (25). Even those who suggest that there is a causal relationship between temporal lobe epilepsy and aggression in some patients recognize that this type of epilepsy is generally not associated with aggressive behavior (25). Male sex, low IQ, lack of religious ties, and a juvenile behavior problem are all more important factors than the epilepsy in the appearance of aggression in epileptic patients (5). Forty-one percent of the group exhibiting aggressive behavior have faced permanent separation from one or both parents before the age of 15 years, and it is often their disruptive behavior, more than their seizures, at an early age that prompts medical attention (5). The patient's age at the onset of his seizure disorder may be more significant in the development of aggressive behavior than the type of seizure disorder he has. Conduct disorders are more likely to appear in disturbed children than are paranoid or depressed behavior, behavior more characteristic of emotionally disturbed adults (5). That these patients with poorly controlled psychomotor seizures are severely disturbed patients is emphasized by the 5 percent incidence of suicide and 2 percent incidence of self-mutilation after temporal lobe surgery for control of the seizures (5). Postoperative depression is a major problem in these patient's with poorly controlled seizures, appearing in about half of the surgically treated patients (5).

Encephalitis and Aggression

The acute onset of aggressive behavior is sometimes a sign of progressive brain disease, such as that developing with viral encephalitis. With an encephalitis that has a predilection for classical limbic structures, such as the hippocampus, amygdaloid nucleus, fornix, cingulate gyri, and mammillary bodies, suspiciousness, impulsivity, and depression may follow an early impairment of memory (13, 27). Paroxysmal temporal lobe abnormalities may be a prominent electroencephalographic findings in viral encephalitis from agents, such as *Herpes simplex,* that attack these limbic structures; but depression is a more likely affective disorder with this disease than aggression (27). Patients recovering from the acute viral encephalitis usually have substantial intellectual and motor deficits as well as behavior problems that necessitate institutionalization (28). Some kinds of viral encephalitis produce affective changes early in the course of the disease that may be misconstrued as violent or aggressive. This is true of rabies encephalitis. The violent, maniacal patient exhibiting an inexplicable fear of water with rabies encephalitis is largely mythical, but patients with rabies do have anxiety, apprehensiveness, and paroxysms of rage or terror. The most typical course for the patient with this type of viral encephalitis involves the development of anxiety, malaise, fever, anorexia, and headache for several days before the development of paresthesias about the site of the animal bite (18,29–31). Profound hyperactivity may follow this nondescript malaise, and a precipitate deterioration into coma is likely (30). Brief paroxysms of intense sadness develop between the attacks of rage in the rabid individual (18). Eighty percent of affected individuals have dysphagia, hydrophobia, and pharyngeal spasms. Other acute viral encephalitides occasionally evoke agitated behavior. Patients with the acute viral encephalitis of encephalitis lethargica (von Economo's encephalitis) had premorbid aggressive and hyperkinetic activity associated with lesions in the anterior hypothalamus (19).

As discussed in the section on dementia, kuru, the slow-viral disease of the Fore islanders produced frankly aggressive behavior relatively early in the course of the illness (32). Victims of this disease became suspicious, angry, and abusive long before any dementia was apparent. They randomly assaulted relatives and strangers who inadvertently passed within striking distance. This combativeness generally yielded to a longer-lasting depression, but its appearance during the course of a viral encephalopathy was additional evidence that assaultive behavior in a previously passive individual might result from viral disease even when it was not a fulminant illness.

Neoplasms rarely produce assaultive behavior, but aggression may occur with hypothalamic tumors (6). Other signs of hypothalamic disease, such as diabetes insipidus, labile affect, and excessive appetite, suggest a destructive lesion in the brain. Rage reactions and aggressive behavior in both man and animals have also been reported with damage to the ventromedial thalamus (33).

Psychosurgery for Aggression

Surgical techniques directed at eliminating aggressive behavior have been widely employed, but there is no consensus on which, if any, techniques are effective and appropriate. Thalamotomy to destroy the lamella medialis or the centre medianum nucleus of the thalamus has allegedly decreased emotional lability, destructive behavior, and anxiety in as many as half of the patients treated (4,7,34). Bilateral ablation of the amygdala has decreased restlessness and destructiveness in patients with behavior disorders associated with epilepsy or a history of encephalitis (6). Patients with postencephalitic aggression had improvement in 75 percent of cases after amygdala surgery, and patients with epilepsy and aggressiveness responded to amygdalotomy with improved behavior in 90 percent of cases (6,19). Destruction of various hypothalamic structures and lesions in the cingulate gyrus, which lies on the mesial face of the cerebral hemisphere, have also been alleged effective in reducing aggressive behavior (8,19). Pathologic suspiciousness may remit after temporal lobectomy, and violent, antisocial behavior invariably remits with hemispherectomy (25). Surgical disruption of many brain structures can effectively alter behavior, but the long-term consequences of such procedures remain to be assessed. Where structural central nervous system disease is apparent, aggressive behavior may actually be secondary to dementia or disorientation, rather than being the primary problem (19).

APATHY

The previously active, ambitious person who abruptly or insidiously becomes apathetic may have a structural lesion in the central nervous system or an endocrine disorder affecting brain function as the basis for his change in temperament. Apathy is a somewhat imprecise description of the usual change in affect, since the patient often has more a blunting of his emotional response than a true indifference to his environment. Initiative is often lost in association with this emotional blunting, and some individuals complain that they are unable to enjoy activities that they customarily found enjoyable, a symptom often referred to as anhedonia (Table 7.2). Frontal lobe damage is especially likely to produce these changes in affect, but thalamic lesions, hypothyroidism, and hyperthyroidism may also produce this personality change. Central nervous system infections, such as general paresis from syphilis, occasionally produce marked apathy as a transient phenomenon, but it is not a prominent characteristic of most infectious disorders (35). After severe head injury, many individuals go through a period of unaccustomed inactivity and lack of initiative, but this too is usually a transient phenomenon (36). The loss of initiative and lethargy that develop with head trauma are not specifically related to frontal lobe or thalamic damage.

Frontal Lobe Damage

The classic example of a personality change following frontal lobe damage is Phineas P. Gage, a railroad foreman who mellowed considerably after

Table 7.2. Causes of Emotional Blunting

Frontal lobe damage (tumor, contusion, demyelination)
Thalamic lesions
Thyroid disease
Postconcussion syndrome

he suffered a penetrating frontal lobe wound from a crowbar. An iron bar, 3 7″ × $1\frac{1}{4}$″, was driven through his forehead during a blasting accident (1). The accident occurred in 1878; and, despite negligible medical intervention beyond removal of the foreign object, Mr. Gage survived for 12 years and provided considerable information on the affective changes with static frontal lobe lesions (37). Most obvious in this gentleman was a general lack of interest in his customary activities. He became irreverent, profane, stubborn, vacillating, and capricious in a decidedly childish way. Minor distractions interfered with his concentration on most tasks (1). Mr. Gage suffered damage to the left frontal lobe extending from the mesial surface just above the orbital roof to the precentral frontal cortex over the convexity of the brain. Most patients with this type of injury have little spontaneity. Initiative disappears entirely; anhedonia, the inability to enjoy anything, is prominent (14,38).

With frontal lobe damage, what is often interpreted as a profound depression is actually a disorder of psychomotor activity. This becomes evident when the patient suffering frontal lobe damage transiently loses his blunted affect and enters a period of apparent euphoria (1). He uses pretentious language, makes lewd remarks, and is caustic or facetious (1). This facetiousness is called "Witzelsucht", and it is often associated with socially inappropriate activities, such as exhibitionism and public urination and defecation (1,37,38). More constant than the precise character of the patient's mood is the profound impairment in decision making that appears with these frontal lesions. Individuals who were previously decisive become unable to make a decision (33). If the orbital surface of the frontal lobe is exclusively involved by the lesion, there is usually no intellectual defect despite the marked personality change (1,33). Cognitive dysfunctions develop in more than half of the cases suffering more extensive frontal lobe damage (37). With an orbital surface lesion, the personality traits appearing include shallow affect, substantial irritability, and heightened distractibility. Patients with this type of damage become angry and aggressive with little provocation (33). The aggressiveness is short-lived, and the provocation is quickly forgotten.

Patients with frontal lobe damage usually have a combination of three affective changes: (*1*) apathy; (*2*) depression with apparent dementia and incontinence; and (*3*) transient euphoria with subsequent restlessness, irritability, and facetiousness (1). Regardless of the basic personality changes, most patients exhibit inappropriate emotional responses to emotionally charged stimuli (1). These affective changes are seen with slowly evolving neoplasms, such as meningiomas, as well as with traumatic injuries to the frontal lobes (Figure 7.1) (33,38). A rapidly evolving lesion, such as an intracerebral bleed, more commonly causes stupor and confusion than subtle personality changes (37). Neurosyphilis probably produces transient apathy in patients with general paresis by direct damage to the frontal lobes by the invading organisms (35).

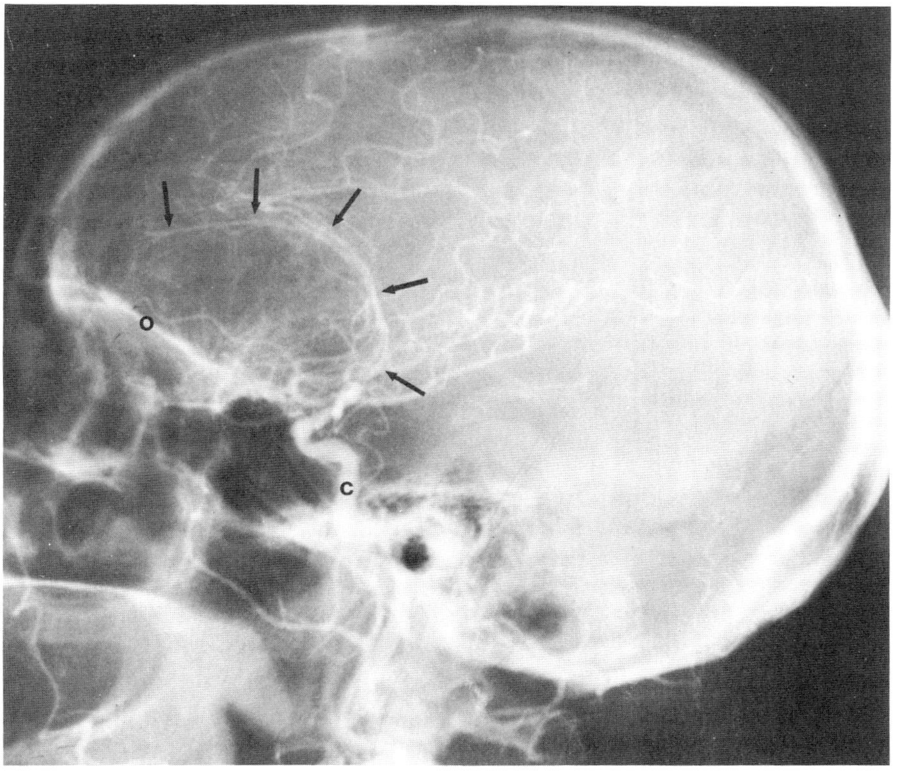

Figure 7.1. This 72-year-old man was referred for neurologic evaluation when his family noticed that he was becoming increasingly confused, disoriented, sloppy, and apathetic. Neurologic examination revealed no focal deficits other than a snout reflex and a rooting reflex. An arteriogram outlined a massive subfrontal tumor, which proved to be a meningioma. The internal carotid artery (c) branches are stretched over the tumor (arrows). The roof of the orbit is labeled **o** (courtesy of Drs. J. Loh and W. Hotson).

Treatment of the personality change must include treatment of the underlying lesion. If the responsible lesion is a meningioma, the tumor must be removed; if neurosyphilis is responsible, high dose penicillin treatment is indicated. In all patients with affective disorders developing with structural lesions in the frontal lobe or, for that matter, anywhere in the brain, the personality disorder does not resolve immediately upon correction of the underlying lesion. Abnormal moods and behavior may persist for weeks or months after treatment of the lesion, and some individuals will have permanent personality changes or affective disorders despite successful treatment of the destructive lesion. Presumably some of the damage caused by the intracranial disease is irreversible in patients with permanent affective changes.

Postconcussion Syndrome

Head trauma often causes blunting of affect and loss of initiative, but many other kinds of personality change also occur with cerebral concussion or contusion. Even when there is no obvious structural damage associated with the trauma, the patient may exhibit emotional lability, depression, euphoria, or unprovoked anger (36). Typical of the loss of initiative is a laxity in personal habits that develops. Individuals characteristically restrained in speech and behavior often develop uninhibited language and sexual behavior (36). Even if the patient appears to be aware of the inappropriateness of the behavior he exhibits, he often compensates with denial, confabulation, or obsessive behavior. Hysterical or paranoid traits not apparent before the trauma may surface transiently after the head injury (36).

Anxiety and irritability develop as part of the postconcussion syndrome after significant head trauma. Even in patients with little evidence of focal structural damage, there may be profound changes in behavior. Patients with head trauma producing transient loss of consciousness have protracted and often incomplete recovery of social interests (42). These individuals are much less motivated after the head trauma than they were before the injury. They interact less with their friends and families and even spend less time at their favorite leisure activities than they did before the head injury (42). This impaired social recovery is not from depression and is not a problem as far as the patient is concerned. The anatomic and physiologic basis for this social apathy are unknown. Recovery may occur after months of limited social initiative. The severity of the affective changes associated with head trauma is to some extent inversely related to the severity of the head injury, substantial "traumatic neurosis" being more typical of minor head injuries than of major head trauma (36). This is also discussed in the section on cognitive disorders associated with head injuries.

Other Structural Causes of Apathy

Intrinsic tumors of the thalamus are also associated with a lack of drive and initiative (1,39). Unlike patients with frontal lobe lesions, patients with thalamic lesions are not aggressive or caustic when provoked. Dementia, or at least a slowing of intellectual performance, often develops with the affective disorder when the dorsomedial nucleus of the thalamus is the site of the lesion (1,39). Flattening of affect and irritability are also well documented with temporal lobe damage, especially in patients who have temporal lobe seizures associated with the structural lesion (40). This emotional blunting develops with temporal lobe gliomas even when no other psychotic features evolve (41). Placidity, that is, an extreme indifference to customarily arousing or irritating stimuli, is one of the principal features of the Klüver-Bucy syndrome, a behavior disorder appearing after bilateral temporal lobe lesions in man (18). The tranquilizing effect of prefrontal leucotomy is probably related to interruption of the fibers connecting the anterior cingulate gyrus, the cortical tissue on the mesial aspect of the hemisphere, with the prefrontal area (18). What feature shared by these diverse cortical and subcortical structures produces the blunted affect characteristically seen when they are damaged is unknown.

Systemic Causes of Apathy

Several systemic diseases may cause affective disorders characterized by apathy, lack of initiative, or just flat affect. Chronic infections, such as unsuspected tuberculosis, can induce subtle personality changes over the course of weeks before other signs of the disease become evident. The insidious personality changes preceding more dramatic signs, such as altered consciousness, may mislead the family into thinking that the patient has a basically psychiatric problem. Patients with unrecognized diabetes mellitus often report no symptoms other than polyuria and polydipsia until after their metabolic problem is recognized and treated. On insulin, they occasionally realize that they were decidedly unmotivated before their treatment. The personality change with correction of the metabolic problem will provide the first evidence that the patient had any defect in initiative before. Hepatic failure, hyponatremia, hypercalcemia, uremia, and many other systemic problems can induce apathy in isolated cases, but the one systemic disorder that most commonly induces profound personality changes is hypothyroidism. With impaired thyroid function, the patient's activities narrow; his affect becomes flat, and his movements are slowed. Although there are usually signs of anxiety and depression, the overall picture is one of an apathetic, withdrawn, often demented individual (43,44). The severity of the affective changes are not correlated with the severity of the hypothyroidism (43).

Treatment of hypothyroidism may be hindered by the personality disorder induced by the endocrine disorder. Thyroid supplements make the patient feel "pushed," driven to become active, pressured to interact. This feeling of duress leads to poor compliance. The hypothyroid patient refuses to take thyroxine despite his apparent understanding of the importance of the hormone. This poor compliance can usually be circumvented by starting the patient on a negligible dose of the replacement hormone and increasing the dosage slowly. Hypoadrenalism, that is, Addison syndrome, also may present with apathy, and like hypothyroidism this endocrine disorder is often characterized by depression and fatigue, as well as lack of initiative and seclusiveness (45). As the adrenal dysfunction progresses the patient will develop impaired memory, irritability, impaired sensory function, delirium, and ultimately obtundation (45). Objective signs of neurologic dysfunction will be subtle until the disease is well advanced. When the psychiatric symptoms are prominent, the electroencephalogram of the hypoadrenal patient will reveal diffuse, high amplitude, slow wave activity (45). Correction of the psychiatric disorder depends upon replacement of the corticosteroid hormones deficient as a result of the hypoadrenalism.

DEPRESSION

An estimated 15 to 30 percent of adults have depressive episodes, most of these episodes having no demonstrable neurologic basis (46–48). Structural or physiologic problems may be responsible for some of these apparently psychogenic depressions, but investigations into these areas have yielded little concrete information. Patients with obvious structural lesions in the brain, such as strokes, have a high incidence of depression (Table 7.3). Thirty-seven percent will have recurrent attacks of depression even if they are treated as effectively as possible for their structural lesions (49). The role of several neurotransmitters, including norepinephrine, in the development of despondent moods is still unclear, and even the nature of the difference betweeen psychotic depressions and normal emotional responses is controversial (46,48). What is accepted by both neurologists and psychiatrists is that a clinically significant mood disturbance is one that results in disturbed sleep, loss of appetite, depressed libido, abnormal gastrointestinal activity, aberrant autonomic function, withdrawal from customary social contacts and activities, suicidal thoughts or gestures, and disturbed reality testing with delusions, hallucinations, or confusion (46). Whether the depression is associated with a major loss in the patient's life, with an endocrine disorder, such as hyperthyroidism, or with a degenerative disease, such as Wilson disease, the risks are the same. One percent

Table 7.3. Nonpsychiatric Causes of Depression

Thyroid disease
Electrolyte abnormalities
Hyperparathyroidism
Adrenal disease
Oral contraceptive pills
Parkinson disease
Wilson disease
Huntington disease
Cerebral vasculitis
Multiple sclerosis
Limbic encephalitis
Herpes encephalitis

of patients with acute depression and 15 percent with recurring depressions commit suicide (46).

Limbic Encephalitis

Inflammatory lesions of the temporal lobe and structures classically considered part of the "limbic lobe" may produce acute depression (27). This so-called limbic encephalitis is often manifested by anorexia, loss of sexual interest, insomnia, psychomotor retardation, irritability, incontinence, and delusions. With progression of the brain dysfunction, the patient may exhibit sexual indiscretions, such as unconcealed masturbation, catatonia, lip smacking and chewing movements, and hallucinations (29). This disorder is routinely confused with involutional melancholia, catatonic schizophrenia, or paranoid schizophrenia, until the deficits progress; seizures, coma, or focal signs make it apparent that the patient has a destructive central nervous system disease (29).

Most patients with limbic encephalitis appear to have an unidentified viral encephalitis, but this disorder also develops in patients with cancer who have no apparent viral infection. Even in these cancer victims, the cause of the central nervous system disease will probably prove to be a virus of some sort. There is no treatment for limbic encephalitis even when it is identified early in its evolution. The primarily psychologic manifestations may evolve for as long as 2 months before the other signs of organic brain disease appear. Once the patient has been hospitalized with seizures or obtundation, his survival is usually limited to a few weeks.

Depression may also develop with the more commonly occurring encephalitis due to *H. simplex*. There is good reason for the similarity between the affective disorders with limbic encephalitis and with herpes simplex encephalitis since many of the same structures are damaged in the two infections. With herpetic disease lesions are more limited to the temporal lobe than in typical cases of limbic encephalitis, but damage to adjoining limbic structures may be extensive (50). This is a grave illness with fatality rates in excess of 60 to 80 percent and with neuropsychiatric deficits usually prominent in those who survive the illness. As already discussed, aggression may be an early and prominent sign of the encephalitis. Although a fulminant encephalitis with seizures and the rapid evolution of a hemiparesis or coma may be fatal within 1 to 2 weeks of its appearance, some patients will have a premonitory personality change with an acute depression and suicidal thoughts as much as 1 week before other signs of the disease (50).

Degenerative Diseases

Degenerative diseases, especially those affecting the basal ganglia of the brain, commonly produce depression as an early affective change. Parkinson disease routinely involves depression that abates somewhat with effective control of the movement disorder (51). Huntington disease is often first recognized when a patient with suicidal tendencies develops the chorea typical of the later stages of this disease. Patients with Wilson disease often succeed in their suicide attempts before the disease is diagnosed or even suspected. Treatment of the depression in each of these degenerative diseases is often frustrated by the progression of the central nervous system disease, but the clinical approach to the depression in these disorders is basically the same as that in psychogenic depressions. The only difference is that the underlying disease is treated if that is feasible. In Parkinson disease, the treatment of the movement disorder is palliative, but it is often effective against the depression. The tricyclic antidepressant imipramine has an anticholinergic effect, and, consequently, it alleviates some of the bradykinesia and rigidity as well as acting against the affective disorder. Wilson disease can be largely reversed with penicillamine treatment, and antidepressant treatment may be unnecessary. In Huntington disease, the basal ganglia and cerebrocortical degeneration progress inexorably and frustrate all efforts to reverse the depression. All of these degenerative diseases are discussed in detail in the sections on movement disorders and on cognitive disorders.

Neoplasia and Vascular Disease

Depression rarely develops with intracranial tumors. Temporal lobe neoplasia occasionally causes a depressive disorder, but seizures or a memory disorder are more typical of these lesions (18). Vascular disease, however, can produce fairly typical "endogenous" depression. This is especially common in patients with systemic lupus erythematosus; the personality change may precede other signs of the disease by years (52). These patients develop progressive withdrawal, ideas of reference, and even catatonia when there is an exacerbation of the underlying collagen vascular disease (52). High dose corticosteroids may reverse the depression in patients with either neoplasia or vasculitis, but this response is inconsistent in both conditions. Treatment of the tumor or the vasculitis, even when it is highly effective, does not necessarily abolish the affective disorder. Antidepressant therapy is often appropriate in these patients long after they are asymptomatic for the tumor or vascular disease.

Multiple Sclerosis

Although patients with multiple sclerosis are often depicted as inappropriately euphoric or optimistic, 18 percent of these patients are severely depressed and up to 3 percent commit suicide (53). Much of what was previously viewed as euphoria was actually a masked depression manifested by unrealistic or excessively optimistic attitudes (54). Victims of this demyelinating disease often exhibit diurnal mood changes with feelings of guilt and suicidal ideation appearing during the depressed periods. Concealed depression is more common than overt depression; but, as the disease progresses and the patient becomes more disabled, the depression becomes more overt (54). This depression is not just a reactive depression to the neurologic disease, since patients with other equally disabling neurologic diseases do not exhibit this affective disorder (53). In fact, patients with multiple sclerosis have an inordinately high incidence of depression preceding the appearance of the demyelinating disease (53). Occasionally, a frank bipolar (manic-depressive) psychosis will appear coincidentally with the multiple sclerosis, a complication that actually does not have substantial impact on the therapeutic approach. Depressed patients with multiple sclerosis should be treated in much the same way as patients without neurologic damage (53). Antidepressant medication and psychotherapeutic intervention with these patients are reasonable and effective. Electroconvulsive treatment is inadvisable.

Endocrine Disorders

Endocrine disorders often cause depression associated with more strictly neurologic signs. Hyperparathyroidism, hypothyroidism, hypoadrenalism (Addison disease), and hyperadrenalism (Cushing disease) are the endocrine disorders most often implicated in patients with an organic basis for their depressions (44). As already mentioned, the depression associated with hypothyroidism is usually less striking than the apathy and lethargy developing in this disease. Severe hypothyroidism produces intellectual problems which are more prominent than the affective problems (44). With hyperthyroidism, a psychotic depression may occur, but extreme anxiety is much more commonly the predominant mood disturbance (44). Cushing disease and Addison disease also have cognitive defects appearing in the disease that overshadow the affective changes, but, at least with Cushing disease, the depression developing with the adrenal disorder is often substantial (44). More common, but less severe, depressive episodes develop with oral contraceptive use. An estimated 10 percent of women using these oral hormone supplements develop depression or irritability significant enough to warrant discontinuation of the contraceptive (45).

Hyperparathyroidism

With hyperparathyroidism, the patient may be anxious, confused, disoriented, obsessive-compulsive, or even catatonic (55). What should suggest hyperparathyroidism is the association of the psychiatric disorder with amnestic states or a more diffuse dementia (56). Depression, fatigue, and lethargy are prominent in these patients. Florid paranoid psychoses with hallucinations and recurring catatonic stupors may persist for months with little additional evidence of an organic basis for the disorder. Weight loss and constipation are routinely present. Gait difficulty may be the only sign suggesting a neurologic dysfunction in the hyperparathyroid patient who is acutely depressed, suicidal, or mute (55). The gait is often shuffling or stiff with decreased arm swing.

The most obvious metabolic consequence of hyperparathyroidism is an elevated serum calcium, and the psychiatric changes in hyperparathyroidism worsen as the serum calcium level rises (44,57). Serum calcium levels between 12 and 15 milliequivalents per deciliter usually produce severe depression; hypercalcemia with levels in excess of 15 milliequivalents per deciliter produces a profound dementia with associated paranoia (44). Coma intervenes as the serum calcium exceeds 19 milliequivalents per deciliter (57). Hemodialysis will reverse the intellectual and emotional disturbances as it clears the excess calcium from the blood.

These neuropsychiatric signs of hyperparathyroidism are not rare. Forty-two percent of patients with primary hyperparathyroidism have psychiatric and neuromuscular signs, with neuropsychiatric signs dominating the clinical picture in 12 percent (55). Weakness, absent tendon reflexes, slurred speech, ataxia, and even transient aphasia establish the organic basis for the neuropsychiatric problems when the serum calcium is markedly elevated (57). If the calcium level rises high enough, seizures may occur. Aside from an elevated serum calcium, the diagnosis may be suspected with a "salt and pepper" appearance on skull x-rays obtained in seeking an explanation for the dull headaches that commonly develop (56). Elevated serum calcium levels increase the rate of water excretion substantially, and so patients are obligated to urinate and drink water excessively. This polyruria and polydipsia may raise suspicions of self-induced water intoxication, but this will be readily dismissed when the hypercalcemia is found. The electroencephalogram in patients with hypercalcemia usually exhibits diffuse slowing of the background rhythm, as well as intermittent rhythmic slow activity in the frontal region (57). All of these signs generally remit after parathyroid resection and return of the serum calcium to more normal levels.

Cushing Syndrome

Prominent psychiatric disturbances are more common in hyperadrenalism than in any other endocrine disorder (45). The commonest psychiatric symptom in hyperadrenalism, or Cushing syndrome, is depression (45). Typical of this depression is pessimism, self-reproach, and loss of interest (44). Some patients attempt suicide, and many display a bipolar affective disorder with typical manic phases characterized by grandiose delusions, hyperactivity, insomnia, and forced speech (44). Poor concentration, irritability, hallucinations, memory impairment, and paranoid delusions occur fairly commonly (45). Five to 20 percent of patients with hyperadrenalism present with an acute psychosis, occasionally resembling schizophrenia (45).

If the hyperadrenalism is secondary to problems in the pituitary gland or the hypothalamus, the patient is even more likely to have a mood disturbance than when the adrenal gland itself is the primary source of the endocrine disorder (45). Iatrogenic Cushing syndrome, such as that seen in the patient on chronic high dose prednisone, has less depression and more hypomania or euphoria than the naturally occurring hyperadrenalism (44). The psychiatric symptoms in Cushing syndrome from any of these sources usually change rapidly: the depression may abruptly yield to paranoid delusions and hallucinations.

What causes the affective changes in adrenal disorders is not known. Cortisol, the principal steroid made in the adrenal gland, increases the reuptake of norepinephrine by neurons in the central nervous system. Most current theories connect depression with depletion of central nervous system norepinephrine, and so the reuptake of this neurotransmitter in hyperadrenalism must lead to increased catabolism and functional depletion if these theories are correct (44). There is some evidence that adrenocorticotrophic hormone (ACTH) is instrumental in the development of depression secondary to adrenal disease, but this is not established (44). This role for adrenocorticotrophic hormone fits with the observation that patients with iatrogenic Cushing syndrome, that is, those given high dose steroids that suppress pituitary release of adrenocorticotrophic hormone, have euphoria, rather than depression, in most cases (45).

Hypothyroidism

Hypothyroidism produces many cognitive deficits that have already been discussed in the section on cognitive disorders, but this endocrine disorder also produces affective disorders. The most common and obvious affective disorder developing with a hypoactive thyroid gland is depression (45). This depression has distinctly paranoid features. A more unusual personality trait associated with hypothyroid depression is excessive facetiousness, the witzelsucht also seen with frontal lobe damage (45). Neurologic signs associated with the psychiatric manifestations of the hypothyroidism include paresthesias, focal weakness, auditory abnormalities, ataxia, tremor, poor coordination, and carpal tunnel syndrome (45). Why an underactive thyroid gland causes any of these problems is unknown, but a disturbance in cerebral blood flow, a depression in cerebral oxygen consumption, and a general slowing of neuronal interactions probably all play roles in the neuropsychiatric signs that develop (45).

Objective signs of neurologic dysfunction may be few until the disorder is well advanced. The electroencephalogram slows, and nerve conduction speeds are decreased in well-established cases, but patients with little more than depression may go undetected. The psychomotor slowing that develops as the endocrine disorder worsens is ascribed to worsening of the depression, and the endorcine problems may be overlooked even when more neurologic signs appear. Thyroid function studies will establish the diagnosis, and thyroid hormone replacement will correct the deficits.

Hyperthyroidism

Hyperthyroidism also may produce an acute depression serious enough to prompt a suicide attempt. Depression develops less commonly in hyperthyroid patients than does anxiety, emotional lability, or a delusional psychosis, but elderly individuals with overactive thyroids show a special vulnerability to depressive reactions. These elderly thyrotoxic individuals become withdrawn, apathetic, and anorectic and are said to have apathetic hyperthyroidism (45). Most individuals with thyroid disease and prominent psychiatric symptoms associated with that endocrine disorder will have restlessness, sleep disturbances, and tremor (45). Neither thyroid disease nor a neurologic reaction to hyperthyroidism may be suspected until the depressed patient has an acute exacerbation of the thyroid disorder and becomes delirious or obtunded during thyroid storm (45). This endocrine disorder is especially easy to overlook because the depression often follows a severe emotional strain, and the psychologic reaction exhibited by the patient is reasonably interpreted as a reactive depression (45). Elevated serum thyroxine or triiodothyronine levels usually establish the diagnosis, and suppression of thyroid overactivity will usually be paralleled by resolution of the neuropsychiatric signs.

Electrolyte Disorders

Hyponatremia, hypokalemia, hypercalcemia, and hypomagnesemia can all lead to depression. The severity of the affective disorder is usually more related to the rapidity of the development of the electrolyte disturbance than to its magnitude (57). Depression itself may lead to electrolyte disorders by disposing the patient to adopt poor dietary habits, but in most cases the electrolyte problem is the cause, rather than the result, of the depression.

Hyponatremia produces apathy, lethargy, withdrawal, anorexia, and tearfulness when it is not severe (57). Severe sodium depletion causes hallucinations, convulsions, or coma. The first signs of the low serum sodium level may be little more than headache, nausea, and vomiting. Concentration and memory are mildly impaired and the patient becomes disoriented. Emotional lability develops and a careful neurologic examination will usually reveal mild papilledema, ataxia, and weakness (57). With more severe hyponatremia, the electroencephalogram has irregular, high amplitude slow wave activity. The normal background alpha wave activity is lost (57). Psychogenic polydipsia, that is excessive, voluntary water drinking, can cause hyponatremia, but inappropriate secretion of antidiuretic hormone is a more common explanation. In psychiatric patients phenothiazine administration may be responsible for the inappropriate antidiuretic hormone secretion (57).

A mildly low serum potassium level occasionally causes personality changes that include depressive symptoms. The patient with hypokalemia becomes tearful, suicidal, hopeless, and fatigued (57). This is not usually the most prominent neurologic sign of recurrent hypokalemia. Diffuse muscle weakness is more typical.

Hypercalcemia produces irritability, withdrawal, anhedonia, anorexia, and loss of initiative, whether the hypercalcemia is from hyperparathyroidism, Addison disease, vitamin D toxicity, prolonged immobility, or sarcoidosis (57). Suicide is a rare complication of this metabolic encephalopathy, but depression is common. Intellectual defects, such as poor concentration and impaired memory, develop if the hypercalcemia persists for years, a situation especially likely in hyperparathyroidism (45). When the serum calcium level reaches very high levels, that is, in excess of 16 milliequivalents per deciliter, the patient will develop an acute organic psychosis with disorientation, paranoid ideas, and hallucinations (45). The patient becomes comatose at serum calcium levels in excess of 19 milliequivalents per deciliter (45). Correction of the serum calcium level corrects the affective disorder with a lag measurable in hours or days.

A low serum magnesium develops with protracted vomiting, diarrhea, malabsorption, or diuretic abuse and causes restlessness, irritability, depression, and more profound personality changes in association with muscle cramps, vertigo, seizures, nystagmus, and tremors (57). All of these electrolyte problems are readily corrected with intravenous electrolyte therapy, and with correction of the electrolytes the patient returns to a normal affect. This is a problem with diagnosis rather than therapy.

Neurologic Side Effects of Antidepressant Therapy

Lithium

Medication and electroconvulsive therapy intended to alleviate depression may inadvertently cause neurologic problems. The widespread use of lithium in manic-depressive illness (bipolar type) has familiarized most psychiatrists with its untoward neurologic side effects (46,47). With lithium intoxication, most patients become dysarthric, tremulous, confused, and mildly obtunded (58–60). As the serum lithium level rises, seizures and myoclonus develop, and coma intervenes. Tendon reflexes are usually hyperactive; plantar responses, extensor; and muscle tone, increased (58). An awake patient may complain of paresthesias and generalized weakness. The narrow therapeutic range of lithium results in the frequent appearance of at least some of these signs of toxicity (61). A level, checked 12 hours after the last dose, that exceeds 1.5–2.0 milliequivalents per liter will usually be associated with signs of neurologic dysfunction. That sign may be little more than a coarse tremor or it may be stupor (62). At therapeutic levels, the patient usually has a fine tremor, but there should be none of the muscle twitching, clumsiness, and lassitude that develop at toxic levels. Memory loss, confusion, incoherent speech, and other signs of dementia are prominent in some toxic patients. Involuntary movements and cogwheel rigidity develop with this drug but much less readily than with the phenothiazines and butyrophenones.

The mode of action of lithium in the brain is controversial, but it probably acts at synapses utilizing norepinephrine for neurotransmission. Lithium chloride increases norepinephrine deamination and thereby decreases the overall level of brain norepinephrine (19). At least in experimental animals, a role for norepinephrine in affective behavior is well established, although in most cases norepinephrine appears to inhibit behavior antagonistic to rage (19).

Objective evidence of a lithium overdose in the absence of lithium levels includes generalized slowing on the electroencephalogram (61). Altered nerve conduction velocities develop along with a generalized peripheral nerve dysfunction induced by toxic levels of lithium (63). Cerebrospinal fluid protein may exceed 100 milligrams per deciliter (58). Systemic signs associated with the neurologic dysfunction include nausea, vomiting, cramps, and diarrhea. Cardiac arrhythmias and hypotension develop in severely toxic patients.

Treatment of the overdose centers on speedy clearance of the drug from the blood. Dialysis will help eliminate some of the drug, but just increasing the sodium chloride load in the blood will induce normal kidneys to increase their rate of lithium clearance (61). When an acute overdose is suspected, gastrointestinal lavage to limit the amount of drug available for absorption is advisable. Ideally, recovery from toxic levels of lithium will occur over 5 to 7 days, but permanent central nervous system damage may appear even when the elevated serum levels are brought back to normal without much delay (61). Persistently slurred speech, staggering gait, clumsiness, and nystagmus may appear as late effects of lithium intoxication (63). These persistent signs reflect central nervous system damage. This is probably because brain levels of lithium may remain elevated longer than serum levels, thereby exposing the central nervous system to a more prolonged toxic dose than that experienced elsewhere in the body (58).

Tricyclic Antidepressants

Tricyclic antidepressant drug overdosage can produce a syndrome indistinguishable from that induced by anticholinergic drugs, such as atropine, scopolamine, benztropine, and trihexyphenidyl. This anticholinergic effect is manifest as confusion, short-term memory loss, hallucinations, slurred speech, staggering gait, agitation or euphoria, insomnia, and mannerisms (47,60,64). The hallucinations may be visual, auditory, or tactile; and the insomnia may yield to stupor and coma. Delayed ejaculation and urinary hesitancy appearing as side effects of the drug are likely to increase the patient's overall anxiety considerably (47). These neurologic signs appear in the setting of prominent flushing, nausea, vomiting, and constipation. Ten percent of patients on tricyclic antidepressants have fine, rapid tremors of the arms at therapeutic levels (60). Visual complaints may develop from paralysis of accomodation or from ophthalmoplegia, that is, a paralysis of the muscles moving the eyes (64,65). Postural hypotension and palpitations are relatively uncommon side effects of these drugs (46,47). Increased sweating is fairly common (46). With cessation of the drugs, these milder signs will resolve within 12 to 24 hours (64). More severe signs of toxicity may require several days off medication to resolve.

Monoamine Oxidase Inhibitors

Monoamine oxidase inhibitors also may have an anticholinergic effect, but their most serious side effect is hypertensive encephalopathy from toxic interaction with other substances (46). Dry mouth, loss of appetite, insomnia, blurred vision, and urinary retention are likely. Postural hypotension is more likely with these drugs than with the tricyclic antidepressants, but most anticholinergic side effects are less prominent with the monoamine oxidase inhibitors than with the tricyclics (47,66). Dairy products, wines, pickled herring, or chocolate, eaten in combination with monoamine oxidase inhibitors, may produce restlessness, hypertension, or coma (46,60,66).

Electroconvulsive Therapy

Electroconvulsive therapy for depression commonly produces transient memory loss, but this usually clears completely within 1 week (46). A variety of techniques have been developed to minimize the intellectual dysfunction likely to attend electroconvulsive therapy. Whether the duration of the stimulus, the area of the brain most directly stimulated, or the intensity of the stimulus is most important in determining the severity of the cognitive disorder is controversial (67). Memory is the intellectual function most consistently disturbed by the shock, and the retrograde, as well as slight anterograde, amnesia that develops shrinks over the course of days. There may be some persistent memory gaps, similar to those seen in postconcussion amnesia. Retention of new information is clearly defective transiently, but even this disorder clears within a few weeks. A unilateral shock to the nondominant hemisphere will disturb memory less than dominant hemisphere stimulation (67). Most practitioners currently believe this unilateral approach is as effective as other electroconvulsive techniques and may be more desirable because of its slighter impact on cognitive function (67). There is no increased incidence of epilepsy after electroconvulsive therapy in depressed patients who do not have seizures before the shock treatments (68). There is no consensus on the wisdom of using electroconvulsive therapy for epileptic patients with severe depression; the substantial risk of precipitating status epilepticus in these individuals makes electroconvulsive therapy justifiable only as a last resort, if at all, for epileptic patients.

Amphetamine Abuse

Some patients abuse stimulants in a covert attempt to deal with depression (69). Such individuals often have a family history of bipolar affective disorders and suicide attempts. Individuals abusing amphetamines often report that the euphoria, increased confidence, and sense of well-being developed with the drug use are tainted by vague fears, poor concentration, and restlessness (70). Paranoid misinterpretations, auditory or visual hallucinations, and delirium will develop in some abusers (70). Although this drug-induced psychosis may clear within a week of stopping the drug, the patient may attempt suicide during the withdrawal period (70). Seizures occasionally develop with protracted abuse, and barbiturates seem to aggravate the agitation when they are used in an attempt to counteract the amphetamine effect. Stimulants, including amphetamines and methylphenidate, may be useful in antidepressant therapy by increasing the serum levels of tricyclic antidepressants, but their high abuse potential limits this application (47). The most effective treatment for an acute overdose is probably haloperidol given intramuscularly in 5 milligram doses repeated hourly for as long as needed to contain the floridly delusional patient (70).

AGITATION

A variety of drugs and chemicals, intentionally or accidentally introduced into the body, can produce agitation with little else manifested as the initial sign of the toxin. One of the more common causes of pathologic agitation is amphetamine abuse. Anxiety, restlessness, an increased startle response, and an inability to concentrate are all likely with this type of drug abuse (70). Toxic confusion and delirium appear with high doses of amphetamine, but the level of drug required to induce this varies from person to person. Chronic amphetamine abuse may precipitate a paranoid psychosis that is indistinguishable from a paranoid schizophrenia (60). Rather than just chronic agitation, these individuals have auditory hallucinations, paranoid ideation, stereotyped behavior, and occasional euphoria (60). Loose associations and flat affect are not characteristic of this toxic psychosis. As the thought disorder becomes more chronic, the patient becomes withdrawn and apathetic. Systemic signs of amphetamine abuse include an increased heart rate, body temperature, and blood pressure. Aside from stopping the drug and dealing with systemic problems as they occur, there is little specific treatment for this drug toxicity. Treating the patient with barbiturates, on the assumption that these drugs will antagonize the stimulant effect of the amphetamines, often increases the agitation and produces clumsiness (70). Chloral hydrate has a similar effect when combined with amphetamines.

The toxin responsible for the mad hatters of Louis Carroll's era was inorganic mercury. Mercuric nitrate was used in the manufacture of felt until 1941 (71). Individuals exposed to this agent for years often became tremulous and easily startled. The appearance of chronic agitation with mercury poisoning is reinforced by occasional coarse jerks, which increase on intentional movements (71). This is a diagnostic consideration only when the agitated patient has had industrial exposure to the heavy metal. Mercury poisoning can occur when food, such as fish, is contaminated through environmental pollution, but the regional character of this type of problem minimizes the diagnostic difficulty. Much of the damage done to the nervous system with heavy metal poisoning is irreversible.

Agitation also occurs without an apparent toxic or physiologic basis. Some individuals experience episodic agitation that is best described as a panic attack (59). During these attacks, the patient has a sudden fear or horror. They react as if their lives were in danger, and yet they cannot explain what triggered the feeling of danger. Autonomic symptoms, including rapid breathing, tachycardia, and excessive sweating, are apparent (59). Patients routinely complain of palpitations, vertigo, pins-and-needles sensations, hot and cold flashes, internal shaking, shortness of breath, and chest pain during these attacks (48). Many of these patients take benzodiazepines for chronic anxiety, and withdrawal from these drugs may contribute to the more organic features of the panic attack (59). In most cases there is no explanation for the profound, abruptly appearing agitation experienced by these individuals. Highly repressed psychologic conflicts are probably responsible for the panic attacks experienced by most individuals.

EUPHORIA

Euphoria, or a feeling of well-being, is relatively uncommon with organic brain disease. The notion that the patient with multiple sclerosis is typically euphoric is wrong (72). Euphoria, along with denial of illness, is occasionally seen in patients with demyelinating disease, but this is usually in a significantly demented individual. Affective changes with demyelinating disease vary with the type of patient involved and the severity of the disease. Young adults with multiple sclerosis for months or for only a few years typically exhibit denial or distress (72). With progression of the disease, some patients become depressed and exhibit excessive concern for their bodily functions. Symptomatic depression and inappropriate euphoria are equally rare in patients with multiple sclerosis (72).

Table 7.4. Causes of Labile Affect

Minimal brain dysfunction (of childhood)
Alzheimer disease
Pick disease
Parkinson disease
Hyperthyroidism
Amyotrophic lateral sclerosis
Progressive supranuclear palsy
Multi-infarct dementia
Neurosyphilis (general paresis)
Disturbed methionine metabolism
Postconcussion syndrome
Electrolyte disturbances
Wilson disease

EMOTIONAL LABILITY

Violent swings in mood developing with organic brain disease are usually more apparent than real. What changes abruptly is the affective display, rather than the actual emotion. The patient will laugh or cry independently of the emotions he is actually feeling. This is referred to as emotional lability whether the emotions are actually labile or the affective display is labile. The most common neurologic causes of emotional lability are degenerative brain diseases (Table 7.4).

Pseudobulbar Affect

Uncontrollable weeping or laughing, recurring independently of the emotions associated with this affective display, are usually from diffuse cerebral disease, in which case it is called pseudobulbar affect (73). The patient laughs or cries with trivial stimuli (33). Unprovoked laughing and, more rarely, crying may be part of a seizure; but the other elements involved in the seizure should indicate the cause of the abnormal affect (18). Occasionally, this emotional lability and affective incontinence will be a sign of depression, but this is less likely an explanation when the emotional lability occurs in an elderly patient (49). This pseudobulbar affect is presumed to develop with damage to centers important in the inhibition of emotional expression (18,73). It is often confused with dementia, but may occur independently of any intellectual deficits. Excessive facial expression may be elicited by nonspecific stimuli, a reaction suggesting impaired voluntary control of the affective display associated with a variety of emotions (18).

In patients acutely affected by laughing or crying attacks, psychiatric problems or intoxication are most likely responsible (18). Patients with manic-depressive illness (bipolar type) occasionally have exaggerated expressions of affect. Unlike victims of diffuse neurologic disease, these psychiatric patients also have pressure of speech (60). In true pseudobulbar palsy from central nervous system disease, the excessively labile affect is often associated with indistinct, dysarthric speech and masked facies. With neurologically impaired individuals, the affective display can be abruptly altered by changing the focus of the patient's attention or by simply shifting to a different topic of conversation. Other features of pseudobulbar palsy are more variable. The palpebral fissures are often kept widely open and blinking is reduced, both giving the impression that the patient is staring. Drooling and difficulty swallowing add to the impression that the patient has a brainstem lesion at the level of the pontine and medullary nuclei, but the actual lesion responsible for the disorder seems to be an upper motor neuron lesion (33). Uncontrollable crying is more common than excessive laughing when the underlying disease is a disorder of the extrapyramidal system (Parkinson disease, progressive supranuclear palsy) or of the motor system (amyotrophic lateral sclerosis) (18). Pathologic laughing or crying may develop with subcortical white matter lesions adjacent to the basal ganglia, and a combination of laughing and crying develops in some of the rare patients with bilateral thalamic lesions (18).

A variety of central nervous system disorders will produce pseudobulbar affect with varying regularity (Figure 7.2). Metabolic encephalopathy, such as that developing with a low serum sodium concentration, can cause a labile affect, but usually does not (57). Meningovascular syphilis occasionally produces emotional lability as one of its early symptoms, but with the decline in the incidence of neurosyphilis this is a rarely observed complication of this central nervous system infection (35). Bilateral cerebral strokes may dispose an occasional patient to develop a pseudobulbar affect, but progressive supranuclear palsy, a degenerative disease producing dementia and ocular palsies, will routinely leave the patient with this organic affective dysfunction (74). Amyotrophic lateral sclerosis, a disease of the motor neurons, and multiple sclerosis, a disease with motor and sensory involvement, both may be associated with pseudobulbar affect (73). Pathologic facial expressions, that is, unprovoked smiling and frowning, also occur frequently with bulbar amyotrophic lateral sclerosis and progressive supranuclear palsy (18). Other brainstem diseases affecting facial musculature may elicit this excessive facial activity.

Little is available to treat this disorder, although treatment is often desparately sought by affected individuals. The outbursts of laughing or weeping are extremely embarrassing and puzzling for the mentally competent patient. Antipsychotic drugs and sedatives are totally ineffective against this affective disorder. Levodopa may provide some control over these episodes, especially in patients not suffering from Parkinson disease (73). Patients with Parkinson disease usually have a pseudobulbar affect that is unresponsive to levodopa.

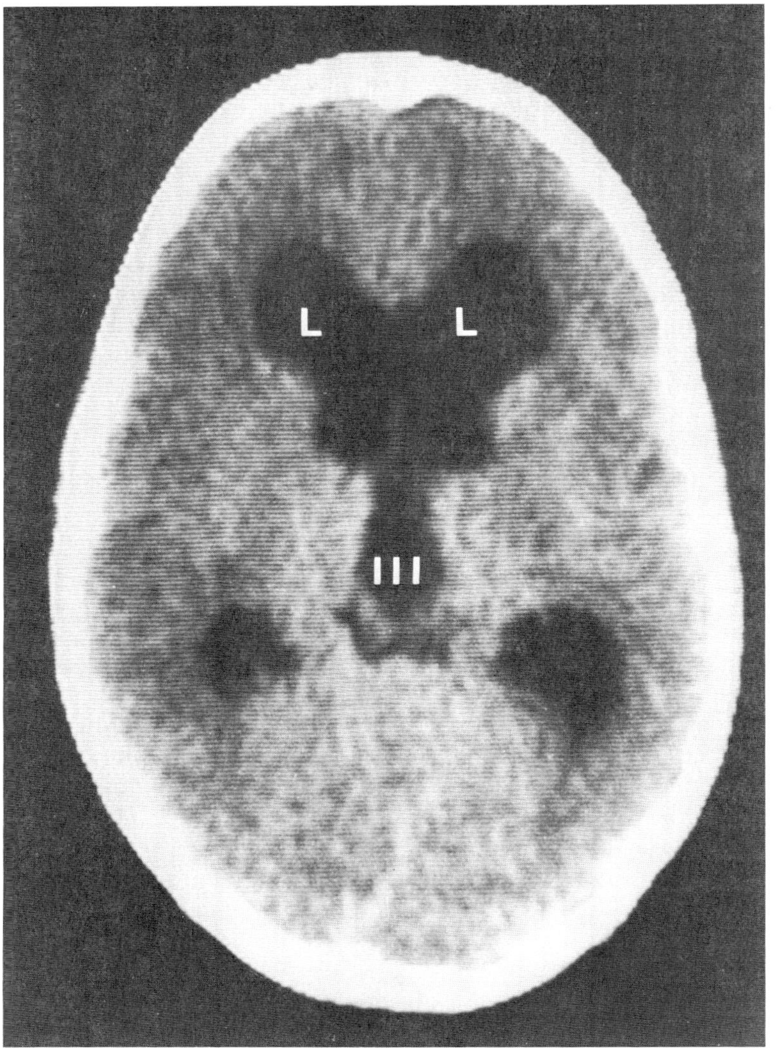

Figure 7.2. An adolescent girl was investigated for mild headaches and a labile affect. Although her school performance had not deteriorated significantly and her neurologic examination was unremarkable, except for slightly full optic discs (early papilledema), this computed tomogram of her brain revealed marked hydrocephalus. The lateral ventricles (L) and the third ventricle (III) are much larger than normal. Gyri and sulci are not apparent at the surface of the brain because the increased intraventricular pressure is pressing the cortex against its meningeal lining. No lesion was found that explained the hydrocephalus (courtesy of Drs. J. Loh and W. Hotson).

Fou Rire Prodromique

Fou rire prodromique is an extremely rare affective disorder that begins apoplectically with pathologic laughter, often associated with headache, tinnitus, and upward deviation of the eyes (18,75). The patient may laugh for hours, until he is breathless and exhausted. This bizarre behavior usually precedes a deepening coma and death (75). There is no treatment to alter the course of the syndrome.

REFERENCES

1. Blumer D, Benson DF: Personality changes with frontal and temporal lobe lesions, in Benson DF, Blumer D (eds): *Psychiatric Aspects of Neurologic Disease.* New York, Grune & Stratton, 1975, p 151.
2. Hypoglycaemia and personality. *Br Med J* 2:134, 1974.
3. Alberts JR, Friedman MI: Olfactory bulb removal but not anosmia increases emotionality and mouse killing. *Nature* 238:454, 1972.
4. Andy OJ: Thalamotomy in hyperactive and aggressive behavior. *Confin Neurol* 32:322, 1970.
5. Taylor DC: Aggression and epilepsy. *J Psychosom Res* 13:229, 1969.
6. Balasubramaniam V, Ramamurth B: Stereotaxic amygdalotomy in behavior disorders. *Confin Neurol* 32:367, 1970.
7. Hassler R, Dieckmann G: Stereotaxic treatment of compulsive and obsessive symptoms. *Confin Neurol* 29:153, 1967.
8. Ballantine HT Jr, Cassidy WL, Flanagan NB, et al: Stereotaxic anterior cingulotomy for neuropsychiatric illness and intractable pain. *J Neurosurg* 26:488, 1967.
9. Broca P: Anatomie comparée des convolutions cerebrales: Le grand lobe limbique et la scissure limbique dans la série des mammifères. *Revue d'Anthropologie* 1:385, 1878.
10. Papez JW: A proposed mechanism of emotion. *Arch Neurol Psychiatry* 38:725, 1937.
11. Livingston KE, Escobar A: Anatomical basis of the limbic system concept. *Arch Neurol* 24:17, 1971.
12. Aird RB: Clinical syndromes of the limbic system. *Int J Neurol* 6:340, 1968.
13. Valenstein E, Heilman KM: Emotional disorders resulting from lesions of the central nervous system, in Heilman KM, Valenstein E (eds): *Clinical Neuropsychology.* New York, Oxford University Press, 1979, p 413.
14. Teuber HL: Prospects for research on schizophrenia: Effects of focal brain lesions. *Neurosci Res Program Bull* 10:381, 1972.
15. Sweet WH: Treatment of medically intractable mental disease by limited frontal leucotomy—justifiable? *N Engl J Med* 289:1117, 1973.
16. Schwartz GE, Davidson RJ, Maer F: Right hemisphere lateralization for emotion in the human brain: Interactions with cognition. *Science* 190:286, 1975.
17. Galin D: Implications for psychiatry of left and right cerebral specialization. *Arch Gen Psychiatry* 31:572, 1974.
18. Poeck K: Pathophysiology of emotional disorders associated with brain damage, in Vinken PJ, Bruyn GW (eds): *Handbook of Clinical Neurology.* New York, American Elsevier, 1969, vol 3, p 343.

19. Goldstein M: Brain research and violent behavior. *Arch Neurol* 30:1, 1974.

20. Hart EJ, Carter S: Minimal brain dysfunction, in Downey JA, Low NL (eds): *The Child with Disabling Illness.* Philadelphia, WB Saunders, 1974, p 255.

21. Maletzky BM: The episodic dyscontrol syndrome. *Dis Nerv Syst* 34:178, 1973.

22. Pincus JH: Can violence be a manifestation of epilepsy? *Neurology (NY)* 30:304, 1980.

23. Blumer D: Temporal lobe epilepsy and its psychiatric significance, in Benson DF, Blumer D (eds): *Psychiatric Aspects of Neurologic Disease.* New York, Grune & Stratton, 1975, p 171.

24. Bach-Y-Rita G, Lion JR, Climent CE, et al: Episodic dyscontrol: A study of 130 violent patients. *Am J Psychiatry* 127:1473, 1971.

25. Stevens JR: Interictal clinical manifestations of complex partial seizures. *Adv Neurol* 11:85, 1975.

26. Falconer MA: Reversibility by temporal-lobe resection of the behavioral abnormalities of temporal-lobe epilepsy. *N Engl J Med* 289:451, 1973.

27. Corsellis JAN, Goldberg GJ, Norton AR: "Limbic encephalitis" and its association with carcinoma. *Brain* 91:481, 1968.

28. Whitley RJ, Soong S-J, Hirsch MS, et al: Herpes simplex encephalitis. *N Engl J Med* 304:313, 1981.

29. Glaser GH, Pincus JH: Limbic encephalitis. *J Nerv Ment Dis* 149:59, 1969.

30. Kramer M: Dream disturbances. *Psychiatr Ann* 9:50, 1979.

31. Plotkin SA, Koprowski H: Phobia of hydrophobia justified. *N Engl J Med* 300:620, 1979.

32. Hornabrook RW: Kuru—A subacute cerebellar degeneration. The natural history and clinical features. *Brain* 91:53, 1968.

33. Sherwin I, Geschwind N: Neural substrates of behavior, in Nicholi AM (ed): *The Harvard Guide to Modern Psychiatry.* Cambridge, Belknap Press, 1978, p 59.

34. Poblete M, Palestini M, Figueroa E, et al: Stereotaxic thalamotomy (lamella medialis) in aggressive psychiatric patients. *Confin Neurol* 32:326, 1970.

35. Lishman WA: *Organic Psychiatry.* London, Blackwell, 1980.

36. Sisler GC: Psychiatric disorder associated with head injury, in Hendrie HC (ed): *The Psychiatric Clinics of North America.* Philadelphia, WB Saunders, 1978, vol 1, p 137.

37. Hecaen H, Albert ML: Disorders of mental functioning related to frontal lobe pathology, in Benson DF, Blumer D (eds): *Psychiatric Aspects of Neurologic Disease.* Grune & Stratton, New York, 1975, p 137.

38. Ruff RL, Russakoff LM: Catatonia with frontal lobe atrophy. *J Neurol Neurosurg Psychiatry* 43:185, 1980.

39. Botez MI, Barbeau A: Role of subcortical structures and particularly of the thalamus in the mechanisms of speech and language. *Int J Neurol* 8:300, 1971.

40. Slater E, Beard AW: The schizophrenia-like psychoses of epilepsy. I. Psychiatric aspects. *Br J Psychiatry* 109:95, 1963.

41. Malamud N: Psychiatric disorder with intracranial tumors of limbic system. *Arch Neurol* 17:113, 1967.

42. Oddy M, Humphrey M: Social recovery during the year following severe head injury. *J Neurol Neurosurg Psychiatry* 43:798, 1980.

43. Jain VK: Affective disturbances in hypothyroidism. *Br J Psychiatry* 119:279, 1971.

44. Sachar EJ: Psychiatric disturbances in endocrine disease: Some issues for research, in Plum F (ed): *Brain Dysfunction in Metabolic Disorders.* New York, Raven Press, 1974, p 239.

45. Ettigi PG, Brown GM: Brain disorders associated with endocrine dysfunctions, in Hendrie HC (ed): *The Psychiatric Clinics of North America.* Philadelphia, WB Saunders, 1978, vol 1, p 117.

46. Klerman GL: Affective disorders, in Nicholi AM (ed): *The Harvard Guide to Modern Psychiatry*. Cambridge, Belknap Press, 1978, p 253.

47. Shopsin B, Waters B: The pharmacotherapy of major depressive syndrome. Part 1: Treatment of acute depression. *Psychosomatics* 21:542, 1980.

48. Task force on nomenclature and statistics, American Psychiatric Association: *Diagnostic and Statistical Manual of Mental Disorders (Third Edition)*. Washington, DC, American Psychiatric Association, 1980.

49. Post F: Dementia, depression, and pseudodementia, in Benson DF, Blumer D (eds): *Psychiatric Aspects of Neurologic Disease*. New York, Grune & Stratton, 1975, p 99.

50. Koenig H, Rabinowitz SG, Day E, et al: Post-infectious encephalomyelitis after successful treatment of *Herpes simplex* encephalitis with adenine arabinoside. *N Engl J Med* 300:1089, 1979.

51. Brown E, Brown GM, Kofman O, et al: Sexual function and affect in parkinsonian men treated with L-DOPA. *Am J Psychiatry* 135:1552, 1978.

52. Bennett R, Hughes GRV, Bywaters EGL, et al: Neuropsychiatric problems in systemic lupus erythematosus. *Br Med J* 4:342, 1972.

53. Whitlock FA, Siskind MM: Depression as a major symptom of multiple sclerosis. *J Neurol Neurosurg Psychiatry* 43:861, 1980.

54. Baretz RM, Stephenson GR: Emotional responses to multiple sclerosis. *Psychosomatics* 22:117, 1981.

55. Karpati G, Frame B: Neuropsychiatric disorders in primary hyperparathyroidism. *Arch Neurol* 10:387, 1964.

56. Gatewood JW, Organ CH, Mead BT: Mental changes associated with hyperparathyroidism. *Am J Psychiatry* 132:129, 1975.

57. Webb WL Jr, Gehi M: Electrolyte and fluid imbalance: Neuropsychiatric manifestations. *Psychosomatics* 22:199, 1981.

58. Brust JCM, Hammer JS, Challenor Y, et al: Acute generalized polyneuropathy accompanying lithium poisoning. *Ann Neurol* 6:360, 1979.

59. Drugs for psychiatric disorders. *Med Lett Drugs Ther* 22:77, 1980.

60. Marsden CB, Tarsy, D, Baldessarini RJ: Spontaneous and drug-induced movement disorders in psychotic patients, in Benson DF, Blumer D (eds): *Psychiatric Aspects of Neurologic Disease*. New York, Grune & Stratton, 1975, p 219.

61. Jefferson JW, Greist JH: Lithium intoxication. *Psychiatr Ann* 8:458, 1978.

62. Klawans HL: Levodopa induced psychosis. *Psychiatr Ann* 8:447, 1978.

63. Uchigata M, Tanabe H, Hasue I, et al: Peripheral neuropathy due to lithium intoxication. *Ann Neurol* 9:414, 1981.

64. Dysken MW, Merry W, Davis JM: Anticholinergic psychosis. *Psychiatr Ann* 8:452, 1978.

65. Mladinich EK, Carlow TJ: Total gaze paresis in amitriptyline overdose. *Neurology (NY)* 27:695, 1977.

66. Monoamine oxidase inhibitors for depression. *Med Lett Drugs Ther* 22:58, 1980.

67. Williams M: Memory disorders associated with electroconvulsive therapy, in Whitty CWM, Zangwill OL (eds): *Amnesia. Clinical, Psychological and Medicolegal Aspects*, ed 2. London, Butterworths, 1977, p 183.

68. Blackwood DHR, Cull RE, Freeman CPL, et al: A study of the incidence of epilepsy following ECT. *J Neurol Neurosurg Psychiatry* 43:1098, 1980.

69. Pope HG: Drug abuse and psychopathology. *N Engl J Med* 301:1341, 1979.

70. Angrist BM: Toxic manifestations of amphetamine. *Psychiatr Ann* 8:443, 1978.

71. Markowitz L, Schaumburg HH: Successful treatment of inorganic mercury neurotoxicity with N-acetyl-penicillamine despite an adverse reaction. *Neurology (NY)* 30:1000, 1980.

72. Peyser JM, Edwards KR, Poser CM: Psychological profiles in patients with multiple sclerosis. *Arch Neurol* 37:437, 1980.

73. Wolf JK, Santana HB, Thorpy M: Treatment of "emotional incontinence" with levodopa. *Neurology (NY)* 29:1435, 1979.

74. Steele JC, Richardson JC, Olszewski J: Progressive supranuclear palsy. *Arch Neurol* 10:333, 1964.

75. Féré MC: Le fou rire prodromique. *Rev Neurol (Paris)* 11:353, 1903.

8
Sexual Dysfunction and Urinary Problems

Adult sexual activity involves complex interactions within the nervous system, as well as between the nervous system and various structures instrumental in sexual excitement, intercourse, and satisfaction. Psychologic factors are much more important in sexual activity than in most other biologic activities, but they are obviously not the only determinants of sexual activity. Regardless of the psychologic factors entering into sexual interest and performance, sexual function requires the integrity of several parts of the central and peripheral nervous system. Sexual dysfunctions caused by nervous system problems are considerably less diverse in their expression than the sexual disorders that may develop with psychiatric problems. Familiarity with the sexual problems that may develop with specific diseases of the nervous system simplifies the investigation of patients complaining of disturbed sexual activity.

Normal sexual function depends on autonomic reflexes in the pelvis and lumbosacral spine, hypothalamic–endocrine interactions, and cerebral activity (1). In this context, normal refers only to the individual's ability to perform, not to the type of sexual activity he or she prefers. Each element in the system contributing to adult sexual behavior can operate largely isolated from the others, but sexual behavior is generally considered normal only when all the elements work effectively in concert. The ability of paraplegic men with genital anesthesia to have erections and ejaculations despite the transection of cerebrospinal pathways to the lumbosacral cord demonstrates how independently these elements of sexual activity can function. Even the integrity of the genitalia is not a prerequisite for sexual activity. Excitement and orgasm are possible after extensive resection of the vulva and the penis (1). The purely structural elements of sexual intercourse can function independently of the emotional components of sexuality, and emotional sexual responses may be quite unrelated to strictly genital activity.

All of the structures contributing to the development and maintenance of adult sexual activity are yet to be defined, but some central nervous system structures have well-established importance. The hypothalamus is one of the brain structures with unequivocal importance in the elaboration of sexual behavior. The maturation of sexual organs requires intact hypothalamic functioning. Disease of the posterior hypothalamus, or even of just the mammillary bodies, is occasionally associated with precocious puberty (1). Sexual function, as well as development, is apparently influenced quite directly by brain function. Stimulation of the septal region will produce penile erection in animals (1). The hypothalamus is sensitive to a variety of stimuli originating outside the central nervous system. Steroidal hormones produced in the reproductive organs themselves clearly have a substantial effect on the hypothalamus. These hormones affect more than just subsequent patterns of gonadotropin secretion by the hypothalamic-pituitary system (2). In some animals, gonadal steroids act on the central nervous system during fetal or perinatal development to influence sexual behavior when the animal matures (2–4). Male patterns of sexual behavior seem to be imprinted in these animals even before they are born (3). That this occurs to any extent in humans is controversial (4).

The current consensus is that social, cultural,and psychiatric factors play pivotal roles in determining patterns of sexual behavior in humans (3). Hormones are generally viewed as secondary in importance, but the issue is far from settled. A relatively large population of individuals raised as girls despite male chromosome patterns changed sexual identities at puberty (3). These children had ambiguous genitalia, and their true sex was only realized when unexpected secondary sexual characteristics started developing at puberty (5). In this situation, social pressure did not force these individuals to change their gender roles, and yet almost all of them did (5). Hypogonadism in a boy often leads to passivity, shyness, apathy, and lack of drive in the affected individual when he reaches maturity, but factors responsible for the poor gonadal development may play a direct role in the evolution of these personality traits (4). Nonetheless, testosterone replacement in the individual before he reaches maturity increases the likelihood of his developing a more assertive personality (4). Other observations in humans have prompted speculation that abnormal hormone levels in the perinatal period may be responsible for some patterns of homosexual behavior (2). Some homosexual men secrete luteinizing hormone in response to estrogen exposure (6). This abnormal pattern of luteinizing hormone secretion may be the result of low serum androgen levels in the affected individual at the time of his birth. Observations in adults indicate that hormones clearly play much less important roles in the preservation of sexual behavior than they do in the development of sexual behavior.

AROUSAL AND ORGASM

Sexual arousal has mechanical and psychologic aspects in both men and women. Genital stimulation will produce reflex changes in the pelvic organs that allow sexual intercourse in normal individuals unless this arousal is inhibited by cerebral activity. The strictly mechanical elements of sexual intercourse function effectively even when they are isolated from the brain. Spinal cord transection in a man or woman does not block the physiologic changes in the genitalia that characterize arousal. Erection and ejaculation by men and vaginal lubrication and penile accomodation by women require a fairly intact lower spinal cord, but they occur with upper spinal cord or brain damage.

Erection is a reflex involving pelvic nerves, sacral spinal cord, and vascular responses in the genitalia. The autonomic nervous system, the part of the nervous system that makes adjustments in the body without consciously registering the required behavior, has central importance in erection and many other aspects of male and female sexual activity (7). Both the sympathetic and parasympathetic components of the autonomic nervous system are needed for the full range of normal sexual activity, but only the parasympathetic nerves are essential for erection. Stimulation of the glans penis is perceived by sensory receptors in the skin, and the signals are transmitted along pelvic nerves to spinal cord segments S-2, S-3, and S-4 (1). Parasympathetic nerves from these sacral segments induce dilatation of blood vessels in the penis and obstruction of vascular channels draining the penis. Consequently, the highly vascular corpora cavernosa of the penis become engorged with blood, and the penis increases in size and decreases in flexibility (1). Parasympathetic impulses also increase prostatic secretions from the prostate gland (1). Ejaculation involves a nerve supply to the pelvic organs distinct from that involved in erection. These nerves originate primarily in the lower thoracic and upper lumbar segments of the spinal cord. They are sympathetic nerves carried in the pelvic plexus from their origin in the hypogastric plexus and lumbar ganglia to their destinations in the seminal vesicles, ejaculatory ducts, and blood vessels of the corpora cavernosa. Impulses carried along these sympathetic nerves produce ejaculation by causing contractions in the innervated structures (1). The sympathetic system for ejaculation is relatively remote from the parasympathetic system for erection, and so individuals with partial spinal cord transection between L-3 and S-2 segments can have erection without ejaculation (1).

The nerves responsible for normal sexual function in women are largely the same as those responsible for normal sexual activity in men. Tactile stimuli to the nipples of the breast may cause more reflex sexual excitement initially than stimuli to the genitalia, but with excitation by whatever route the parasympathetic nerves initiate several genital changes (7). The labia majora flatten and separate, and the labia minora increase in size. Vascular engorgement is responsible for much of the structural change with arousal in women, as well as in men. Parasympathetic activity increases vaginal secretion, and, in fact, at a strictly physiologic level this is the first pelvic response to sexual stimulation (1). Sympathetic nerve fibers play a role in further elements of arousal and orgasm.

Spinal cord damage can interfere with orgasm in both men and women, but hormonal changes are relatively unimportant. If the anterolateral tracts in the thoracic or lumbar spinal cord are cut, both erection and ejaculation are usually lost, at least temporarily. Similar spinal cord lesions in women that cause analgesia of the vulva will abolish the individual's ability to have an orgasm (1). Arousal in men and women is unrelated to any change in sex hormone levels in the blood. During sexual intercourse, serum androgen levels in men do not change, but threshold levels of androgen must be present for normal heterosexual behavior (1). Elevated serum prolactin may interfere with potency, but if the man with hyperprolactinemia can achieve an erection, he can have an orgasm.

HYPOSEXUALITY

Impaired sexual performance or limited sexual interest occasionally develops with disease of the nervous system, but problems of hyposexuality are most commonly secondary to psychologic conflicts. In allegedly happily married couples not seeking help for sexual problems, 40 percent of the men report problems with erection or ejaculation, and 63 percent of the women complain of problems with arousal or orgasm (8). The most common functional complaint in men is premature ejaculation; 77 percent of women lack interest in sexual activity or have trouble relaxing when their spouses initiate the sexual encounter (8). Even when there is no physiologic problem or psychologic complaint, 15 to 17 percent of women allege that they are unable to have an orgasm while having intercourse (8). All of these sexual dysfunctions are largely independent of age: the only dysfunction that correlates with age is erectile problems in men (8). With so high an incidence of sexual difficulties and dysfunctions in "normal" adults it is not surprising that sexual problems often surface in patients questioned specifically about these areas as part of an investigation of psychiatric or neurologic disease.

At least in men, sexual interest and activity will continue largely unchanged despite substantial changes in androgen levels (4). Only the most severe androgen deficiency states will produce impaired libido and impotence. Administering estrogens to sexually active men will inhibit their potency and sexual interest, but men exposed to these agents are usually aware of their exposure and are not anxious about their altered sexual behavior (4). This presumed independence of sexual interest from androgen levels is probably overstated since even in women sexual interest seems to be partly related to androgen levels (4). Severe sexual dysfunction appears rarely in cerebral disorders that produce no intellectual problems. Patients with epilepsy occasionally complain of poor sexual performance, but even in this group the affected individuals belong to a fairly circumscribed set of epileptics. Most with complaints of hyposexuality have psychomotor (complex partial) seizures (12).

Sexual Dysfunction in Epilepsy

Severely limited sexual activity or interest is the most common sexual complaint in patients with psychomotor seizures, but some have transvestitism, fetishism, and hypersexuality (1,9,13–15). These are probably more accurately described as dysfunctions, rather than as complaints, since most of the affected individuals express little or no concern over their behavior. Compulsive or public masturbation, masochism, and self-mutliation also occur, but they are rare (9). If the psychomotor epilepsy developed before or at puberty, the patient is likely to report rare, if any, sexual arousal (1). Two-thirds of the epileptics with poor heterosexual function have little sexual drive. These patients do not complain of loss of libido because they never had the libido to lose (9). In patients with temporal lobe seizures that can only be controlled with surgical resection of the temporal lobe, hyposexuality is prominent in 58 percent (10). Sexual desire and ability return to normal, if they were ever present, in 12 percent of patients with poorly controlled psychomotor seizures after resection of the temporal lobe in which the seizures arose (1,9,10). Indeed, hypersexuality may be a transient phenomenon in these patients postoperatively (10). Compulsive masturbation after temporal lobectomy is the most common manifestation of this hypersexuality; true heterosexual hypersexuality is rare (9). If anticonvulsants successfully suppress the psychomotor seizures, sexual arousal may tend toward normal even without temporal lobe surgery (1). Lesions over the convexity of the frontal lobe also show an association with impaired arousal and poor sexual function, but this hyposexuality is invariably in the setting of a diffuse loss of initiative.

Hyposexuality with Chronic Pain

Chronic pain, especially that developing in the absence of an apparent organic lesion, usually has a devastating effect on sexual interest and activity. When one member of a married couple has chronic pain, there is a consistent deterioration in sexual activity after the onset of the pain complaint, and this is associated with a perceived deterioration in the marriage by the unaffected spouse (11). The spouse with pain usually reports that the marriage is as strong as ever, but this misconception probably develops from the "sick" partner's dependence on the family (11). Sixty to 70 percent of patients with chronic pain have significantly decreased sexual activity, and 16 percent have no sexual activity (11). This change in sexual behavior is usually ascribed to the increased pain suffered by the affected individual during intercourse.

There are obviously complex issues involved in this change in sexual behavior. In some cases, the pain provides a justification for avoiding sexual activity with an unexciting or conflict ridden partner. Women with chronic pain complain that they never reach orgasm during intercourse in 40 percent of cases, but 16 percent never reached orgasm even without the pain (11). Even though arousal in men should involve little pain-provoking activity, 28 percent of men with chronic pain report the new onset of problems with getting or keeping an erection (11). Neurologic lesions that can cause sexual problems and pain do not account for these statistics.

Hyposexuality and Psychoactive Drugs

Impaired libido and difficulties with achieving orgasm occasionally develop as side effects of psychoactive drugs. Women on monoamine oxidase inhibitors, such as phenelzine and tranylcypramine, may have problems with achieving climax (16). Phenothiazines and antidepressants can cause impotence (17). Men on thioridazine occasionally have problems with ejaculation (18). Even when a psychiatric problem is apparent, impaired sexual activity cannot be ascribed to the psychologic conflict automatically. The patient's psychiatric problem increases his risk of being exposed to drugs that can affect sexual interest and performance.

IMPOTENCE AND IMPAIRED AROUSAL

Neurologic bases for sexual dysfunction aroused considerable speculation in medical circles even before neurology was recognized as a distinct discipline. Remarkable interpretations of brain and spinal cord injuries associated with impotence appeared in leading medical journals from the early nineteenth century onward (19,20). For several decades, the cerebellum was ascribed major importance in the function of sexual organs and the generation of sexual interest. This is a difficult notion to justify retrospectively, since if any part of the nervous system has nothing to do with sexual function it is the cerebellum. Nonetheless, in 1839 Dr. Fisher of Boston felt he had settled the question of cerebellar importance in sexuality with several well-documented cases of impotence following posterior fossa injuries. A typical patient "made the discovery that he had lost the desire and physical power for sexual intercourse . . . from the time he was wounded" (19). It took no less a figure than the famous nineteenth century neurologist Brown-Sequard to refute this localization of sexual function after it had been accepted for about 4 decades (20). Brown-Sequard's claim that cerebellar injury produced no neurologic sign except for blindness did nothing to convince skeptics that his views on impotence were accurate (20). Although the role of the brain in sexual function was controversial, no one could doubt the importance of spinal cord function. The loss of sexual function with traumatic spinal cord injuries made it clear that the cord was involved in at least the transmission of sexual intent to the genitalia. Penile erection at the time of cord transection in men executed by hanging provided more evidence that the spinal cord played some role in sexual function.

It is now recognized that impotence can occur on the basis of neurologic disease, and that disease may be in either the central or peripheral nervous system (Table 8.1). Distinguishing psychiatric from neurologic and iatrogenic bases for impotence is often difficult, especially since impotence may develop as a side effect of drugs, such as phenothiazines, that are routinely used in patients with psychiatric disorders. Roughly 90 percent of the patients complaining of impotence have psychologic bases for their sexual dysfunction (21). In men younger than 50 years old, impotence usually develops from emotional conflicts, depression, fear of erectile failure, poor health, or simple fatigue (4,22). Despite an apparent psychiatric explanation for the impotence, disease in the brain, spinal cord, autonomic nerves, and other peripheral nerves should be considered before the problem is attributed to strictly psychologic problems. The 10 percent of impotent patients without psychogenic sexual dysfunction suffer from vascular diseases, endocrine dysfunctions, metabolic disorders, traumatic injuries, surgical injuries, and medication effects, as well as neuromuscular diseases (21). Features that suggest that psychologic conflicts are responsible for the sexual dysfunction include the patient's admitting normal erections and ejaculations with unfamiliar women or during homosexual encounters and the patient's observation of an erection when awakening from a dream. Men normally have penile erections during dreaming, even when the dream is not erotic. With erotic dreams nocturnal emissions may

Table 8.1. Characteristics of Impotence

Psychogenic	*Neurogenic*
Acute onset common	Slowly progressive deficit common
Nocturnal erections preserved	Erection always absent
Libido variable	Libido usually intact
Intact testicular sensitivity	Impaired testicular sensitivity
Intact bladder dynamics	Abnormal bladder dynamics
Absent associated symptoms	May develop Charcot joints, neuropathic ulcers, diarrhea, retinal disease, etc.

occur, thereby establishing the integrity of the ejaculatory system in the patient complaining of impotence (22). If an erection can occur during dreaming, then it is clear that neural and vascular structures essential for the erection are intact.

Spinal Cord Disease

Spinal cord disease will cause impotence, especially if the sacral cord is damaged (1). As already noted, transection of the spinal cord above the lumbar spine levels will not interfere with erections developing in response to genital stimulation. However, when a man complains of progressive difficulty with erections and deteriorating control of bladder function, a spinal cord lesion should be suspected. When neurosyphilis occurred in epidemic proportions before the introduction of penicillin, tabes dorsalis, the form of neurosyphilis causing dorsal spinal root and posterior column damage, routinely produced impotence (23). Men with multiple sclerosis have demyelination in the spinal cord producing impotence in 26 percent of affected individuals (21). Impotence is the principal symptom of neurologic disease in 3 percent of all men with multiple sclerosis (21,23). Both men and women with multiple sclerosis note a change in their sex lives after the onset of the disease. About half complain of unsatisfactory sexual activity or admit to having no sexual activity (21). Only 20 percent of the men with multiple sclerosis report fully adequate erections (21). Thirty-three percent of the women affected are unable to have an orgasm, and 27 percent say they have no libido (21). Reflecting the separation of sexual functions in the spinal cord, multiple sclerosis patients with impotence may have orgasms with ejaculation despite the absence of an adequate erection (21). Penile implants have been of some help in solving the problem of erection in men sexually impaired by demyelinating diseases.

Diabetes Mellitus

Disease of the autonomic nervous system commonly causes impotence, and diabetes mellitus is the most common disease to produce an autonomic neuropathy. Damage to the cauda equina or parasympathetic nerves in the pelvis may eliminate penile erection, but substantial signs of bladder and bowel dysfunction are usually associated with this. Diabetes mellitus will occasionally cause impotence as the initial symptom of the disease or as the only obvious neurologic sign of the disease (17). Postural hypotension usually develops soon after the appearance of the impotence in these diabetic individuals (24). Up to 60 percent of men with some type of diabetic neuropathy develop problems with erection (23,17). Bladder function is invariably imparied in these diabetic men with impotence, but the bladder problem may be so slight that it is only apparent if a cystometrogram is performed (17). Squeezing the testicles ordinarily causes intense pain, but men with diabetic neuropathy lose this testicular sensitivity partly or completely. This is a useful sign in defining the cause of unexplained impotence. Patients with poorly controlled diabetes may develop transient impotence that can be reversed with better nutrition and better diabetic control, but the impotence that develops from a true diabetic neuropathy is irreversible (17).

Women with diabetes mellitus do not develop the severe sexual dysfunctions commonly occurring in men (17). This is especially difficult to understand since they are just as vulnerable to autonomic neuropathies as male diabetics. Libido and frequency of orgasms are relatively unchanged by this endocrine disease, although about 35 percent of diabetic women report that they do not have orgasms. This problem with orgasms does not correlate with the severity of the diabetes, the duration of the disease, the dose of insulin the patient must take, or the severity of complications of the diabetes, including peripheral neuropathy (17). Recurrent vaginal infections seem to be the principal sexual complication of the disease in women.

Brain Damage

Although erections do occur with complete transection of the thoracic spinal cord, patients with cerebral damage may develop impotence. The brain is not essential for potency, but a damaged brain may interfere with potency. Two out of three men with temporal lobe (complex partial) seizures report impotence (23,25). Damage to or abnormal activity in this part of the cerebral cortex has a special effect on sexual potency; impotence does not develop after frontal leucotomy or with other types of epilepsy (23,25). Indeed, sexual activity may increase after frontal leucotomy (23). Patients with structural lesions in the temporal lobes commonly have impotence preceding the appearance of the seizures. Uncontrolled complex partial epilepsy exacerbates the impotence, and good seizure control often restores potency (23). This is not simply a problem with sexual interest. Quite often, libido is normal in patients with structural lesions in the temporal lobes, but erections are poor or lost prematurely (23). Some degenerative diseases of the cerebral cortex, such as Alzheimer disease, will lead to impotence, but the changes associated with these diffuse degenerative diseases are usually so dramatic in cognitive areas that sexual dysfunction is not a complaint. When the autonomic nervous system is affected preferentially, impaired sexual function is likely to be an early and significant complaint.

Shy-Drager Syndrome

A degenerative disease of the nervous system with special impact on the autonomic nervous system is Shy-Drager syndrome. Impotence is commonly the first sign of this disease (24,26). Men in their thirties to sixties are most often affected, and the disease progresses slowly over the course of a decade. Problems with bladder control, including enuresis, develop soon after impotence in men (24). Loss of libido is one of the most common initial signs in both men and women with Shy-Drager syndrome. If the patient develops urinary incontinence early in the progression of the disease, a spinal cord or autonomic lesion is often suspected (26). Intolerance of heat, easy fatigability, and orthostatic hypotension appear early in the disease (24). Additional signs include parkinsonism, fecal incontinence, hyperreflexia, dysarthria, ophthalmoplegia, tremor, poor rapid alternating movements, and wasting of distal musculature (26). Intellectual function remains normal throughout the disease (24).

Endocrine Disorders

Hormones can dramatically affect sexual function. Increased levels of androgen at puberty are essential for the development of normal libido and potency (22). Of course, men and women may exhibit fairly intact libido for some time after the removal of their gonads (22). Men who never developed normal gonads and have negligible levels of androgen are characteristically passive, hypokinetic, timid, and apathetic (22). Androgens seem to be important in female sexual drive as well as male sexual drive. Adrenalectomy and hypophysectomy in women lead to loss of libido (22). Men and women with elevated serum prolactin levels from pituitary tumors or idiopathically commonly have loss of libido (27,28). Men with hyperprolactinemia may also be impotent (28). Both of these deficits will be reversed within 4 to 12 weeks of starting treatment with the prolactin-depressing drug bromocriptine (27).

Chronic alcoholism usually leads to hypogonadism with loss of libido and potency (17,29). This appears to be due to alcohol-induced gonadal injury, rather than to central nervous system injury, but there is some alcohol-associated hypothalamic-pituitary dysfunction. Alcoholic men have elevated serum prolactin levels (29). This effect of alcohol on sexual performance is somewhat paradoxical since sexual interest is provoked by alcohol in many individuals (30). This sexual arousal may be related to a surge in serum levels of luteinizing hormone that occurs secondary to alcohol suppression of serum androgen levels (30). Women have decreased sexual responsiveness with moderate exposure to alcohol, but they, like men, report increased sexual arousal with increasing intake of alcohol (30). Despite this provocative role in sexual interest, sexual performance by men is consistently impaired by excessive alcohol consumption. Alcohol abuse is a leading cause of impotence (30).

Antihypertensive Drugs

Because hypertension is so common a problem in the United States, any patient complaining of impotence must be questioned on his antihypertensive use. Many patients are not aware that the drugs they are taking are antihypertensives and that these drugs can cause impotence. If the patient is taking antihypertensive medication, but the drugs do not explain the sexual dysfunction and there is ambiguous evidence of bladder dysfunction, such as enuresis or stress incontinence, then more specific investigations of spinal cord function should be considered. When there is striking evidence of sensory and motor deficits in the legs associated with the sexual dysfunction, the appropriate course of investigation includes electromyographic studies of leg muscles and radiographic studies, including a myelogram. Possible causes of impotence include spinal cord tumors and cysts. These are treatable lesions.

Pain on Intercourse: Dyspareunia

Problems with sexual function often develop if the patient has pain on sexual intercourse. This is called dyspareunia, and it can interfere with sexual activity in both men and women. Dyspareunia is common in women after the climacteric, when vulvar and vaginal epithelia thin and vaginal secretions decrease (4,22). Even before menopause, considerable pain may occur on attempted intercourse if there is persistent spasm of the musculature of the outer third of the vagina. This is called functional vaginismus when the spasms are involuntary and recurrent (31). Spasticity in perineal muscles is a rare cause of dyspareunia in women with multiple sclerosis. The woman's resisting penetration of the vagina by her male partner or the man's attempting to penetrate into her vagina before she is aroused and secreting lubricants can produce considerable pain on intercourse for both individuals involved in the attempt.

Men have dyspareunia with a blunt erection, such as that developing in Peyronie syndrome (32). This was first described by Peyronie, the court physician for Louis XIV, in 1743, and is due to a plaque of fibrous tissue in the penis in and around the corpora cavernosa and spongiosum (32). This and other structural abnormality will cause poor erections or pain on attempted vaginal penetration.

Any superficial lesion on the genitalia may cause dyspareunia in men or women. Herpes genitalis is a common nonneurologic cause of painful intercourse. Even before vesicles appear on the penis or on the labia, the victim of this viral infection may have severe burning, itching, tingling, or sharp pain in the area of the lesions with this discomfort increasing on attempted intercourse (33). Pain occasionally radiates down the legs or into the buttocks (33). The pain is maximal during the first 2 days that the lesion appears and it declines rapidly, but the discomfort experienced with the lesions and the fear of recurrence of the lesions may inhibit sexual activity considerably. In women, at least, psychologic stress can play a substantial role in the recurrence of the genital lesions (33). This is a problem affecting generally young adults, with the average age of occurrence in women being 23 years of age (33). This is an especially serious cause of dyspareunia in this sexually active group, since the average duration of vulnerability to recurrent lesions is $3\frac{1}{2}$ years (33).

Sexual Conflicts with Impaired Arousal and Impotence

Stress may prompt changes in sexual activity, but in some cases it is the change in sexual activity that introduces considerable stress into the relationship between two people. With heterosexual couples, impotence arouses concerns about the male partner's virility. The affected man may be much more preoccupied by this than is his sexual partner, but his preoccupation alone often serves as a very disruptive force in the relationship. Diabetic men find it especially perplexing that their ability to have erections is abating, while their interest in sexual activity is stable or increasing. Libido is commonly unaffected in neurologic conditions causing impotence. With couples who are reticent about their sexual activity, the impotent man's partner may become concerned that infidelity is responsible for the change in sexual behavior. If dyspareunia is responsible for the altered sexual relationship, the unaffected partner quite reasonably feels rejected.

There are many ways to minimize the sexual conflicts that develop with impaired arousal and impotence. If there is a nonpsychologic basis for the sexual dysfunction, a simple explanation of the organic problem to both the affected individual and his or her partner may relieve a great deal of the tension that has developed between the two people. Common misconceptions must be dispelled before the couple can relax and enjoy their sexual relationship again, if in fact they did enjoy it before the problem developed. It is important that failure to achieve an erection not be misconstrued as a lack of interest in sexual activity or even as an inability to have sexual satisfaction. The concepts of potency and virility must be separated. Techniques for minimizing dyspareunia and sexual frustration should be described in explicit terms. Obviously, some couples use the sexual problem as an explanation for longstanding animosity towards each other. In such cases the affected individuals will be reluctant to change their unsatisfying sexual techniques and discard the sexual conflict to which they ascribe all their problems.

HYPERSEXUALITY

Excessive or inappropriate sexual behavior is an unusual manifestation of brain dysfunction. Obviously, hypersexuality is defined relative to the social norm, and older reports of indiscriminate mating by patients with seizure disorders arouse little suspicion of sexual dysfunction in these patients when viewed in the perspective of current views on normal sexual behavior. Hypersexuality as a pathologic sign must refer to an atypical or inappropriate increase in sexual activity for the individual patient. Sexual exhibitionism may develop postictally in some seizure patients not ordinarily disposed to indiscriminate sexual display (1). Occasional patients report an unprovoked feeling of sexual arousal in the postictal period (1,13). With cerebrocortical lesions from deep-seated frontotemporal tumors, diencephalic damage from encephalitis lethargica, or diffuse cerebritis from rabies, patients may exhibit transient hypersexuality (1). Lesions in the frontal lobe in the supraorbital region often cause gross sexual misconduct, such as public masturbation or indiscriminate attempts at sexual intercourse (1). Patients may have seizures triggered by sexual intercourse or masturbation, and unexpectedly this may lead to hypersexual behavior because the seizure itself may provide a pleasurable sensation (1).

Increased sexual interest and activity is unequivocally present in patients with Parkinson disease treated with levodopa (34). About 30 percent of patients treated with this dopamine precursor exhibit a change in sexual behavior, but men are more affected by this than women by a ratio of three to one (34). The men with the most dramatic increase in sexual activity on levodopa are those with no complaints of impotence before the introduction of the antiparkinsonian medication. Why women do not have this improved libido is unknown, but it may be related to the more profound changes in the endocrine system that occur in women at menopause. Most women with Parkinson disease are postmenopausal and probably do not have as active a hypothalamic-pituitary-gonadal axis as men with preserved potency in advanced age. Luteinizing hormone may be increased by the dopamine produced by the patients receiving levodopa, and elevation of this hormone may be involved in the relative hypersexuality appearing in these parkinsonian patients.

Kleine-Levin Syndrome

Adolescent men exclusively exhibit the Kleine-Levin syndrome of hypersexuality and episodic hypersomnia. These patients have episodes lasting days or weeks during which they sleep excessively, eat excessively, and exhibit inappropriate sexual behavior (35,36). Visual and auditory hallucinations occasionally develop, and the electroencephalographic pattern shows generalized slowing of background activity. No cause is known. It most commonly develops idiopathically, but it occasionally reflects damage from trauma, tumors, or encephalitis (15). No treatment is available, but the episodes cease by the time the patient reaches 30 years of age (36).

Klüver-Bucy Syndrome

Klüver and Bucy described changes in monkeys after bilateral ablation of the anterior temporal lobes, which included heightened distractibility, increased docility, and visual agnosia, as well as disturbed sexual behavior with excessive masturbation and indiscriminate mounting of other monkeys, whether they be male or female (15,37,38). The animals explored all objects in their environment by mouthing and smelling them (39). The responsible lesions appeared to be those involving the amygdaloid complex, hippocampus, and pyriform cortex of the temporal lobes (15). Similar behavior develops occasionally in patients after bilateral temporal lobectomies. These patients have profound memory loss if the lesions extend posterior to the amygdala, and they are likely to be extremely apathetic rather than just docile (15,40).

The full Klüver-Bucy syndrome only appears in primates and includes: (*1*) placidity, (*2*) hypersexuality and aberrant sexual behavior, (*3*) compulsive attention to every object in sight, (*4*) disturbed memory, (*5*) disturbed visual discrimination, (*6*) increased mouthing of all objects, and (*7*) changes in dietary patterns (41,42). These patients have massive oral grasping, and they seem to use their hands only as adjuncts to their mouths. Even dangerous items, such as razors, will be put in the mouth (41). Abnormal sexual behavior includes uninhibited conversation on sexual topics, indiscriminate verbal advances, attempts at kissing anyone nearby, compulsive masturbation, and public masturbation (39,41). Previously heterosexual individuals may become decidedly homosexual in behavior (42). Neurologic signs unrelated to the aberrant sexual behavior include stereotyped movements and repetitive imitation. Easy distractibility is prominent. All these abnormalities are likely to subside as the lesions in the temporal lobes become more chronic.

The pathologic basis for this syndrome when it appears acutely in humans is probably bilateral mesiobasal temporal lobe damage (41). This may develop with surgical resection of these areas or with Alzheimer disease, Pick disease, bilateral infarctions, toxoplasmosis encephalitis, viral encephalitis, demyelinating disease, or hypoglycemic brain damage (39,42). What the basic cognitive defect is that produces this extraordinary behavior pattern is unknown.

Persistent Erections: Priapism

Persistent penile erection (priapism) develops with spinal cord disease, especially if the damage is from trauma and the lesion is in the cervical or thoracic spinal cord (1). This is not easily confused with psychogenic erections since the lesion producing priapism must generally transect the spinal cord. As other signs of spinal shock subside, the priapism may persist or recur episodically for minutes or hours at a time (1). Much less commonly, priapism may be observed in patients with psychomotor seizures, but a history of amnestic episodes or frank convulsions should suggest the etiology of this sexual phenomenon.

Nonneurologic causes of priapism include sickle cell trait, anticoagulant treatment, and leukemia. In these hematologic disorders the cause of the priapism is unknown (32). The erections may last for weeks and may be painful. A bypass procedure to drain blood from the corpus spongiosum may be necessary, but with this procedure or with spontaneous resolution of the priapism the patient is often left impotent (32).

BLADDER CONTROL

Urinary Incontinence

Problems with bladder control in alert individuals are usually from local disease. Bladder reflexes or bladder sphincters may fail in numerous structural lesions in the pelvis. Occasional stress incontinence is espcially common in women after multiple vaginal deliveries. Men undergoing transurethral resection of the prostate because of urinary retention secondary to prostatic enlargement may find bladder control impaired after the surgery because of intraoperative injury to the bladder sphincter. Bladder infections in women are routinely associated with freqquency and urgency of urination, and occasional incontinence develops. More neurologic bases for bladder dysfunction include denervation and spasticity. The bladder with an impaired nerve supply, such as that seen with diabetic autonomic neuropathy, will fill beyond its capacity and inadvertently spill urine as an overflow phenomenon. This neurogenic bladder disorder is often called a flaccid bladder, and the unintentional voiding of urine by this type of bladder is called overflow incontinence. Spinal cord lesions affecting the sacral cord may also produce a flaccid bladder, but damage higher in the spinal cord usually produces a spastic bladder that empties reflexively even when the volume of urine in it is well below the real capacity of the bladder. Patients with multiple sclerosis routinely develop spastic bladders if they have other evidence of spinal cord demyelination. Treatments of these types of bladder dysfunction are usually directed at the primary lesion responsible for the bladder involvement. With untreatable diseases, such as multiple sclerosis, the patients usually require training in intermittent self-catheterization or surgical revisions of the

Table 8.2. Causes of Urinary Incontinence and Dementia

Hydrocephalus
Chronic subdural hematoma
Alzheimer disease
Neurosyphilis
Frontal lobe tumor
Machiafava-Bignami disease

urinary system to minimize the disability that arises with persistent urinary incontinence.

Demented patients often have poor personal hygiene, and poor toilet habits may be part of this problem with self-care. Whenever urinary incontinence and dementia develop together, however, certain brain diseases should be considered and sought (Table 8.2). Frontal lobe lesions, hydrocephalus, and chronic central nervous system infections can all produce intellectual impairment and poor bladder control, but other signs of neurologic disease are usually associated with these problems.

Enuresis

Urinary incontinence occurring during sleep is usually from nocturnal seizure activity or impaired bladder control if it occurs after early childhood. Episodes of enuresis occurring during the first few years after toilet training are not unusual and should not be viewed with excessive concern. These childhood lapses in bladder control during sleep generally do not have a pathologic basis. Normal adults may also have a rare episode of enuresis when they are aroused from slow wave (stage IV) sleep (43). Prolonged periods of confusion and terror are likely to accompany the enuresis during this arousal. As discussed in the section on sleep disorders, enuresis, as well as sleep-talking, sleep-walking, and night terrors, occur predominantly in stage-IV sleep, regardless of the associated pathology (43). The pathology associated with the enuresis may be a spinal cord tumor, but this is relatively rare (44). More commonly, the enuresis is idiopathic and follows a familial pattern along with other abnormal motor activities during sleep. Sixty-two percent of adult somnambulists have a history of enuresis, and in 38 percent that history extends to a family history of enuresis (45).

Urinary incontinence may result from sleep-related seizure activity. Sleep is so provocative an agent in patients with seizure disorders that fits may occur in some patients only when they are asleep. The patient is usually unaware of the seizure unless he bites his tongue or urinates in bed, and then he may seek help for that isolated symptom. The simplest way to determine if enuresis is actually a sign of nocturnal seizure activity is to do an electroencephalogram while the patient is asleep. Although an overt seizure may not occur, abnormal electrical activity can often be detected on the sleep recording. Anticonvulsant medication will stop the enuresis if epilepsy is responsible.

A spinal cord lesion, such as a tumor or cyst, causing enuresis will usually produce other signs and symptoms of spinal cord dysfunction. Impotence in men and impaired sexual response in women may be early problems associated with enuresis. As the cord lesions evolve, gait difficulty and daytime incontinence usually appear. A cystometrogram to assess bladder function by its response to an increasing volume of fluid will demonstrate bladder dysfunctions indicative of upper or lower motor neuron disese. If the history and cystometrogram suggest spinal cord pathology, a myelogram will help settle the issue.

Uncomplicated idiopathic enuresis is usually short-lived, but it may be very disturbing to the patient. For those patients concerned about the incontinence and for those with chronic enuresis, imipramine may provide some relief. The anticholinergic action of this tricyclic antidepressant on the muscles of the bladder wall is generally viewed as central to its effectiveness in inhibiting enuresis (44). It must be used on a daily basis to be effective against nocturnal incontinence. Imipramine will not affect the enuresis if it is a seizure phenomenon (46).

Urinary Retention

Problems with urinary control include an inability to initiate urination or to effectively empty the bladder. Patients with urinary retention often seek medical attention because of abdominal discomfort, but occasionally the only symptom of this bladder dysfunction will be a mass in the abdomen created by the greatly distended bladder (47). Structural damage to the neck of the bladder or abnormal sphincter activity can produce retention that lasts days and requires catheterization to relieve the pain produced by the bladder distention. Urinary tract infections can also produce retention by irritating the urethra and causing pain on attempted urination. Neurologic diseases that can produce urinary retention include lesions of the afferent (sensory) nerves from the bladder to the spinal cord, lesions of the spinal cord itself, and lesions of the efferent (motor) nerves from the spinal cord to the bladder. Infections, such as poliomyelitis, can produce transient urinary retention, but more permanent bladder dysfunctions are usually from diabetes mellitus, spinal cord tumors, cauda equina tumors, spinal cord cysts (syringomyelia), and pelvic trauma (47). With each of these neurologic disorders there are usually other signs of the disease besides the bladder problem. Diabetes usually produces sensory deficits in the feet if there is bladder dysfunction, and spinal cord lesions will routinely produce weakness or numbness in the legs. Damage to the cauda equina, the collection of spinal roots extending from the lowest portion of the spinal cord, produces fecal incontinence along with urinary retention. If the bladder dysfunction is an isolated problem, structural disease in the urinary tract must be sought.

Although there are several structural and physiologic bases for urinary retention, some individuals develop substantial retention and profound bladder distention despite the absence of any organic disease (Table 8.3). Urinary retention developing acutely in patients without obvious bladder infection, urethral defect, or neurologic disease is usually secondary to emotional problems (47,48). Additional symptoms in these patients routinely include low back pain, headache, and chronic gastrointestinal

Table 8.3. Causes of Urinary Retention

Psychogenic urinary retention
Urinary tract infection
Bladder obstruction
Diabetes mellitus
Infectious polyneuritis
Trauma
Syringomyelia
Spinal cord tumor
Cauda equina tumor
Combined system disease
Periarteritis nodosa

complaints (49). The retention will develop with stress, and individuals reacting in this way to stress often have a history of enuresis during childhood or adolescence. Women are more likely to have psychogenic urinary retention than are men (47). The typical patient is overtly seductive or depressed, relates the onset of her urinary problem to physical or emotional trauma, and routinely has undergone numerous gastrointestinal or gynecologic surgical procedures (49). The initiating trauma is usually gynecologic surgery, but sometimes the patient dates the problem to childbirth, an episode of marital conflict, the termination of a love affair, or the appearance of a systemic illness. Thirty-five percent of the women suffering from the suprapubic discomfort, frequency, and dysuria that characterize urinary retention have obvious psychiatric symptoms, such as extreme anxiety or auditory hallucinations (49). Psychiatric evaluation will reveal gross psychopathology in more than half, and up to 32 percent are overtly psychotic with schizophrenic or depressive psychoses (49). The nonpsychotic individuals usually have hysterical conversion reactions as the basis for their urinary retention. Men affected by this idiopathic urinary retention commonly admit to impotence and enuresis when specifically asked about these symptoms (48).

Both men and women with this problem usually have fairly obvious secondary gain from the disability. The abdominal discomfort associated with the fluid retention provides justification for avoiding sexual activity, as well as other types of physical activity. Numerous urologic procedures designed to relieve the functional obstruction by altering the neck of the bladder or dilating the urethra generally produce no lasting improvement (49). Retention of urine will occur periodically over the course of years, usually in concert with recurrent psychic trauma. Without treatment, the retention will abate after a few days or weeks (49).

REFERENCES

1. Blumer D, Walker AE: The neural basis of sexual behavior, in Benson DF, Blumer D (eds): *Psychiatric Aspects of Neurologic Disease*. New York, Grune & Stratton, 1975, p 199.
2. Sexual behavior and the sex hormones. *Lancet* 2:17, 1979.
3. Wilson JD: Sex hormones and sexual behavior. *N Engl J Med* 300:1269, 1979.
4. Ettigi PG, Brown GM: Brain disorders associated with endocrine dysfunctions, in Hendrie HC (ed): *The Psychiatric Clinics of North America*. Philadelphia, WB Saunders, 1978, vol 1, p 117.
5. Imperato-McGinley J, Peterson RE, Gautier T, et al: Androgens and the evolution of male-gender identity among male pseudohermaphrodites with 5-alpha-reductase deficiency. *N Engl J Med* 300:1233, 1979.
6. Dörner G, Rohde W, Stahl F, et al: A neuroendocrine predisposition for homosexuality in men. *Arch Sex Behav* 4:1, 1975.
7. Masters WH, Johnson VE: *Human Sexual Response*. Boston, Little, Brown and Company, 1980.
8. Frank E, Anderson C, Rubinstein D: Frequency of sexual dysfunction in "normal" couples. *N Engl J Med* 299:111, 1978.
9. Taylor DC: Sexual behavior and temporal lobe epilepsy. *Arch Neurol* 21:510, 1969.
10. Blumer D: Hypersexual episodes in temporal lobe epilepsy. *Am J Psychiatry* 126:1099, 1970.
11. Maruta T, Osborne D, Swanson DW, et al: Chronic pain patients and spouses: Marital and sexual adjustment. *Mayo Clin Proc* 56:307, 1981.
12. Mignone RJ, Donnelly EF, Sadowsky D: Psychological and neurological comparisons of psychomotor and non-psychomotor epileptic patients. *Epilepsia* 11:345, 1970.
13. Mohan KJ, Salo MW, Nagaswami S: A case of limbic system dysfunction with hypersexuality and fugue state. *Dis Nerv Syst* 36:621, 1975.
14. Waxman SG, Geschwind N: Hypergraphia in temporal lobe epilepsy. *Neurology (NY)* 24:629, 1974.
15. Sherwin I, Geschwind N: Neural substrates of behavior, in Nicholi AM (ed): *The Harvard Guide to Modern Psychiatry*. Cambridge, Belknap Press, 1978, p 59.
16. Monoamine oxidase inhibitors for depression. *Med Lett* 22:58, 1980.
17. Ellenberg M: Sexual function in diabetic patients. *Ann Intern Med* 92(part 2):331, 1980.
18. Drugs for psychiatric disorders. *Med Lett Drugs Ther* 22:77, 1980.
19. Fisher JD: Contributions illustrative of the functions of the cerebellum. *Am J Med Sci* 23:352, 1839.
20. Brown-Sequard CE: Lectures on the diagnosis and treatment of the various forms of paralytic, convulsive, and mental affections, considered as effects of morbid alterations of the blood, or of the brain or other organs. *Lancet* 2:515, 1861.
21. Massey EW, Pleet AB: Penile prosthesis for impotence in multiple sclerosis. *Ann Neurol* 6:451, 1979.
22. Martin JB, Reichlin S, Brown GM: *Clinical Neuroendocrinology*. Philadelphia, FA DAvis, 1977.
23. Hierons R, Saunders M: Impotence in patients with temporal-lobe lesions. *Lancet* 2:761, 1966.
24. Shy GM, Drager GA: A neurological syndrome associated with orthostatic hypotension: A clinical-pathologic study. *Arch Neurol* 2:511, 1960.
25. Blumer D: Temporal lobe epilepsy and its psychiatric significance, in Benson DF, Blumer D (eds): *Psychiatric Aspects of Neurologic Disease*. New York, Grune & Stratton, 1975, p 171.

26. Ziegler MG, Lake CR, Kopin IJ: The sympathetic-nervous-system defect in primary orthostatic hypotension. *N Engl J Med* 296:293, 1977.
27. Parkes D: Bromocriptine. *N Engl J Med* 301:873, 1979.
28. Martinez AJ, Lee A, Moossy J, et al: Pituitary adenomas: Clinicopathological and immunohistochemical study. *Ann Neurol* 7:24, 1980.
29. Van Thiel DH: Feminization of chronic alcoholic men: A formulation. *Yale J Biol Med* 52:219, 1979.
30. Mendelson JH, Mello NK: Biologic concomitants of alcoholism. *N Engl J Med* 301:912, 1979.
31. Task force on nomenclature and statistics, American Psychiatric Association: *Diagnostic and Statistical Manual of Mental Disorders (Third Edition)*. Washington, DC, American Psychiatric Association, 1980.
32. Blandy J: Sexual problems in urology, in Crown S (ed): *Psychosexual Problems: Psychotherapy, Counselling and Behavioural Modification*. New York, Grune & Stratton, 1976, p 367.
33. Guinan ME, MacCalman J, Kern ER, et al: The course of untreated recurrent genital Herpes simplex infection in 27 women. *N Engl J Med* 304:759, 1981.
34. Brown E, Brown GM, Kofman O, et al: Sexual function and affect in parkinsonian men treated with L-DOPA. *Am J Psychiatry* 135:1552, 1978.
35. Kleine W: Periodische Schlafsucht. *Monatsschr Psychiatr Neurol* 57:285, 1925.
36. Chiles JA, Wilkus RJ: Behavioral manifestations of the Kleine-Levin syndrome. *Dis Nerv Syst* 37:646, 1976.
37. Klüver H, Bucy PC: Psychic blindness and other symptoms following bilateral temporal lobectomy in rhesus monkeys. *Am J Physiol* 119:352, 1937.
38. Klüver H, Bucy PC: An analysis of certain effects of bilateral temporal lobectomy in the rhesus monkey, with special reference to psychic blindness. *J Psychol* 5:33, 1938.
39. Powers JM, Schaumberg HH, Gaffney CL: Klüver-Bucy syndrome caused by adrenoleukodystrophy. *Neurology (NY)* 30:1131, 1980.
40. Glaser GH, Pincus JH: Limbic encephalitis. *J Nerv Ment Dis* 149:59, 1969.
41. Poeck K: Pathophysiology of emotional disorders associated with brain damage, in Vinken PJ, Bruyn GW (eds): *Handbook of Clinical Neurology*. New York, American Elsevier, 1969, vol 3, p 343.
42. Marlowe WB, Mancall EL, Thomas JJ: Complete Klüver-Bucy syndrome in man. *Cortex* 11:53, 1975.
43. Roth N: Sleep and motility. *Dis Nerv Syst* 38:778, 1977.
44. Pearlman CA, Greenberg R: Medical-psychological implications of recent sleep research. *Psychiatry Med* 1:261, 1970.
45. Karacan I, Moore CA: Genetics and human sleep. *Psychiatr Ann* 9:11, 1979.
46. Rodin EA: Psychosocial management of patients with complex partial seizures. *Adv Neurol* 11:383, 1975.
47. Plum F: Bladder dysfunction, in Williams D (ed): *Modern Trends in Neurology*. London, Butterworths, 1962, vol 3, p 151.
48. Berlin RM, Carvell MC, Noori SS, et al: Psychogenic urinary retention in a man. *Psychosomatics* 21:607, 1980.
49. Larson JW, Swenson WM, Utz DC, et al: Psychogenic urinary retention in women. *J Am Med Assoc* 184:697, 1963.

9
Movement Disorders

Abnormal movement or immobility develops with psychologic stress or neurologic disease and may prompt psychiatric evaluation of an otherwise normal individual. An uncharacteristic pattern of movement occasionally worries the victim of the disorder enough to seek medical attention, but more typically the individual with abnormal movements is unaware of or unconcerned by his symptoms. Often the gradually progressive gait difficulty, tremors, clumsiness, or posturing arouse concern in those familiar with the patient when the patient himself is unaware of the problem, and these concerned friends or family members compel the patient to see a physician. The disturbance of movements coupled with the patient's apparent indifference to the movement disorder reinforces the casual impression that he has a psychologic problem. Even when the patient is aware of the movement disorder, he may volunteer the suspicion that the basic problem is just "nerves," a curious reaction to daily stress (Table 9.1). Because many movement disorders do have a psychologic basis, physicians are often inclined to minimize the significance of a peculiar movement or activity. Irrepressible limb jerks, "tics," involuntary grimacing, head tilting, and painful jaw clenching may be ascribed to an anxiety neurosis or a conversion reaction by the medical practitioner or mental health professional initially evaluating the patient. This misinterpretation of abnormal movements is even more likely when the patient has a well-established psychiatric history. Individuals with obvious mental illness may be misdiagnosed as suffering from an exacerbation of their cognitive or affective disorder, rather than experiencing a new problem. Although the patient with abnormal movements may have a psychiatric basis for his symptoms, degenerative neurologic disease, brain dysfunction precipitated by metabolic disorders, and basal ganglia disorders caused by antipsychotic drugs must also be considered as possible causes of the movement disorder. Movement disorders developing from central nervous system disease usually can be treated and occasionally can be cured.

Psychiatric patients can develop movement disorders on several bases. Abnormal movement, as well as a poverty of movement, can occur as a

Table 9.1. Movement Disorders Misdiagnosed as Stress Reaction

Oromandibular dystonia with blepharospasm (Meige disease)
Essential tremor
Dystonia musculorum deformans
Huntington disease
Chorea gravidarum
Hyperthyroid tremor
Sydenham chorea
Bruxism

feature of psychiatric disorders ranging from schizophrenia to endogenous depression. Those patients with mental illness not developing abnormal motor function on the basis of their psychiatric problems often develop movement disorders as a side effect of their antipsychotic medication. Medications frequently causing movement disorders include the commonly used drugs haloperidol, chlorpromazine, lithium carbonate, and thiothixene. The movement disorder induced may in fact be a diminution in normal motor activity, but whether the patient has increased or decreased movement is less important than that there is an alteration in his normal movement or tone. The absence of movement can certainly be just as worrisome and disabling as an excess of movement. Bradykinesia, a generalized slowing of movements, appears with psychotic depression, as well as with such degenerative nervous system disorders as Parkinson disease. This same slowing of movement develops with the routine use of phenothiazines and butyrophenones. The context of bradykinesia usually leaves little doubt whether it has a neurogenic, iatrogenic, or psychogenic etiology. This is also true for disorders associated with tremors, but not for the less frequent disorders of facial movement and total body movement. Grimacing will develop with neuroleptic drug treatment as part of a tardive dyskinesia, but in the absence of a drug history the patient may have a habit spasm or a degenerative disease. There are criteria for deciding whether or not dyskinesias are a result of treatment, habit, or progressive disease, just as there are ways to distinguish contrived jerking movements of the limbs from the involuntary limb jerks of Huntington disease and the clumsy limb movements of multiple sclerosis. Once the etiology of the disorder is defined, the appropriate treatment can be initiated.

Sorting out the bases for movement disorders in psychiatric patients is more complicated than diagnosing disturbed movement in nonpsychiatric cases. The psychiatrist faces patients with movement disorders both as a manifestation of abnormal behavior and as a consequence of accepted psychiatric therapy. To further complicate the distinction between neurologic and psychiatric movement disorders, psychiatric problems develop along with abnormal movements in some neurologic diseases characterized by psychomotor disturbances. Even when psychiatric reactions are not a basic feature of the neurologic disease, some patients will develop profound thought or affective disorders during the treatment of the neurologic disorder. Patients with Wilson disease or Huntington disease, both degenerative diseases of the basal ganglia of the brain, may be suicidal, and patients treated with levodopa for Parkinson disease may become agitated or euphoric. Movement disorders may be evidence of neurologic or psychiatric disease, and psychiatric disorders may appear at the onset or during the treatment of movement disorders.

DECREASED MOVEMENT

A generalized decrease or slowing of normal movements, whether they be limb, truncal, or facial movements, is called bradykinesia or akinesia. Mild bradykinesia is common in a variety of depressive disorders, and extreme states of limited motion appear in schizophrenia and affective disorders, as already discussed in the chapter on alterations of consciousness (1). Bradykinesia may occur as an isolated sign; but, when the disorder has a neurologic basis, tremor, increased muscle tone, and impaired cognition routinely develop along with the slowing of movements. The most common neurologic disease with prominent bradykinesia is Parkinson disease, a degenerative disease affecting the basal ganglia. Determining whether degenerative disease of the brain or an affective disorder is responsible for bradykinesia is complicated by the frequent development of affective disorders in degenerative nervous system diseases. Patients with Parkinson disease commonly experience depression and bradykinesia before rigidity, tremor, or dementia appear.

Whenever decreased movement or immobility appears coincidentally with a psychotic depression, an organic basis for the psychiatric problem should be vigorously pursued. Suicidal ideation is often associated with the bradykinesia, tremor, and rigidity that characterize the early phases of hepatolenticular degeneration (Wilson disease), a disorder of copper metabolism that leads to cerebral and basal ganglia damage. Suicide is also a leading cause of death in patients with Huntington disease, a dominantly inherited dementing illness that produces increased movements in affected adults but rigidity and decreased movements in some affected children. Bradykinesia and psychosis occurring together are usually explained as the consequence of antipsychotic treatment in a psychiatric patient, and this is, in fact, the most common reason for concurrence of the two problems. Bradykinesia is a predictable side effect of most antipsychotic medications used in chronic, as well as acute, cognitive, and affective disorders. Because the symptoms appearing secondary to antipsychotic medication are similar to those appearing with idiopathic Parkinson disease, the patient is described as parkinsonian or as exhibiting parkinsonism.

Because parkinsonian signs develop with several diseases that damage the basal ganglia, determining the initial injury in patients with psychiatric as well as neurologic deficits may be no simple task. Parkinsonism arising with phenothiazine use is indistinguishable from that arising as a late sequela of influenza encephalitis. A thorough history is the best tool for distinguishing between drug-related, postinfectious, metabolic, degenerative, and other kinds of parkinsonism. The psychotic patient with bradykinesia and rigidity presents a complicated diagnostic situation if there is no history to clarify the setting in which the movement disorder first appeared. A parkinsonian patient treated with bromocriptine may exhibit a psychosis and movement disorder indistinguishable from the psychosis and movement disorder of the schizophrenic patient treated with haloperidol. The sequence of events and the various elements involved in the evolution of the psychiatric and neurologic problems determine the course of treatment appropriate for the psychotic patient with a movement disorder.

PARKINSON DISEASE

Clinical Features

Parkinson disease is characterized by bradykinesia, tremor, rigidity, and dementia (2). These four basic features appear separately or in various combinations during the evolution of the disease, but each feature assumes a fairly stereotyped form. The bradykinesia is evident in gait, limb movement, facial expression, and truncal movement. Both the initiation and the performance of movements are slowed. Standing from a seated position may be so slowed that the patient can never rise without considerable assistance. A failure to smoothly shift the center of gravity as the trunk is eased out of a chair will force the patient to fall repeatedly back into the chair. Routinely associated with this bradykinesia is a profound reluctance to be at all active. The patient is afraid of being injured during an attempt to be more active. Other signs may precede or follow the bradykinesia. Tremor is commonly a complaint annoying enough to induce the patient to seek medical attention, even if it is much less a problem than a coincidental bradykinesia. The tremor is fine, often limited to flexion-extension movements of the fingers at 4 to 6 cycles per second when the limb is in a stationary position (2). "Pill-rolling" tremors, so called because the patient seems to be rolling a pill between his thumb and index finger, and other static tremors disappear when the patient uses the tremulous limb. Tremors may also involve the face or neck muscles. Tone in the limbs with or without tremor is increased. Resistance to movement is constant, regardless of the speed or amplitude of the passive movement, very much like the resistance felt on bending a lead pipe. An intermittent change in the resistance to movement will appear at some joints during manipulation of the limb. This rhythmic alteration in rigidity is often called "cogwheeling." The dementia in Parkinson disease was long unrecognized, and James Parkinson originally contended that patients with the "shaking palsy" do not have intellectual deterioration (3,4). Dementia is common in the elderly group most often affected by Parkinson disease, but the incidence of progressive dementia is too high in this degenerative disease to be explained by "senility" (2). At least 55 percent of patients dying with Parkinson disease have a significant dementia (3). Orientation, construction, and memory are particularly impaired, with social behavior, language, and manipulation of old information less impaired (3). Thought processes slow in much the same way movements slow. Questions may be answered accurately but only after an inordinate delay. More commonly, the patient fails to answer or gives an inaccurate answer.

Affective, as well as intellectual, function is impaired in Parkinson disease. This is most commonly manifest as a depression out of proportion to the neurologic deficits (2). Some patients develop emotional lability, but this is usually difficult to disentangle from inappropriate reactions induced by the intellectual problems. If depression does occur, it will make the dementia appear more severe than it actually is and, accordingly, may discourage an energetic approach to the patient's other symptoms.

Either depression or dementia is often the initial sign of Parkinson disease. Fifty percent of patients with Parkinson disease develop a significant depression at some time in the illness (5). The psychomotor retardation developing during the depressive phase of manic-depressive psychosis is indistinguishable from the bradykinesia or "bradyphrenia" of Parkinson disease (1). Both patients will have little facial expression, slow motor performance, and soft monotonous speech. The history of the illness will distinguish the progressive, degenerative nervous system disorder from the episodic, remitting affective disorder.

Other signs occurring with Parkinson disease include more extensive neurologic and systemic dysfunctions. The patient has little spontaneous facial movement and this produces the poverty of facial expression usually described as "masked facies." Blinking is reduced, and there is a prominent stare. A normal individual told not to blink when the glabellar area on the forehead between the eyes is repeatedly tapped will stop blinking, but the parkinsonian patient will have the Meyersen sign of persistent blinking on glabellar tapping. Parkinsonian patients also have a characteristic dysarthria. Speech volume is poorly controlled: words taper off to a hurried, unintelligible whisper. When he tries to walk, the patient seems stiff and mechanical, because the normal swing of his arms is lost. His steps are short and shuffling with a tendency to increase in speed (propulsion) as he walks. His trunk is bent forward; and stopping, as well as initiating walking, is difficult. Patients often resist all efforts to get them to walk because of an almost obsessive fear of being unable to stop themselves once they have started taking steps. They commonly complain that they will fall if they are forced to walk, even though they have never actually suffered a fall because of the gait problem. Turns are made with the head and trunk turning together as if fused into a single block. This is called turning *en bloc*, and it is usually accomplished with several shuffling steps. Any change in direction may destabilize the patient sufficiently to produce a fall. Just sitting or standing in a fixed position may be complicated by a tendency to fall backwards (retropulsion). Smooth eye movements, characteristic of normal visual pursuit, are lost, and the steplike saccadic eye movements retained are short or hypometric. Seborrhea gives the masked, staring face an oily appearance. Despite the patient's disabled appearance, mentation may be relatively intact until late in the disease. Dementia is often a prominent component of Parkinson disease, but it is not necessarily present just because the patient moves slowly. Profound bradykinesia may occur with largely intact intellectual function.

Pathogenesis

Any patient with this set of signs and symptoms is called parkinsonian or a victim of parkinsonism. He has Parkinson disease only if his movement disorder results from an idiopathic degeneration of his basal ganglia characterized by prominent loss of neurons and pigment in the substantia nigra, a collection of pigmented neurons in the midbrain (Figure 9.1). Inclusion bodies, called Lewy bodies, in the basal ganglia neurons are also typical (3). Patients may have parkinsonism and not have Parkinson disease if autopsy reveals degeneration of other basal ganglia structures, such as the globus pallidus, with sparing of the substantia nigra. Parkinsonism refers to a set of traits, not to a diagnosis or etiology. Parkinson disease is a discrete pathologic entity developing sporadically in individuals of all races and ancestries.

The basic defect in Parkinson disease is presumed to be degeneration of a system of neurons essential to the regulation of movements that uses the neurotransmitter dopamine (6). Dopamine is a neurotransmitter or local hormone in several areas of the brain, including the hypothalmus, pituitary gland, prefrontal cortex, and brainstem areas, as well as the basal ganglia (7). In Parkinson disease, the major pathologic changes are found in the pigmented midbrain component of the basal ganglia, the substantia nigra. Pigmented neurons in the substantia nigra are lost; these cells convert levodopa to dopamine. Dopamine in this system is actually active in the deep brain structures above the substantia nigra in the aggregates of neurons called the putamen and caudate or the striatum. Dopamine is a largely inhibitory neurotransmitter in these subcortical or diencephalic structures (6). The loss of dopamine in the striatum produces levels less

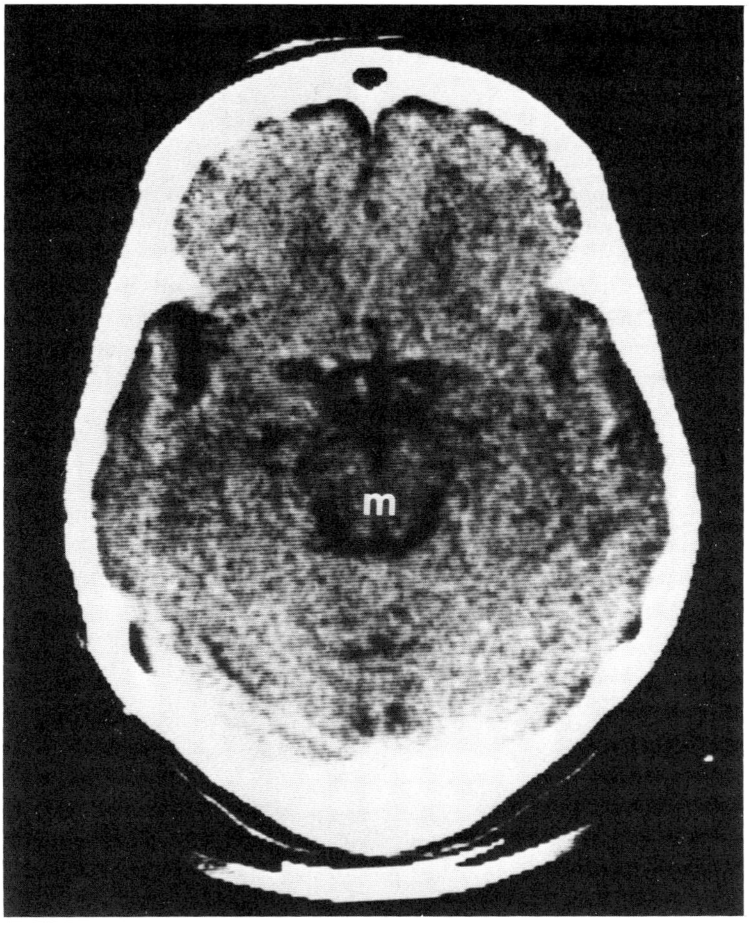

Figure 9.1. The substantia nigra is a collection of pigmented neurons in the ventral half of the midbrain (m). This structure is too small to be seen clearly on a computed tomogram, and atrophy of the substantia nigra will cause no change in the radiographic appearance of the midbrain. The two humps on the dorsal aspect of the midbrain (below the "m") are the superior colliculi.

than 20 percent of normal in patients with autopsy-proven Parkinson disease (6). The basal ganglia regulate body movements according to cues provided by several neurotransmitter systems. Just as important as the dopamine system is the acetylcholine-utilizing or cholinergic system. An imbalance in the effectiveness of dopaminergic and cholinergic systems is the theoretical basis for parkinsonism and other movement disorders (8). A relative excess of cholinergic activity results from the loss of dopamine transmitting neurons. According to this hypothesis, Parkinson disease should respond to either an enhancement of the dopamine system or a reduction of the acetylcholine activity in the striatum.

Treatment: Psychiatric Complications

Dopamine does not cross the blood-brain barrier, and so any attempts to compensate for a deficiency in this neurotransmitter must provide this material to the brain indirectly or provide other substances that will offset the dopamine deficiency. Drugs have had to be devised to induce excess dopamine formation or reduce dopamine destruction. Actually, most of the substances first effectively used in the treatment of parkinsonism were directed at the cholinergic system. Drugs depleting acetylcholine or interfering with its action are still often adequate treatment for Parkinson disease.

Anticholinergic Drugs and Other Early Approaches. Systemic effects of anticholinergic drugs, such as trihexyphenidyl and benztropine, include flushing, dry mouth, nausea, vomiting, dry eyes, constipation, urinary urgency and hesitancy, and occasional cardiac arrhythmias (9). These systemic effects are less often the basis for discontinuing the anticholinergic treatment than are the undesired neurologic and psychiatric effects (Table 9.2). In addition to suppressing the rigidity, tremor, and bradykinesia of parkinsonism, these atropine-like drugs may produce pupillary dilatation, disorientation, short-term memory loss, dysarthria, clumsiness, insomnia, or excessive drowsiness (9). All these unwanted effects reflect actions of the drug on muscarinic receptor sites in the central nervous system. Anticholinergics compete with acetylcholine for receptor sites and thereby block the action of acetylcholine itself (9). Psychiatric manifestations of anticholinergic medications include hallucinations, euphoria, agitation, inappropriate affect, stereotypy, mannerisms, and delusions (8,9). These affective and cognitive disorders develop in about 30 percent of patients treated with benztropine, trihexyphenidyl, and other atropinic drugs (8). Anticholinergics used in combination with neuroleptics and antidepressants may produce undesirable side effects independently of the antipsychotic drug or by interacting with the antipsychotic drug. The threshold for tricyclic antidepressant toxicity is lowered by anticholinergic medication (9). All signs of anticholinergic drug overdose related to the nervous system will resolve within 24 hours of discontinuing the drugs (9).

Other drugs used primarily before the introduction of levodopa include amphetamines, monoamine oxidase inhibitors, tricyclic antidepressants, and amantadine. For each there was a rationale and empirical improvement to justify its use. Amphetamines and methylphenidate increase monoamine neurotransmission, and presumably thereby increased motor activity (8). Monoamine oxidase inhibitors, such as tranylcypramine and isocarboxazid, retard catabolism of biogenic amines and, at least, ameliorated the depres-

Table 9.2. Neurologic and Psychiatric Side Effects of Antiparkinsonian Drugs

Medication	*Neurologic Side Effects*	*Psychiatric Side Effects*
Anticholinergics	Disorientation Memory impairment Insomnia Dysarthria Drowsiness Clumsiness Urinary retention	Agitation Delusions Euphoria Inappropriate affect Hallucinations Stereotypy Mannerisms
Amantadine		Disorientation Delusions Hallucinations
Levodopa	Choreoathetosis Akathisia Orofacial dyskinesia Nausea and vomiting Insomnia On-off effect	Agitation Delusions Euphoria Obsessional behavior Vivid dreams Hallucinations Stereotypy Impaired judgment
Bromocriptine	Choreoathetosis Orofacial dyskinesias	Delusions Nocturnal confusion Hallucinations Aggression

sion commonly associated with Parkinson disease. Tricyclic antidepressants, such as imipramine and amitriptyline, have an anticholinergic effect and relieve bradykinesia, rigidity, and depression (8). Amantadine was developed as an antiviral agent and has been found to ameliorate parkinsonism for months at a time. Both amantadine and amphetamines appear to act presynaptically rather than postsynaptically (7).

Prominent psychiatric complications are likely to develop with several of these drugs. Amphetamines can precipitate profound cognitive disorders or agitation. Both amphetamines and methylphenidate increase the incidence of schizophrenic symptoms in treated patients, presumably by pathways affected by increased dopamine activity in the basal ganglia (10). Amantadine occasionally produces delusional and confusional states (8). It can induce or exacerbate hallucinations, especially if the patient has renal disease and can not effectively eliminate the drug (10). Complications resulting from the use of these drugs in Parkinson disease have been considerably less of a problem since the introduction of the potent antiparkinsonian drug levodopa.

Levodopa. Levodopa (L-dopa) is converted in the brain to dopamine and presumably compensates for the dopamine deficiency in the basal ganglia developing with Parkinson disease (2). This drug may reduce tremor, rigidity, and bradykinesia, but, at the same time, it may induce abnormal involuntary movements (6). Denervation of the striatal receptor cells in this degenerative disease probably produces hypersensitivity to dopamine. The patient may have writhing movements or exhibit an inability to sit still. Choreoathetosis and akathisia, as they are called, most often occur at peak levels of serum levodopa, at least initially (8). Levodopa-induced orofacial and tongue movements, also called levodopa dyskinesias, develop in 39 to 80 percent of parkinsonian patients treated with the drug for more than 5 years (11,12). Involuntary head movements, grunting, and limb choreoathetosis also develop (11). Patients commonly have nausea and vomiting, insomnia, agitation, orthostatic hypotension, and transient tachycardia initially; but, with continued use of the levodopa, these signs decrease (8).

Ten to 25 percent of patients on long-term levodopa treatment will develop significant psychiatric symptoms (2,13). These typically include affective disorders and hallucinations. A levodopa psychosis will appear soon after the start of treatment in patients with a history of mental disease, but a frank psychosis does not usually develop in the previously well patient until the drug has been administered for months or years (10). With a past history of schizophrenia, recurrence of the antecedent psychosis routinely occurs within a few weeks of levodopa administration (10). This commonly observed exacerbation of quiescent psychosis is a major reason why levodopa is not an appropriate drug for treating the drug-induced parkinsonism of the mentally ill patient on phenothiazines or butyrophenones. Recurrence of an old psychosis induced by levodopa may not subside for months (10). Stereotypy, the repetitive, purposeless limb or truncal movement seen in schizophrenia, develops in some patients with Parkinson disease treated with levodopa (1). The restlessness and anxiety routinely appearing on starting levodopa may progress to severe agitation with episodic hypomania, poor judgment, euphoria, or paranoid delusions (2,8). One-third of all patients on levodopa for more than 2 years develop recurrent visual and, less commonly, auditory hallucinations (10,12,13). These usually occur at night, are not threatening, and, in over 65 percent of cases, are associated with levodopa-induced dream abnormalities (10). Remarkably vivid, coherent, and factual dreams are reported by one-fourth of all patients treated with levodopa (12). Night terrors and nightmares develop in 10 percent of treated patients (10). Stereotyped obsessional behavior or an acute delirium will rarely appear.

If a frank psychosis occurs, it will include a paranoid delusional system with little or no other evidence of cognitive dysfunction (10). This will develop in about 3 percent of levodopa-treated patients after 2 years of drug use (10). Patients with paranoid psychoses in their past, unrelated to drug use, are more likely to have significant confusion as part of their drug-induced psychoses. These psychotic disorders subside readily with termination of the levodopa. A drug holiday, that is, a cessation of all treatment for 5 to 7 days, is especially effective in treating the psychiatric complications of levodopa use (13). After the holiday, the patient requires a lower dose of levodopa to improve the movement disorder and the psychiatric problems are the least likely of all the levodopa-induced side effects to recur (13).

Institution of low dose phenothiazine treatment is unavoidable in some cases to help the patient weather the psychosis as it abates (8,10). Depression is characteristically relieved on levodopa treatment, but rare patients become more depressed and attempt suicide (2,8). Antidepressant treatment is often helpful in patients with Parkinson disease, both to increase the patient's level of activity and to minimize the possibility of self-destructive behavior. Tricyclic antidepressants, such as imipramine, are the drugs of choice. Monoamine oxidase inhibitors are contraindicated because they may precipitate a hypertensive crisis when used in combination with levodopa (14).

There is some loss of the patient's customary inhibitions when he is treated with levodopa, and this may account for the observed increase in sexual activity (2,5,8). Increased sexual interest and activity develop three times as commonly in parkinsonian men treated with the drug as in parkinsonian women, with as many as one-half of the levodopa-treated men exhibiting this change in sexual pattern (5). Speculation to explain this rather specifically male-related effect of levodopa treatment has included theories that the catecholamine acts on hypothalamic-pituitary-gonadal systems that are not so active in postmenopausal women as they are in senescent men. Consistent with this endocrinologic explanation is the observed maximum effect on sexuality in parkinsonian men who are not impotent before the introduction of the levodopa (5). Apparently, the drug increases sexual interest and activity most in men who still have some sexual function despite the other disabilities arising with the Parkinson disease. There is no correlation between the effect of levodopa on sex drive and its effect on locomotor function in either men or women (5).

Dopa-Decarboxylase Inhibitors. Dopa-decarboxylase inhibitors, such as carbidopa, are combined with levodopa to reduce conversion of the drug to dopamine outside the central nervous system. This decreases both the dose of levodopa needed and systemic side effects. Nausea and vomiting, the principal limitations to the use of high dose levodopa, are decreased without sacrificing effectiveness against signs of parkinsonism (15). Combination of levodopa with a dopa-decarboxylase inhibitor does not decrease the incidence of psychiatric disturbances or choreoathetoid movement disorders developing with levodopa treatment alone (8). Patients also continue having levodopa-induced dyskinesias and the bizarre motor phenomenon referred to as the "on-off" effect, in which the medication abruptly, but transiently, seems to lose all its effectiveness (7,11,15).

Patients often have a progressive decline in their response to antiparkinsonian medication. After 3 to 4 years on levodopa or other antiparkinsonian medications, the patient may have increasing signs of parkinsonism despite increases in the dosage of drugs previously effective in controlling their movement disorder (12). Drug-related side effects become more severe Dyskinesias, violent limb jerks (myoclonus), on-off phenomena, hallucinations, and more complex psychoses all appear as the patient enters this refractory phase of his disease. The most effective approach to this drug failure is stopping all antiparkinsonian medications. After 1 week off all drugs, the patient usually has a good response to medication when it is restarted (13).

Bromocriptine. Efforts to avoid the unwanted side effects of levodopa led to the use of dopamine agonists, that is, drugs presumed to work at the dopamine receptor in place of dopamine. Dopamine agonists currently in clinical use include the ergot alkaloids (6,15). These drugs appear to act at the dopamine receptor as if they were an alternative to dopamine itself, but some dopamine activity must be present in the brain for these agonists to ameliorate the signs of parkinsonism (16). If dopamine synthesis or storage is inhibited, the ergot alkaloids are ineffective in suppressing the abnormal motor phenomena of Parkinson disease (7). There is some evidence that these ergot derivatives decrease the rate of synthesis and release of acetylcholine, thereby compensating for a relative insufficiency of dopamine in the basal ganglia (1). With less acetylcholine available in the system, the limited dopamine available can more effectively modulate movements. Receptor sensitivity after denervation is also an important factor in determining the efficacy of these drugs. There may, in fact, be several mechanisms involved in the action of ergot alkaloids in Parkinson disease.

Bromocriptine is the ergot alkaloid most widely used in the treatment of Parkinson disease, but results with this drug have been disappointing (17). Some patients with poorly controlled parkinsonism while on levodopa will show improvement on bromocriptine; but problems with bromocriptine include gastrointestinal disturbances, mental changes, and orthostatic hypotension. These are, in fact, more of a problem with bromocriptine than with levodopa; abnormal involuntary movements may be just as much of a problem for patients treated with levodopa (15). Ten milligrams of bromocriptine are usually as effective as the combination of 100 milligrams of levodopa with 10 milligrams of carbidopa (7). This would place an effective dose of bromocriptine in most parkinsonian patients at under 100 milligrams, but some patients require as much as 200 milligrams daily of bromocriptine to elicit a good response. Improvement in the motor abnormalities in Parkinson disease will appear within a few days of starting treatment (7). Although combining levodopa and bromocriptine occasionally improves the therapeutic results, most patients responding poorly to levodopa will respond poorly to bromocriptine (7). The "on-off" effect seen with long-term levodopa treatment is not so common with bromocriptine, but choreiform and dystonic movement disorders induced by levodopa will also appear with bromocriptine treatment (7,17).

Altered behavior and awareness develop in 20 to 35 percent of all patients with Parkinson disease given bromocriptine (7). Psychiatric disorders occurring with bromocriptine also include visual and auditory hallucinations, delusions, and personality changes (6). These disturbances are not dose-related and are, in fact, the most common adverse effects of bromocriptine (15,18). The type of psychiatric problem developing with bromocriptine depends largely upon the patient's personality or prevailing mental state (18). Paranoid or aggressive behavior and nocturnal confusion are fairly common (18). Despite initial hopes that bromocriptine would produce fewer psychiatric complications than levodopa, the changes in awareness and behavior produced with this dopamine agonist are more frequent and more lasting than those produced by an equivalently antiparkinsonian dose of levodopa (18). Thought disorders often persist 2 to 6 weeks after the drug has been stopped (15).

POSTENCEPHALITIC PARKINSONISM

Parkinsonism may develop in some patients after they have had a viral encephalitis. The symptoms developing with this postencephalitic parkinsonism are indistinguishable from those occurring with idiopathic Parkinson disease. Postencephalitic parkinsonism is not a rare disorder. It is especially common in children surviving several different viral encephalitides, including those caused by influenza viruses. Although the structural damage to the brain suffered during the viral infection occurs primarily during the acute phase of the encephalitis, the parkinsonian signs that appear after the illness may progress over the course of weeks or months (19). Associated with the rigidity, tremor, and bradykinesia typical of postencephalitic parkinsonism are intellectual problems of varying severity. Children who develop postencephalitic parkinsonism often exhibit hyperkinetic behavior, with excessive restlessness and purposeless activity paradoxically superimposed upon the parkinsonism (19). These children have the psychomotor slowing typical of parkinsonism along with the easy distractibility of minimal brain dysfunction. Abstract thinking is the intellectual function most consistently impaired with postencephalitic parkinsonism (19).

Some patients may insidiously develop bradykinesia and rigidity without any antecedent episodes consistent with encephalitis. This parkinsonism may be unrecognized as postencephlitic until after autopsy examination of the brain reveals changes typical of viral damage to the basal ganglia. Parkinsonian signs developed in many individuals who lived through the encephalitis lethargica epidemic occurring after 1918, even though they did not have clearly documented episodes of encephalitis. Presumably, the encephalitis may be relatively minor before the development of parkinsonism, but a history of headache, altered consciousness, and, occasionally, seizures can usually be obtained on careful questioning. These signs and symptoms help establish that the patient had a viral encephalitis and that the insidiously progressive movement disorder is postencephalitic parkinsonism. This disease presents a special diagnostic problem, because the movement abnormalities developing with postencephalitic parkinsonism are indistinguishable from the motor manifestations of schizophrenic catatonia (1).

Pathologic changes are concentrated in the basal ganglia. As in idiopathic Parkinson disease, dopamine activity in the basal ganglia is deficient and acetylcholine activity is intact (10). Treatment of the disease is the same as that for idiopathic Parkinson disease. Levodopa and bromocriptine are both effective agents for reducing the rigidity, tremor, and bradykinesia (7).

NEUROLEPTIC-INDUCED PARKINSONISM

Parkinsonism develops as a side effect of treatment with reserpine, phenothiazines, butyrophenones, and thioxanthines (1,20). In fact, parkinsonism is the most common neurologic side effect in the early stages of neuroleptic treatment (21). Rigidity, tremor, abnormal postures, and bradykinesia appear to a variable extent with each of these drugs. Reserpine will produce these signs in as many as 29 percent of patients on high dose treatment, but this drug is no longer widely used as either an antipsychotic or an antihypertensive and so is less likely to be responsible for drug-induced parkinsonism than are the other neuroleptics (1). Careful examination of patients on a butyrophenone, such as haloperidol, or a piperazine phenothiazine, such as trifluoperazine, will reveal some sign of parkinsonism in over 90 percent of patients on these antipsychotics, with obvious signs of parkinsonism developing in about 15 percent (1). Tricyclic antidepressants and lithium are only rarely associated with parkinsonism, the most common sign of disturbed motor activity with these drugs being a fine, rapid tremor in the arms (1).

Parkinsonism is usually apparent within 2 to 4 weeks of starting the patient on neuroleptic drugs (20). Haloperidol and piperazine phenothiazines will induce the parkinsonism most rapidly. The piperidine class of phenothiazines, which includes thioridazine and clozepine, is least likely to produce signs of parkinsonism (1,20). Thioxanthines, such as thiothixene, are derivatives of the phenothiazines and so share the same likelihood of producing parkinsonism (1). Drug-induced parkinsonism usually subsides when the neuroleptic is stopped; the interval between the cessation of all antipsychotics and the disappearance of all parkinsonian signs is frequently 4 months and is, occasionally, 9 months (22).

Clinical Features

Bradykinesia is the earliest sign of parkinsonism induced by neuroleptic drugs. It is often the only sign appearing, but it may be prominent even in the absence of rigidity nd tremor. Rigidity with cogwheeling usually develops days or weeks after the appearance of bradykinesia. The postural abnormalities characteristic of parkinsonism, such as stooped posture, will develop only after the increase in tone if they develop at all. The least common extrapyramidal sign developing with neuroleptics is the static tremor. Static tremors and rigidity are usually greater on one side of the body than the other in patients with idiopathic Parkinson disease; this asymmetry of parkinsonian signs is not at all typical of drug-induced parkinsonism (1). Kinetic tremor, that is, a tremor that increases in severity with voluntary movement of the affected limb, occurs in occasional patients with idiopathic Parkinson disease, but it is observed more frequently in patients with drug-induced parkinsonism. Akathisia, an irresistible urge to be in constant motion, appears soon after the introduction of some neuroleptics (23). The patient usually complains of muscle discomfort preceding the restlessness. The impulse to move elicits no specific pattern of motor activity and may just induce the patient to move his limbs purposelessly. Antiparkinsonian medication is usually effective against this symptom, as well as the others induced by neuroleptics.

The development of parkinsonian signs secondary to neuroleptic drugs is usually rapid, if the patient is at all susceptible. Fifty to 75 percent of the patients ultimately affected will be symptomatic within 1 month of starting the drugs; 90 percent will be symptomatic within 3 months (1). With piperazine phenothiazines, the development of parkinsonian signs may be so rapid that the patient is mute and immobile within 48 hours of starting antipsychotic treatment (1).

Pathophysiology

How neuroleptics cause parkinsonism is not known, but some neurochemical effects of the drugs suggest a few reasonable mechanisms. Both phenothiazines and butyrophenones increase the rate of synthesis and release of the neurotransmitter acetylcholine in the basal ganglia (1). Presumably this could produce a relative deficiency of dopamine in the basal ganglia. These neuroleptics could also produce parkinsonian signs by inhibiting the presynaptic release of dopamine or by blocking dopamine receptors (1,24). Which mechanism, or combination of mechanisms, is responsible for the movement disorder developing in patients on phenothiazines and butyophenones is controversial.

Treatment of Drug-Induced Parkinsonism

Parkinsonian signs usually clear within 3 weeks of stopping treatment with neuroleptic drugs, but parkinsonism will occasionally persist for months. Stopping the responsible drug is, obviously, not always an option. Antipsychotics are generally administered when the patient has serious cognitive problems, and stopping the drugs because of the movement disorder induced may cause substantial psychologic deterioration. A more reasonable course is to suppress the movements while continuing the neuroleptics. The variety of antiparkinsonian drugs available suggests that this should be fairly simple, and in practice it generally is. The treatment of drug-induced parkinsonism is similar to the treatment of idiopathic and post-encephalitic parkinsonism with the notable exception of levodopa use. Levodopa cannot be used to treat psychotic patients with neuroleptic-induced parkinsonism, because it will invariably exacerbate the psychotic symptoms. Anticholinergic drugs, such as trihexyphenidyl and benztropine, are usually given to patients developing rigidity and bradykinesia while on phenothiazines or butyrophenones, because these drugs do not usually cause recurrence of a dormant psychosis. Benztropine mesylate, 1 to 6 milligrams per day, or trihexyphenidyl hydrochloride, 2 to 15 milligrams per day, should minimize drug-induced parkinsonism (20). The usefulness of bromocriptine in drug-induced parkinsonism has not yet been established (7).

The advantage of developing a neuroleptic drug that does not produce extrapyramidal (parkinsonian) side effects has long been recognized, but efforts to produce such a drug have been consistently unsuccessful. A recently developed class of neuroleptics, structurally related to the tricyclic antidepressants, is associated with a low incidence of parkinsonian side effects. These are the dibenzodiazepines, which include the drug clozapine. Their clinical feasibility remains to be demonstrated.

Neuroleptic Malignant Syndrome

An idiosyncratic, but devastating, reaction to antipsychotic drugs is the neuroleptic malignant syndrome (24). In this syndrome, patients taking phenothiazines, thioxanthines, or butyrophenones develop severe parkinsonian signs with potentially lethal autonomic disturbances. Affected patients are rigid and bradykinetic to a greater degree than usually seen with drug-induced parkinsonism, and they develop high fevers. This hyperthermia is followed within hours or days by excessive sweating and salivation, tachycardia, rapid breathing, and unstable blood pressure. The autonomic problems always develop after the parkinsonism, but the autonomic difficulty is what makes this syndrome malignant, that is, potentially lethal. Oculogyric crisis, involuntary posturing, seizures, or choreiform movements appear as part of the syndrome in some patients; but, regardless of the specific features exhibited by the patient during the acute phase of the disorder, the syndrome will take weeks to resolve, if the patient survives. Twenty-five percent of patients developing the neuroleptic malignant syndrome die from it (24). The immediate cause of death is usually severe dehydration or renal failure secondary to myoglobinuria. The myoglobinuria is a complication of muscle breakdown.

The cause of this syndrome is unknown, and the only treatment available is discontinuation of the neuroleptic drugs. Because the syndrome occasionally develops in patients who have recently stopped taking levodopa, current theories favor an overwhelming blockade of dopamine receptors as the basic disorder leading to the malignant syndrome (24). There is no structural or physiologic evidence to prove or discredit this theory. The brain has no consistent abnormalities at autopsy; the cerebrospinal fluid is unremarkable while the patient is alive; and the electroencephalogram is normal or nonspecifically slow when the patient is acutely ill (24). This syndrome is similar to lethal catatonia, a disorder of consciousness already discussed in the chapter on altered consciousness, but the patient's drug history often helps distinguish between the two problems.

WILSON DISEASE (HEPATOLENTICULAR DEGENERATION)

Hepatolenticular degeneration is a hereditary disease producing abnormal movements and altered mentation. Inheritance follows an autosomal recessive pattern, and the severity of the disease in affected individuals is variable. This is a multisystem disorder. The initial presentation of the disease may be a neurologic, psychiatric, hepatic, renal, or hematologic disorder (25). Liver or brain diseases are the most common reasons for the patient's seeking medical attention.

Psychiatric Signs

The initial symptom of Wilson disease may be emotional lability with severe depression, sometimes leading to suicide (Table 9.3) (25). Even patients who are brought to medical attention for liver or kidney disease often have a history of slowly progressive personality changes or unreported psychotic episodes. A comprehensive family history commonly reveals that a not very distant relative suffered from insanity and died in early adult life. The circumstances surrounding the death of a mentally ill cousin or grandfather may be unknown, especially if the affected ancestor was institutionalized for psychotic behavior or profound dementia. Rather than making family members more concerned about aberrant behavior in another relative, the prior experience with mental illness in the family often makes them complacent. The affective or intellectual disorder evolving in another member of the family is appropriately considered hereditary, but inappropriately dismissed as hopeless. Fortunately, most families at risk for Wilson disease are not familiar with the

Table 9.3. Psychiatric Features in Diseases with Parkinsonism

Degenerative Disease	*Psychiatric Abnormalities*
Parkinson disease	Depression Emotional lability
Wilson disease	Depression Emotional lability Suicide attempts Manic disorder Schizoaffective psychosis Schizophreniform psychosis
Shy-Drager syndrome	Diminished libido

details of past psychiatric problems in the family and do exhibit considerable concern when the member with Wilson disease becomes extremely dependent or self-destructive. It is usually at this fairly advanced stage of the disease that the patient is brought to a physician, that physician often being a psychiatrist. Indeed, more patients who become symptomatic for Wilson disease are referred initially to psychiatrists than to neurologists, internists, or pediatricians (25).

Psychiatric problems are usually directly from brain damage, but they occasionally develop secondary to systemic problems that cause brain dysfunction. Extensive liver disease will cause hepatic failure and, consequently, hepatic encephalopathy. Damage to the kidneys causes electrolyte problems, and the patient will develop a metabolic encephalopathy from acidosis or hyperkalemia. Degenerative changes occur in the brain from deranged copper metabolism in the central nervous system. Exactly how this neuronal damage is expressed varies. Although a psychotic depression is fairly typical early in the evolution of psychiatric problems, patients with this brain disease also have manic, schizophreniform, and schizoaffective disorders; rare patients have little more than an anxiety neurosis (25). Neurologic signs will eventually develop in all of these psychologically disturbed patients, these nonpsychiatric signs usually developing between 12 and 32 years of age.

Neurologic Signs

Parkinsonism is prominent early in this degenerative disease and throughout the untreated course. Initial neurologic signs commonly include rigidity, tremor, and bradykinesia. Incoordination, dysarthria, masklike facies, excessive salivation, and trouble swallowing are often associated with these simpler extrapyramidal signs. Unlike the tremor in Parkinson disease, the tremor in Wilson disease is both a kinetic and a resting tremor; that is, the tremor is present when the limb is inactive and increases when purposeful movements are attempted. This tremor involves the arms proximally, as well as distally, and may extend to the head and tongue. Some patients have an arm tremor that originates in the upper arm, appears coarse on casual observation, and is made more prominent by abducting the arms at the shoulders. This is called *Fliegelschlappen*, or wing-beating tremor. Dystonic posturing and spasticity are late signs of the neurologic disease (25). Speech difficulty progresses to slurred speech, then low volume speech, and ultimately aphonia. The patient with irreversible brain damage caused by this disease may have writhing or choreoathetoid movements involving all of his limbs (25). Coma occasionally develops before parkinsonian signs are prominent, but this change in consciousness is generally secondary to hepatic or renal damage.

Metabolic Features

Hepatic disease is more common than neurologic or psychiatric disorders as the primary manifestation of Wilson disease in children who become symptomatic at between 6 and 14 years of age (25). Neurologic involvement may be entirely occult in these young patients (26). A rapidly progressive or chronic active hepatitis is occasionally the initial manifestation of the hepatolenticular degeneration (26). A liver biopsy will reveal elevated liver copper with cirrhosis. The patient typically has an enlarged spleen and a small liver (26). Hemolytic anemia may develop with the liver disease (25). Kidney disease can produce marked elevation of serum potassium levels with a resultant hyperkalemic paralysis. When this weakness occurs, the patient is invariably acidotic because of renal tubular acidosis. Urinary copper excretion is routinely elevated in Wilson disease, and the excess copper is presumed to cause the renal damage.

Pathology

Patients dying with this disease in the past, either as a result of the systemic disorder or by way of suicide, have had degeneration in the brain affecting several different systems. There is some loss of cerebrocortical neurons to account for the psychiatric manifestations, but most of the damage is found in the basal ganglia. The putamen and globus pallidus, the so-called lenticular nuclei, have prominent neuronal loss, and this early observation led to naming the disease hepatolenticular degeneration. Damage to the liver, rather than the brain, often causes death from hepatic failure secondary to cirrhosis.

Diagnostic Studies

The simplest ways to diagnose Wilson disease are by looking at the eyes for changes in the cornea and examining the blood for low levels of the protein ceruloplasmin. Copper deposits at the periphery of the cornea will appear as a brownish-green ring on the internal aspect of the cornea. These deposits are in the membrane that lines the inner face of the cornea.

A slit lamp is usually needed to see this Kayser-Fleischer ring. A low serum concentration of the copper-containing protein ceruloplasmin is another manifestation of disordered copper handling. Ceruloplasmin binds copper in the same way that hemoglobin binds iron. It is not responsible for copper transport or storage, but it is apparently quite sensitive to disturbed copper metabolism. A liver biopsy specimen will reveal a noninflammatory fibrosis and increased liver copper content. The level of copper in the urine will also be increased. Studies of renal function generally reveal several abnormalities, including renal tubular acidosis and proteinuria.

Additional clinical signs of Wilson disease include increased pigmentation over the anterior aspects of the lower legs and bluish-green lines running transversely across the fingernails. Most patients have several manifestations of the disease when they are first recognized. Brain, liver, and kidney damage progresses over the course of years if the patient is not treated.

Treatment

Chelating agents, drugs that bind copper and remove it from the body, are currently used to treat all patients with Wilson disease. The first commonly used drug, BAL (British anti-Lewisite), had the major disadvantage that it had to be given by injection. Although this drug is still occasionally used, most patients are first given a trial of penicillamine. Penicillamine is an effective chelating agent that can be taken orally, but about 25 percent of patients will develop adverse reactions to the drug. This is usually just a skin rash, but even this rash may be so severe that continued use of the drug is not possible. With treatment, the neurologic and psychiatric signs of the disease will subside if irreversible brain damage was not already present when the treatment was started. Liver and kidney damage may be averted or even partially reversed if penicillamine is introduced early in the evolution of the disease.

SHY-DRAGER SYNDROME

An uncommon cause of parkinsonism associated with orthostatic hypotension is Shy-Drager syndrome. This degenerative disease of the nervous system may be encountered by psychiatrists dealing with middle-aged men developing impotence and diminished libido (27). The first sign of the disorder is often a problem with sexual function, which may persist as the most substantial manifestation of the disease for months or years. As the disease progresses, the patient, who is usually a man 40 to 60 years of age, develops urinary and fecal incontinence, rigidity, tremor, impaired sweating, heat intolerance, dizziness, and orthostatic hypotension (27,28). The iris of the eye will atrophy, and the distal musculature in the limbs will waste. Clinically, the patients general appearance resembles that seen with

Parkinson disease, but intellectual function does not deteriorate, as it so often does in Parkinson disease (27).

Pathologic changes in the nervous system in patients with Shy-Drager syndrome are distinct from those seen in Parkinson disease. There is cell loss in the substantia nigra, which probably accounts for the parkinsonian symptoms developing with the disease, but there are also lesions in the cerebellar cortex, the inferior olivary nuclei, and the locus coeruleus of the pons. What causes changes in these central nervous system structures is unknown.

Survival is measured in years. The most life-threatening problem the patient must deal with is the postural hypotension. There is no effective treatment.

OTHER CAUSES OF PARKINSONISM

Changes characteristic of Parkinson disease will appear in a variety of structural and metabolic problems affecting the brain (29). With manganese poisoning, the cause of the parkinsonism is usually apparent from the history of occupational exposure to the metal poison. In hyperparathyroidism, the metabolic problem inducing rigidity and gait difficulty may be unsuspected until an elevated serum calcium is detected. Severe dementia will evolve early in the course of progressive supranuclear palsy, a degenerative disease of the central nervous system (30). The earliest sign of this degenerative disease is difficulty with vertical gaze, specifically with downward gaze. As the disease evolves, affective and intellectual problems become just as prominent as the signs of parkinsonism that often cause this disorder to be misdiagnosed as Parkinson disease.

INCREASED MOVEMENT

Purposeless involuntary movements cause considerable disability. Patients without psychiatric problems often find the excessive movement of a body part or of the entire body is an intolerable burden and seek psychiatric assistance to deal with their handicap. When the movement disorder develops in a patient with existing psychiatric problems, treatment of the individual is greatly complicated. Abnormal facial movements are the most common involuntary movement disorders psychiatrists encounter, but incidental abnormal movements, often producing considerable anxiety, include tooth-grinding, tremors, tics, muscle jerks, and involuntary limb movements. In some cases there is an obvious relationship between the movement disorder and coincidental psychiatric problems, such as the tremor and anxiety in hyperthyroidism. Treating the underlying disorder will abolish both the neurologic and psychiatric symptoms. In other instances, the coincidence of dramatic psychiatric and neurologic symptoms may be inexplicable, such as in the case of coprolalia and tic in Tourette's syndrome, even though treatment abolishes both of the signs. In rare cases, movement disorders occur strictly in the setting of psychosis, but, whenever an abnormal movement occurs, a neurologic explanation should be sought.

ABNORMAL FACIAL MOVEMENTS

Facial movements are more distressing than many other forms of abnormal muscle activity simply because they are impossible to conceal. Grimacing, excessive blinking, tongue thrusting, and other types of inappropriate facial activity may change an individual's entire lifestyle. Embarrassment caused by the facial movements often causes self-imposed isolation. The victim of the movement disorder shuns all but his most intimate acquaintances. This obviously causes considerable psychologic difficulty, but the irony of abnormal facial movements is that most are caused by psychiatric intervention. The majority of patients with excessive or inappropriate facial activity develop the disorder after taking major tranquilizers or other antipsychotic drugs. Those not caused by psychiatric intervention are often labeled stress-related, and the victim of the unexplained facial movement is referred to a psychiatrist for evaluation or treatment. Recognizing which facial movements have an organic basis and which are induced by psychologic conflicts is a complex task; but, even if the cause of the abnormal facial movement is determined, the treatment may be extremely unsatisfying. This means that patients with neurologic disturbances causing abnormal facial movements often have a permanently disfiguring movement disorder. The stress associated with this uncontrollable facial activity routinely causes substantial psychologic difficulty for the patient and commonly justifies psychiatric intervention.

The facial movements developing with neuroleptic drug use fall into two major categories, the acute dyskinesias and the tardive dyskinesias. Tardive dyskinesias are a more enduring problem than acute dyskinesias, but predicting which facial movements will be transient and which will be persistent is impossible. Observation of the patient for a few weeks determines which type of dyskinesia the facial activity is. Involuntary facial movements largely indistinguishable from tardive and acute dyskinesias also occur independently of drug use. These are called idiopathic orofacial dyskinesias and include some discrete syndromes, such as Meige syndrome and buccolingual dyskinesia of the elderly. Diagnostic approaches and treatment differ for each of these dyskinesias.

Before any effort is made to treat a facial dyskinesia, the physician must be confident that facial dyskinesia is actually the cause of the abnormal facial movement. Focal seizure activity, habit spasm, posttraumatic facial nerve dysfunction, and idiopathic hemifacial spasm can all be confused with facial dyskinesia. A careful history and neurologic evaluation will usually establish the precise nature of the movement disorder, but occasionally more invasive diagnostic tests are appropriate. Most of these non-"dyskinetic" facial movement disorders do respond to treatment.

Dyskinesias

Dyskinesia is a movement disorder characterized by grimacing, mouth opening, neck muscle spasms, and, occasionally, spasmodic arching of the back (opisthotonus). Facial distortion during bouts of such involuntary movements may be extreme. This is almost always a disorder of facial or neck muscle activity, but the uncoordinated muscle activity need not be limited to the face and neck. Excessive involuntary movements occasionally involve the trunk and limbs as well, resulting in writhing or jerking movements and abnormal postures (31). The purposeless contractions of facial muscles, often called dystonic contractions, are generally symmetrical, and the frequency of spasms ranges from several times per hour to several times per minute (31). Forceful diaphragmatic contractions can produce grunting or gasping noises (20). Relaxation may decrease the movements, and sleep will abolish them; but they are never under voluntary control (31).

Dyskinesias usually develop after long-term neuroleptic use, but some individuals develop the abnormal facial activity after a single dose of antipsychotic medication, and rare patients develop a typical dyskinetic syndrome with no exposure to neuroleptic drugs whatsoever (32,33). An idiosyncratic facial dyskinesia appears in some individuals after short-term antihistamine use, but this is less likely to be persistent than the dyskinesia developing with neuroleptics (34). Orofacial dyskinesia is not usually a feature of psychotic disorders, but movement similar to dyskinetic movements may develop in schizophrenic patients or patients with bipolar affective psychoses (22,35). A diagnostic problem arises in the schizophrenic patient previously treated with neuroleptics because stereotyped or manneristic movements may develop either as a withdrawal phenomenon or as a symptom of the schizophrenia (36). Drug manipulation may help settle the issue; the movements will abate when the antipsychotics are restarted if they were a withdrawal phenomenon.

Dyskinesia develops from disordered basal ganglia function. There are several theoretic neurophysiologic explanations for the dysfunction, but there is no established pathophysiology (11,20). The most popular explanation for neuroleptic-induced dyskinesias is that with prolonged phenothiazine or butyrophenone use dopamine receptors develop denervation hypersensitivity. The antipsychotic drug produces this receptor hypersensitivity by effectively blocking dopamine transmission. Stopping the neuroleptic will induce excessive movements, even if there is no rebound of brain dopamine levels to higher than normal, simply because the normal dopamine released after the antipsychotic is withdrawn faces an excess of dopamine receptors. An alternative explanation is that there is simply an imbalance between dopamine and acetylcholine systems in the basal ganglia (11). Consistent with this is the improvement in some tardive dyskinesias when physostigmine is used. Physostigmine is an acetylcholinesterase inhibitor that increases acetylcholine activity, presumably thereby compensating for any increased dopamine activity (32).

Acute Dyskinesia

Dyskinesias may appear when the patient starts taking neuroleptic drugs or when the drugs are stopped. The abnormal movements or postures that develop as an idiosyncratic reaction to the introduction of phenothiazines or butyrophenones are often called dystonias, not because the tone of the facial or neck muscles is increased, but simply to distinguish this movement disorder from the more common disorder appearing with drug withdrawal. Dystonia is also used to refer to more generalized disorders of posture. Signs of an acute dyskinesia or dystonia include oculogyric crisis, excessive blinking (blepharospasm), grimacing, slurred speech, torticollis, neck arching (retrocollis), jaw clenching, and aversive eye movements (1). Acute dystonic reactions are discussed in detail in the section on abnormal posturing later in this chapter.

Twenty percent of young adults treated with butyrophenones or phenothiazines develop facial dyskinesias and abnormal limb movements when the neuroleptics are stopped (22). This withdrawal-emergent dyskinesia occurs even more commonly in patients under 12 years of age, but in these children the dyskinetic movements are more generalized and may appear as a remarkable clumsiness (22). Up to 50 percent of children on neuroleptics will have a transient dyskinesia that subsides within 5 weeks after the drug is stopped (22). If the acute dyskinesia subsides within 6 to 12 weeks with no treatment, the reaction is considered nothing more than a withdrawal phenomenon. This movement disorder is not the only neurologic problem associated with neuroleptic withdrawal. Seventeen to 75 percent of patients will have nausea, vomiting, restlessness, sleep difficulty, headache, dizziness, and excessive sweating within 1 to 2 weeks of discontinuation of the drug (22). These signs and the withdrawal-emergent dyskinesias are generally considered evidence of a transient excess in brain dopamine, as the previously impaired dopamine system rebounds to a level of activity above normal. The phenothiazines with the greatest anticholinergic activity exhibit the strongest tendency to elicit transient dyskinesias. Chlorpromazine and thioridazine are the two most commonly used neuroleptics associated with a high incidence of withdrawal-emergent dyskinesias (22). Treatment is unnecessary and inadvisable. If the movements persist more than 12 weeks, the diagnosis must be reconsidered.

Tardive Dyskinesia

Prolonged phenothiazine or butyrophenone use in the treatment of psychotic patients may produce a dyskinesia that persists long after the neuroleptic drugs have been stopped (21,23). In elderly patients, especially those on high doses of antipsychotic medications, the movement disorder is more likely to develop and is more often irreversible (23). This late-appearing movement disorder is generally called tardive dyskinesia. Three to 6 percent of patients in mental hospitals and 20 percent of the elderly in custodial or chronic care facilities treated with antipsychotics develop tardive dyskinesia (1,23). Tardive dyskinesia is as common a sequela of long-term neuroleptic use as drug-induced parkinsonism is a complication of short-term use (37). In fact, there appears to be some correlation between the development of drug-induced parkinsonism and the susceptibility to tardive dyskinesia. Severe tardive dyskinesia most commonly develops in the patient with severe parkinsonism while on neuroleptics (21). Despite their propensity to occur in the same patients, these two movement disorders do not usually occur simultaneously (21). There is some overlap in the presentation of the signs, but this is minimal: the tardive dyskinesia usually begins to appear before the parkinsonian signs have fully subsided. This transition from one movement disorder to another invariably occurs days or weeks after the neuroleptics have been discontinued.

Clinical Features. Tardive dyskinesia is a chronic problem. It is distinct from the acute dystonic reactions that may develop while a patient is being treated with phenothiazines or butyrophenones (31). The earliest sign of a tardive dyskinesia may be little more than writhing movements of the tongue on the floor of the mouth (1). Unlike the acute dystonias, the upper face usually does not exhibit abnormal movements regardless of how severe the abnormal facial movements become in tardive dyskinesia. Forceful, random movements of the mouth and jaw are especially typical of tardive dyskinesia. Rhythmic, involuntary movements of the tongue, mouth, or surrounding face may produce intermittent tongue protrusion, mouth puckering, or chewing movements (23). Patients occasionally puff out their cheeks or develop tic-like movements of the lips and eyes. Forceful, involuntary, muscle jerks (myoclonic jerks) occasionally develop in the limbs, but these are notably rare (23). Involuntary trunk movements and ballistic limb movements also occur occasionally (1). Abnormal postures, such as opisthotonus or tortipelvis (hip tilt), are rarely the dominant elements in tardive dyskinesias in adult life; and, if they appear at all, they will characteristically develop in patients under 50 years of age (1). In adults, oral and facial movements are the most common manifestations of the dyskinesia; in children, the mouth and face are much less frequently affected (1,23). Repetitive writhing movements of the limbs are more likely in this younger group of patients (23).

Tardive dyskinesia usually develops insidiously and may be apparent even while the patient is still taking antipsychotic medications. The movements increase dramatically when the neuroleptic is stopped. Exposure to the responsible drug is often measured in years before the movement disorder appears (31). The minimum exposure to an antipsychotic that will induce tardive dyskinesia is 3 to 6 months (1). Piperazine phenothiazines and butyrophenones are the neuroleptics most likely to cause tardive dyskinesia.

Diagnostic Considerations. Anticholinergic drugs used to decrease the parkinsonian signs developing with neuroleptic use may confuse the clinical picture by inducing a reversible oral dyskinesia (31). The tricyclic antidepressant amitriptyline can also produce an oral dyskinesia that is more persistent than that appearing with anticholinergic use (31). The most confusion with tardive dyskinesias arises with the transient "withdrawal" dyskinesia that may develop when the antipsychotics are stopped (31). This withdrawal phenomenon has none of the treatment problems inherent in a true tardive dyskinesia (36). The movement disorder usually clears completely and spontaneously. This is also true of the tardive dyskinesias developing in children. After discontinuing the neuroleptic, the child with a tardive dyskinesia will invariably be free of all abnormal movements and postures by 1 year after cessation of drug treatment (1).

Pathophysiology. Tardive dyskinesia characteristically involves an increased sensitivity to dopamine, although no consistent pathologic or neurochemical deficits in the basal ganglia have been established as the basis for this disorder (1). That the movements usually develop after a neuroleptic is stopped suggests dopamine receptor hypersensitivity (38). Efforts to treat tardive dyskinesia have reflected the observed sensitivity to dopamine and the theoretic hypersensitivity of receptors in the basal ganglia in all dyskinesias as already discussed (1).

Treatment. Frequent drug holidays reduce the risk of developing tardive dyskinesia, but only slightly (20). Because the movement disorder is thought to result from excessive dopamine activity or dopamine receptor hypersensitivity, the most logical approach to treatment is administration of a dopamine antagonist. This logic is sound, but, in practice, it can produce additional problems for the patient. Dopamine antagonists used to treat the dyskinesia include haloperidol and a variety of phenothiazines, drugs often responsible for the disorder initially (32). Obviously, treating the problem with a drug that causes the disorder should be avoided whenever alternative methods are available (20). Haloperidol treatment may suppress the movements while the patient is on high doses, but the tardive dyskinesia may reemerge with even more violence when the dose of the neuroleptic is simply decreased. Unfortunately, other approaches to treatment have been fairly unreliable. This failure to develop an effective and safe therapy for tardive dyskinesia may reflect gross flaws in current theories explaining the disorder. Contrary to generally accepted theoretic assumptions, apomorphine and bromocriptine, dopamine agonists, may decrease the movements (16). Drugs that increase brain acetylcholine have had little effect on the dyskinesia. Physostigmine occasionally decreases the movements presumably by way of its central cholinesterase inhibiting activity (32). Reserpine, 1 to 5 milligrams per day, may help, but its depressant effects often cause new psychiatric problems (20).

Deanol, a drug commonly used to suppress skeletal muscle spasticity, increases brain acetylcholine content, but reports of its effectiveness in suppressing tardive dyskinesia have been quite inconsistent (11,32,36). Some report improvement in 40 percent of patients on 500 to 1,000 milligrams per day of deanol while others find no advantage over placebo (11,32). Deanol has also been reported effective in 75 percent of patients with levodopa-induced dyskinesia (11). Its presumed mode of action is by increasing choline levels, thereby providing more substrate for the production of acetylcholine (36). Another choline precursor is lecithin, and trials with this substance have met with some success in reducing dyskinetic movements in tardive dyskinesia (39). Choline itself is about as effective as lecithin, but most find it unpleasant to take orally.

Because depression frequently accompanies the onset of tardive dyskinesia, some clinicians have used lithium and tricyclic antidepressants in the management of the disorder (38,39). Surprisingly, 58 percent of patients treated with these drugs have reduced movements (38). Recently developed dopamine receptor blockers, called sulpiride and oxiperomide, promise to be more selective in their site of action and may prove quite effective in improving tardive dyskinesias (40).

Evaluating drugs for tardive dyskinesia is complicated by the observed irregularities in the course of the disease. Spontaneous fluctuations in the abnormal movements are routinely seen and may be quite dramatic (121). The dyskinesia resolves completely in forty percent of victims within fifteen months (36). Remission of signs is more likely to be complete when the patient is a young adult, rather than elderly.

Meige Disease (Oromandibular Dystonia with Blepharospasm)

Dyskinesia may develop independently of levodopa therapy, neuroleptic withdrawal, or chronic neuroleptic use. One form of idiopathic dyskinesia associated with no intellectual, coordination, or sensory problem is Meige disease (41). Abnormal facial movements are a prominent feature in this movement disorder, and neuroleptic use is often suspected because this disorder is strikingly similar to tardive dyskinesia in its clinical appearance. Unlike the facial movements developing initially with tardive dyskinesia, prominent eye blinking is an early sign. Otherwise, the grimacing, lip puckering, neck movements and tongue thrusting that develop are indistinguishable from the facial movements in tardive dyskinesia.

Meige disease appears late in adult life and usually worsens with age. It is commonly confused with neurotic behavior, because the patient routinely presents with excessive, anxiety-related blinking (blepharospasm) or tooth-grinding (bruxism). The blepharospasm may become so constant and severe that the patient loses functional vision (40). His eyes open and close so often and so strenuously that he cannot perform acts requiring visual attention. Visual acuity when the eyes are held open is no worse than before the blepharospasm. Stress and fatigue will increase the blinking; this symptom may appear years before or after jaw movements. With the fully developed syndrome, the patient will have uncontrollable grimacing, jaw movements, and tongue movements. Muscles ordinarily used for chewing will be greatly hypertrophied, and the constant jaw movements will grind down or break teeth over the course of years (40).

The etiology of this disorder is unknown (40). Presumably, the dopamine system in the basal ganglia is overactive, but there is no chemical or anatomic proof of this. There is no satisfactory treatment. Patients with Meige disease only occasionally show temporary improvement with haloperidol treatment (41). Consistent with the presumed dopamine system defect underlying this disease is the observed increase in involuntary movements when patients are given levodopa (40). The anticholinergic drugs likely to exacerbate tardive dyskinesia are often beneficial in controlling the movements in Meige disease (41). Inconsistent with a dopamine system defect as the cause of the disease is the observed improvement in some patients on the acetylcholine precursor deanol (40). That anticholinergics may be beneficial, cholinesterase inhibitors may be deleterious, and acetylcholine precursors are occasionally helpful underlines the limitations of any theories that view cholinergic and dopaminergic influences in the basal ganglia as acting only antagonistically. Acetylcholine has an enhancing effect on dopamine mechanisms in the basal ganglia of some animals (41). All these factors greatly complicate any rational approach to treatment of this disorder. Meige disease usually persists regardless of treatment.

Depression-Dependent Dyskinesias

Although orofacial dyskinesias may develop with antipsychotic drug use, these abnormal facial movements may arise directly from the psychotic disorder under treatment. This is often difficult to ascertain since several different types of drugs used incidentally in the treatment of psychotic patients can produce orofacial dyskinesias. These include barbiturates and antihistamines (42). The psychotic disorder producing orofacial movements most indistinguishable from drug-induced dyskinesias is manic-depressive psychosis (35). Oral, buccal, lingual, and more generalized dyskinetic movements develop in some patients with this bipolar affective disorder during the depressive phase of the illness. Patients most at risk are those with a rapidly cycling bipolar psychosis (35). This orofacial dyskinesia clears during the manic phase of the illness and sometimes improves after electroconvulsive treatment.

Distinguishing between the movement disorder associated with depression and the dyskinesia developing as a response to drug treatment is difficult, if not impossible. Recognition of a depression-dependent movement disorder is usually a retrospective judgment. The patient's dyskinesia improves as his depression abates, even though his medication is not changed. Susceptibility to drug-induced dyskinesias may, in fact, be exaggerated in patients with depressive mood disorders. Neuroleptic-induced dyskinesias are slightly more common in patients with bipolar affective disorders than in patients with other diagnoses (35). Treatment of the depression is the treatment of choice for the dyskinesia.

Focal Motor Seizures

Abnormal facial movements generally do not develop as the most prominent symptom in a patient with focal seizure activity; but, if the facial movement is limited to one side of the face and there is ipsilateral arm or hand movements, focal motor seizure activity must be considered. Persistent facial movement can occur with epilepsia partialis continua, a devastating epileptic disorder characterized by incessant seizure activity limited to a circumscribed area in the cerebral cortex. An electroencephalogram will establish epilepsia partialis continua as the cause of the facial movements if it is in fact responsible. Focal epileptiform activity will appear on the brain wave recording. This diagnosis can generally be dismissed if both sides of the face are equally involved by the abnormal movements. If focal motor seizure activity is responsible, anticonvulsant therapy is advisable, but often ineffective.

Hemifacial Spasms

Abnormal facial movements may be limited to one side of the face and appear independently of any drug use. Paroxysmal activity in the muscles innervated by the facial nerve will produce hemifacial twitching or distortion (43,44). The patient appears to have a facial twitch or painful tic. There is little of the mouth puckering and tongue thrusting that is typical of the facial dyskinesias. This disorder also involves more than just the twitching about the eye of essential blepharospasm, a facial disorder often developing in individuals under psychologic stress. Both the lower and upper face will be involved in the paroxysmal contractions. This idiopathic facial movement disorder is called hemifacial spasm; and, despite the name, the tonic-clonic contractions of the facial muscles occasionally generalize and become bilateral (44). Most patients are accused of having a "nervous twitch" or a bizarre facial habit spasm. Because the hemifacial contractions increase in frequency and force when the patient is agitated or depressed, many patients conclude inaccurately that they are suffering from a psychiatric problem and consult a psychiatrist or psychologist for help with their involuntary facial activity. The psychiatrist will routinely discover that the patient's personality is not at all typical of the individual susceptible to conversion reactions and that much of the social difficulty the patient complains of developed after the appearance of the facial movements.

One-third of all patients with hemifacial spasm have evidence of some facial weakness, even though they have no apparent facial nerve damage (43). Synkinesis, that is, an inappropriate spread of muscle activity on attempted limited movements of the face, is seen in all patients with hemifacial spasm (43,44). When the patient blinks, the corner of his mouth will retract, or, when he smiles, his eye will close. Synkinesis normally develops in patients with Bell's palsy, an idiopathic facial weakness that develops over the course of a few hours or a few days, and with obvious facial nerve injuries. Although synkinesis is generally considered a sign of facial nerve damage, there is no slowing of conduction in the facial nerve in patients with hemifacial spasm.

Any patient with this paroxysmal grimacing should be investigated for a structural lesion at the base of the brain, because this type of facial movement occasionally develops with lesions impinging upon the facial nerve. Lesions producing such movements as isolated phenomena are generally fairly benign, but they do include arteriovenous malformations, cerebellopontine angle tumors, and posterior fossa aneurysms (43). Focal motor seizures are easily distinguished from hemifacial spasm on the basis of an electroencephalogram; there are no brain wave abnormalities with hemifacial spasm.

The cause of hemifacial spasm is unknown. Theoretic explanations for this abnormal facial movement include transaxonal spread of nerve impulses from one fiber in the facial nerve to another as a result of occult damage (43). Current opinion favors a vascular etiology for the problem, with vascular compression of the nerve, rather than ischemic injury to the nerve, being the most popular theory. Which posterior fossa artery is in a position to press upon the facial nerve is variable from individual to individual. The posterior inferior cerebellar artery often has a loop that swings superiorly to impinge upon the facial and auditory nerves. Even more commonly, the anterior inferior cerebellar artery lies against the seventh cranial nerve as it emerges from the brainstem. That these vessels play a role in hemifacial spasm was suggested by the relief obtained by surgically separating the overlying artery from the facial nerve. Some relief from hemifacial spasm occurred in every case treated with this type of surgery (44). Referring all patients with hemifacial spasm for this surgery is still premature. This is substantial neurosurgery and is still an experimental approach to this type of movement disorder. There is no established treatment for this disorder. Spontaneous remissions and recurrences are common (43).

Facial Myokymia

Facial myokymia is an involuntary movement disorder clinically manifest as continuous, fine, undulating movements of the facial muscles (43). Synkinesis does not occur as a feature of this abnormal facial activity. The movements are usually limited to one side of the face and are most often caused by an intrinsic brainstem lesion (43). The clinical phenomenon may be evident months before a destructive brainstem lesion, such as a glioma, can be defined on computed tomograms of the brain or with arteriographic studies. Lesions producing this type of muscle activity are occasionally static, but the patient should be investigated rigorously to define a treatable lesion. The electromyogram has a characteristic picture in this disorder, a diagnostic point of considerable importance, since such lethal disorders as bulbar amyotrophic lateral sclerosis can be eliminated as possible causes of the facial muscle activity if the typical myokymic pattern is found (Figure 9.2). There is no treatment for the clinical phenomenon other than treating any underlying disease found on investigation of the movements.

Habit Spasms

Some individuals develop facial twitches or "tics" as a habit spasm. Implicit in this designation is that the movement has no pathologic basis and the

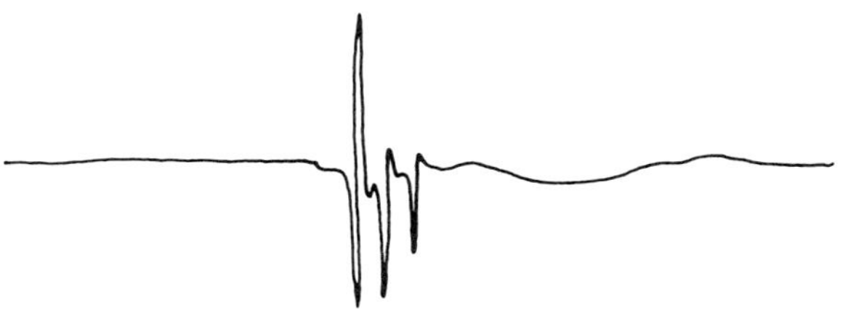

Figure 9.2. Clustering of motor potentials into triplets of this sort is typical of electromyographic recordings from muscles exhibiting myokymia.

movements are entirely normal. This may be an overstatement of the voluntary character of such facial habit spasms. It is true that the patient can voluntarily suppress the grimacing, eye blinking, or platysmal contractions that constitute the facial tic, but with prolonged suppression the patient complains of increasing tension. The paroxysmal activity is irresistible, and the patient's sense of increasing tension can only be relieved by following through with the habit spasm. With stress or anxiety, the frequency of the facial tics will increase, but the character of the facial movements will remain fairly consistent. Patients with compulsive eye blinking do not develop paroxysmal lip retractions with stress. Habit spasms involving the face may be transient, especially if they develop in children. All neurodiagnostic studies will fail to explain the movement disorder. Autopsy examination of the brain will uncover no structural lesions to explain the tics. Efforts to suppress the movements with sedative or antianxiety drugs are routinely unsuccessful.

Buccolingual Dyskinesia of the Elderly

Buccolingual dyskinesia syndrome of the elderly is an idiopathic facial movement disorder that involves predominantly tongue and lip movements (41). Victims of this disorder frequently have senile dementia, as well as abnormal facial movements. The prominent dementia, the absence of a lifelong history of facial tics, the age of the patient, and the stereotypical character of the mouth movements all distinguish this facial movement disorder from facial habit spasms (16). These movements are similar to those appearing in edentulous individuals; individuals without teeth often smack their lips or chew as compulsive responses to not feeling a solid resistance between the mandible and the maxilla. Dentures will suppress the abnormal movements if a poor dental occlusion is the only problem. Buccolingual dyskinesia of the elderly persists with good dentures or good teeth.

Buccolingual dyskinesia is improved by cholinergic drugs, such as physostigmine and choline salts, and is exacerbated by anticholinergic drugs, such as trihexyphenidyl and benztropine (41). Bromocriptine has been used with some success in this disorder, but the high incidence of psychiatric reactions with this drug limits its usefulness (16). Efforts to treat the involuntary movements are reasonable when the patient has adequately intact mentation to be disturbed by the unrelenting movements. Family members may seek therapy that will suppress the dyskinesia in individuals who are not adequately competent to recognize that they are exhibiting this facial activity. Such situations involve the physician in largely cosmetic therapy. The drugs used to suppress these movements expose the patient to too many risks to justify their use when the patient himself is not disturbed by the facial movements.

TOOTH GRINDING (BRUXISM)

Tooth grinding or gnashing is so common that it is probably not appropriate to call it a movement disorder. Its appearance usually raises considerable concern in those around the person exhibiting this behavior, but the individual with the movements is usually unaware of them. This is because bruxism most often occurs during sleep. About 10 percent of the general population has nocturnal tooth grinding (45). In most cases, there is no apparent cause. Malocclusion of the teeth is occasionally responsible, but an idiosyncratic central nervous system trait is probably more important in most patients.

Bruxism may develop in children or adults and usually occurs early in sleep. Episodes last seconds or minutes and are especially likely during stage two of NREM (non-rapid eye movement) sleep (45). The noise produced by the tooth grinding often wakes the patient's bed partner but does not wake the patient. Alcohol may increase the likelihood of exhibiting tooth grinding and the duration of episodes of nocturnal bruxism in some individuals, but it certainly does not play a role in most children affected (45). Tooth grinding during sleep is occasionally so forceful that dental work is damaged or gums and other supporting structures are traumatized. The affected individual occasionally awakens with bleeding gums or sore jaws. Over the course of years, this movement disorder may wear down molar and premolar teeth considerably.

Occasionally, bruxism occurs in awake patients. It may develop as the initial sign in Meige disease or as a late sign in progressive metabolic brain diseases (40). Meige disease is a reasonable consideration only if the patient is over 50 years of age when the problem first appears. A variety of storage diseases causing damage to the central nervous system can precipitate bruxism associated with profound mental retardation in childhood. Phenothiazine and butyrophenone intake should also be considered as possible causes of the jaw movements in adults or children exposed to these drugs. Tardive dyskinesia can appear initially as little more than bruxism.

Any patient with nocturnal bruxism may seek psychiatric help because of the common suspicion that unconscious conflicts are producing the disturbing behavior. Appropriate in the initial evaluation of these patients is a careful assessment of the dental occlusion and temporomandibular joint function. Also worth considering are nocturnal seizures provoked by sleep and manifested by limited motor activity including jaw clenching and movements. If these dental and neurologic bases are not the explanation, then further medical investigations are not warranted unless the bruxism is occurring while the patient is awake. Drug toxicity or a slowly evolving movement disorder must be suspected when the bruxism is unrelated to sleep. Treatment of the underlying disorder is appropriate in these situations. Idiopathic nocturnal bruxism is usually unaffected by sleep medications or other relaxants. A bite plate or other dental device can interfere with the occlusion necessary for bruxism, and such a device may prove essential in the chronic tooth-grinder to limit tooth destruction.

TREMORS

Tremors are rhythmic, oscillatory movements generally affecting the limbs or the head. An axial tremor, that is, an oscillatory movement of the trunk or head up-and-down or side-to-side, is called titubation. Tremors in the limbs are much more common than titubation and may develop in individuals with no apparent central nervous system pathology to explain the abnormal movement. In fact, in some cases appendicular tremors are normal phenomena. A fine tremor in the hands developing with stress is normal. A tremor is pathologic when it reflects structural damage to or physiologic disturbance of the nervous system (Figure 9.3). Pathologic tremors occur at rest, during movement, or during sustained postures.

There are three principal kinds of pathologic tremor: these are usually called static, kinetic, and end-point intentional (Table 9.4) (20). The static tremor appears when a limb is at rest, with no substantial force being exerted across any joint to maintain the posture. It may be fine or coarse,

Table 9.4. Tremors

Type	*Context*	*Characteristics*	*Conditions*
Static	Resting	Rapid May disappear on movement of the limb	Parkinson disease Drug-induced reserpine phenothiazines butyrophenones Wilson disease
Kinetic	Movement Sustention	Slow Low amplitude	Benign essential tremor Drug-induced caffeine isoproterenol lithium tricyclic antidepressants amphetamines alcohol withdrawal opiate withdrawal Hyperthyroidism Mercury poisoning Wilson disease
End-point	Movement	Slow Amplitude increases as target approached	Cerebellar disease

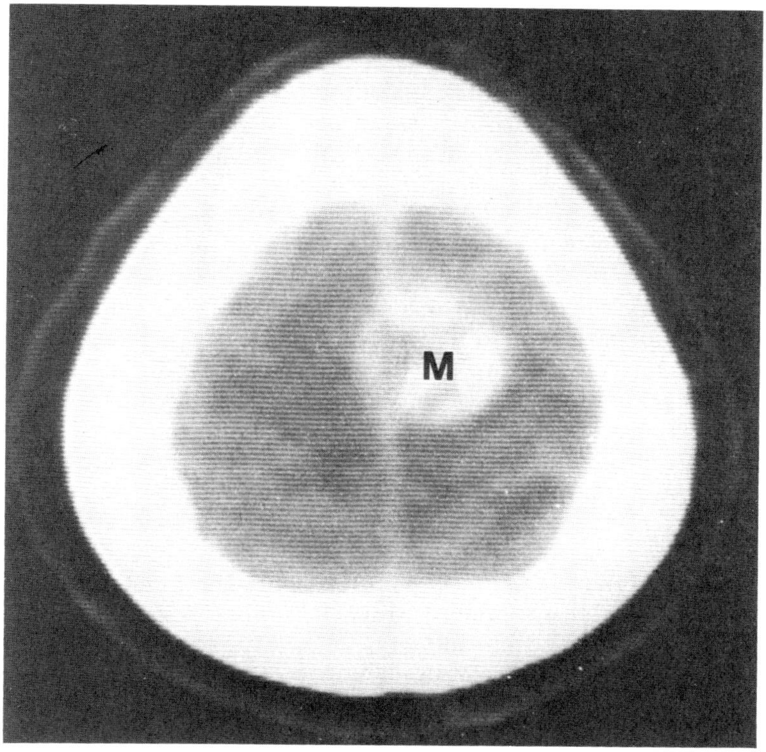

Figure 9.3. A 64-year-old woman sought medical attention for recurrent shaking of her right leg. The episodes of leg shaking had been increasing in frequency over the course of 3 years. A computed tomogram of her head revealed a calcified meningioma (M) growing off the falx cerebri. Underlying the tumor there was substantial edema involving much of her superior right cerebral hemisphere (courtesy of Drs. J. Loh and W. Hotson).

but in most conditions causing static tremors it is relatively fine. It disappears with sleep, increases with stress, and may appear in the neck, jaw, or tongue, as well as the limbs. This is the "pill-rolling" tremor of parkinsonism and the fine resting tremor of hyperthyroidism. In parkinsonian patients, the tremor disappears entirely when the patient uses the involved part, regardless of how coarse the tremor is when the limb, head, or tongue is at rest. Kinetic tremors appear when the limb is moving or involved in maintaining a position against resistance (20). That resistance need be no more than gravity. The activity that elicits the kinetic tremor determines whether it is called a postural sustention or action tremor. The wing-beating tremor of Wilson disease is a sustention tremor, the movement appearing or increasing on maintaining the arms in an abducted posture. Action and postural tremors occasionally develop with hyperthryroidism and extreme anxiety, but they are more regularly seen as a side effect of various drugs, such as caffeine, lithium, tricyclic antidepressants, and amphetamines (20). In severe cases, these same drugs can produce a tremor that is both static and kinetic. Kinetic tremors are typically fairly coarse and by definition are not at all apparent when the limb is at rest. Sustaining a posture or attempting to perform fine tasks will exacerbate the movement disorder. Mercury poisoning was a common cause of this tremor when mercury nitrates were used in the manufacture of felt hats for men (20). The movements and affective disorder induced by the neurotoxic mercury provided the basis for the general view that "hatters" often became "mad hatters." Alcohol and opiate withdrawal also produce this type of tremor. The picture is confused in alcoholics by the peculiar abnormality of tone called asterixis exhibited by these individuals. On maintaining extensor positions of the hands and fingers, irregular lapses in the tonic muscle contractions produce an irregular, tremorlike movement. A special form of kinetic tremor, often viewed as a separate disorder, is the end-point intentional or end-point kinetic tremor. This tremor is coarse, slightly irregular, associated with limb movement, and increasing in amplitude as the limb approaches the intended target (20). Such tremors may be prominent when the limb is nearly fully extended, in which case they are often called terminal. Cerebellar disease characteristically produces this kind of tremor.

Although some diseases produce more than one type of tremor, each of these major tremor categories represents a movement disorder with a distinct pathophysiologic basis. The physiologic problem responsible for static tremors is thought to be decreased activity of the dopamine utilizing system in the basal ganglia of the brain (20). Consistent with this hypothesis is the observed development of this tremor with drugs, such as reserpine, haloperidol, and chlorpromazine, that interfere with dopamine activity in the basal ganglia (20). Most kinetic tremors seem to develop because of excessive activity in one of the neurotransmitter systems that uses catecholamines acting on beta-adrenergic receptors (20). Consistent with this is the observed induction of kinetic tremors by isoproterenol, a beta-adrenergic receptor stimulator. End-point intentional tremors develop with damage to feed-back systems used for directing complex movements. This type of tremor occurs with structural, rather than neurochemical, disturbances.

Tremor with Anxiety

Fear, stress, and anxiety elicit uncontrollable shaking in normal individuals. If the disturbing stimulus is transient, the tremor is acute. When the stress is more chronic, the tremor may become more chronic. This stress-related tremor is in no sense pathologic. Even when the shaking is severe, it is a normal phenomenon. The tremor developing with excessive anxiety, whether it is acute or chronic, is nothing more than an exaggerated physiologic tremor (46). The normal, or generally unnoticed, tremor in individuals with no movement disorder has a frequency of about 7 to 10 hertz, precisely the same frequency range as the tremor observed in acutely anxious individuals (46). The amplitude of the tremor is what makes it apparent in the anxious individual. With chronic anxiety, the tremor is still within the physiologic frequency range, but it tends to have a slightly higher frequency than that seen with acute anxiety (46). An increased level of circulating catecholamines is usually held responsible for the increased amplitude of the physiologic tremor in anxious individuals (46). Stress-related tremor is not a conversion reaction: the patient usually recognizes that anxiety or fear are producing the tremor, and he usually knows what is causing his anxiety or fear. Resolution of the stressful situation will abolish the tremor.

Hysterical Tremor

Tremor is not a common conversion reaction, but this is probably because it does not represent a very serious disability. A patient developing hysterical deficits is more inclined to complain of dramatic deficits, such as a sensory loss over one side of the body or complete blindness. Hysterical tremors are quite variable in character when they do occur. The amplitude and frequency of the tremor will constantly shift, and the abnormal activity will often abate completely when the patient believes he is not being observed. The arms are most often involved by the movement, and, if both arms are simultaneously involved, the tremors in each arm will have different characteristics. If the tremor affects an arm and a leg, the periodicity of the movement in the limbs will typically be out of synchrony. Occasionally, the tremor will appear in an arm on one side of the body and a leg on the other side. The severity of the tremor is often highly responsive to suggestion. Mild sedation, a maneuver that exacerbates several types of pathologic tremors, characteristically decreases the severity of the tremor in hysterical patients. The only effective treatment for this hysterical movement disorder is resolution of the underlying psychiatric problem.

Cerebellar Disease

Tremor is a common sign of cerebellar disease, and it is usually quite prominent in patients with cerebellar lesions, but it is not the most common or even the earliest sign of posterior fossa disease in most patients with cerebellar damage. Focal or diffuse cerebellar lesions usually cause gait difficulty, rather than tremor, as the initial sign of disease (47). When tremors do develop with cerebellar damage, they are almost always kinetic, are often associated with uncoordinated (ataxic) movements of the affected limbs, and are invariably associated with disease in the ipsilateral cerebellar hemisphere. The tremor is coarse and in a horizontal plane. To test for the abnormal movment the examiner asks the patient to keep his arm immobile while it is outstretched. The tremor will be apparent on trying to maintain this position, but it will become even more prominent if the patient tries to touch a target placed at arms-length from his body. The outstretched arm will oscillate about the target with increasingly wider excursions as the object moves away from the patient.

Pastpointing often appears as an additional sign of cerebellar dysfunction in patients with kinetic tremors. The defect appearing with pastpointing is more one of calculating position in space than of directing movements in a coordinated manner. This simply means that the patient with pastpointing inaccurately reaches for a stationary object even if movement at the arm joints in minimized. Dysmetria, a phenomenon characterized by inaccuracies in the rate, force, and trajectory of limb movements, also develops with cerebellar disease (47). Although pastpointing may be present when the arm is moved only at the shoulder joint, dysmetria involves inaccurate movements at several joints simultaneously.

Patients exhibiting the combination of tremor, pastpointing, and dysmetria invariably have cerebellar damage or damage to cerebellar pathways. These signs often appear abruptly, such as with cerebellar infarction or hemorrhage, and occasionally resolve with time. Other systems in the brain are able to compensate at least at a gross level for loss of cerebellar structures. The most commonly encountered nervous system disease producing kinetic tremor and other signs of cerebellar dysfunction is multiple sclerosis (47). Deficits characteristically remit and recur with this demyelinating disease; but kinetic tremors, dysarthria, and gait ataxia are often remarkably stable problems for years in patients with multiple sclerosis (48). Although multiple sclerosis is the most common explanation for these clinical signs, it is certainly not the only explanation. Abruptly appearing kinetic tremors in adults should raise concern for cerebellar tumor or infection. In the elderly, hemorrhages or infarctions in the cerebellum may cause kinetic tremor initially, but progressive obtundation will signal the gravity of the condition (49).

Computed tomography of the posterior fossa can clarify the nature of most focal cerebellar lesions. When this radiographic procedure is ambiguous, posterior fossa arteriography may help define the lesion. If both of these procedures are unrevealing, a lumbar puncture may reveal an acute or chronic infection disturbing cerebellar function. Mumps and Epstein-Barr virus infections are especially likely to produce cerebellar dysfunction. Congenital anomalies, such as adult Chiari malformations, may require pneumoencephalography to establish the anatomic characteristics. Kinetic tremors and gait difficulty may first appear in these patients in middle-age (50). The clearest indication of the anomaly will be low-lying cerebellar tonsils.

Essential Tremor

The physiologic tremor appearing with stress in normal individuals may be greatly amplified in some elderly individuals, producing the fine oscillations of essential tremor. This is often familial and is routinely aggravated by stress (33). Although this tremor appears at rest, it is not suppressed on movement and may be quite disabling or embarrassing. The apparent increase in tremor or amplitude with anxiety often leads to the patient's or his family's misconstruing this movement disorder as a psychiatric problem. Alcohol often suppresses the tremor, and chronic dependence on alcoholic beverages may reinforce the impression that the patient's problem is basically emotional. The tremor may extend to involve the head and neck as well as the arms (51). It is occasionally so severe that it interferes with reading, writing, and eating.

A consistent history of slowly evolving tremor over the course of decades is the most reliable evidence of this relatively benign disorder. Usually other family members have been affected and the patient knows his movement disorder is not from a life-threatening disease. The drug of choice for this disorder is propranolol, the beta-receptor blocking agent, with effective doses ranging from 100 to 200 milligrams daily in divided doses (33). Some clinicians believe that the more selective beta-adrenoceptor blocker metoprolol may be more effective than propranolol (51,52). There are no consistent pathologic changes in the brains of patients with essential tremor.

Hyperthyroidism

Anxious patients with fine limb tremors, rapid heart rates, emotional lability, and poor concentration should be evaluated for hyperthyroidism. Tremor often appears before the development of affective disorders, such as depression with suicide attempts; but the tremor may remain uninvestigated because the patient does not complain about it and those around the patient focus on the personality change caused by the thyroid disease. Mood and thought disorders developing with this endocrine disease are, in fact, more serious problems than the movement disorders that the hyperthyroidism can cause. Treatment of the overactive thyroid will suppress the tremor.

MYOCLONUS

Myoclonic movements are brief and shocklike, with most movements affecting the limbs. The paroxysmal muscle activity causing the myoclonic movement is always involuntary and often disturbing to the patient. A normal myoclonic movement that occasionally arouses concern in anxious patients is the massive, myoclonic jerk that occurs as the individual is falling asleep. Anxious patients are no more susceptible to these sleep-related movements than relaxed individuals, but the anxious individual may be excessively concerned with body functions; previously unnoticed phenomena may arouse grim suspicions of a crippling disease. In fact, myoclonic jerks do occur with several neurologic disorders, but jumping movements of the limbs may be voluntary in individuals with conversion reactions. These voluntary actions are often mistaken for myoclonus.

Most neurologic diseases associated with myoclonus are lethal. A notable exception is myoclonic epilepsy, a rare seizure disorder that may affect adolescents and occasionally produces myoclonic limb movements forceful enough to throw the patient to the ground. This myoclonic activity may be suppressed with the anticonvulsant clonazepam. Myoclonus in some individuals appears only when movement is voluntarily initiated in the limb involved. This is called intention myoclonus, and it may involve the face as well as the limbs (53). It is invariably idiopathic and is presumed to involve impaired brain serotonin production (53). Use of the serotonin precursor L-5-hydroxytryptophan with the decarboxylase inhibitor carbidopa helps control the movements but occasionally produces scleroderma (53). More lethal causes of myoclonus include subacute sclerosing panencephalitis, a progressive degenerative disorder of the nervous system developing in children after measles infections, and Unverricht-Lafora disease, an idiopathic neuromuscular disorder producing marked dementia and myoclonus. Myoclonic movements of the palate occasionally develop with Wernicke disease, the thiamine deficiency disease of the brain, but these movements are too rhythmic in most cases to be considered authentic myoclonus. Victims of severe cerebral hypoxia occasionally develop involuntary limb movements within days or weeks of the brain damage, a sequela often called posthypoxic myoclonus. Eighty-four percent of patients with Creutzfeldt-Jakob disease will have myoclonus at some time during the course of their illness, but in most cases it is near the end of this invariably lethal, slow-viral illness (54). Psychiatric patients developing myoclonus should be investigated for progressive degenerative disease of the brain, unless the abnormal movement is an obvious consequence of drug therapy. Toxic levels of lithium will produce myoclonus.

TICS

Movements under voluntary control, but occurring irresistibly at frequent intervals are called tics or habit spasms. Motor tics are abrupt, rapid, repetitive movements of a stereotyped nature performed apparently involuntarily (55). As already mentioned, many habit spasms take the form of abnormal facial movements. Hand gestures, head turning, kicking movements, and shoulder shrugging may also occur frequently enough to be recognized as habit spasms. Vocal tics include throat clearing, grunts, squeals, snorts, and recurrent obscenities (55). These abnormal movements and sounds need not have a purely psychologic basis, but psychologic factors play a role in the frequency of their occurrence. When the patient with a tic is under stress, the tic will occur more often and may be more obvious. It invariably subsides with sleep, and the patient can voluntarily prevent the tic for several seconds or minutes. Suppressing the tic produces a progressive feeling of tension that is relieved when the tic is allowed to appear.

Tics are generally benign phenomena reflecting no apparent structural disease in the central nervous system and evolving into no more than an embarrassment. There are notable exceptions (Table 9.5). Compulsive shouting (klazomania) and obscene remarks (coprolalia) may develop after an epidemic encephalitis (56). Minor brain damage or a toxic reaction to medication occasionally leads to tic phenomena. Tics without any associated vocalization occur in about 1 percent of children treated with methylphenidate for minimal brain dysfunction (57). Rarely, a benign tic evolves into a more complex tic syndrome, such as tic de Gilles de la Tourette (57). Most of these habit spasms are transient, the total duration of the movement disorder not exceeding 1 year (58). Vocal tics are an exception; they usually last years or remain for life.

Idiopathic Tics

There are a few distinct types of idiopathic tics (59). The most common tic is the transient tic of childhood, also known as acute simple tic. This is a habit spasm that appears at one time or another in about 12 percent of all children (60). It is usually little more than excessive blinking (blepharospasm) or a minor facial twitch. Boys are affected more often than girls

Table 9.5. Tics

Type	*Onset*	*Duration*
Simple tics		
Transient	Early childhood	Up to 1 year
Chronic	Before age 15 or after age 30	Until death
Subacute	Childhood or adolescence	Ends by end of adolescence
Multiple tics		
Transient and subacute	Same as simple	Same as simple
Tourette syndrome (chronic)	90% symptomatic before 11 years old	10–70 years

(58). Movements invariably involve the eyes, mouth, nose, head, neck, or arms, and their frequency, as well as their severity, generally fluctuates for the duration of the tic disorder. Symptoms last for as little as a week or as much as a year (60). Stress will clearly exacerbate the tic, and parental pressure to "break the bad habit" they see the child developing usually makes the tic noticeable for a longer time by introducing more stress. Although there has been considerable speculation that there is a psychologic basis for the disorder, none has been established (60). The cause of transient tics is unknown. Because most tics are transient and benign, treatment is usually not warranted, but the movements can be suppressed with butyrophenones.

A simple tic occasionally persists throughout life, in which case it is called a chronic simple tic (59). The movements do not progress over the course of years, but they do not subside either. These tics may begin before 15 years of age, but many of the individuals developing the movements are free of tics until their fourth, fifth, or sixth decades of life (60). As with the more common transient tics, no pathology is known to correlate with the disorder, and no treatment is warranted.

Intermediate between the transient tics of childhood and the chronic tics of later life are the subacute simple or multiple tics of childhood and adolescence (59). The only trait distinctive in this group of tics is that the disorder, which starts in childhood or adolescence and persists for more than a year, invariably subsides by the end of adolescence (60). Obviously, distinguishing between a chronic tic and a subacute tic is a retrospective judgment. If a simple tic persists and evolves into multiple tics, the patient may prove to have the tic syndrome of Gilles de la Tourette.

Gilles de la Tourette Syndrome

A movement disorder not yet assigned to strictly neurologic or psychologic causes is the Gilles de la Tourette syndrome. This is called a tic syndrome, but the symptomatology is much more complex than that ordinarily seen with a severe habit spasm (Table 9.6). The affected patient usually develops symptoms during childhood, the average age of onset being 7 years old (56). Ninety percent of the patients who will develop this syndrome have unequivocal signs of the disorder by $10\frac{1}{2}$ years of age (60). A single tic may be the only symptom initially, this taking the form of an eye twitch, head jerk limb jerk, or grimace. Stammering, stuttering, throat clearing, or obscene shouts (coprolalia) are less common initial manifestations, but appear regularly as the syndrome evolves. As the child grows, massive involuntary contractions of the muscles of the face, neck, trunk, limbs, and respiratory tract will produce bizarre movements and noises. The young adult may flail his arms purposelessly or hiss (61). Fifty-six percent of affected patients will develop complicated tics with jumping and stamping (56). These tics are often dismissed as just bad habits or transient

Table 9.6. Psychiatric Phenomena in Tourette Syndrome

Coprolalia
Obscene gesturing
Exhibitionism
Self-destructive behavior
Sociopathic behavior
Obsessive-compulsive behavior

tics of childhood (56). Supporting this impression is the disappearance of all signs during sleep. Adults with this disorder also stop being symptomatic with intense sexual arousal (56). As symptoms become more complex, they are less likely to be ascribed to an obsessive-compulsive neurosis or a borderline state.

Although the syndrome was named after Georges Gilles de la Tourette, a French physician who described nine patients with multiple tics, the disorder was first described by Itard in 1825 (62). Its essential features and significance have been debated since Gilles de la Tourette tried to establish that there was a syndrome of chronic multiple tics with associated behavior disorders in 1885 (60,63). There is no longer controversy that this is a distinct entity and that it has some familial features. Early studies indicated that about 43 percent of affected individuals were descendants of eastern European Jews, but the discovery of this disorder in a variety of ethnic groups has cast doubt on the significance of these statistics (55). The prevalence of Tourette's syndrome is one to five cases per 10,000 individuals in the United States (58). There is no doubt that the two sexes are affected differently: men are affected three times as often as women (60). Although a family history of some type of tic can be found for 28 percent of children randomly selected, the incidence of family members with tic or Tourette syndrome is significantly higher in children with the disorder than those in the general population (60). Despite this increased familial incidence, there is no clear pattern of transmission (55).

Clinical Features

Initially, the patient may have a waxing and waning course after a very insidious onset (57). Half the patients have a single tic as their first symptom, and this usually involves the eye (60). A definite diagnosis of Gilles de la Tourette syndrome rests on four features (55): the presence of multiple motor and vocal tics; symptom onset before 14 years of age; waxing and waning course; and repeated changes in the symptomatology with old manifestations being supplanted by new features.

Sixty percent of the affected children have coprolalia, and the types of tics exhibited by the children routinely change over the course of years (59). These children have a high incidence of sleep disturbances, learning problems, self-destructive behavior, inappropriate sexual activity, and antisocial behavior. Exhibitionism is reported by one-third of affected individuals (55). Obscene gesturing commonly develops as just another tic (59). Tic-like movements may also imitate movements of other individuals coming in contact with the victim of Tourette syndrome. Obsessive-compulsive behavior appears in two-thirds (55).

Formal psychologic tests suggest organic deficits in 68 percent of those with the syndrome and consistent with this is the 71 percent incidence of electroencephalographic abnormalities in children with Tourette syndrome (59,60). Delta wave sleep is decreased in affected individuals, and sleep is usually disturbed (55). This sleep disturbance is not caused by the tic movements since they subside with sleep. Minor motor abnormalities, such as limb drift, mirror movements, and chorea, can be detected in more than half the patients carefully examined (59). Intellectual deterioration generally does not occur.

Pathophysiology

Psychologic conflicts, especially in the realm of sexuality, were given central importance in the etiology of this disorder for several decades, but, currently, opinion is divided over whether this is a strictly psychologic or strictly neurologic problem (59, 60). Vocal and motor tics clearly can develop with structural damage to the brain. Such tics were well described after the epidemic encephalitis of von Economo (59). The rare autopsies on patients with Tourette syndrome have revealed no structural damage (59).

There is no consistent neuropathology associated with this syndrome. Those who believe it is a neurologic problem with a discrete etiology suggest it is a neurotransmitter disturbance perhaps involving acetylcholine, but no neurotransmitter in inappropriate levels has yet been found (61,64). Choline, a neurotransmitter precursor, is increased in the red blood cells of affected individuals, but abnormal acetylcholine levels in the brain have not been established (61). Tic frequency is inconsistently increased by levodopa administration, an observation lending little support to the notion that there is a dopamine problem basic to this disease (59). Other dopamine agonists may actually decrease the frequency of tics (59).

Treatment

Whatever the etiology of Tourette syndrome, it is a treatable condition. Haloperidol in doses as low as 5 milligrams daily suppresses most, if not all, of the symptoms (55). The response to haloperidol is best in individuals with a family history of Tourette syndrome. The decrease in deltawave sleep observed in these patients is also reversed by haloperidol treatment. The dose of haloperidol required usually decreases with time. Stress may exacerbate the symptoms and appropriately increased haloperidol doses may be necessary to deal with transient problems (55). Tetrabenazine, a drug that impairs catecholamine storage in the central nervouse system, is effective at doses of 100 milligrams per day in some patients responding poorly to high dose haloperidol treatment. Phenothiazines, especially those in the piperazine group (fluphenazine and perphenazine), are also effective in controlling the symptoms of Tourette syndrome (59). Pursuing the notion that this is an acetylcholine deficiency, some investigators have used oral lecithin, a precursor of acetylcholine (64). Mentation and tics improved in the few patients treated in this way (64).

CHOREA AND ATHETOSIS

Purposeless, more or less fluid, movements of the limbs and trunk are called chorea. Although the clinical term means "dance," the patient may have jerking or writhing movements rather than the organized limb excursions suggestive of a dance. Rare choreiform movements may be incorporated by the patient into semipurposeful gestures, such as raising a hand to the face or scratching a leg with the foot. These efforts to conceal the involuntary movements will be ineffective when the movements are more frequent or more pronounced. Those observing the patient will often conclude that the movements are voluntary or just "tics" because they disappear during sleep (65). Children with the movement disorder are dismissed as just restless, unless the movements become so forceful that purposeful activity is largely impossible. Because chorea occurs in disorders of the central nervous system that almost invariably also cause intellectual or affective disorders, most adults developing the movements will not seek medical attention on their own. Concerned family members usually initiate the medical or psychiatric consultation. Psychiatrists are often the first physicians consulted because the patient often denies that he has a movement disorder even when it becomes severe.

The most common setting for chorea is the child with rheumatic fever, but endocrine disorders, such as thyrotoxicosis and Addison disease (hypoadrenalism) are also associated with chorea (65,66). In young adults this movement disorder raises the possibility of systemic lupus erythematosus or encephalitis (67,68). In fact, chorea is the most common movement disorder developing in systemic lupus erythematosus (68). The development of these abnormal movements is not always a grave sign. There are a few benign conditions in which chorea may be prominent, but these are generally not associated with any cognitive or affective disorders. Healthy individuals developing transient chorea include pregnant women. Chorea appearing during pregnancy is probably an abnormal response to normal endocrine changes. This chorea gravidarum stops when the pregnancy ends.

Structural damage in the central nervous system from stroke, hypoxia, vitamin deficiencies, and even chronic subdural hematomas may also produce chorea (29). When there is no clear precipitating event or deficiency associated with the development of the jerking movements, degenerative disease of the central nervous system must be suspected. Choreiform movements are occasionally the first sign of Creutzfeldt-Jakob disease, a slow-viral infection leading to profound dementia and death within months of the appearance of the abnormal movements. Chorea is usually a problem affecting both sides of the body simultaneously, but one side of the body may have abnormal movements while the other is free of chorea, a clinical situation occasionally appearing with congenital hemiatrophy of the brain or a chronic subdural hematoma (69,70). The chorea developing with structural damage to one side of the brain is usually contralateral to the damage. When the structural lesion is a chronic subdural hematoma, removal of the blood clot or residual fluid does not necessarily abolish the movements. In such chronic situations, haloperidol may be required to suppress the chorea. Presumably, the pressure of the fluid overlying the brain produces vascular insufficiency in the thalamic, subthalamic, or basal ganglia structures responsible for the movement disorder (69).

Individuals who abuse amphetamines occasionally develop chorea that is closely linked to the drug abuse (71). Stopping the drug stops the chorea. This same type of stimulant-induced movement disorder also occurs in children given pemoline mesylate or methylphenidate as part of the treatment of minimal brain dysfunction (71). In both the drug abuser and the hyperactive child who develop chorea, a preexisting brain lesion is presumed to exist (71). Classically, this reaction to amphetamines has been attributed to their dopamine agonist action (72). The stimulant drug uncovers a susceptibility to movement disorders that might have gone undetected without the drug use.

A type of chorea often confused with minimal brain dysfunction is called Prechtl's choreiform syndrome (73). This develops in children who are often quite intelligent and have good coordination. The affected child has his normal movements unpredictably interrupted by jerking movements. These children are not hyperactive or easily distracted, but some are mistakenly treated with stimulants that can exacerbate the movement disorder. Some children with this type of chorea develop Tourette syndrome, but in most cases it is transient and benign.

Choreoathetosis

Purposeless limb and trunk movement with more continuity and fluidity than the characteristically abrupt, jerking motion of chorea is called athetosis. There is a writhing quality to this movement, but its separation from choreiform movements is so arbitrary that clinicians will often describe such movement disorders as choreoathetoid (Table 9.7). Both chorea and athetosis may develop after a stroke that caused hemiplegia or a persistent hemisensory deficit (74). Unlike most choreiform movements,

Table 9.7. Common Causes of Choreoathetosis

Sydenham chorea (rheumatic fever)
Chorea gravidarum
Huntington disease
Systemic lupus erythematosus
Encephalitis
Hyperthyroidism
Hypoadrenalism
Ischemic or hypoxic brain damage

the constant motion in the affected limb of stroke victims may continue into sleep. Damage in patients with this stroke-induced movement disorder and with most choreiform movements on other bases is in the basal ganglia. However, athetosis or choreoathetosis does not always indicate structural or degenerative central nervous system damage. Hyperthyroidism produces choreoathetosis that subsides completely with treatment of the thyroid disorder (66). Loss of position sense in the limbs may lead to erratic, spontaneous movements at rest or with a fixed posture. This is more accurately referred to as pseudoathetosis since the underlying problem is a sensory, rather than motor, deficit (74). Chronic alcoholics, vitamin deficient patients, and juvenile diabetics may develop peripheral neuropathy severe enough to precipitate pseudoathetosis. The movements appear when virtually all position sense is lost.

Purposeless movements may also extend to total body movements, pacing, or running. This inability literally to sit still is called akathisia and is distinct from choreoathetosis. It develops with idiopathic and postencephalitic parkinsonism, as well as with neuroleptic treatment (1). About 20 percent of the patients on piperazine phenothiazines will develop this restlessness; the first sign of the akathisia is shuffling or tapping of the feet, rocking, or a constant complaint of tension relieved by movement (1). This movement disorder may develop within a few days of starting neuroleptic medication. Fifty percent of those who will be symptomatic have the disorder within 1 month of starting the drugs. Ninety percent will develop symptoms within 2 months (1). The basis for this disorder is unknown. Patients of all ages are equally susceptible, and, although the akathisia is likely to remit spontaneously after weeks or months, it is resistant to anticholinergic and antihistamine drugs. Amphetamines decrease akathisia in some patients.

Stereotypy and Mannerisms of Schizophrenia

Schizophrenic patients with purposeless, repetitive, fragmented movements, called stereotypy, may be misdiagnosed as suffering from chorea or dyskinesias (Table 9.8) (1). These stereotyped movements may be fairly

Table 9.8. Movement Disorders in Schizophrenics

Stereotypy	*Dyskinesias*
DISTINCT FEATURES	
Unrelated to drug use (occasionally seen with anticholinergic drugs and levodopa treatment)	Usually associated with phenothiazine or butyrophenone use
Incorporated into purposeful acts as mannerisms	No consistent incorporation into purposeful acts
Ritualistic repetition of movement	Random recurrence of the movements
SHARED FEATURES	
Variable, brief head, neck, tongue, limb, and trunk movements	

complex, and, when relatively fluid limb or trunk movements occur, they may be indistinguishable from choreoathetosis. When the stereotypy is incorporated into a goal-directed activity, the resulting movement sequence leading to the performance of a generally pointless act is called a mannerism (1). The inclusion of the stereotypy in purposeful acts is ritualistic, unlike the inclusion of dyskinetic or choreiform movements in purposeful acts, which is totally random. The schizophrenic patient will stereotypically repeat the unnecessary movement, whether it be leg lifting, rocking, skipping, or grimacing whenever he engages in a specific activity. These mannerisms and stereotypies are often more complex than involuntary dyskinetic movements, but they are too common and variable to recognize on the basis of the character of the movements alone.

As much as 24 percent of catatonic schizophrenics exhibits stereotypy (1). This movement disorder usually appears early in the course of the mental illness and persists for years. Regardless of whether or not the associated psychotic disorders have a biochemical etiology, these movements probably do have a neurochemical basis. Pimozide, a drug that blocks the activity of dopamine, abolishes stereotypy in some patients (1). Alternatively, giving levodopa to patients with Parkinson disease may induce movements indistinguishable from schizophrenic stereotypy (1).

Patients exhibiting stereotypy and mannerisms generally do not exhibit chorea, athetosis, or dyskinesias. Choreoathetosis was quite often described in schizophrenics of various types in early articles on this thought disorder, but these patients probably had significant cognitive disorders associated with degenerative neurologic disease, rather than simply psychiatric disease (1). True chorea and athetosis are, in fact, rare in purely psychiatric illness.

Sydenham Chorea

Children and young adults developing personality disorders associated with chorea are likely to have Sydenham chorea. This disorder is usually recognized as an encephalopathy because of the antecedent group A streptococcal infection or the concurrent rheumatic fever found with it (67,75). About three-fourths of the patients developing this transient chorea are 7 to 12 years of age, and 65 percent of the adolescents (11 to 17 years of age) developing the chorea are women (67). Key clinical features are the gradual onset and seasonal character. Initially, the child simply appears restless or "fidgety," symptoms usually dismissed as a transient behavior problem. More florid movements and altered mentation may ensue in days or weeks. These symptoms appear in the springtime in one-third of patients (67). As the movements evolve, the chorea will usually be generalized, rather than limited to one side. Ten percent of patients have a pronounced personality change, disorientation, confusion, emotional lability, or delirium (67,75). One-third will have associated cardiac disease. About 40 percent have dysarthria (67). Speech is occasionally halting and explosive (75).

The cause of this movement disorder is unknown. It is presumed that a central dopaminergic system becomes reversibly defective and that this system is sensitized by female sex hormones. Serum immunoglobulins (IgG antibodies) in the patients with chorea react with cytoplasmic antigens from the caudate and subthalamic nuclei of the brain (75). The chorea that develops presumably reflects the action of dopamine on sensitive striatal receptors or the excessive production of dopamine in damaged presynaptic neurons (75). There are no pathologic changes in the brain, and any slow or fast activity developing on the electroencephalogram during the episode of chorea subsides with remission of the movement disorder. Although the movement disorder subsides, the encephalopathic features may persist to some extent. Behavioral difficulties in these adolescents are an occasional sequela. Chorea rarely lasts longer than 3 to 4 months.

Treatment is not advisable. Neuroleptics, such as chlorpromazine, will suppress the movements, but the child may develop dystonic posturing in response to the drug. Reserpine also may suppress the chorea in some individuals, presumably by depleting presynaptic dopamine supplies (75). This drug has adverse effects of its own which make it as undesirable a therapeutic agent as the phenothiazines and butyrophenones. The chorea may be reactivated with pregnancy, contraceptive use, or phenytoin therapy. Recurrence of the chorea occurs in 20 percent of cases (67). A progressive decrease in the incidence of Sydenham chorea over the past 15 years is well documented but unexplained. This movement disorder no longer routinely accompanies the other manifestations of rheumatic fever.

Huntington Disease

Huntington disease is a degenerative disorder of the central nervous system characterized by abnormal movements and thought or affective disorders. That psychiatric problems are a prominent feature of this disease was recognized in the earliest descriptions. George Huntington characterized the disease as "insanity with a tendency to suicide" (76). Chorea is the movement most often observed with this disorder. The dancing movements may be brisk and interrupted, giving the appearance of myoclonic jerking rather than fluid motion. The disease is inherited as an autosomal dominant trait with complete penetrance (11,77,78). Most families carrying the genetic abnormality can be traced back to the offspring of a British woman. Elizabeth Wanne, a confessed witch from Suffolk, England, produced numerous progeny with the disease trait before being tried and punished for her sacrilege (79). Cases occasionally appear in families not previously recognized as carrying the trait, but careful family histories will usually reveal psychiatric diseases, unexplained suicides, or involuntary movement disorders in close relatives of the Huntington disease victim.

Both the degree and progression of dementia and chorea vary from individual to individual (79,80). Even the age of onset of the disease is extremely variable. Signs of neurologic dysfunction may appear in childhood or may be inapparent until the fifth decade of life. When the disease appears in childhood or adolescence, there is little chorea and much rigidity (81). In most patients, a mild personality disorder is the initial sign of the disease. The patient becomes apathetic, careless, slovenly, and erratic in his treatment of family and friends. That this is the first evidence of an emerging psychosis will usually go unsuspected even if the patient consults a psychiatrist. The slowly progressive personality disorder is usually dismissed as a "functional" problem until more cognitive and affective deficits develop (79).

Clinical Features

All patients with Huntington disease will develop a profound dementia. The severity of this dementia depends primarily on the duration of the disease (79). Intellectual problems often appear before any movement disorder develops, the initial manifestation of cognitive dysfunction being impaired problem solving. Subtle defects in intellectual function routinely develop months or years before a definite dementia can be appreciated on clinical interview. WAIS scores for performance tests will fall in asymptomatic individuals who ultimately develop the disease (79). When symptoms, such as the personality changes, do develop, the patient will become grossly inattentive, vague, obtuse, and repetitious. With progression of the dementia, verbal test scores fall on the WAIS, and the patient becomes less communicative and more inactive.

Later neurologic signs of the degenerative disease include dysarthria and gait difficulty. Juvenile Huntington disease occasionally causes seizures (81). Tremors of the face and hands, lurching gait, and poor coordination develop in many adult patients (81). Half of the patients with Huntington disease lose fast saccadic eye movements and have poor upward gaze (78). Signs notably absent include aphasia, cortical blindness, ataxia, apraxia, agnosia, and the catastrophic memory disorder of Korsakoff psychosis (79). Patients with Huntington disease do, however, have word-finding problems and difficulty with abstraction.

The course of the disease is invariably progressive. Patients never stabilize after a few signs and symptoms have developed. The patient's life expectancy is shortened by decades, with the terminal episode resulting from a suicide attempt or from uncontrollable systemic infections. Diffuse trauma sustained because of the involuntary movements reduces the patient's ability to resist infection, and his unwillingness to eat or drink contributes to the malignancy of any infection. The patient may die in an akinetic state, bedridden, mute, and incontinent. Dehydration, aspiration, and malnutrition are all likely to play a role in his death. Survival averages 16 years from the onset of the patient's first symptoms (79). Some patients survive for 25 to 30 years.

Fertility is unaffected by the disease, and serious illness rarely develops before the patient has the opportunity to have children. Genetic counseling is certainly appropriate in families exhibiting this disorder, but its usefulness in actually decreasing the size of families with affected members is questionable. Individuals advised that half of their children will be affected by the disease may react by having more children to increase the likelihood that some of their children will be normal.

Psychiatric Signs and Symptoms

Problems with recall, calculations, and comprehension develop early in the course of Huntington disease, but more consistent and bothersome are the psychiatric manifestations of this disease (Table 9.9) (81). Paranoia, irascibility, irritability, and limited concentration are prominent traits in the mildly demented patient (81). Profound depression is the most common affective disorder seen with this disease, that depression often preceding all other symptoms (81). The patient will readily admit to

Table 9.9. Psychiatric Abnormalities in Huntington Disease

Irritability
Irascibility
Irrational guilt
Apathy
Aggression
Paranoid delusions
Psychotic depression
Suicide attempts
Hallucinations

suicidal thoughts and successful suicides are the cause of death in 7 percent of nonhospitalized individuals (79,81). Outbursts of anger, physical assaults on family members, and progressive withdrawal from social contacts often isolate the patient early in his disease course. The affective disorder resembles a manic-depressive psychosis; hallucinations and well-structured delusions occur infrequently (79). Psychomotor retardation appears with irrational feelings of guilt, poverty, loss, or offensiveness. The depressive episodes may last months and recur over the course of years. As in typical bipolar psychoses, manic episodes occur, but these are relatively brief. Antidepressants and electroconvulsive treatments help with the depressive episodes, but the manic bouts are not manageable (79). Patients complaining of delusions of control, feelings of persecution, and recurrent auditory or tactile hallucinations may be misdiagnosed as paranoid schizophrenic.

Pathogenesis

Huntington disease is a degenerative disease of the brain. Neurons and associated neural structures deteriorate as the disease progresses. The basal ganglia are the sites of some of the more dramatic changes, and problems with neurotransmitter activity in this part of the brain is currently considered responsible for many of the signs evolving with the disease.

Because chorea was often considered the alternative to parkinsonism, patients with Huntington disease were classically assumed to have excess dopamine activity, just as patients with Parkinson disease were assumed to have decreased dopamine activity. Dopamine excess or dopamine receptor hypersensitivity is also an attractive hypothetical basis for any disease causing progressive psychotic disorders, disorders often responsive to dopamine-activity blocking neuroleptics. Unfortunately, recent studies of the basal ganglia in patients dying with Huntington disease indicate a more complex neurotransmitter problem (80).

Although levodopa administered to these patients does exacerbate the movement disorder, enzymes unrelated to dopamine synthesis or breakdown are also affected (11,82). Choline acetyltransferase, an enzyme important in the manufacture of acetylcholine, is lower than normal in the putamen and caudate (striatum) of Huntingtonian patients; but probably even more important than abnormal acetylcholine production are reduced levels of glutamic acid decarboxylase, an enzyme essential for the production of the inhibitory neurotransmitter gamma-aminobutyric acid (GABA) (81–83). This inhibitory transmitter is decreased in the caudate, putamen, globus pallidus, and substantia nigra of Huntington disease victims (83). Deficiencies of both gamma-aminobutyric acid and acetylcholine may be responsible for the loss of neurons in these structures.

The neurotransmitter imbalances long invoked as the explanation for Huntington disease may be real, but their cause and character are unclear. Microscopic examination of the caudate and putamen of the basal ganglia reveals a loss of small neurons with proliferation of astrocytes (80). Despite these histologic changes, the dopamine content of the striatum is normal (80).

A normal dopamine content in a neuron-depleted structure may mean that nerve cells are being exposed to excessive neurotransmitter simply because there is more available for individual cells. This produces an imbalance in the dopaminergic, cholinergic, GABAnergic systems in the basal ganglia and perhaps in the cerebral cortex as well.

Treatment

Efforts to slow the course of this disease have been largely unsuccessful. Steroids do nothing to improve the affective and movement disorders (84). Tetrabenazine, a synthetic benzoquinolizine resembling reserpine, improves some patients' symptoms (80). Presumably, this drug depletes central nervous system dopamine and other monoamines (83). Unfortunately, it produces drowsiness, akathisia, and insomnia (80). Lecithin, a precursor of acetylcholine, also has some beneficial effects on the movement disorder in this acetylcholine-deficiency or dopamine-excess disease (39). Haloperidol and phenothiazines are used to counteract the relative overactivity of the dopaminergic neurons, but these drugs provide only inconsistent relief of the abnormal movements (81). Based upon the observed inhibition of gamma-aminobutyric acid degradation by isoniazid, the antimicrobial agent used in treating tuberculosis, treatment of Huntington disease patients with isoniazid has been attempted in a few uncontrolled trials (81). The majority of patients display striking improvement in movement and affective disorders, but the antidepressant effect of isoniazid may be tied more closely to its metabolites acting as monamine oxidase inhibitors than to its specific activity against gamma-aminobutyric acid degradation (81). Supporting this notion is the ineffectiveness of sodium valproate in altering the depression in these patients (81). Sodium valproate, an anticonvulsant, also inhibits the degradation of gamma-aminobutyric acid. Those patients responding to isoniazid treatment show no improvement in strictly cognitive functions, such as recall and calculations. Another disadvantage of the isoniazid is the high dose necessary (12 to 18 milligrams per kilogram per day) and the high risk of liver disease and systemic lupus erythematosus with use of this drug.

Definitive Diagnosis

Diagnosis relies upon autopsy confirmation of the disease in a family member. Before death, the disease may be presumed responsible for dementia and chorea if the head of the caudate nucleus is atrophied. The caudate lies along the lateral wall of the lateral ventricles, and loss of the normal concave shape anteriorly in this ventricle indicates caudate atrophy (Figure 9.4). This is readily assessed by computed tomography of the head

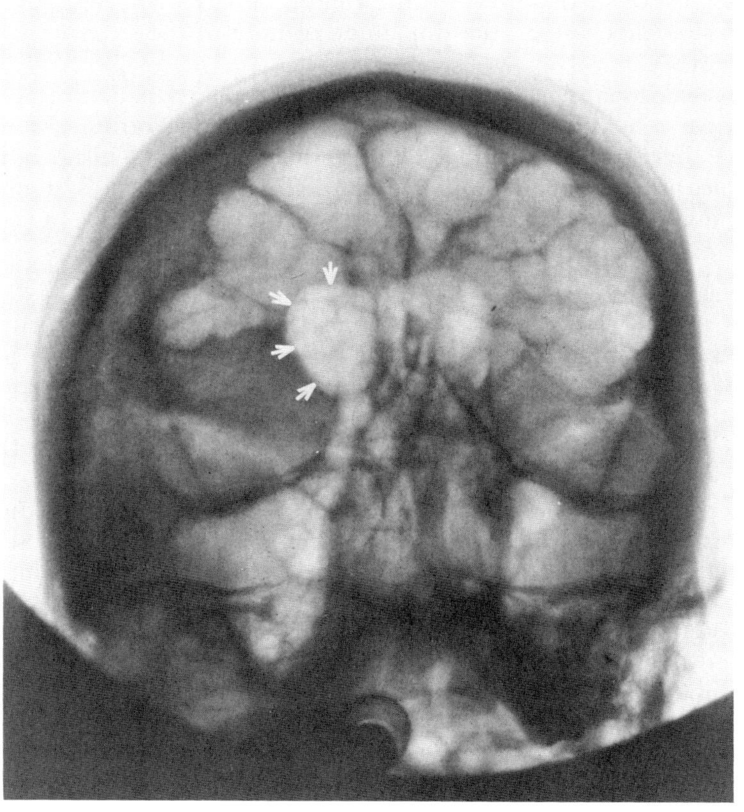

Figure 9.4. The frontal horn of the lateral ventricle is filled with air in this pneumoencephalogram. The patient had signs and symptoms typical of Huntington disease, and the air study was performed to confirm the diagnosis. The white arrows indicate the lateral and superior margins of the lateral ventricle. The head of the caudate nucleus, which normally bulges into the lateral wall of this part of the lateral ventricle, is completely absent. This much atrophy of the caudate nucleus is usually seen only in nearly terminal Huntington disease patients.

or by pneumonencephalography. These anatomic changes are not usually apparent until the dementia and movement disorders are well advanced (78).

Diagnosis of Huntington disease gene carriers may be feasible in the near future because of a generalized abnormality in cell membrane structures that is probably detectable before the disease is symptomatic (85). The obvious advantage of such early detection is to allow counseling of the affected individual before he decides whether or not to have children. Some indication of the probability that an individual will develop Huntington disease may be provided by a provocative levodopa test (78).

Some investigators have given asymptomatic individuals at risk for the disease test doses of levodopa. There was good correlation between the development of chorea with the drug and subsequent development of the disease (77). This is still investigational, and the risk of prematurely inducing active disease with this provocative test is unknown. Currently, there is no reliable method for detecting presymptomatic victims of Huntington disease (78).

Chorea Gravidarum

Chorea occasionally develops with pregnancy or estrogen use. Initially, this may be manifest as increasing restlessness and anxiety, followed by jerking movements of the arms or legs within days or weeks (86). If the movements develop during pregnancy, the disorder is called chorea gravidarum. The involuntary movements in women with chorea gravidarum are usually asymmetric, producing a hemichorea, that is, a movement disorder affecting only one side of the body. Choreiform movements developing during pregnancy may be so forceful that they interfere with walking and sleeping. Involuntary mouth and tongue movements also develop and interfere with eating and drinking.

This same kind of movement disorder occassionally develops in women taking birth control pills. With contraceptive use, the chorea is likely to appear within weeks of starting the hormone and evolve slowly. Estrogen-induced chorea is not necessarily associated with chorea gravidarum, the movement disorder of pregnancy, but patients with either estrogen-induced or pregnancy-induced chorea have a past history of chorea in 50 percent of cases (72). More than 40 percent have had prior episodes of Sydenham chorea, the movement disorder developing with rheumatic fever (72). Even with this history of a prior episode of chorea, these women are often considered hysterical. The impression that this behavior is simply from poor adjustment to pregnancy or contraceptive use is strengthened by the personality change commonly associated with the movement disorder. The development of dysarthria with the personality disorder and the chorea usually alerts the patient or her family to the more organic nature of this problem (72). Unfortunately, chorea developing during pregnancy or with contraceptive use is not always from a benign lesion (Table 9.10). The movement disorder and agitated personality may be the first signs of systemic lupus erythematosus or Huntington disease, both diseases that occasionally surface during pregnancy (86).

The cause of chorea gravidarum is unknown. It is presumed that there is structural damage in the basal ganglia, which is usually silent until hormone levels change. The sex hormones are presumed to alter the sensitivity of the basal ganglia to normal levels of a neurotransmitter, perhaps dopamine (72). The fundamental change in the brain may in fact be hormone-induced changes in neurotransmitter levels. Supporting this

Table 9.10. Disorders Producing Chorea During Pregnancy

Idiopathic chorea gravidarum
Sydenham chorea
Systemic lupus erythematosus
Huntington disease

hypothesis is the well-established influence estrogen has on catecholamine turnover in the brain (86).

Treating these women is usually unnecessary. Discontinuing the estrogen supplement or awaiting the conclusion of the pregnancy is preferable to using neuroleptic drugs, such as haloperidol, to suppress the movements. The incidence of chorea gravidarum and estrogen-induced chorea has been declining over the past few decades (86). The reason for this change is unknown.

Rare Causes of Chorea

Senile Chorea

Elderly patients with no prior history of a movement disorder occasionally develop slowly progressive choreiform movements over the course of weeks or months. Associated with the jerking movements of the body will be a mood change, best characterized as anxiety. The family often attributes both the abnormal movements and the affective disorder to irrational nervousness or senility and seeks medical attention only when the chorea is so marked that it interferes with walking or eating. The cause of this chorea is unknown. In some cases it is apparently Huntington chorea with a remarkably late onset. If the patient does not have an autopsy and there is no family history of Huntington disease, it may be impossible to prove that this is the cause of the movement disorder. With radiographic procedures alone, no obvious lesions will be found in the brain, and no metabolic problems will surface as the movement disorder evolves. Some patients with senile chorea respond briskly to small doses of haloperidol. Both the movements and the associated anxiety may abate on only a few milligrams daily of this butyrophenone.

Chorea with Acanthocytosis

Chorea need not be associated with dementia or affective disorders. There is a rare, but well-described, recessively-inherited degenerative disease of the basal ganglia that produces a movement disorder identical to that in Huntington disease, but without the mental changes characteristic of Huntington disease (82). Jerking movements and a prominent orofacial dyskinesia develop by the third decade of life; and within 15 years, the patient is unable to walk, speak, or feed himself because of the constancy and severity of the chorea. Psychometric testing will reveal little or no deterioration in cognitive function as the disease evolves. Depression and suicide are not a significant feature of this illness. Red blood cell changes are usually seen in this disorder. The outline of the erythrocytes is spurred or thorny, a phenomenon called acanthocytosis (82).

The pathology of this disease is indistinguishable from Huntington disease, but the altered activity in the glumatic acid decarboxylase and choline acetyltransferase, characteristic of Huntington disease, are not present (82). This disorder has never been successfully treated and affected patients die of infections or inanition.

Paroxysmal Dystonic Choreoathetosis

Episodes of disabling purposeless movement developing with stress are routinely considered hysterical but may be from a neurogenic choreoathetosis (87). Disorders associated with paroxysmal choreoathetosis include multiple sclerosis, asphyxia, hypoparathyroidism with hypocalcemia, and thyrotoxicosis (66,88). Paroxysmal choreoathetosis also appears as a primary problem in some patients without any of these diseases. Idiopathic posturing or writhing limb and trunk movements appear primarily in two groups of patients (66). One has a familial incidence of the movement disorder that follows an autosomal dominant pattern of inheritance (89). The other is nonfamilial. The familial or Mount-Reback type is usually symptomatic when the patient drinks whiskey, exerts himself, or becomes emotionally upset (87,88). In the nonfamilial type, abnormal postures, choreiform jerks, and athetoid movements are precipitated by normal, but often abrupt, movement (87). Tension, anxiety, or embarrassment is likely to trigger grimacing, arm extension, slurred speech, gait difficulty, or flapping of the arms.

Each attack of the nonfamilial type will last about 15 to 30 seconds and may recur several times a day (87). Quite often this choreoathetosis will be part of a startle reaction (79). Attacks will first appear in childhood or adolescence and are often attributed to a developmental maladjustment. This suspicion is reinforced by the emotional setting of the attacks and the patient's ability to inhibit some attacks by holding the initially affected limb (87). The neurologic examination in this nonfamilial paroxysmal choreoathetosis is invariably normal, and an electroencephalogram performed during the attack will be normal or inconsistently abnormal (87,89); but the choreoathetosis does abate when the patient is given phenytoin or a barbiturate (88). Autopsy studies on patients with this paroxysmal kinesigenic choreoathetosis have revealed no abnormalities in the brain (88).

The types of movements exhibited by patients with the familial (Mount-Reback) form of paroxysmal choreoathetosis are the same as in the nonfamilial form. Attacks last longer in the familial type, often extending to hours rather than seconds. Patients are symptomatic early in life, with the first abnormal movements occurring in some individuals during infancy (89). Caffeine or alcohol may precipitate an attack of posturing or choreiform movements (88). Attacks recur several times daily or only a few times monthly (89). In addition to choreoathetosis, patients with the Mount-Reback syndrome have involuntary posturing or dystonia with the attacks. This dystonia may be heralded by an abnormal sensation in the hand or at the corner of the mouth, but more commonly the patient simply feels "nervous" just before the dystonic reaction occurs (88). The dystonic attack itself may produce a unilateral flexor spasm or an inability to move. The patient is quite often mute during the attack, and the disorder may be mistaken for petit mal epilepsy. A normal electroencephalogram during the attack rules out this diagnosis (88); the patient is alert throughout the attack. Clonazepam, 2 milligrams three times a day, often abolishes the paroxysmal movement disorder; but, despite this response to an anticonvulsant, autopsy studies on affected patients have failed to reveal any structural disease in the brain (88).

The familial and nonfamilial paroxysmal choreoathetoses are probably different entities at the level of structural or chemical lesions in the brain, although the pathophysiologic bases for both of these disorders are unknown. The autosomal dominant pattern of inheritance and the character of the movements often lead to the familial paroxysmal choreoathetosis being misdiagnosed as Huntington disease (89). This is especially unfortunate since the paroxysmal dystonic choreoathetoses are not associated with dementia, affective disorders, or shortened lifespans. These forms of choreoathetosis are very difficult to distinguish from focal motor epilepsy, and some investigators, in fact, believe these are forms of reflex epilepsy even though electroencephalographic changes are not apparent during the attacks (87). Dystonic seizures similar to those appearing in the Mount-Reback syndrome also develop in patients with cortical scars, multiple sclerosis, and basal ganglia disease (88). Associated signs and absence of a family history should clarify the etiology of the paroxysmal dystonic choreoathetosis in these situations (88).

The paroxysmal choreoathetosis developing in rare patients with hyperthyroidism resembles the nonfamilial "kinesigenic" disorder (66). Attacks of grimacing and tonic limb posturing may last seconds or minutes and are likely to occur several times daily. During these episodes, the electroencephalogram will reveal little more than diffuse slowing (66). Distinctive and unexplained in this movement disorder is the close association between the frequency of choreoathetoid paroxysms and the level of serum thyroxine. As the hyperthyroidism is treated and the serum thyroxine decreases, the movements will disappear. Propranolol, the beta-adrenergic receptor blocker, and haloperidol, the dopamine antagonist, will both inhibit the paroxysmal choreoathetosis developing with hyperthyroidism, but the mechanism of action of these drugs is unknown (66).

The neurophysiologic basis for this reversible choreoathetosis is also unknown.

ABNORMAL POSTURING

Abnormal postures or eccentric gaits, especially when they develop in children, are often ascribed to psychologic difficulties. Occasionally, the organic basis for the abnormal posture is recognized when a responsible drug is discontinued, but the exacerbation of symptoms in both drug-induced and idiopathic posturing with emotional stress commonly prompts psychiatric evaluation of the patient. Whether the abnormal posturing involves several limbs or only a single muscle, it is usually called a dystonia.

Focal Dystonias

Focal dystonias are spasms of specific muscles, such as the sternomastoid muscle in torticollis ("wry neck") or the orbicularis oculi muscles in blepharospasm (60). Writer's cramp (graphospasm) may be a focal dystonia, although psychologic conflicts surrounding the disability raise suspicion of a conversion reaction (90). These focal dystonias are not familial, and they may start during or after middle age (60). If the focal dystonia involves several groups of muscles, the abnormal posturing is called a segmental dystonia (60). Unfortunately, these generally benign focal or segmental dystonias occasionally progress to become a generalized dystonia, called dystonia musculorum deformans or idiopathic torsion dystonia. Irregular, sustained involuntary movements produce abnormal postures in this torsion dystonia that range from recurrent inversion of the foot while walking to dramatic contortions of the limbs and trunk. The affected individual seems to writhe slowly. Attempts to suppress focal dystonias with drugs, nerve sections, and muscle surgery have been largely unsuccessful.

Dystonia Musculorum Deformans

Idiopathic torsion dystonia assumes two major forms, both of which are frequently misdiagnosed as conversion reactions at their onsets. The more common form appears in children between the ages of 4 and 16 years, especially those of eastern European Jewish descent (91). These children have normal perinatal and developmental histories, and careful examination will reveal no intellectual sensory, motor, or coordination deficits

(91). The initial symptom is usually a peculiar gait, which may be interpreted by parents as just an idiosyncrasy or behavior problem. Legs and arms are progressively involved by the abnormal posturing, and the patient may be wheelchair bound by adolescence. This disorder has been ascribed classically to an autosomal recessive gene, but recent studies indicate the disease is transmitted in an autosomal dominant pattern with variable penetrance (91).

The other form of idiopathic torsion dystonia generally appears in non-Jews and starts during adult life. Unlike the juvenile dystonia, postural problems affect the axial, rather than limb, muscles initially, and torticollis is often a presenting symptom. The adult dystonia progresses slowly and may be associated with blepharospasm or graphospasm (91). It is generally not seen in black Americans. Inheritance is typically autosomal dominant with complete penetrance. Both the juvenile and adult forms of dystonia musculorum deformans are assumed to result from disturbed brain catecholamine function, but this has not been proven (91).

No effective treatment has been found for either form of torsion dystonia. The severe disability caused by these dystonias has prompted some neurosurgeons to attempt controlling the abnormal posturing by placing stereotactic lesions in the thalamus (92). Improvement after this kind of surgery has been inconsistent.

Acute Dystonic Reactions

As already mentioned in the section on acute dyskinesias associated with antipsychotic treatment, neuroleptic drugs occasionally produce a reversible dystonia, which may be focal or generalized (23). An acute dystonic reaction to neuroleptic drugs will develop in 2.5 to 5 percent of all patients started on these antipsychotic medications (1). The reaction begins within 48 hours of drug administration in 50 percent of those who do develop abnormalities and within 5 days in 90 percent (1). The abnormal posturing is of sudden onset. Muscle spasms about the face, head, and neck are especially common, and spasms about the jaw and in the tongue may be adequately forceful to interfere with speaking, swallowing, and even mouth opening (23). Grimacing is usually the most obvious movement disorder, but abnormal posturing of the head, neck, or trunk, called torticollis, retrocollis, and opisthotonus respectively, also develop in some cases (23). The muscle reaction is usually not so diffuse that the patient is wheelchair-bound, but back and leg muscles are sufficiently involved by the involuntary spasms in some patients to produce a gait abnormality. Disordered postures and truncal involvement are more characteristic of acute dystonic reactions in children. The child may develop arching of the body (opisthotonus), tilting of the pelvis (tortipelvis), or lateral curvature of the spine (scoliosis). Occasional patients complain of problems with eye movements, especially in the vertical plane (20). This complaint is called oculogyric crisis when the eyes are tonically deviated upwards and pain accompanies the involuntary upward gaze. Oculogyric crises usually last minutes to hours (23).

Dystonia occurring in children under 15 years of age is often generalized, whether the dystonia is drug-induced or is a manifestation of a progressive neurologic disease, such as dystonia musculorum deformans (1). Adults typically have dystonic reactions limited to their neck, face, and arms. In both children and adults with acute dystonic reactions, the posturing may be continuous or intermittent. Acute dystonic reactions involving the face and limbs often last hours to days if no treatment other than discontinuation of the drug responsible is attempted.

Piperazine phenothiazines and butyrophenones are the antipsychotics most likely to produce acute dyskinesias; but, regardless of the drug responsible, if the dose administered was not massive, the dystonia does not usually persist for more than several hours or a few days (1). Drug-induced dystonia is most common in young adults given prochlorperazine for vomiting, and in adults started on neuroleptics for psychiatric problems (20). A reversible dystonia develops in some psychiatric patients within the first days or weeks of phenothiazine treatment (88). This acute dystonia may develop after only one dose of neuroleptic drug, and it usually appears within 24 to 48 hours of starting or changing the dose of a neuroleptic (20,23). This reaction is more common in young people than in old people, and it develops in men more often than in women (23).

The cause of this dystonic reaction is unknown. Idiosyncratic sensitivity to the neuroleptic clearly plays a role, but there is no way to predict which patients will have this untoward reaction (23). Presumably, introduction of the neuroleptic causes an acute functional deficiency in basal ganglia systems that normally inhibit aberrant movements and postures. An acute excess of brain acetylcholine developing secondarily to the dopamine blocking agents may be the neurochemical basis for the disorder. Consistent with this is the observed usefulness of anticholinergic drugs, such as benztropine and trihexyphenidyl, in suppressing this acute reaction to neuroleptics (20). Diphenhydramine given intravenously will usually rapidly abolish the signs of the acute dystonia (93). Unfortunately, the dystonia may recur after it subsides.

Torticollis

Undirectional rotation of the head or unilateral flexion of the neck is called torticollis. This abnormal posturing of the head may be constant or intermittent; when it is intermittent, it is called spasmodic torticollis. Patients with torticollis have a family history of torticollis or a related movement or postural disorder in 17 percent of cases (94). Occasionally, the torticollis is followed by other disorders of posture, and a fully developed torsion dystonia will appear (90,91). Fortunately, there is no progression in most patients. The cause of this head deviation is unknown, and the course is exceedingly variable. Speculation in the past ascribed this movement disorder to a conversion reaction associated with unresolved conflicts (90). Spasmodic torticollis seemed especially common in cases of marital discord. Current opinion is leaning away from this psychiatric explanation and favoring a more neurochemical explanation.

Fluctuation in the severity of the symptom is common. This makes the evaluation of any therapy more difficult, but none has had a dramatic effect on the torticollis, despite the possibility of spontaneous improvement while the patient is being treated. Treatment with rhizotomy (spinal root cutting), myotomy (neck muscle section), thalamotomy, anticholinergic drugs, diazepam, doxepin, fluphenazine, haloperidol, prochlorperazine, and bromocriptine have all been unsuccessful (17). Electromyographic feedback techniques have worked in some patients, but there is no consensus that this is a reliable therapy (94). Some neurologists have also reported control of the posturing with a combination of L-glutamine, isoniazid, pyridoxine, and diazepam (94). This pharmocologic approach was based on the assumption that gamma-aminobutyric acid was depleted in the basal ganglia of patients with this disorder. Both the treatment and the presumed etiology are speculative.

Writer's Cramp

Painful or immobilizing cramps developing in the hand while the patient is trying to write usually develops in individuals with obsessive-compulsive personality types (90). This is called writer's cramp or graphospasm, and it results from contraction of both agonistic and antagonistic muscles in the hand and forearm. It is apparently involuntary, but its common occurrence in individuals dependent upon their writing skills raises the possibility that it is a symptom of a conversion reaction (90). This idiosyncratic and relatively minor complaint is generally totally disabling for the individuals susceptible to it. Without their writing or drawing ability, these individuals are unable to conduct their normal occupation, and so all their energy becomes focused on overcoming the inappropriate hand activity. Reinforcing the impression that writer's cramp is a symptom of psychologic conflicts is the observation that victims of writer's cramp are especially likely to suppress or deny emotions (90). There is no effective treatment.

TRANSIENT CLUMSINESS

Transient signs of clumsiness in the arms or legs usually reflect disease of the cerebellum or brainstem, if they do, in fact, have an organic basis (47).

The most common cause of transient clumsiness in elderly patients is vascular disease in the vertebrobasilar system. Demyelinating disease and metabolic disease are less often responsible, but these will cause problems in younger people and so are more likely to be misconstrued as hysteria. Regardless of the underlying disease, limb clumsiness or ataxia is rarely an isolated sign. Other signs of brainstem damage or cerebellar disease will invariably surface when a careful neurologic evaluation of the patient is performed. These signs include ocular motor abnormalities, disturbed hearing, impaired facial movements, and tremors. If none of these additional signs is present, the final diagnosis may prove to be hysteria. Because there are so many subtle and obscure diseases causing transient clumsiness, a diagnosis of conversion reaction should always be considered suspect or tentative. Even if the patient has obvious psychologic problems surfacing with the attacks of clumsiness, the underlying disease may be unequivocally organic. Emotional stress and anxiety-related hyperventilation often precipitate attacks even in cases of structural cerebellar disease (95).

With impaired perfusion of the vertebrobasilar artery, the patient will develop problems with limb strength or coordination lasting minutes to hours. The signs developing with decreased blood flow will be determined by the blood vessel most involved. When the basilar artery is impaired, numerous cranial nerve signs are likely to appear. When a branch to the cerebellum is selectively involved, the patient may have little more than unilateral tremor, limb clumsiness (ataxia), and gait difficulty. Although emboli arising in the heart rarely travel to the vertebrobasilar system, cardiac arrhythmias may cause symptoms by decreasing the effective blood pressure in the partially occluded vertebrobasilar arteries. Treating the underlying vascular or cardiac problem is the only feasible approach to this recurrent ataxia.

Patients with multiple sclerosis may have attacks of dysarthria, ataxia, and gait problems lasting seconds to minutes recurring several times a day (48,95,96). Each attack is similar to the next. If speech is slurred with one episode of clumsiness it is usually slurred with all episodes. The frequency of the attacks, sometimes approaching 40 to 50 daily, in a relatively intact individual raises suspicions of hysteria. The unlikely explanation of seizure disorder is ruled out once an electroencephalogram is obtained during the attack. Emotional stress will increase the severity and frequency of the attacks in patients with multiple sclerosis. The patient may subsequently have major episodes of demyelination, which clarify the diagnosis, but, even when the diagnosis is recognized, physicians may misinterpret the transient ataxic episodes as signs of psychologic stress. That this is an organic problem is supported by the observed decrease in attack frequency when the patient is given adrenocorticotrophic hormone intramuscularly (95).

HICCOUGHS

Hiccoughs may develop as a nervous habit or tic; but, occasionally, persistent hiccoughs reflect central or peripheral nervous system disease. Episodes may last days or months if the underlying problem is brainstem damage or phrenic nerve irritation. Processes disturbing the brainstem and triggering the disorder include syringobulbia, tabes dorsalis, encephalitis, meningitis, tumor, infarction, and demyelination (97). Phrenic nerve irritation may be caused by peritonitis, myocardial infarction, gastrointestinal hemorrhage, or a subphrenic abscess. Systemic disorders, such as uremia, alcohol intoxication, and general anesthesia, can also induce persistent hiccoughing (97). Fortunately, most cases have a psychogenic basis, and the individual episodes will be limited to a few hours or days.

The mechanism producing nonpsychogenic episodes of hiccoughing is not known. Presumably, centers in the hypothalamus, medulla, and cervical spinal cord are responsible for this respiratory reflex. With no apparent basis for the disorder, the treatment has been limited. Phenothiazines, phrenic nerve section, quinidine, and carbamazepine have all been tried with inconsistent results (97). Cases related to emotional conflicts will show improvement as the conflicts abate with psychiatric intervention.

GAIT DISORDERS

Impaired or abnormal gait develops with disease in many parts of the nervous system, but it may also be a sign of muscle weakness or joint disease. Disturbed gait is the initial sign in some cases of cerebral, cerebellar, or basal ganglia damage. With significant disease of the labyrinth in the ear, the patient cannot walk because of balance impairment. Weakness in the muscles of the hip girdle interferes with the stability of the legs, and the affected individual is obliged to walk with a broad-based gait. Pain in the hip joint from arthritis, metastatic disease, or other local problems will alter the normal pattern of walking. Many individuals with profound gait disorders have no apparent disease to explain the aberrant gait. Such individuals are often referred for psychiatric evaluation.

Damage at almost any point in the nervous system can directly or indirectly produce an abnormal pattern of walking. The pattern that develops is usually characteristic of the part of the nervous system injured. Cerebellar damage produces a wide-based, staggering gait; basal ganglia damage leads to short, shuffling steps. A demyelinating lesion involving the corticospinal tracts in the spinal cord usually produces a stiff-legged gait, with the affected leg circumducted at the hip with each step. Peripheral nerve damage may require the patient to lift his foot unnaturally from the ground with each step, either to overcome a foot drop or to compensate for lost position sense. What is consistently true for these neurologically derived gait disorders is that each step exhibits the same problem as the prior step. The pattern of the deficit does not change as the patient tries to walk. This is a valuable trait in distinguishing hysterical gait disorders from neurologic gait disorders.

Even minor gait problems are usually associated with other signs or symptoms that clarify their origins. Patients with weakness in the muscles of the hip girdle will have difficulty getting out of chairs or getting off the toilet. The problem with walking may become most pronounced after the patient has tried to climb a flight of stairs. Spinal cord damage may cause relatively little change in the pattern of walking, but the legs may become extremely stiff for protracted intervals. Problems with bladder and bowel control often appear with spinal cord lesions, and sometimes the first complaint of the spinal cord disease will be sexual dysfunction. The impotent patient may incidentally note that his gait has changed along with his sexual function. Patients with staggering gait from cerebellar disease also frequently have slurred speech. Whatever the nature of the gait problem, the signs and symptoms associated with the altered gait should suggest the pathology responsible for the problem.

Psychogenic Gait Disorders: Astasia Abasia

Psychogenic gait disorders can assume several forms. Some patients simply insist that they are totally unable to stand or walk. This usually causes little confusion, because the patient will have normal leg movements despite his insistence that he has no power or coordination in the legs. Other patients adopt the gait disorders they perceive in handicapped individuals who play significant roles in their lives. The physical examination in such patients will be inconsistent with the apparent deficit. Patients with typically spastic gaits will have no increased tone in the legs. A staggering gait will be unaffected by depriving the patient of visual cues. Many of these psychogenic gait disorders will improve when the patient is not under obvious scrutiny.

Patients with psychogenic gait difficulty frequently exhibit astasia abasia, a constantly shifting pattern of motor and coordination deficits that effectively limits walking. Steps will be taken only after a dramatic display of fear and exertion. Leg movements will be erratic, with some steps being short and others long. The patient commonly walks on the outside of the foot or twists the ankle into awkward positions while walking. Excessive tripping is common, but injury as a result of any falls suffered is rare. If the patient falls, it will routinely be into the arms of someone standing nearby. When assisted with minor support, the gait may improve dramatically. These patients are usually highly suggestible, and they may accept the suggestion that with their kind of problem walking backwards is preserved (98). If the patient can walk backwards with no difficulty and struggles to walk forward, then the diagnosis of an hysterical gait disorder is confirmed and further investigations are inadvisable. Occasionally, an anxious or dependent patient will elaborate on minor gait difficulties arising with organic disease of the nervous system; but, even when the problem is confused by this psychogenic overlay, objective neurologic deficits should help direct the investigation of the gait disorder.

Astasia abasia usually demands considerable strength and coordination. A patient with significant nervous system disease cannot produce the exaggerated stumbling movements of this hysterical gait disorder without actually falling. Support and psychotherapy are often helpful in gradually reducing the gait difficulty. Confronting the patient with his true gait abilities never reduces the disability.

Shuffling and Magnetic Gaits

A shuffling gait may be the initial and, for many months, sole manifestation of Parkinson disease in patients with this degenerative disease of the basal ganglia. As described in the section on movement disorders, the patient takes small steps on a narrow base and tends to shuffle as he walks. This is also called a festinating gait. Characteristically, the patient is very unstable and often falls forward or backward with very little provocation. Arm swing is eliminated, and turning is performed much more slowly than walking. Falls frequently occur when the patient tries to turn. Poor control of initiation and cessation of walking causes additional problems for the patient, and many victims of this disorder are so terrified of walking that they become wheelchair bound long before their actual functional deficits warrant such a limitation. A four-legged walker often improves the patient's gait dramatically, largely because he is less worried about his ability to stabilize himself while walking.

The anxiety associated with a highly unstable festinating gait will exacerbate the gait difficulty. Some patients also notice that any anxiety introduced by an unfamiliar environment or by acute stress will increase gait difficulty considerably. The parkinsonian individual may be totally unable to walk without assistance when he comes to a physician's office, even though he has no substantial gait problem while he is at home. Parkinsonian patients are at great risk while crossing streets because they frequently freeze when they see oncoming traffic. The patient's extraordinary fear of falling is not at all unreasonable. If the patient falls, it may be virtually impossible for him to stand without considerable assistance.

Patients with frontal lobe disease may exhibit a shuffling gait similar to that of the parkinsonian patient. With each step, the patient seems to be struggling against a force that holds his feet to the ground. This is called a magnetic gait because of the apparent exertion required to lift the feet off the ground. The steps may be of fairly normal length and turning will not present problems. The affective changes characteristic of frontal lobe lesions help distinguish a magnetic gait from the festinating gait of parkinsonism.

Spastic Gait

Damage to motor neurons or their axons above the level of the spinal cord anterior horn cells often causes increased tone in the muscles innervated by the injured neurons. The abnormal tone increases in severity when an affected limb is passively moved quickly. The variable tone exhibited by the affected muscles is called spasticity. This is discussed in further detail in the chapter on weakness. Spasticity from an upper motor neuron lesion may be very subtle. Before objective changes in the tone of a limb become apparent, a patient with spasticity may develop characteristic gait abnormalities. Typically, arm swing on the affected side is damped, and the spastic leg is bent less than appropriately at the knee and circumducted slightly at the hip. The amount of circumduction and stiffness in the leg movements will be dictated by the degree of spasticity on the involved side. The slight change in gait that develops with mild spasticity may cause pain at the hip or knee joints. A traumatic arthritis develops because of the altered gait pattern. Patients commonly complain of leg pain before they realize that they actually have a gait problem.

Severely spastic gaits most often develop after cerebrovascular accidents. Demyelinating disease, such as multiple sclerosis, may cause severe or mild spasticity; but a spastic gait is not usually the initial sign of multiple sclerosis. Degenerative diseases of the motor system, the most common being amyotrophic lateral sclerosis, also produce spasticity associated with atrophy of muscles and fine, involuntary muscle activity, called fasciculations. Whenever spasticity appears, a central nervous system lesion should be sought. The lesion may be in the brain or in the spinal cord.

Steppage Gait

Impaired position sense at the ankle or substantial weakness of the dorsiflexor of the foot will produce a slapping gait. The foot is raised an exaggerated distance off the ground to avoid tripping over it. This so-called steppage gait frequently developed when neurosphilis was common. The problem in these patients with tabes dorsalis was absent position sense. Impaired position sense still appears in patients with combined system disease from vitamin B_{12} deficiency, but the spasticity that always accompanies this spinal cord disease routinely impairs the gait long before the position sense problems appear. This high-stepping gait usually appears with peripheral neuropathy, such as that caused by diabetes mellitus. The peripheral nerve damage interferes with information on the position of the ankle. A spinal root lesion also produces a steppage gait in some individuals who develop severe tibialis anterior muscle weakness. With impaired strength in this muscle the patient has considerable difficulty with dorsiflexion of the foot. If the patient does not lift his foot well above the ground, he is likely to trip or twist his ankle as the toe catches prematurely on the ground. Efforts to set the heel on the ground securely may be so faulty or erratic that a destructive arthritis develops at the ankle joint. When foot dorsiflexor weakness alone is involved, a brace to keep the foot from dropping when the lower leg is lifted may improve the gait considerably. With position sense deficits, such local appliances are not helpful.

Staggering Gait: Gait Ataxia

A staggering, wide-based, unstable gait is usually a sign of cerebellar or labyrinthine dysfunction (Figure 9.5). This gait ataxia can occur independently of individual limb ataxia and may be transient or permanent. It usually appears with other coordination problems, but it may be the initial sign of a progressive central nervous system lesion.

Alcohol is the most common cause of transient gait ataxia. Chronic alcoholics will have enduring gait ataxia; the occasional drinker may be unable to walk during an acute intoxication but have no residual gait difficulty as serum alcohol levels fall. The lesion with alcohol is in the cerebellum and probably reflects damage from two processes. The transient ataxia with alcohol intoxication derives from alcohol's interference with cerebellar neuron function. Permanent damage and its attendant gait ataxia develops from thiamine deficiency damaging the superior cerebellar structures. Gait problems with alcoholism may develop gradually or precipitately. Once established, the gait ataxia of chronic alcoholism is usually unresponsive to thiamine treatment.

Idiopathic cerebellar degeneration presents with gait ataxia in most forms of this disorder (47). Staggering gait and repeated falls in a child are the signs most often detected initially by parents in cases of recessively inherited cerebelloparenchymal degeneration. These children and adults with olivopontocerebellar atrophy usually become wheelchair bound after several years of deteriorating gait. The pathology need not be in the cerebellum itself. The most common form of hereditary ataxia is Friedreich disease, a progressive degenerative disease of young adults with primarily spinal cord damage. This disorder is untreatable.

The anticonvulsant phenytoin is toxic to cerebellar Purkinje cells and produces a drug-induced gait ataxia. A serum phenytoin level in excess of 25 micrograms per milliliter often causes a staggering gait, and, as the phenytoin level goes higher, the patient will become completely unable to stand or walk. Slurred speech, problems with eye movements, and mild confusion reinforce the impression that these patients are drunk. Lowering the serum phenytoin level reverses the gait ataxia.

Disease of the labyrinth of the ear will produce an ataxic gait largely indistinguishable from the staggering gait of cerebellar disease, but the ataxia is more likely to be transient and associated with vertigo. The patient has difficulty walking, partly because of illusory movement in the environment. Balance, rather than limb coordination, is primarily affected

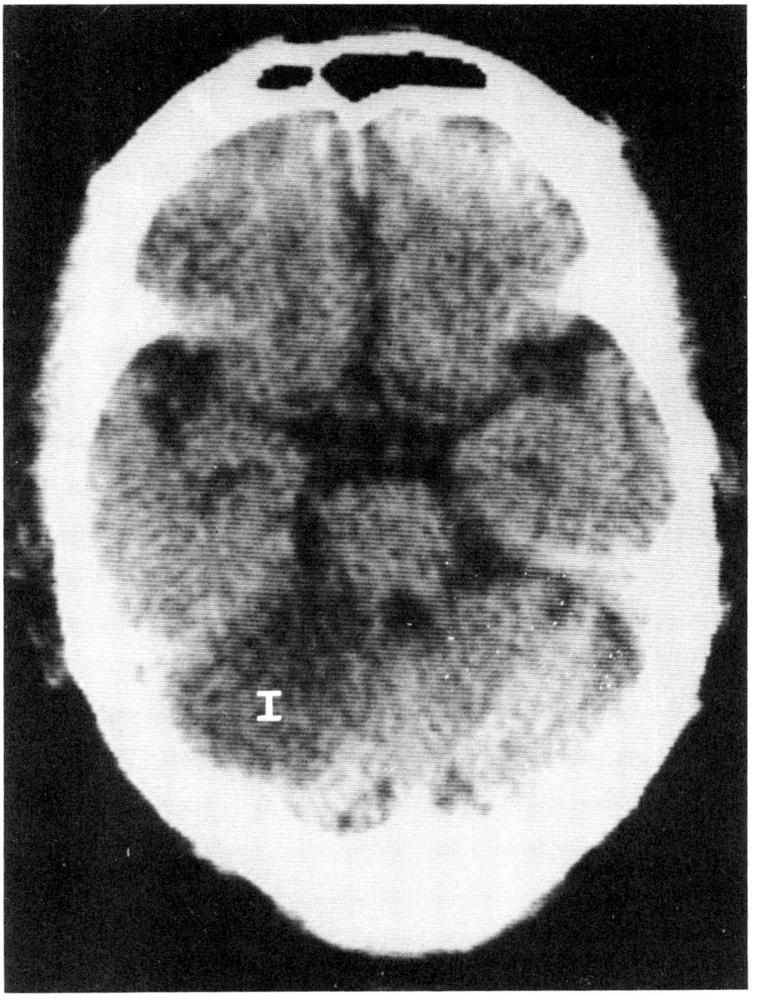

Figure 9.5. A 73-year-old man abruptly developed a severe right-sided headache over the frontal and pareital areas. On neurologic examination, he had slurred speech, a staggering gait, and clumsiness. Nausea, vomiting, and vertigo appeared at the sam- time as the headache. A computed tomogram of the posterior fossa revealed cerebellar infarction (I) (courtesy of Drs. J. Loh and W. Hotson).

in this inner ear disturbance. Degenerative or inflammatory diseases of the labyrinth or labyrinthine nerve are most commonly responsible for this balance problem. Treatment of the inner ear disease will improve the patient's gait. Even if the labyrinth is completely destroyed, gait difficulty will usually subside as other central nervous system elements compensate for the defective balance system.

REFERENCES

1. Marsden CB, Tarsy D, Baldessarini RJ: Spontaneous and drug-induced movement disorders in psychotic patients, in Benson DF, Blumer D (eds): *Psychiatric Aspects of Neurologic Disease*. New York, Grune & Stratton, 1975, p 219.
2. Mental changes in parkinsonism. *Br Med J* 2:11, 1974.
3. Boller F, Mizutani T, Roessmann U, et al: Parkinson disease, dementia, and Alzheimer disease: Clinicopathological correlations. *Ann Neurol* 7:329, 1980.
4. Parkinson—Physician, oryctologist, and social reformer. *J Am Med Assoc* 184:58, 1963.
5. Brown E, Brown GM, Kofman O, et al: Sexual function and affect in parkinsonian men treated with L-DOPA. *Am J Psychiatry* 135:1552, 1978.
6. Lieberman A, Kupersmith M, Estey E, et al: Treatment of Parkinson's disease with bromocriptine. *N Engl J Med* 295:1400, 1976.
7. Parkes D: Bromocriptine. *N Engl J Med* 301:873, 1979.
8. Yahr MD, Duvoisin RC: Drug therapy of parkinsonism. *N Engl J Med* 287:20, 1972.
9. Dysken MW, Merry W, Davis JM: Anticholinergic psychosis. *Psychiatr Ann* 8:452, 1978.
10. Klawans HL: Levodopa induced psychosis. *Psychiatr Ann* 8:447, 1978.
11. Casey DE: Deanol in the management of involuntary movement disorders: A review. *Dis Nerv Syst* 39:7, 1977.
12. Weiner WJ, Koller WC, Perlik S, et al: Drug holiday and management of Parkinson disease. *Neurology (NY)* 30:1257, 1980.
13. Koller WC, Weiner WJ, Perlik S, et al: Complications of chronic levodopa therapy: Long-term efficacy of drug holiday. *Neurology (NY)* 31:473, 1981.
14. Monoamine oxidase inhibitors for depression. *Med Lett Drugs Ther* 22:58, 1980.
15. Fahn S, Cote LJ, Snider SR, et al: The role of bromocriptine in the treatment of Parkinsonism. *Neurology (NY)* 29:1077, 1979.
16. Delwaide PJ, Hurlet A: Bromocriptine and buccolinguofacial dyskinesias in patients with senile dementia. *Arch Neurol* 37:441, 1980.
17. Juntunen J, Kaste M, Iivanainen M, et al: Bromocriptine treatment of spasmodic torticollis. *Arch Neurol* 36:449, 1979.
18. Parkes D: Mechanisms of bromocriptine-induced hallucinations. *N Engl J Med* 30:1479, 1980.
19. Lucas AR, Goodlund LS: Clinical management of children with brain disorders, in Hendrie HC (ed): *The Psychiatric Clinics of North America*. Philadelphia, WB Saunders, 1978, vol 1, p 179.
20. Goetz CG, Dysken MW, Klawans HL Jr: Assessment and treatment of drug-induced tremor. *J Clin Psychiatry* 41:310, 1980.
21. Crane G: Pseudoparkinsonism and tardive dyskinesia. *Arch Neurol* 27:426, 1972.
22. Gardos G, Cole JO, Tarsy D: Withdrawal syndromes associated with antipsychotic drugs. *Am J Psychiatry* 135:1321, 1978.
23. Freedman DX: Neurological syndromes associated with antipsychotic drug use. *Arch Gen Psychiatry* 28:463, 1973.
24. Henderson VW, Wooten GF: Neuroleptic malignant syndrome: A pathogenic role for dopamine receptor blockade. *Neurology (NY)* 31:132, 1981.
25. Cartwright GE: Diagnosis of treatable Wilson's disease. *N Engl J Med* 298:1347, 1978.
26. Fitzgerald MA, Gross JB, Goldstein NP, et al: Wilson's disease (hepatolenticular degeneration) of late adult onset. *Mayo Clin Proc* 50:438, 1975.
27. Shy GM, Drager GA: A neurological syndrome associated with orthostatic hypotension: A clinical-pathologic study. *Arch Neurol* 2:511, 1960.

28. Ziegler MG, Lake CR, Kopin IJ: The sympathetic-nervous-system defect in primary orthostatic hypotension. *N Engl J Med* 296:293, 1977.

29. Bae SH, Vates TS Jr, Kenton EJ III: Generalized chorea associated with chronic subdural hematomas. *Ann Neurol* 8:449, 1980.

30. Steele JC, Richardson JC, Olszewski J: Progressive supranuclear palsy. *Arch Neurol* 10:333, 1964.

31. Jacobson G, Baldessarini KJ, Manschreck T: Tardive and withdrawal dyskinesia associated with haloperidol. *Am J Psychiatry* 131:910, 1974.

32. Tarsy D, Bralower M: Deanol acetamidobenzoate treatment in choreiform movement disorders. *Arch Neurol* 34:756, 1977.

33. Winkler GF, Young RR: The control of essential tremor by propranolol. *Trans Am Neurol Assoc* 96:66, 1971.

34. Barone DA, Raniolo J: Facial dyskinesia from overdose of an antihistamine. *N Engl J Med* 303:107, 1980.

35. Cutler NR, Post RM, Rey AC, et al: Depression-dependent dyskinesias in two cases of manic-depressive illness. *N Engl J Med* 304:1088, 1981.

36. Tarsy D: Deanol in tardive dyskinesia. *N Engl J Med* 291:1416, 1974.

37. Wolf JK, Santana HB, Thorpy M: Treatment of "emotional incontinence" with levodopa. *Neurology (NY)* 29:1435, 1979.

38. Rosenbaum AH, Maruta T, Dune DD, et al: Tardive dyskinesia in depressed patients: Successful therapy with antidepressants and lithium. *Psychosomatics* 21:715, 1980.

39. Barbeau A: Lecithin in neurologic disorders. *N Engl J Med* 299:200, 1978.

40. Casey DE: Pharmacology of blepharospasm-oromandibular dystonia syndrome. *Neurology (NY)* 30:690, 1980.

41. Tolosa ES, Lai C: Meige disease: Striatal dopaminergic preponderance. *Neurology (NY)* 29:1126, 1979.

42. Thach BT, Chase TN, Bosma JF: Oral facial dyskinesia associated with prolonged use of antihistaminic decongestants. *N Engl J Med* 293:486, 1975.

43. Auger RG: Hemifacial spasm: Clinical and electrophysiologic observations. *Neurology (NY)* 9:1261, 1979.

44. Auger RG, Piegras DG, Laws ER Jr, et al: Microvascular decompression of the facial nerve for hemifacial spasm: Clinical and electrophysiologic observations. *Neurology (NY)* 31:346, 1981.

45. Hartmann E: Alcohol and bruxism. *N Engl J Med* 301:333, 1979.

46. Tyrer PJ, Lader MH: Tremor in acute and chronic anxiety. *Arch Gen Psychiatry* 31:506, 1974.

47. Gilman S, Bloedel JR, Lechtenberg R: *Disorders of the Cerebellum*. Philadelphia, FA Davis, 1981.

48. McAlpine D, Lumsden CE, Acheson ED: *Multiple sclerosis. A Reappraisal.* Baltimore, Williams & Wilkins, 1972.

49. Ott KH, Kase CS, Ojemann RG, et al: Cerebellar hemorrhage: Diagnosis and treatment. *Arch Neurol* 31:160, 1974.

50. Dobkin BH: The adult Chiari malformation. *Bull Los Angeles Neurol Soc* 42:23, 1977.

51. Britt CW, Peters BH: Metoprolol for essential tremor. *N Engl J Med* 301:331, 1979.

52. Ljung O: Treatment of migraine with metoprolol. *N Engl J Med* 303:156, 1980.

53. Sternberg EM, Van Woert MH, Young SN, et al: Development of a scleroderma-like illness during therapy with L-5-hydroxytryptophan and carbidopa. *N Engl J Med* 303:782, 1980.

54. Brown P, Cathala F, Sadowsky D, et al: Creutzfeldt-Jakob disease in France: II. Clinical

Characteristics of 124 consecutive verified cases during the decade 1968–1977. *Ann Neurol* 6:430, 1979.

55. Nee LE, Caine ED, Polinsky RJ, et al: Gilles de la Tourette syndrome: Clinical and family study of 50 cases. *Ann Neurol* 7:41, 1980.

56. Shapiro AK, Shapiro E, Wayne HL: The symptomatology and diagnosis of Gilles de la Tourette's syndrome. *J Am Acad Child Psychiatry* 12:702, 1973.

57. Golden GS: The effect of central nervous system stimulants on Tourette syndrome. *Ann Neurol* 2:69, 1977.

58. Task force on nomenclature and statistics, American Psychiatric Association: *Diagnostic and Statistical Manual of Mental Disorders* (*Third Edition*). Washington, DC, American Psychiatric Association, 1980.

59. Sweet RD, Bruun RD, Shapiro AK, et al: The pharmacology of Gilles de la Tourette's syndrome (chronic multiple tic), in Klawans HL Jr (ed): *Clinical Neuropharmacology*. New York, Raven Press, 1976, vol 1, p 81.

60. Shapiro AK, Shapiro ES, Bruun RD, et al: *Gilles de la Tourette Syndrome*. New York, Raven Press, 1978.

61. Hanin I, Merikangas JR, Merikangas KR, et al: Red cell choline and Gilles de la Tourette syndrome. *N Engl J Med* 301:661, 1979.

62. Itard JMG: Mémoire sur quelques fonctions involontaires des appareils de la locomotion, de la préhension, et de la voix. *Arch Med Gen* (*Paris*) 8:385, 1825.

63. Gilles de la Tourette G: Étude sur une affection nerveuse caracterisée par l'incoordination motrice accompagnée d'écholalie et de coprolalie. *Arch Neurol* (*Paris*) 9:19, 158, 1885.

64. Barbeau A: Cholinergic treatment in the Tourette syndrome. *N Engl J Med* 302:1310, 1980.

65. Heffron W, Eaton RP: Thyrotoxicosis presenting as choreoathetosis. *Ann Intern Med* 73:425, 1970.

66. Fischbeck KH, Layzer RB: Paroxysmal choreoathetosis associated with thyrotoxicosis. *Ann Neurol* 6:453, 1979.

67. Nausieda PA, Grossman BJ, Koller WC, et al: Sydenham chorea: An update. *Neurology* (*NY*) 30:331, 1980.

68. Bennett R, Hughes GRV, Bywaters EGL, et al: Neuropsychiatric problems in systemic lupus erythematosus. *Br Med J* 4:342, 1972.

69. Vincent FM: Chorea: A late complication of subdural hematoma. *Neurology* (*NY*) 30:335, 1980.

70. Feit H: A form of chorea that responds to dantrolene sodium. *Neurology* (*NY*) 29:1631, 1979.

71. Nausieda PA, Koller WC, Weiner WJ, et al: Pemoline-induced chorea. *Neurology* (*NY*) 31:356, 1981.

72. Nausieda PA, Koller WC, Weiner WJ, et al: Chorea induced by oral contraceptives. *Neurology* (*NY*) 29:1605, 1979.

73. Denckla MB, Heilman KM: The syndrome of hyperactivity, in Heilman KM, Valenstein E (eds): *Clinical Neuropsychology*. New York, Oxford University Press, 1979, p 574.

74. Dooling EC, Adams RD: The pathological anatomy of posthemiplegic athetosis. *Brain* 98:29, 1975.

75. Naidu S, Narasimhachari N: Sydenham's chorea: A possible presynaptic dopaminergic dysfunction initially. *Ann Neurol* 8:445, 1980.

76. Huntington G: On chorea. *Med Surg Reporter* (*Philadelphia*) 26:317, 1872.

77. Klawans HL, Goetz CG, Paulson GW, et al: Levodopa and presymptomatic detection of Huntington's disease—Eight year follow-up. *N Engl J Med* 302:1090, 1980.

78. Klawans HL, Goetz CG, Perlik S: Presymptomatic and early detection in Huntington's disease. *Ann Neurol* 8:343, 1980.

79. McHugh PR, Folstein MF: Psychiatric syndromes of Huntington's chorea: A clinical and phenomenologic study, in Benson DF, Blumer D (eds): *Psychiatric Aspects of Neurologic Disease.* New York, Grune & Stratton, 1975, p 267.

80. Toglia JU, McGlamery M, Sambandham RR: Tetrabenazine in the treatment of Huntington's chorea and other hyperkinetic movement disorders. *J Clin Psychiatry* 39:81, 1978.

81. Perry TL, Wright JM, Hansen S, et al: Isoniazid therapy of Huntington disease. *Neurology (NY)* 29:370, 1979.

82. Bird TD, Cederbaum S, Valpey RW, et al: Familial degeneration of the basal ganglia with acanthocytosis: A clinical, neuropathological, and neurochemical study. *Ann Neurol* 3:253, 1978.

83. Schwarcz R, Bennett JP, Coyle JT: Inhibitors of GABA metabolism: Implications for Huntington's disease. *Neurology (NY)* 2:299, 1977.

84. Brown WT, Sanberg PR, McGeer PL: Corticosteroids and chorea. *Arch Neurol* 36:454, 1979.

85. Noronha ABC, Roos RP, Antel JP, et al: Huntington's disease: Abnormality of lymphocyte capping. *Ann Neurol* 6:477, 1979.

86. Ichikawa K, Kim RC, Givelber H, et al: Chorea gravidarum. *Arch Neurol* 37:429, 1980.

87. Kertesz A: Paroxysmal kinesigenic choreoathetosis. *Neurology (NY)* 17:680, 1967.

88. Lance JW: Familial paroxysmal dystonic choreoathetosis and its differentiation from related syndromes. *Ann Neurol* 2:285, 1977.

89. Richards RN, Barnett HJM: Paroxysmal dystonic choreoathetosis. *Neurology (NY)* 18:461, 1968.

90. Meares R: An association of spasmodic torticollis and writer's cramp. *Br J Psychiatry* 119:441, 1971.

91. Korczyn AD, Kahana E, Zilber N, et al: Torsion dystonia in Israel. *Ann Neurol* 8:387, 1980.

92. Young RR, Delwaide PJ: Spasticity. *N Engl J Med* 304:96, 1981.

93. Drugs for psychiatric disorders. *Med Lett Drugs Ther* 22:77, 1980.

94. Korein J: Treatment questioned in familial spasmodic torticollis. *Neurology (NY)* 27:899, 1977.

95. Espir MLE, Watkins SM, Smith HV: Paroxysmal dysarthria and other transient neurological disturbances in disseminated sclerosis. *J Neurol Neurosurg Psychiatry* 29:323, 1966.

96. Harrison M, McGill JI: Transient neurological disturbances in disseminated sclerosis: A case report. *J Neurol Neurosurg Psychiatry* 32:230, 1969.

97. McFarling DA, Susac JO: Hoquet disbolique: Intractable hiccups as a manifestation of multiple sclerosis. *Neurology (NY)* 29:797, 1979.

98. Booker HE: Management of the difficult patient with complex partial seizures. *Adv Neurol* 11:369, 1975.

10 Sleep Disorders

Sleep is essential for normal intellectual functioning and appropriate emotional responses. For some patients with psychiatric problems, it is a burdensome or difficult activity. Getting to sleep, limiting sleep, and avoiding abnormal behavior during sleep can all become major focuses of an individual's day. Many of the disturbing activities that occur during sleep, such as sleep-talking and nocturnal emissions, are normal phenomena; but there are many activities, such as bedwetting, tongue-biting, interrupted breathing, and leg cramps, that may reflect serious neurologic or more general disease. In some cases, what appears to be a psychologic reaction to stress is the result of a sleep disorder: the patient who cannot stay awake for serious discussions or sexual activity may have the sleep disorder called narcolepsy. The individual who loses all muscle tone when frightened and falls to the ground, may have cataplexy, a symptom developing in narcoleptics. Normal sleep phenomena, such as dreaming, occasionally develop pathologic characteristics. Terrifying dreams may awaken the dreamer so frequently that he becomes severely sleep deprived. These and many other sleep-related phenomena can disturb an individual sufficiently to make him seek medical advice. Some patients assume that they have psychiatric problems because they feel well despite the sleep-related disorders. Those who consult internists or neurologists for their problems are often referred for psychiatric evaluation if there are no signs of organic disease.

Sleep disorders are of three types: insomnia or impaired sleep, hypersomnia or excessive sleep, and abnormal phenomena occurring with sleep. The common patterns of normal sleep and sleep-related phenomena are well-defined; but what constitutes, as well as what causes, abnormal sleep is more controversial. Night terrors, enuresis, sleep-walking, sleep-talking, and restless legs are all sleep-related phenomena that are generally viewed as aberrant, but are unsatisfactorily explained by current hypotheses. The traditional view that these are psychiatric problems has largely yielded to more structural or, at least, neurochemical explanations. Even with the redefinition of some sleep disorders as neurologic or metabolic disorders, there are still many disorders of sleep with well-established psychologic etiologies. Character disorders may lead to chronic fatigue states with excessive drowsiness. Depressive illnesses may cause insomnia and altered sleep-wake cycles.

Insomnia and delayed sleep onset are the most common sleep disorders occurring with stress or psychosis, but even these complaints may have simple organic bases. Barbiturate abuse or vascular headache may be the occult basis for a sleep disorder. Even when a personality disorder is apparent in a patient with complaints of disordered sleep, the psychologic problem may be secondary to the sleep disturbance. The patient with sleep apnea may develop a personality disorder as sleep deprivation becomes a chronic problem. Narcoleptics often become depressed and irritable as their excessive sleepiness causes more and more social or employment problems. Treatment of most sleep disorders is feasible, whether the cause is functional or organic. Choosing the appropriate treatment requires some insight into the fundamental character of the sleep disorder.

NORMAL SLEEP STAGES

Defining normal sleep in terms that will not confuse it with other alterations of consciousness was awkward until objective measures of brain activity, such as the electroencephalogram, were introduced into the definition (Table 10.1). Purposeful behavior and reactions to the environment are

Table 10.1. Electroencephalographic Stages of Sleep

Stage 1
Interrupted alpha wave activity
Generalized slowing
Slow eye movements
No spindles
Stage 2
Diffuse slow (theta wave) activity
Spindles and K complexes
Low voltage background activity
Stage 3
High voltage slow waves
Spindles occasionally on slow waves
Delta activity dominating 20–50% of the record
Stage 4
More than half the record dominated by high voltage delta activity (0 to 3 Hz)
REM
Rapid eye movements apparent
Low voltage beta and theta activity

ordinarily absent or altered in sleep, but defining sleep as just this deviation from waking activity is misleading and inaccurate. Akinetic mutism also presents as an absence of purposeful behavior and interaction with the environment, but aside from these traits it has little else in common with sleep. Electroencephalographic studies of sleeping patients and clinical evaluations in different stages of sleep have clarified what physiologic and behavioral changes characterize sleep and are normal in sleep. Electroencephalographic findings and ocular motor changes define two distinct phases of sleep: (*1*) slow wave, or non-rapid eye movement sleep (NREM), and (*2*) paradoxical, or rapid eye movement sleep (REM) (1). In NREM sleep the dominant wave activity recorded on the electroencephalogram becomes progressively slower as the patient becomes more difficult to arouse. Although the individual's arousal threshold continues to rise as he enters REM sleep, this phase of sleep produces a paradoxically awake electroencephalographic picture (1,2). Slow wave sleep is divided into stages 1, 2, 3, and 4, each stage being defined by distinct electroencephalographic patterns. These NREM stages have been viewed as important in recovery from muscular fatigue, whereas REM sleep plays a role in psychologic adjustment to environmental events and learning (1).

Non-Rapid Eye Movement Sleep

NREM sleep ordinarily precedes REM sleep by more than 1 hour (2,3). As an individual becomes drowsy and enters the light sleep of stage 1 NREM, slowing of the overall electroencephalographic pattern will appear (3). The normal waking activity of the electroencephalogram is replaced by widespread low voltage, desynchronized activity (2). Alpha waves are lost and the low voltage mixed frequency waves of waking become less symmetric (2). Normal individuals have brief, shocklike movements, called sleep starts or hypnic jerks, during this stage (4). These are isolated massive contractions of trunk and limb muscles occurring at the start of sleep. The sleeper may report an associated sense of falling, and the convulsive movements may arouse him to a more awake state (4). No epileptic activity appears on the electroencephalogram with these sleep starts. Their origin is unknown.

In stage 2 NREM sleep, 12 to 14 cycles per second sinusoidal wave activity, called sleep spindles, and high voltage vertex sharp waves appear (Figure 10.1). Sharp waves may appear over the occiput at the back of the head, as well as over the vertex of the head, in normal stage 2 sleep. These are quite different from epileptic pattern changes that may appear with sleep (Figure 10.2). In stage 3 NREM, sleep spindles and very slow wave activity will account for 20 percent of the brain wave activity. This increases to 50 percent in stage 4 NREM (3). The slowest wave activity seen in these later stages of NREM sleep is in the delta wave range of 0.5–2.5 cycles per second (2). This slow wave activity is of relatively high

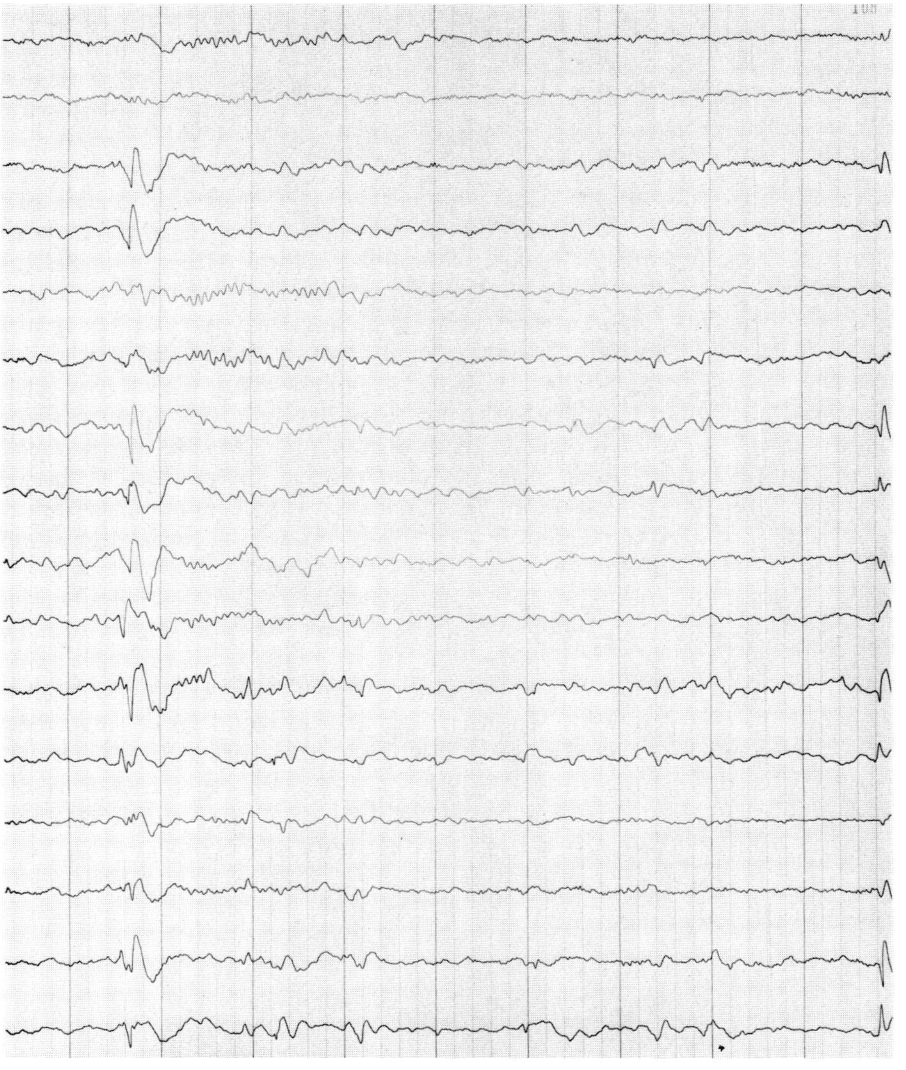

Figure 10.1. The high-voltage sharp waves on this electroencephalogram are normal findings during sleep. These waves are called vertex sharp waves, and on this electroencephalogram they are followed by low-voltage sinusoidal waves, called sleep spindles, that are most obvious in the fifth and sixth lines of this recording. Sleep spindles have a frequency similar to or slightly higher than alpha wave activity and usually first appear in stage-2 NREM sleep.

amplitude and is associated with intact muscle tone (5). Proprioceptive reflexes in the limbs are preserved, and metabolic requirements are minimized (5).

Rapid Eye Movement Sleep

With the onset of rapid eye movement sleep the electroencephalogram changes abruptly to low amplitude fast waves (3,6). Just before these electroencephalographic changes, random electrical activity in skeletal muscles decreases (5). Gross body movements, massive muscle twitches, and minor activity in the limb and facial musculature may still occur but are infrequent. Respiratory and cardiac rates increase and are more variable than during NREM sleep. The patient with ulcers will have increased gastric acid secretion during this stage (1). All boys and men, regardless of age, will have penile erections during REM sleep unless there is peripheral nerve disease or vascular disease interfering with this normal sexual phenomenon (3). The muscles in the neck, chin, and limbs lose their normal tone, becoming totally relaxed and largely immobile as this stage of sleep progresses (5,7). This loss of tone in skeletal and facial muscles occurs even in patients with spasticity in paralyzed limbs (7). Dreams occur primarily, if not exclusively, during this rapid eye movement phase of sleep (8).

Normal sleep has four or five 90-minute cycles of NREM sleep alternating with REM sleep (6). The REM period lasts an average of 15 minutes. The total time spent in REM sleep during an average night is $1\frac{1}{2}$ hours, or 20 percent of sleeping time. Individual REM periods get longer later at night, so that most of the total REM time is in the last third of sleep (2). Most stage 4 NREM sleep occurs during the first third of sleep.

Neurophysiology of Sleep

The central nervous system centers responsible for REM and NREM sleep are fairly distinct both structurally and neurochemically. Sleep is initiated by basal medial forebrain structures and brainstem mechanisms (1). A catecholamine-utilizing system is implicated in the maintenance of normal vigilance. With interruption of the dorsal ascending noradrenergic bundle, cortical arousal is reduced. NREM sleep results from inhibition of the reticular activating system by a serotonin-utilizing system (6). Catecholamine-containing and acetylcholine-containing neurons in the brainstem are involved in the initiation of phasic events in REM sleep (6). These phasic events include the rapid eye movements themselves, irregularities in pulse and breathing rates, and middle ear and laryngeal muscle contractions (6). The locus coeruleus, a collection of pigmented nerve cells in the pons, is vital to suppression of tone and limb movements during REM sleep (9).

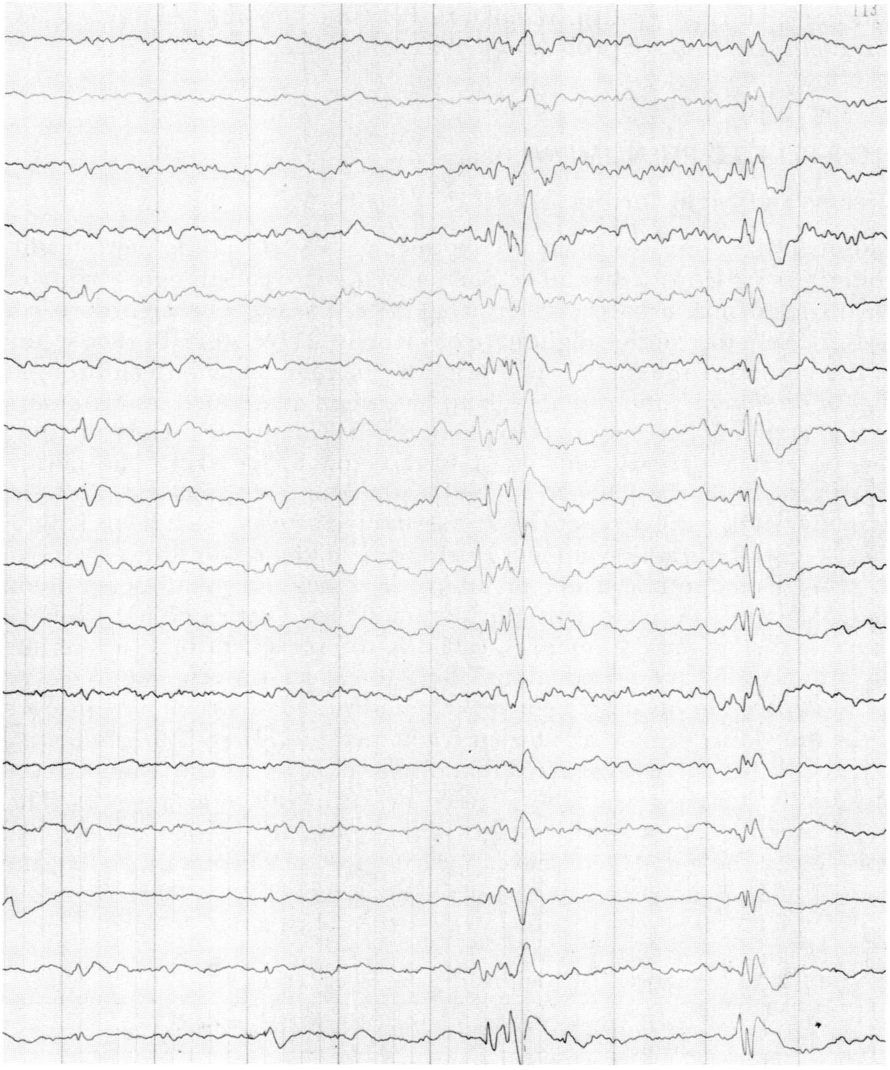

Figure 10.2. This electroencephalogram, recorded from a 5-year-old child with generalized tonic-clonic seizures, reveals obvious spikes. This spike activity was apparent only when the child was asleep. The spike activity on the recording occurred while the patient was not having an apparent convulsion.

Complex hormonal and neuroendocrine changes coincide with the various stages of the sleep cycle. Growth hormone secretion is most prominent during stage 3 NREM sleep (3,10). Prolactin secretion peaks during NREM sleep, most often during the latter half of a night's sleep (3). This all suggests that sleep serves many psychologic and physiologic functions. Normal growth, regular sexual function, and psychologic adjustments to stress are probably all affected by sleep.

SLEEP-RELATED PHENOMENA

Dreams and Night Terrors

Although dreaming normally occurs during REM sleep, the more frightening, less structured dreamlike phenomena, often called night terrors or pavor nocturnus, usually occur during NREM sleep. The night terror is distinct from the routine nightmare or incubus (Table 10.2) (8). The victim of the night terror experiences a brief, frightening image, which prompts him to scream out and often awaken; but, when questioned on the nature of the terrifying perception, the patient is usually amnesic (11). If anything can be recalled it will only be a frightening image (12). The abrupt awakening is not usually associated with clear consciousness, and the individual will exhibit repetitive, perseverative activity, such as picking at the sheets or thrashing about. During the night terror the heart rate increases, the pupils dilate, breathing becomes irregular, perspiration increases, and the electroencephalogram shows a series of high voltage sharp and slow wave complexes, called K complexes. Efforts to calm the individual will have no apparent effect for at least a few minutes. The facial expression invariably conveys the individual's extreme terror, even if the individual cannot recall what frightened him. Even if the individual can recall the horrifying image that awoke him, he usually cannot recall any of the episode when he is fully awake in the morning (12). This phenomenon occurs during stages 3 or 4 of NREM sleep, the initial episode of the night generally appearing 30 to 200 minutes after the patient falls asleep (12). The terror phenomena last 20 to 60 seconds and

Table 10.2. Characteristics of Nightmares and Sleep Terrors

Nightmare (Incubus)	*Sleep Terror (Pavor Nocturnus)*
Frightening dream sequence	Brief, frightening image
No scream on awakening	Scream on awakening
Common in adults	Most common in children
Slight autonomic response	Marked autonomic response
May occur in REM sleep	Occurs in stages 3 and 4 NREM sleep
Good recall of episode in morning	Routinely amnesic for episode
Usually in the late evening	Usually in the early evening
Sexes equally vulnerable	Men more affected than women
Unrelated to antipsychotic use	Increased occurrence with antipsychotics
Unrelated to somnambulism	Often associated with somnambulism

rarely occur more than once nightly (8). Patients with night terrors occasionally exhibit other aberrant sleep phenomena, such as sleep-walking (somnambulism).

The nightmare is a longer, more structured, dreamlike phenomenon. Although some are believed to occur during NREM sleep, others are closer to true dream phenomena and occur during REM sleep (12). Because of this, nightmares commonly occur later in the evening than the typical night terror. Much more often than in the night terror, the patient with a nightmare will recall details of the frightening experience. A common feature in the nightmare is that the patient perceives a growing threat to his safety, and he awakens as the enormity of the threat peaks (12). The panicky scream on awakening so typical of the night terror is not at all common with nightmares. Nightmares can occur at any age.

Children are more likely to have night terrors than are adults (8). One to 4 percent of all children have an episode of night terror at some time before adolescence (12). The terrors usually subside by 12 years of age, and, if they recur, it will generally not be until the third or fourth decade of life (12). Boys and men are more commonly affected than women and girls. Patients under extreme stress, physically exhausted, or medicated with tricyclic antidepressants or neuroleptics are more susceptible to night terrors (12).

Although the elderly are not usually susceptible to night terrors, parkinsonian patients on levodopa are an exception. Five percent of these individuals suffer from night terrors while on levodopa (11). Nightmares also occur in 5 percent of these parkinsonian individuals, but an extraordinary 25 percent report affectively neutral, but extremely vivid, dreams that merge with frank hallucinations (11).

Despite their differences, nightmares and night terrors may share several features. With both, involuntary screams, arousal, and amnesia for the frightening incident may occur. The night terror and the nightmare both can occur in the first one-third of the night's sleep, although this is much more typical for the night terror (8). Two out of three individuals with night terrors will have an episode during the first cycle of NREM sleep in stage 3 or 4 (8). Suppression of stage 4 sleep decreases the incidence of these attacks (8). The likelihood and the intensity of a nightmare or night terror are directly related to the length of the antecedent stage 4 NREM sleep and the amount of delta wave activity apparent in the electroencephalogram during that NREM sleep (8).

Dream Anxiety Attacks

Night terrors and nightmares are distinct from dream anxiety attacks (8). The latter are simply frightening dreams that may awaken the dreamer; and, although the individual may be upset by the dream, she can usually recall more than just a single frightening hallucination. She does not experience the overwhelming anxiety characteristic of the night terror or the sense of impending doom characteristic of the nightmare. Women have dream anxiety attacks three times as often as men, and there is a significant, disturbing life event at the onset of these attacks in 38 percent of cases (8). Unlike the victim of night terrors, the patient with dream anxiety attacks will often complain of insomnia. Fifty-four percent of dream anxiety attacks occur in the last half of a night's sleep, invariably during REM sleep. In contrast to the aberrant sleep phenomena often seen in night terror victims, sleep-walking is unlikely with dream anxiety attacks (8,13). Violent, occasionally self-destructive, behavior accompanies the night terror or nightmare in over 50 percent of affected individuals, a phenomenon also not seen with dream anxiety attacks. Dream anxiety attacks increase with REM sleep deprivation and there is some evidence that they are involved in psychologic adaptation to stressful life events (1,8). Diazepam may relieve all of these dream disorders (8).

Effects of Aging and Stress on Sleep

Normally, sleep duration decreases with age, and many individuals become unduly concerned about such changes in their sleep patterns (3). The time required to fall asleep after relaxing in an appropriate environment, that is, the sleep-onset latency, increases from an average of 8 minutes in the fourth decade of life to 18 minutes in the eighth decade. The duration of stage 3 NREM and stage 4 NREM sleep decrease with aging.

Aging is, however, not the only setting for physiologic changes in sleep. Sleep patterns in individuals of any age can be altered by sleep deprivation (2). The first night of recovery sleep will have more slow wave (stage 3 and 4) NREM sleep in the first hours and an increase in REM in the later hours and subsequent nights (2). Psychologic conflicts routinely interfere with sleep. Quite often the patient with no opportunity to discuss truly stressful issues will develop sleeplessness. Any apparently healthy individual who is excessively concerned about changes in his sleep pattern should be questioned regarding new issues in his life. The preoccupation with sleep may be little more than a justification for seeking medical attention. Employment problems, family conflicts, recent loss, or fear of unrecognized illness may all be the real motivations for the consultation. Unless directly questioned on these matters, most patients will not volunteer the information, even though they may be extremely eager to discuss these stressful issues once they are raised.

INSOMNIA

Decreased sleep duration, delays in falling asleep, and repeatedly interrupted sleep are all forms of insomnia. About 2 percent of individuals over 18 years of age have chronic sleep problems, which they consider insomnia (14). The incidence of sleep problems among individuals seeking medical attention for any type of problem is substantially higher; physicians report significant difficulties with sleep in 17 percent of the patients they see (14). Disorders interfering with sleep may have a psychiatric basis or may cause psychologic problems. Patients often become anxious or depressed because they fear they have a disabling systemic illness; they literally "lose sleep over" their preoccupation with serious illness. Reassurance of the healthy patient is often enough to end the sleep disorder, but some patients have persistent mood disturbances that interfere with sleep even after a medical evaluation has found no organic disease responsible for their symptoms. Anxiety-related insomnia is characterized by considerable difficulty in falling asleep and frequent nocturnal awakenings (3). Before anxiety or depression can be invoked as the cause of a sleep disorder, however, systemic and neurologic illnesses must be excluded. That the patient's symptoms fit with a psychologic sleep disorder does not prove that a treatable systemic illness is not responsible. The pain associated with arthritis will chronically prolong sleep latency, the time it takes the patient to fall asleep once he relaxes in an environment suitable for sleep. Frequent nocturnal awakenings may also be caused by strictly organic illness. Cluster headache routinely awakens individuals with this type of vascular headache from a sound sleep. Both of these circumstances rarely cause diagnostic difficulties, but many diseases interfering with sleep are much less obvious. Occult poisoning may provide considerable diagnostic difficulty until specific effects of the agent are apparent. Thallium can cause insomnia and daytime drowsiness before the seizures or hair loss typical of this type of poisoning develop (15). In most cases, a thorough history and careful physical examination will establish the cause of the insomnia if it does not have a psychiatric basis.

Systemic Causes

Withdrawal from drugs and drug abuse are common causes of insomnia that frequently go unsuspected because the patient and his family are reluctant to volunteer information. The history of drug practices may be fragmented and misleading (16). The high frequency of alcohol abuse in the United States makes it a relatively common cause of sleep complaints. Alcohol disturbs sleep both when the individual abuses it and when he abruptly abstains from it. This drug depresses REM sleep and decreases the latency of sleep onset when the patient is intoxicated, but REM sleep increases when the alcohol is withdrawn (17).

Breathing problems (sleep apnea) with interrupted nocturnal sleep is a more subtle but more readily treatable cause of insomnia. In the sleep apnea syndrome, the patient's constant fatigue associated with sleep deprivation is commonly perceived as a problem with excessive sleep. This is not the only situation in which the patient's complaint does not accurately reflect the real problem that he is facing. Some sleep-related phenomena, such as the restless legs syndrome, may prompt a patient to complain of insomnia even though the real problem is a worrisome symptom appearing during efforts to sleep (5). These phenomena interfering with sleep will be discussed in the section on aberrant behavior during sleep.

If both of the parents in a family complain of insomnia, 48 percent of the offspring will have difficulty falling asleep (18). This decreases to 29 percent if insomnia is a problem for only one parent and to 18 percent if it is a problem for neither parent (18). These figures need not reflect inheritance of a sleep disorder. Children may simply adopt their parents' practices. Individuals who smoke regularly may find nicotine acts as a stimulant; but, more commonly, it is caffeine or alcohol that fragments sleep (3). Prolonged barbiturate excess may cause remarkable sleeplessness when the drug is withdrawn. A patient in barbiturate coma after an overdose may remain awake for as long as 6 days when he recovers from the drug-induced coma (19). Patients chronically taking sleep medications may complain that they are unable to sleep without the medication, but they usually do not recognize that this is a normal drug withdrawal effect.

Depression

Nonpsychotic depression often brings the patient to a physician with complaints of decreased sleep duration, difficulty falling asleep, or early morning awakening (3,16). Eighty to 90 percent of depressed patients have insomnia (20). Not only is the total amount of sleep decreased in depressed individuals, but, at least in severe depressive illness, the pattern of normal sleep is disturbed. Dreaming appears earlier in sleep in these depressed individuals than in normal individuals (2). Muscle tone is maintained at an inappropriately high level while the individual is trying to relax (5). Electroencephalographic studies reveal a decrease in stage 1 and 2 NREM sleep, and sleep shifts from one stage to another after abnormally brief intervals. This causes REM sleep to appear earlier in the evening than in the person free of depression. The significance of REM sleep suppression with antidepressant treatment, such as with imipramine and amitriptyline, is unknown; but this property of tricyclic antidepressants probably plays a therapeutic role in the treatment of the depression since behavioral suppression of REM sleep also improves endogenous depression (3).

All depressions do not have the same effects on sleep. Sleep is more disturbed in an isolated depressive illness than in the depressive phase of a bipolar psychosis (1,16). Termination of a psychotic depression with a manic phase in a bipolar affective disorder is associated with severe REM sleep suppression (1,2). This contrasts with changes in sleep in other psychotic disorders. During an acute schizophrenic episode, the patient will have decreased REM sleep with no excessive increase, as a rebound phenomenon, when the acute psychotic episode is over (1). Chronic schizophrenics have relatively normal sleep patterns (2).

Sleep Apnea

Sleep apnea interferes with nocturnal sleep and produces excessive daytime drowsiness. The patient repeatedly stops breathing during both REM and NREM sleep. This cessation of breathing, or apnea, arouses the patient from sleep as arterial blood gases become abnormal (10). The apnea arises from upper airway obstruction probably because of loss of central nervous system coordination of upper airway musculature during sleep (10). Less commonly the apnea is "central," developing without apparent upper airway obstruction. The affected individual does not make an inspiratory effort. Patients may also demonstrate an initial central apnea followed by temporary upper airway obstruction (21). The patients affected are almost always obese men who are quite often hypertensive and characteristically snore loudly (4,10,21). Pulmonary function tests performed while they are awake are normal (21). Apneic periods disturb both the duration of total sleep and the duration of individual stages of sleep. Stage 3 and 4 NREM sleep are reduced, and about half the time spent in NREM sleep is spent in apnea (21). Apneic periods last from 20 to 150 seconds, and these usually occur in clusters, repeating one after another over 20 to 30 minutes (21). After a run of such apneic periods the patient usually awakens or nears wakefulness. Such arousals occur late at night or in the early morning. After very few days of disturbed sleep, the chronic sleep deprivation leads to excessive drowsiness and repeated naps during the day with a short latency to sleep onset (21).

This sleep disturbance also alters neuroendocrine secretory cycles, but only rarely reflects any structural damage in the brain. Nocturnal prolactin secretion is decreased (10). Normal patterns of growth hormone secretion are lost. Structural lesions causing the sleep disorder do not produce the usual neuroendocrine changes. Sleep apnea may appear with a parietal lobe tumor or with communicating hydrocephalus, but growth hormone and prolactin secretion with these structural lesions are normal (10).

Efforts to treat sleep apnea with hypnotic drugs increase the sleeping difficulty rather than improving sleep duration (21). Indeed, treatment of sleep apnea with a hypnotic can be fatal (14). Current therapy is aimed at eliminating the upper airway obstruction. A temporary tracheostomy may be necessary.

Treatment

Most patients complaining of sleep difficulty do not have an organic basis for the insomnia and are adequately treated with short-term hypnotic medication. About 10 percent of the population in the United States uses some form of medication at some time in their lives to help them fall asleep (3). Although psychiatric visits account for only 3 percent of all office visits, psychiatrists prescribe 23 percent of all the hypnotics used in the United States (14). Thirty-nine percent of the patients using sleep medication are over 60 years of age. Expected turnover rates and effective dose levels may be misleading in this elderly group. The likelihood of an adverse drug reaction increases with both advanced age and diminished renal function (14). An increasing awareness of the complications of excessive sleep medication and the potential for abuse of these drugs has led to a shift away from barbiturate prescribing and toward benzodiazepine use over the past 7 years (14). An additional consideration in the treatment of insomnia is the role of depression in the sleep disorder. If the insomnia is a symptom of a depressive illness, sedatives will simply aggravate the psychiatric disorder and provide little relief from the sleep disorder (16). Antidepressant medication is appropriate for the treatment of insomnia in these depressed patients. If anxiety is playing a prominent role in sleep disruption, chlordiazepoxide may effectively minimize the sleep disturbance (16).

The principal benefit of most hypnotics is reduction of sleep onset time (14). The benzodiazepine currently preferred by most physicians is flurazepam. Fifteen milligrams of flurazepam just before bedtime is usually an effective hypnotic dose. Even at this dose there are limitations to use of the drug. Flurazepam has a cumulative effect with drowsiness, ataxia, and impaired daytime visual motor coordination developing as early as 7 days after the start of nightly use (14). Even if the patient takes flurazepam daily over the course of a few weeks, little tolerance will develop for the drug (16). Metabolites of flurazepam, as well as other benzodiazepines, such as nitrazepam, are psychoactive for up to 8 days after termination of treatment (14). Alcohol in combination with flurazepam or diazepam causes more interference with driving skills than when it is combined with an equivalent dose of barbiturate (14). Both barbiturates and benzodiazepines are tolerated poorly by patients with liver disease (14). A prominent feature in their favor is that the benzodiazepines produce less morning malaise, or "hangover," than the more REM-sleep-suppressing hypnotics, like barbiturates and glutethimide (1). A fairly safe and cheap hypnotic with few of the side effects exhibited by barbiturates is chloral hydrate. Chloral hydrate has little, if any, REM-suppressing activity, a property that may renew enthusiasm for the drug if REM sleep proves valuable for psychologic adjustment to stress experienced during the waking hours (1).

Most hypnotics disturb the normal sleep stages. Stages 3 and 4, as well as REM sleep, are most vulnerable to this disruption (1). Sleep onset is the feature of sleep most directly affected by hypnotics, but with the reduction in time needed to fall asleep there will be an overall increase in the electroencephalographic evidence of sleep spindles and fast wave (13–32 cycles per second) beta activity (3). Stopping most hypnotics after habitual use will produce a rebound insomnia with excessive REM sleep, extraordinary nightmares, and occasional hallucinations (3).

Less conventional hypnotics, which may not have the adverse effects seen with barbiturates and benzodiazepines, include L-tryptophan and aspirin (3). Presumably, the hypnotic effect of L-tryptophan derives from its being a precursor of serotonin, a neurotransmitter implicated in slow wave sleep (3). Aspirin increases free plasma tryptophan, but it is at best only transiently hypnotic. L-tryptophan decreases the sleep onset latency without appreciably altering the sleep stages recorded on the electroencephalogram (3).

Neurologic and Psychiatric Consequences

Insomnia is more than just an inconvenience. Sleep deprivation is a precipitating factor in about 10 percent of patients developing status epilepticus, the seizure disorder in which one fit follows another with potentially fatal results (21). Coordination is routinely impaired with sleep deprivation, and tremors that are not ordinarily present may surface in susceptible individuals. Sleep disorders also produce psychologic disturbances. Mild sleep deprivation impairs intellectual function and resourcefulness. Routine tasks become more difficult to perform and unfamiliar tasks are more difficult to master. The severity of the psychologic disturbance will depend upon the severity of the sleep disturbance. REM sleep deprivation will interfere with character defensive operations (1). Prolonged sleep deprivation leads to ego disorganization, hallucinations, and delusions (2). Obviously, the first step in dealing with any sleep disorder is an attempt to define the causes of the disturbance and eliminate them. When such a therapeutic approach is likely to require a protracted effort before realizing any improvements in sleep, symptomatic treatment is appropriate.

HYPERSOMNIA

Excessive drowsiness and frequent or prolonged periods of sleep often have an organic basis, but psychologic problems may cause these symptoms as well. Dissociative reactions and psychoneurotic fatigue states are associated with hypersomnia, but even in these clearly disturbed patients the sleep disorder should induce the physician to look for an organic etiology (6). The range of organic problems to be considered is not extensive. Aside from obvious metabolic problems, such as hypothyroidism, hyperparathyroidism, and diabetes mellitus, narcolepsy and pickwickian syndrome are the most frequently encountered idiopathic causes of episodic hypersomnia. There is no obvious central nervous system disease in either of these sleep disorders, but cerebral or brainstem disease does occasionally produce excessive sleep. The Kleine-Levin syndrome is a rarely encountered sleep disorder characterized by episodic hypersomnia with obvious cerebral dysfunction, if not destruction, associated with the hypersomnia. A brainstem infarction developing with occlusion of the mesencephalic artery may produce unremitting hypersomnia (22). These infarction victims exhibit profound drowsiness alternating with frank akinetic mutism; the responsible lesion is presumably a disconnection of the thalamus from its reticular activating system inputs (22). Drug abuse is a more common cause of hypersomnia than any of these syndromes, but usually the patient is aware of the basis for his sleep irregularity when drug ingestion is involved. Elderly individuals may exhibit persistent drowsiness with sepsis, dehydration, or anemia (22). These potentially lethal conditions occasionally present with little more than drowsiness in old people, and so the investigation of hypersomnia in the elderly is a medical emergency. Obviously, all nonpsychiatric causes of excessive daytime sleepiness warrant prompt diagnosis and treatment.

Narcolepsy

A common neurologic cause of excessive daytime sleepiness that is not from apparent structural disease in the central nervous system is narcolepsy. The principal characteristic of narcolepsy is recurrent sleep attacks, appearing abruptly and inappropriately. This is an easily recognized disorder. The diagnosis is suggested by the pattern of the sleep attacks and symptoms associated with the attacks. For objective confirmation of the clinical impression, an electroencephalogram obtained during sleep and normal consciousness should show REM onset sleep with each attack. REM sleep appears as soon as the patient dozes. The clinical phenomena associated with the sleep attacks in many individuals are cataplexy, hypnagogic hallucinations, and sleep paralysis (6). Cataplexy is a sudden loss of muscle tone. While laughing or when startled, the patient will abruptly fall to the ground. Hypnagogic hallucinations are visual hallucinations appearing as the patient falls asleep, and sleep paralysis is an inability to perform voluntary movements upon awakening.

Tumors in subcortical structures and destructive lesions in the brainstem may produce hypersomnic states, but these are distinct from narcolepsy by virtue of the gradual onset of the sleep state and the protracted duration of an individual sleep episode (23). Prolonged "sleepy spells" may prove to be a manifestation of continuous cerebral seizure activity (24). These structural and physiologic bases for hypersomnia do not exhibit the other clinical phenomena typical of narcolepsy.

True narcolepsy is a relatively uncommon disorder, appearing in 0.03–0.05 percent of the population (18). Men are more commonly affected than women and a familial occurrence in first degree relatives can be established in 41 percent of patients affected. The associated symptoms of cataplexy, hypnagogic hallucinations, and sleep paralysis are usually more helpful in establishing the diagnosis than are the more objective electroencephalographic studies because sleep-onset with rapid eye movement sleep, the electroencephalographic hallmark of narcolepsy, also can occur in patients with "traumatic" neuroses (1). These psychiatric patients will have REM sleep appearing at or soon after sleep-onset because they are so severely sleep-deprived that REM stage appears whenever they can fall asleep. The patient's age at the onset of the hypersomnia, the association of hallucinations with the disorder of consciousness, and the occasional appearance of loosening of associations with drowsiness may cause difficulty in distinguishing narcolepsy from incipient schizophrenia (6). Psychosis and severe emotional distress are not the only psychiatric problems to consider in patients with episodic hypersomnia. Fatigue states on a psychoneurotic basis can also be difficult to distinguish from narcolepsy (6).

Sleep Attacks

Narcolepsy often appears initially when the patient is having difficulty sleeping at night (6). The frequent naps that occur during the day can be dismissed as just a reaction to excessive fatigue, until these sleep attacks become more chronic and frequent. Typically, the sleep attacks last 15 seconds to 2 hours, but most attacks are less than 20 minutes long and occur two to six times daily (25). The longer attacks occur when the patient is in a position and environment conducive to sleep (6). Patients fall asleep during routine business, eating, sexual activity, athletics, and operating machinery (25). Attacks begin between 10 and 20 years of age in the majority of patients (6). Only 5 percent have sleep attacks before 10 years of age. Twenty-five percent of narcoleptics are over 20 years of age at the onset of hypersomnia. This disorder is not necessarily a constant problem for the patient once it appears. Eighty-seven percent of patients have episodes of recurring and remitting narcolepsy (6).

The daytime sleep attacks are associated with nocturnal sleep disturbances, a pattern reminiscent of sleep apnea. Other features of narcolepsy cause some confusion with more malignant causes of hypersomnia. Sleep attacks indistinguishable from those appearing with idiopathic narcolepsy occasionally develop after encephalitis (6). The dramatic transition to deep sleep during stimulating activities occurs in pickwickian syndrome, the hypersomnia of obese individuals, as well as in narcolepsy. Distinguishing between the sleep attacks of narcolepsy and those of the pickwickian syndrome is complicated by a high rate of obesity in narcoleptic patients (6).

Cataplexy

Only 10 percent of narcoleptics have sleep attacks with all three accessory symptoms of cataplexy, hypnagogic hallucinations, and sleep paralysis (6). The symptom most often associated with sleep attacks in the narcoleptic is cataplexy, the abrupt loss of muscle tone that results in violent falls. Sleep attacks and cataplexy appear together in 70 to 95 percent of patients with narcolepsy (6,9,26). Of course, sleep attacks can occur alone. Patients with REM sleep appearing inconsistently at the onset of the sleep attack usually have only sleep attacks as the manifestation of their narcolepsy (25). If cataplexy develops in the narcoleptic it develops independently of the sleep attacks. Frequent sleep attacks are not necessarily associated with frequent episodes of cataplexy.

Cataplexy is a reversible loss of muscle tone lasting seconds to minutes and appearing abruptly (9). Leg muscles are primarily affected, and, consequently, the patient may be injured during the precipitate fall that occurs if the cataplexy develops while he is standing (25). Extraocular muscles are usually spared, but jaw and neck muscles are routinely affected (25). Breathing is not substantially affected. In mild cases, a sagging jaw, inclined head, or buckling knee may be the only manifestations of the cataplexy (9).

Stress, heavy meals, anger, laughter, or fear may all precipitate the attacks. Rarely, cataplexy appears years before the sleep attacks of narcolepsy, but usually the atonic disorder develops at about 25 years of age, years after the onset of sleep attacks (9). The mechanism underlying this episodic loss of muscle tone probably involves the locus coeruleus of the brainstem. Cataplexy is like the motor inhibition seen with REM sleep: deep tendon reflexes are lost, and eye movements are preserved (6). In normal REM sleep there is loss of tone in the submental and nuchal muscles with dreaming, perhaps to minimize the head movement that would be reflexly associated with scanning eye movements (5). The locus coeruleus plays a central role in inhibiting muscle activity and tendon reflexes in REM sleep (9). A persistently normal electroencephalogram during the cataplectic attack and electromyographic evidence of reflex inhibition (H reflex inhibition) at a spinal cord level attest to the noncortical central nervous system origin of this atonia (9).

Cataplectic attacks may occur repeatedly with little interval between attacks, resulting in a virtually unremitting cataplexy, called status cataplecticus (9). The patient with this problem will be virtually paralyzed. Fortunately, this is very rare. A more common setting for the cataplectic attack is at the onset of a sleep attack (9).

Hypnagogic Hallucinations

Hallucinations with narcolepsy usually appear as the individual falls asleep and are, therefore, called hypnagogic (6). Sleep-related hallucinations occasionally appear as the patient awakens and are then called hypnopompic (23). Hypnagogic hallucinations are analagous to dreams developing in REM sleep and may, indeed, arise by way of the same mechanisms (6). Affected individuals usually report that they see complete scenes, isolated objects, human or animal figures, or just flashes of light and unstructured patterns (27). Patients awakened from a sleepy state by an abrupt noise may see flashes of light coincident with the noise (27). The more structured hallucinations are usually frightening. In fact, they may be auditory, olfactory, or tactile, as well as visual (28). Fourteen to 57 percent of narcoleptics have hypnagogic hallucinations, and 20 to 50 percent have hypnopompic hallucinations (25). Although narcolepsy may appear with both sleep attacks and cataplexy, unassociated with hallucinations, hypnagogic hallucinations often occur together with sleep paralysis (25).

Sleep Paralysis

Sleep paralysis is an inability to move voluntarily on first awakening. Minor external stimuli, such as someone touching or calling the patient, may abruptly release him from this paralysis. Like cataplexy, this is a manifestation of REM sleep-related motor inhibition (6). Presumably, suppression of the REM sleep system during wakefulness is defective (6). It usually lasts only a few seconds, moments during which the patient is terrified. A cholinoceptive (acetylcholine-using) frontobulbar pathway is probably involved in sleep paralysis as well as cataplexy (25). Clearly, the entire tetrad of phenomena of narcolepsy is idiopathic, and that cataplexy and sleep paralysis have a basis separate from the sleep attacks is inferred from the difference in response to drugs used in treating these varied symptoms.

Treatment

Methylphenidate is currently the drug of choice for treating the sleep attacks (25). Amphetamines are also used for decreasing sleep attacks, but cataplexy and sleep paralysis respond to neither of these drugs. Twenty milligrams daily of methylphenidate may be adequate to abolish sleep attacks (9). As already mentioned, early narcolepsy may be difficult to distinguish from incipient schizophrenia, and with amphetamine treatment the patient may develop a paranoid thought disorder so characteristic of schizophrenia that the diagnosis of narcolepsy will be questioned (6). Despite the early effectiveness of methylphenidate and amphetamines, the patient is likely to develep tolerance to the drugs, and abuse is fairly common (6). As well as producing depression, irritability, and paranoid ideation, the amphetamines will disturb nocturnal sleep. Monoamine oxidase inhibitors may be effective in some narcoleptics, but the orthostatic hypotension, edema, impotence, and weight gain occasionally associated with these drugs make methylphenidate a better choice (6). Nocturnal sleep disturbances exacerbated by amphetamines or methylphenidate may be minimized with the addition of nightly diazepam to the drug regimen (6).

Imipramine relieves cataplexy but is not an effective drug for treating sleep attacks (6,26). Seventy-five to 100 milligrams daily usually stop the cataplectic attacks (9). The closely related tricyclic antidepressant clomipramine is more effective than imipramine, but experience with this drug is relatively limited (26). The mode of action of these drugs is unknown, but an anticholinergic effect of the drug is presumed central to its functioning (25). The site of action that relieves the cataplexy is probably in the brainstem median raphe nuclei and descending serotonergic pathways that terminate on the anterior horn cells in the spinal cord (26). Central nervous system 5-hydroxytryptamine is the neurotransmitter most directly affected by these tricyclic compounds (26). Impotence, blurred vision, and urinary retention develop as adverse reactions to imipramine (25). Problems with ejaculation occasionally develop in patients taking clomipramine (26). In status cataplecticus intravenous clomipramine will arrest the atonia (9). Hypertensive episodes may occur with combined tricyclic antidepressants and amphetamine treatment (6). Supporting the connection between REM sleep and cataplexy is the REM sleep inhibiting effect of tricyclic antidepressants (3).

Kleine-Levin Syndrome

Kleine-Levin syndrome is periodic hypersomnia associated with excessive eating, usually developing in adolescent men (23,29–31). The sleep attacks in this syndrome may last 1 to 6 weeks and recur at intervals months or years apart (32). During the sleep attack these patients can be awakened, but they are irritable and often excited at the time of attempted arousal (32). They do not achieve a normal level of consciousness despite their being awake. Actions are slow, time sense is confused, and memory is faulty. Arousal is always limited to brief periods, that is, minutes (23). A protracted sleep attack may be heralded by decreased appetite and listlessness (23). Symptoms associated with the irresistible drowsiness and irritability of these adolescent men include excessive or inappropriate sexual behavior, excessive eating (bulimia), outbursts of abusive behavior, paroxysms of laughing, shouting, or singing, and general hyperactivity (29,33). Visual and auditory hallucinations may occur (33). Marked sweating and drinking are common (29). Some patients have elevated blood sugars. The etiology of this disorder is unknown. The symptoms usually stop by 30 years of age (33). Alcohol may play a role in precipitating some attacks (23).

Although this is generally believed to be a neurologic, rather than a psychiatric disorder, there is little convincing evidence to assign it to one group or the other. The patient's symptoms involve disturbed behavior and consciousness. Depressive disorders are routinely reported in the families of patients with Kleine-Levin syndrome (23). Despite this, the patient's mental and physical health are usually unremarkable before the illness (32). Emotional stress often precipitates the initial episode (33). There is little evidence of an underlying physiologic disorder. The electroencephalogram shows some slowing of the basic alpha rhythm when symptoms are prominent, and sleep-onset rapid eye movements appear in this disorder; but the electroencephalogram during the sleep attack is usually normal (23,29,33).

This is a self-limited disorder. The sleep attacks, excessive intake, and inappropriate sexual behavior remit without treatment (33). Amphetamines have been used with some success in treating the sleep attacks (32). A structural lesion has not been found in victims of this disorder, although similar signs rarely appear in patients who have had severe head trauma or encephalitis (29).

Pickwickian Syndrome

Extremely obese individuals may suffer from bouts of sleep attacks associated with respiratory abnormalities but not with the cataplexy, sleep paralysis, and hallucinations typical of narcolepsy (34). This is called the pickwickian syndrome if the patient has idiopathic hypoventilation and excessive appetite as well as sleep attacks. The name refers to Charles Dicken's *Pickwick Papers* in which a character named Joe exhibited the classical features of this syndrome. In common with narcolepsy is the patient's tendency to fall asleep for brief periods of time during all kinds of activities. Patients will doze off in the middle of a sentence, while eating, or during sexual intercourse.

Features essential to the diagnosis include an elevated arterial P_{CO_2} and a depressed P_{O_2}. The patients will have apparent polycythemia and often have right-sided ventricular hypertrophy of the heart. There is no structural lung disease or obstruction of the airway, but the patient still does not move air as effectively as required for adequate oxygenation of the blood (34). The patient's extraordinary appetite is as much a part of the syndrome as it is a cause of it. The patient has more frequent sleep attacks as he becomes more obese, and with the decreased activity associated with the hypersomnia the patient becomes more obese.

The cause of this syndrome is unknown. Despite this, it can be effectively treated, the treatment being enforced weight loss. All of the symptoms remit as the patient loses weight (34). A dramatic improvement in alertness and activity often appears with a relatively minor loss of weight.

ABERRANT BEHAVIOR DURING SLEEP

Complex activities can occur during sleep. Sleepwalking and sleeptalking are familiar enough to most individuals that their appearance will arouse only modest concern. If the sleepwalker's behavior poses a threat to his own safety or if the sleeptalker's remarks provoke anxiety in those near enough to hear, these phenomena will usually be brought to a physician's attention. Activities interfering with sleep are more consistently the object of a consultation. Nocturnal leg cramps and "restless legs," which interfere with the patient's ability to relax may produce considerable sleep-deprivation. Disturbing motor phenomena, such as tooth-grinding and nocturnal myoclonus, will usually disturb the patient's bed partner, rather than the patient himself. The victim of the aberrant behavior routinely faces the choice of sleeping alone or constantly being awakened by his distraught bed partner. That this behavior is not necessarily pathologic provides little comfort for the individual disturbed by the movements or noise produced during sleep. A commonly concealed nocturnal problem that may prompt a medical or psychiatric consultation by a very worried patient is bed-wetting (enuresis). Many patients are reluctant to discuss this problem until they are directly questioned on the matter. Some admit that the abnormal behavior made them suspect that they were losing their sanity.

Somnambulism

Sleepwalking (somnambulism), as well as sleeptalking (somniloquy) and enuresis, occur primarily in stage 4 of NREM sleep (5). In adults the nocturnal wandering can also appear during stage 2 sleep in the early morning hours. Somnambulists usually have close relatives with the same disorder and with other sleep irregularities. Thirty-eight percent of somnambulists have a family member with nocturnal enuresis (18). Sixty-two percent have a personal history of enuresis (18). The nocturnal wandering in some adults is accompanied by screaming and by irrational acts, such as walking into traffic, that could be fatal. During the somnambulism, the patient's eyes are open and his expression is often fearful (13). The adult sleepwalker exhibits a fast gait, a relatively violent resistance to restraints, and a propensity for multiple episodes in a single night (13). Patients are routinely amnesic for the episode.

This aberrant phenomenon is much more common in children than in adults. Sixty percent of children between 5 and 12 years of age have at least one episode of sleepwalking, the child usually exhibiting a slow gait, a rather docile response to intervention, and a propensity for only one episode during an entire night (13). At least when the sleepwalking occurs in childhood, there is generally no structural lesion or physiologic disturbance responsible for it. The neurologic examination will reveal no focal deficits, and the electroencephalogram in these children will be normal even during the sleepwalking episode. The nocturnal wanderings may be suppressed with a small dose of diazepam given at bedtime (1).

Sleepwalking is more difficult to deal with in adults and may reflect significant central nervous system pathology. Relatively few disorders can mimic somnambulism, but the few that can require vigorous treatment. The most common neurologic disorder misdiagnosed as sleepwalking is the involuntary ambulation occurring during a psychomotor (complex partial) seizure (13). Although adults are not incontinent during sleep walking and show no other signs consistent with a seizure disorder, electroencephalography commonly reveals temporal lobe spikes on both sleep and awake recordings (13). Indeed, sleepwalking and enuresis are the two aberrant sleep-related phenomena most often associated with psychomotor epilepsy (35). Adult somnambulists respond well to phenytoin or carbamazepine treatment, a therapeutic observation supporting the notion that these are nocturnal complex partial seizures in some adults (13).

Enuresis

Bedwetting (enuresis) occurs in stage 4 NREM sleep (5). It rarely has a structural basis, but spinal cord damage and other central nervous system abnormalities must be considered when it appears with no associated family history (1). Problems with bowel control and sexual function should be specifically sought. A slowly progressive spinal cord tumor could cause these sphincter and sexual problems as initial signs of the disease. Diabetes mellitus can disturb bladder function sufficiently to allow incontinence during sleep especially in elderly individuals. Fortunately, most cases of nocturnal enuresis are entirely benign. A high family incidence of the disorder is reassuring, but even without a hereditary disposition to enuresis the patient most probably has idiopathic benign enuresis if there are no other obvious neurologic complaints associated with the aberrant nocturnal phenomenon.

The cause of bedwetting is unknown. One hypothesis ascribes this nocturnal incontinence to an accentuation of normal physiologic events typical of NREM sleep prompted by arousal (5). In normal arousal from stage 4 NREM sleep, an increase in electromyographic activity precedes the disappearance of high voltage slow wave cortical activity (5). The muscles become active before there is a distinct change in the level of consciousness; this could lead to bladder evacuation before the patient awakens. This agrees with the observed tendency for enuresis to occur during arousal from slow wave sleep (2). Whatever the etiology of the sleep irregularity, imipramine at a dose of 75 to 100 milligrams nightly will suppress the enuresis (1). Its mode of action involves an anticholinergic action on the bladder wall (1).

Restless Legs Syndrome

Problems with sleep are occasionally ascribed to irritability limited to the legs (36). The patient has an ill-defined, disagreeable sensation, apparently deep in the legs, whenever he tries to sleep. This "cramping" or "aching" sensation, especially prominent in the calves, is associated with an irresistible urge to exercise the legs (3,4,37). The patient feels compelled to get out of bed and stand or walk. Attacks occur several times weekly (36).

Cramps do not develop in the "restless" muscles, but shocklike jerks often accompany this restless legs syndrome, and these jerks further complicate the task of falling asleep (5,36). Both the disagreeable sensations and the involuntary limb jerks appearing in this syndrome generally occur as the patient is falling asleep, but they may develop when the patient is just relaxing, especially if he is very tired (5). Symptoms usually appear in the evening (37). Individuals developing restless legs syndrome as adults often recall being restless as children when required to sit still for more than a few minutes.

One-third of the patients with restless legs syndrome have relatives with the same problem (3,37). This disorder probably has a hereditary basis that is transmitted in an autosomal dominant fashion. The underlying lesion is probably in the central nervous system, but no structural or neurochemical defect has been found in affected individuals (36). Occasionally, patients evolve signs of motor neuron disease or have uremia, but the majority of affected individuals have a stable benign disorder that disturbs nothing more than their sleep (4,5).

A variety of treatments used in this disorder have been unsuccessful (5). Warm baths, haloperidol, diazepam, and diphenhydramine usually fail to relieve the feelings of restlessness; but even if they are successful in suppressing that symptom, most patients still complain of involuntary limb jerks interfering with their sleep (37). Forceful, involuntary limb jerks, called myoclonic jerks, are normal phenomena in drowsiness, but the myoclonus appearing during stages 1 and 2 of NREM sleep with restless legs syndrome is much more forceful and diffuse than that occurring with drowsiness in normal individuals (37). Clonazepam, a drug closely related to diazepam and flurazepam, suppresses myoclonus in other conditions and because of that action it has been applied to treat restless legs syndrome with some success (36). 0.5 milligrams three times daily may relieve both the myoclonus and dysesthesias completely.

Nocturnal Leg Cramps

Nocturnal leg cramps are distinct from "restless legs." These leg cramps interfere with sleep simply by making the patient so uncomfortable that he cannot relax. They may occur every night when the patient first gets into bed or they may assume a more unpredictable pattern. In most cases, there is no apparent pathology responsible for the painful nocturnal cramps. One situation in which the muscle cramps are partly understood is postdialysis leg cramps. Electrolyte shifts with the dialysis are apparently responsible for the nocturnal cramps. At least in dialysis patients, the muscle cramps will subside with quinine treatment (38). Vitamin treatment has been tried by some patients, but there is no evidence that it is effective. A maneuver that does decrease the development of these leg cramps is stretching the calf muscle just before sleeping. Most muscular disorders interfering with sleep are not so easily treated.

Nocturnal Myoclonus

Repetitive, stereotyped, involuntary movements of the limbs appear during sleep in as much as 13 percent of the population complaining of insomnia (4). These nonepileptic, sleep-related movements are called nocturnal myoclonus or periodic movements of sleep. The actual movement usually involves dorsiflexion of the foot, extension of the great toe, and flexion of the knee and hip. The movements are repetitive, have a duration of 1.5 to 2.5 seconds, and recur every 30 seconds for as long as 1 hour (4). They appear in NREM sleep and are often considered the cause of insomnia by the affected patient. In fact, these periodic movements of sleep appear just as often in patients with hypersomnia and are probably a result of sleep-wake disturbances rather than a cause (4). Both men and women are equally affected and the mean age of the affected patient is 47 years old (4). The cause of the movements is unknown. There is no treatment for this symptom.

Other Aberrant Behavior

Bruxism and head-banging in sleep are occasionally observed in children. These may develop in any stage of sleep. The significance of bruxism is discussed in the section on facial movements in the chapter on movement disorders. In most cases, these apparently self-abusive activities have no significance.

DIAGNOSTIC APPROACHES TO SLEEP DISORDERS

Problems with sleep are common and are usually caused by stress. Most patients with excessive drowsiness do not have narcolepsy and most with insomnia do not have sleep apnea. Evaluating the patient with a sleep-related complaint obviously requires some diagnostic restraint simply because the possible explanations for any sleep disorder are fairly diverse. The first step is a clear and complete history of the problem. If the recurrent drowsiness is associated with unexplained falls and early morning hallucinations, the diagnosis of narcolepsy can be adopted confidently. An electroencephalogram that shows rapid eye movements at the onset of sleep will confirm the diagnosis adequately to justify treatment for narcolepsy. Progressive stupor in an adolescent requires a more aggressive approach. Drug abuse should be excluded as a problem before more extensive tests are performed on the individual. Most patients are unaware of the effect drug or alcohol withdrawal can have on sleep, and many are reluctant to discuss drug abuse unless they are convinced that it is relevant. A careful general physical examination with special attention to the neurologic examination is appropriate in every patient with sleep-related problems, even if there is obvious stress in the individual's life that could account for the sleep disorder. Obvious systemic problems should not be overlooked simply because the patient eagerly volunteers that marital strife has been disrupting his sleep. Progressive stupor presents special problems because the patient must be evaluated quickly, even if the drowsiness later proves transient and recurrent. Although Kleine-Levin syndrome may occasionally explain hypersomnia, a careful examination of serum electrolytes, liver function studies, renal function, and blood cell counts should be obtained on an emergency basis to establish that the problem is not a metabolic encephalopathy or a systemic infection. Even if systemic infection is not apparent, a cerebrospinal fluid examination should be conducted after a computed tomogram of the brain is obtained. The computed tomogram will limit the possibility that a brain tumor is responsible for the sleep disorder and the cerebrospinal fluid examination will determine whether or not there is a central nervous system infection. If the problem is one of a sleep-related phenomenon, such as somnambulism or somniloquy, an electroencephalogram obtained during sleep with nasopharyngeal leads should be obtained to look specifically for temporal lobe seizure activity. Any abnormal activity found on the electroencephalogram should be followed up with a computed tomogram of the brain, with and without contrast enhancement, to look for progressive intracerebral lesions.

REFERENCES

1. Pearlman CA, Greenberg R: Medical-psychological implications of recent sleep research. *Psychiatry Med* 1:261, 1970.
2. Hartmann E: Sleep, in Nicholi AM (ed): *The Harvard Guide to Modern Psychiatry*. Cambridge, Belknap Press, 1978, p 103.
3. Ware JC: The symptom of insomnia: Causes and cures. *Psychiatr Ann* 9:27, 1979.
4. Coleman RM, Pollak CP, Weitzman ED: Periodic movements in sleep (nocturnal myoclonus): Relation to sleep disorders. *Ann Neurol* 8:416, 1980.
5. Roth N: Sleep and motility. *Dis Nerv Syst* 38:778, 1977.
6. Zarcone V: Narcolepsy. *N Engl J Med* 288:1156, 1973.
7. Tauber ES, Coleman RM, Weitzman ED: Absence of tonic electromyographic activity during sleep in normal and spastic nonmimetic skeletal muscles in man. *Ann Neurol* 2:66, 1977.
8. Kramer M: Dream disturbances. *Psychiatr Ann* 9:50, 1979.
9. Guilleminault C, Wilson RA, Dement WC: A study of cataplexy. *Arch Neurol* 31:255, 1974.
10. Clark RW, Schmidt HS, Malarkey WB: Disordered growth hormone and prolactin secretion in primary disorders of sleep. *Neurology (NY)* 20:855, 1979.
11. Klawans HL: Levodopa induced psychosis. *Psychiatr Ann* 8:447, 1978.
12. Task force on nomenclature and statistics, American Psychiatric Association: *Diagnostic*

and Statistical Manual of Mental Disorders (Third Edition). Washington, DC, American Psychiatric Association, 1980.

13. Pedley TA, Guilleminault C: Episodic nocturnal wanderings. Response to anticonvulsant drug therapy. *Ann Neurol* 2:30, 1977.
14. Solomon F, White CC, Paron DL, et al: Sleeping pills, insomnia and medical practice, *N Engl J Med* 300:803, 1979.
15. Prick JJG: Thallium poisoning, in Vinken PJ, Bruyn GW (eds): *Handbook of Clinical Neurology*. New York, American Elsevier, 1979, vol 36, p 239.
16. Drugs for psychiatric disorders. *Med Lett Drugs Ther* 22:77, 1980.
17. Mendelson JH, Mello NK: Biologic concomitants of alcoholism. *N Engl J Med* 31:912, 1979.
18. Karacan I, Moore CA: Genetics and human sleep. *Psychiatr Ann* 9:11, 1979.
19. Bird TD, Plum F: Recovery from barbiturate overdose coma with a prolonged isoelectric electroencephalogram. *Neurology (NY)* 18:456, 1968.
20. Klerman GL: Affective disorders, in Nicholi AM (ed): *The Harvard Guide to Modern Psychiatry*. Cambridge, Belknap Press, 1978, p 253.
21. Guilleminault C, Eldridge FL, Dement WC: Insomnia with sleep apnea: A new syndrome. *Science* 181:856, 1973.
22. Segarra JM: Cerebral vascular disease and behavior I. *Arch Neurol* 22:408, 1970.
23. Bonkalo A: Hypersomnia. *Br J Psychiatry* 114:69, 1968.
24. Goldensohn ES, Gold AP: Prolonged behavioral disturbances as ictal phenomena. *Neurology (NY)* 10:1, 1959.
25. Karacan I, Moore CA, Williams RL: The narcoleptic syndrome. *Psychiatr Ann* 9:69, 1979.
26. Schachter M, Parkes JD: Fluvoxamine and clomipramine in the treatment of cataplexy. *J Neurol Neurosurg Psychiatry* 43:171, 1980.
27. Lessell S, Cohen MW: Phosphenes induced by sound. *Neurology (NY)* 29:1524, 1979.
28. DeVaul RA, Hall RCW: Hallucinations, in Hall RCW (ed): *Psychiatric Presentations of Medical Illness*. New York, SP Medical and Scientific Books, 1980, p 91.
29. Sherwin I, Geschwind N: Neural substrates of behavior, in Nicholi AM (ed): *The Harvard Guide to Modern Psychiatry*. Cambridge, Belknap Press, 1978, p 59.
30. Kleine W: Periodische Schlafsucht. *Monatsschr Psychiatr Neurol* 57:285, 1925.
31. Levin M: Periodic somnolence and morbid hunger: A new syndrome. *Brain* 59:494, 1936.
32. Duffy JP, Davison K: A female case of the Kleine-Levin syndrome. *Br J Psychiatry* 114:77, 1968.
33. Chiles JA, Wilkus RJ: Behavioral manifestations of the Kleine-Levin syndrome. *Dis Nerv Syst* 37:646, 1976.
34. West JB: Disorders of regulation of respiration, in Thorn GW, Adams RD, Braunwald E, et al (eds): *Harrison's Principles of Internal Medicine*, ed 8. New York, McGraw-Hill, 1977, p 1374.
35. Aird RB: Clinical syndromes of the limbic system. *Int J Neurol* 6:340, 1968.
36. Boghen D: Successful treatment of restless legs with clonazepam. *Ann Neurol* 8:341, 1980.
37. Boghen D, Peyronnard J-M: Myoclonus in familial restless legs syndrome. *Arch Neurol* 33:368, 1976.
38. Danielli HW: Simple cure for nocturnal leg cramps. *N Engl J Med* 301:216, 1979.

11 Weakness

Weakness, developing abruptly or evolving slowly, usually indicates disease of the central nervous system, the peripheral nerves, or the skeletal muscles. It is a relatively uncommon symptom of conversion hysteria and a rarely misconstrued symptom in chronic depression. Problems in evaluating weakness do not occur when a 60-year-old hypertensive man complains of a suddenly developing left arm and leg paresis; the difficulty arises when a 25-year-old woman with no history of prior illness complains that she tires easily and cannot lift relatively light objects over her head. A cautious physician might consider myasthenia gravis or a hereditary myopathy as possible causes of the young woman's difficulty; but, if there is no consistent pattern of weakness, most physicians would appropriately suspect a psychiatric basis for the impaired strength. Edrophonium tests for myasthenia gravis, muscle biopsies for hereditary myopathy, and nerve conduction studies for peripheral neuropathy are unpleasant and, occasionally, hazardous procedures. Deciding which patients should be subjected to such studies requires careful evaluation of all the signs and symptoms experienced by the patient, as well as an objective assessment of the psychologic factors entering into the patient's complaints.

UNILATERAL WEAKNESS: HEMIPARESIS

Cerebrovascular accidents are the most common cause of unilateral weakness or paralysis and are almost always the cause of hemiparesis in elderly patients. These vascular accidents are caused by occlusion of a blood vessel or bleeding from a blood vessel that supplies the brain or spinal cord. An atherosclerotic plaque in the wall of an artery often provides a site for blood clot formation. The resulting clot may gradually or abruptly occlude the lumen of the blood vessel, or it may fragment and occlude small blood vessels distal to the atherosclerotic vessel. Some vessels are temporarily narrowed by spasm of the regulatory muscles in the blood vessel wall. In susceptible individuals the spasm may evolve into permanent occlusion of the vessel; this may be the basis for strokes developing with complicated migraine headaches. An even rarer cause of vascular occlusion in the nervous system is invasion of the blood vessel by a fungus, such as *Actinomyces*, which extends through the blood vessel wall and may produce bleeding from the vessel as well as obstruction. Coagulation disorders occasionally produce thrombi in cerebral blood vessels, and some bacterial infections, including syphilis, can elicit inflammatory changes in blood vessel walls that narrow or obstruct intracranial vessels.

Smaller vessel occlusion may develop with longstanding hypertension. The walls of small arteries thicken until blood flow is impaired. Blood clots carried to the brain from diseased heart valves or diseased neck vessels will produce occlusion of arteries in the brain, the extent of damage being determined largely by the size of the blood clot (embolus) involved. The deficits appearing with the infarction will reflect the area supplied by the vessel occluded. Bleeding from defective blood vessels (aneurysms, arteriovenous malformations) will cause focal neurologic deficits determined by the area of the brain into which the bleeding occurs. The expanding blood clot destroys brain tissue and impairs the function of intact tissue by crushing it. These are all fairly dramatic incidents producing sudden changes in patients with diseased blood vessels. A young woman with a history of rheumatic heart disease and longstanding evidence of valvular heart disease who suddenly develops a dense hemiparesis would be considered a victim of an embolic stroke and would be treated with anticoagulation medication to decrease the likelihood of additional strokes unless a problem other than the valvular disease was found to be responsible for the stroke. An elderly man with several years of high blood pressure is assumed to have had an intracerebral bleed when he develops a hemiplegia, that is, complete paralysis of one side of his body, unless there are other obvious factors that could more simply explain his deficits. If he was struck on the head before developing the paralysis, a subdural hematoma must be considered. All possible causes of hemiplegia or hemiparesis must be considered in any patient developing these deficits, but the patient's history and presentation will make certain explanations much more probable and, therefore, much more appropriate for immediate attention.

Young Adults with Hemiparesis

Young adults developing unilateral weakness with no antecedent neurologic or systemic disease to explain their sudden change in strength are more difficult diagnostic problems than middle-aged or older adults simply because the likelihood of hypertensive or atherosclerotic vascular disease in the young group is unlikely and no other etiology is excessively prevalent. If a young person has an acutely appearing hemiplegia, a number of possible causes must be considered. Probable causes include lupus cerebritis with systemic lupus erythematosus, Todd's paralysis following an unobserved seizure, intracerebral hemorrhage from an arteriovenous malformation, or hemorrhage into an occult tumor, such as a malignant melanoma. Systemic lupus eythematosus can produce brain disease indirectly by damaging the heart valves, thereby providing a source for emboli to the brain; this valvular heart disease is called Libman-Sacks endocarditis. A hemiparesis may develop rapidly with some encephalitides that produce little more than personality changes before the appearance of the focal motor deficits. *Herpes simplex* virus commonly produces unilateral weakness because of its tendency to induce substantial swelling in a temporal lobe. Hematologic disorders, such as sickle-cell disease, can produce strokes when there are abrupt changes in the flow characteristics of the blood, but these generally appear in children with already recognized blood dyscrasias.

Many causes of hemiparesis in younger people require fast decisions to avoid permanent loss of function. The adolescent with no known head trauma may have an epidural or subdural hematoma. The young woman with no recent illness other than a mild viral syndrome may have a brain abscess. Fortunately, most serious causes of acute hemiparesis in young adults are not that puzzling. Hemiplegia associated with fever and a heart murmur is likely to be from embolic complications of an infectious heart disease, subacute bacterial endocarditis. Progressive weakness associated with a visual field cut in a patient with recurrent inner ear infections is likely to be from a brain abscess. These are dangerous situations, but the patient's evident systemic illness leaves little doubt that a neurologic catastrophe has developed as a complication of the initial illness. Of more importance to the psychiatrist is the situation in which the authenticity of the patient's complaint is questioned. Hemiparesis or hemiplegia as a sign of hysteria or malingering is not rare. Usually careful attention to inconsistencies on the physical exam will clarify whether or not the weakness is from neurologic or psychologic problems.

Hysterical Signs

Immediately after the development of weakness in an arm or leg, tone is usually depressed in the affected limb. Passive movement of the weak limb will reveal this increased plasticity. A truly paralyzed limb will fall wherever it is placed, even if it is placed over the patient's face or over a hard surface. When the paralysis is contrived, the patient will usually avoid any threatening movements of the affected limb. This is an unreliable sign though, because too often the patient with no real weakness will allow his hand to hit his face or will allow his foot to land on a hard surface. Facial paralysis is difficult to feign, and so it is a fairly reliable indicator of a true hemiparesis. If facial paresis is not present, weakness on turning the head away from the paralyzed side will also help establish the authenticity of the weakness. Most patients are not adequately familiar with the function of neck muscles to realize that the right sternocleidomastoid muscle turns the head to the left. The patient with a contrived right-sided weakness will have intact strength on turning the head to the left and impaired strength on turning it to the right. Hoover's sign is also a useful indicator of factitious leg paralysis. Placing one hand under the heel of an allegedly paralyzed leg, the examiner can feel the normal downward pressure by the abnormal leg when the normal leg is actively lifted off the bed.

Investigation of a Hemiparesis

Rapid evaluation of an acutely evolving hemiplegia is feasible where computed tomography of the head and cerebral angiography are available. Care must be taken in some patients with suspected hematologic disorders, such as those with sickle-cell disease. Patients with this hemoglobin disorder may develop more cerebral blood flow problems when their red cells are exposed to the contrast material used in these radiographic techniques. In this situation, a hematologic evaluation would logically precede any invasive studies, including a postcontrast computed tomogram. Patients with complicated migraine headaches are also at increased risk because the contrast material used during angiography may cause more vasospasm. A brain abscess will usually appear as an area of decreased density on the computed tomogram of the head; with contrast enhancement, this decreased density will be surrounded by a faint ring. Bleeding into an occult tumor will be indistinguishable from bleeding developing in an arteriovenous malformation or with rupture of an aneurysm. Both will appear as highly dense areas on the computed tomogram displacing normal brain structures. Arteriography in these cases will clarify the cause of the bleed. The aneurysm or arteriovenous malformation will usually be clearly defined by an arteriogram, and abnormal vessels feeding a hemorrhagic tumor may be apparent.

Transient Weakness

Hemiparesis or hemiplegia lasting only minutes or hours is more difficult to assess than persistent weakness. The character of the weakness is usually determined only through history supplied by the patient alone. What the patient describes as "weakness" may actually be numbness or pain in the affected parts of the body. If indeed the transient symptom was limb or facial weakness, the physician must determine whether or not the complaint warrants further investigation. Hysteria is impossible to establish in this situation, since even if a transient episode occurs while the physician is present, the fluctuating nature of the deficit and the patient's agitation during the episode may compromise the value of the examination. Whether the weakness is authentic or not, the patient often elaborates on the

Table 11.1. Causes of Transient Weakness

Transient ischemic attacks
Focal motor seizure activity
Hemiplegic migraine
Hysterical conversion reaction
Local trauma (brachial plexus injury)
Transient electrolyte abnormalities
Neuromuscular junction poisons

deficits. An improbable distribution of weakness does not prove the weakness is spurious. Complaints of transient weakness must be fully explored for possible neurologic bases (Table 11.1).

Transient Ischemic Attacks

Elderly patients and patients with valvular heart disease often have transient weakness as a manifestation of a transient ischemic attack (Table 11.2). Ischemia is a decrease in the supply of blood to part of the brain. Impaired blood flow to the spinal cord also does occur, but it is much less common and is often difficult to distinguish from intracranial ischemia. Ischemia of the eye or optic nerve is discussed in the chapter on visual abnormalities. Inadequate perfusion of any of these regions of the nervous system will produce signs of neurologic dysfunction that are determined by the part of the nervous system denied adequate blood flow. Ischemia to specific parts of the brain produces characteristic patterns of neurologic dysfunction. Impaired blood flow through the middle cerebral artery will produce weakness and sensory impairment involving the face and hand more than the leg. If the left middle cerebral artery is the site of difficulty, the patient will usually become aphasic. Vertebrobasilar insufficiency is more likely to cause vertigo, double vision, and slurred speech (Figure 11.1). When the neurologic dysfunction is slight, the site of the ischemia

Table 11.2. Diseases Associated with Transient Ischemic Attacks

Hypertension
Diabetes mellitus
Valvular heart disease
Peripheral vascular disease
Hyperlipidemia
Cervical spondylosis (vertebrobasilar only)
Carotid or vertebrobasilar occlusion
Anemia
Polycythemia

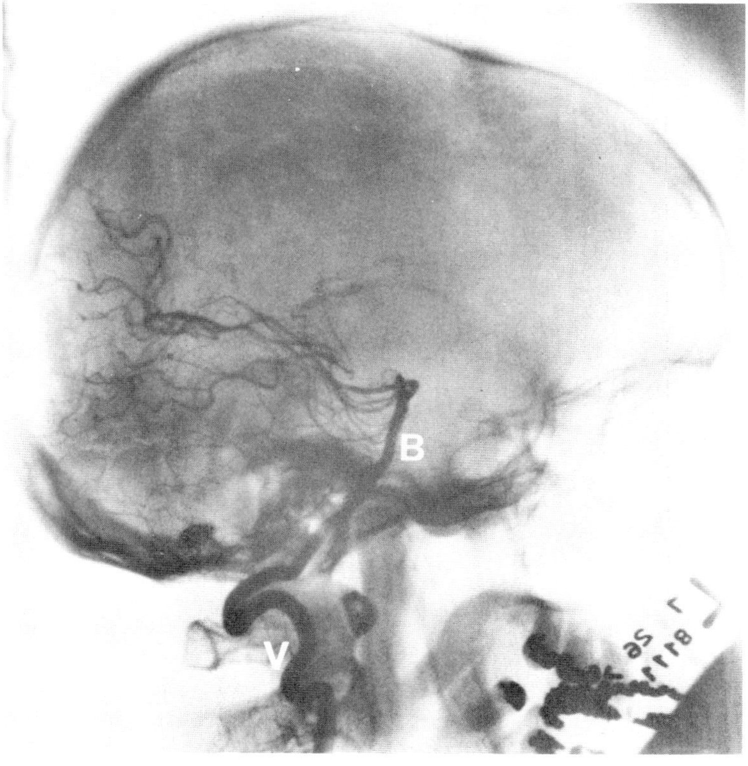

Figure 11.1. This normal arteriogram shows the vertebrobasilar system on lateral view. The vertebral artery (V) becomes the basilar artery (B) at the level of the pons. Ischemia in the distribution of these arteries produces signs of brainstem and cerebellar dysfunction, with incoordination arising with cerebellar ischemia often being overshadowed by the more disabling sensory and motor signs of brainstem dysfunction. Transient amnesia may occur with these ischemic attacks because part of the temporal lobe involved in memory is supplied by the vertebrobasilar vessels (courtesy of Dr. M. Tenner).

may be inapparent. Limb weakness can develop with poor perfusion of a middle cerebral artery or a vertebrobasilar artery branch.

If the blood flow returns to a level adequate for normal function before the brain tissue is irreversibly damaged, the ischemic attack is said to be transient. Blood flow to limited areas of the brain may be interrupted by transient thrombus build up in the vessel, spasm of the blood vessel walls, inflammation in or around the vessel, pressure from a mass or swelling overlying the vessel, or by recurrent emboli discharged from the heart or neck vessels (1). Whether or not there is a history of rheumatic or other valvular heart disease, the patient with transient neurologic deficits must be investigated for cardiac disease. Careful auscultation of heart sounds and an echocardiogram to define mitral and aortic valve integrity are usually adequate in the examination of an otherwise healthy person. If valvular heart disease is found, chronic anticoagulation or valve replacement may be necessary to stop the transient ischemic attacks and avoid a completed stroke. Intracranial masses can produce transient neurologic deficits by transiently impairing blood flow, and so, victims of transient ischemic attacks should be evaluated for possible brain tumors or subdural hematomas. Complicated migraine produces transient neurologic deficits that occasionally become permanent perhaps because they have a combination of vasospasm and coagulation disorders. Giant cell arteritis, such as that occurring with temporal arteritis, usually causes persistent ischemia and stroke when the patient develops neurologic signs, but the ischemic attack with this type of disease is occasionally transient.

Transient ischemic attacks (TIAs) will be followed by a completed stroke in as much as one-fourth of the patients affected (2). The risk of a stroke is greatest during the first few weeks after the transient ischemic attack, with 24 percent of those who will have a stroke succumbing within the first month after the transient episode (3). About one-third of those ultimately suffering strokes will develop the fixed deficit within 3 months of a transient ischemic attack (3). The type of stroke developing will depend upon the area supplied by the occluded vessel, the permanent deficits usually following the same pattern as the transient deficits. Transient ischemic attacks in the areas supplied by the carotid artery are about twice as common as those in the areas supplied by the vertebrobasilar vessels, but survival after a stroke involving either system is equally likely (3). Misdiagnosis of a transient ischemic attack is more likely with suspected vertebrobasilar attacks because syncope or vertigo may be a feature of the vertebrobasilar transient ischemic attack. Physicians often attribute isolated cases of syncope or vertigo to these transient ischemic attacks, but such transient problems, with no associated clumsiness, slurred speech, double vision, or facial weakness are not likely to represent vertebrobasilar circulation attacks (4). Dizziness or vertigo will be present in 90 percent of patients with vertebrobasilar insufficiency, but visual disturbances will also be present in 55 percent and other cranial nerve signs in 20 percent (5). With carotid artery disease, the transient symptoms may be more isolated. The patient may have selective loss of vision in one eye, called amaurosis fugax, or a transient aphasia. In most patients, the transient ischemic attack looks like a stroke until the signs start to clear. In most cases, all deficits resolve within 1 or 2 hours. In all cases, they resolve by 24 hours. By definition, if the deficits persist for more than 24 hours, the episode is not a transient ischemic attack. It is a stroke. Signs and symptoms resolving completely within a few days are often called reversible ischemic neurologic deficits (RINDs); but, regardless of how complete the resolution of the signs is, the episode cannot be considered a transient ischemic attack if it lasts more than 24 hours.

Most transient ischemic attacks classically have been attributed to recurrent emboli from atheromatous plaques in the carotid or vertebral arteries or from diseased heart valves (1,5). Transient thrombosis, that is, blood clot formation causing occlusion, of various sized arteries has also been considered a likely cause of many transient ischemic attacks in some individuals, but more recent blood flow studies suggest that problems with autoregulation of cerebral blood vessels is much more important in most patients than any of these other mechanisms (5). There are, of course, special circumstances, such as with cervical spondylosis or aortic valve disease. Cervical spondylosis, an arthritic disorder of the cervical spine, can cause transient ischemic attacks by compromising flow through the vertebral arteries. Valvular heart disease will send emboli from the heart to the brain. Problems with autoregulation may develop with embolic or thrombotic disease, but the importance of the physiologic deficit is supported by the failure of treatments that act on anatomic lesions.

Treatment of Transient Ischemia

Transient ischemic attacks must be treated with reference to their cause. If valvular heart disease is playing a role, valve replacement or anticoagulation may stop the attacks. If a lipid disorder is involved, corrective dietary measures may eliminate the attack. Surgery on plaques in major arteries to the head has been disappointing (3). In fact, the number of infarcts developing in patients with transient ischemic attacks in some series was greater in the group submitting to endarterectomy, the surgical removal of atheromatous plaques in the blood vessel wall (2). Carotid endarterectomy to increase blood flow for patients with vertebrobasilar insufficiency is not effective (6). Clearly there are some instances in which endarterectomy is useful and appropriate. Patients developing transient ischemic attacks after they have had a major artery occlusion may profit from endarterectomy even though they have suffered a completed stroke if they are having recurrent transient ischemic attacks (7). Presumably, these patients develop emboli above the occluded vessel, and these reflux into viable areas of the brain. In patients with severe atherosclerotic disease but no valvular heart disease, surgery, anticoagulation, and no treatment all provided similar long-term rates of stroke and stroke deaths in large numbers of patients (2). Regardless of the treatment, 23 percent of the patients suffering transient ischemic attacks die of heart disease, rather than of cerebrovascular disease (2). Myocardial infarctions or arrhythmias are the principal causes of death in these patients.

STROKE

A stroke is structural damage to the brain or spinal cord caused by vascular disease (Table 11.3). If there is occlusion of a blood vessel and neural tissue dies from the inadequate blood flow, the lesion is an infarction. If a blood vessel bursts and the surrounding neural tissue is crushed by the expanding blood clot, the lesion is a hemorrhage. Psychiatrists usually are not involved in the evaluation and care of individuals suffering these vascular catastrophes except when the nature of the event is not obvious from the symptoms that develop. Aphasia and altered consciousness are two of the more common situations in which a psychiatric opinion may be sought to assess the basis for the patient's problem. Other symptoms caused by strokes that may not be readily interpreted as such are discussed in other sections of this book.

Psychiatric involvement with the stroke patient usually occurs during the recuperative phase of the illness. A protracted hospitalization to deal with complications of the stroke or to allow rehabilitation occasionally precipitates an acute psychosis, especially in elderly patients. Presumably, the combined stress of a major illness and unfamiliar surroundings may provoke paranoid delusions, disorientation, visual and auditory hallucinations, and combativeness. Minimizing the stress the patient must face and keeping him surrounded by familiar people may help considerably in the management of the psychotic phenomena. Antipsychotic medication should be avoided if at all feasible, but in many cases the cognitive disorder is so disturbing to the patient that neuroleptics must be used. Small doses of haloperidol or a phenothiazine are usually sufficient to suppress destructive behavior. Diazepam and other benzodiazepines are often used to deal with these stroke patients, but the sedation that they produce may mask the progression of stroke complications and may cause a paradoxical excitement. The sleep-wake cycle is commonly disturbed in stroke patients and mild sedation may spare the patient considerable sleep deprivation; but any sedation given must be administered cautiously because of the confusion that a drug reaction would cause in management of any patient soon after a stroke. It is wisest to delay any type of sedation for at least 10 days after the acute appearance of a fixed neurologic deficit. If the stroke is going to evolve, it will usually produce new signs within 7 to 10 days of the initial signs (Table 11.4).

Table 11.3. Causes of Stroke in Young Adults

Coagulation disturbances
Complicated migraine
Hormone-related (birth control pills, pregnancy)
Subacute bacterial endocarditis
Libman-Sacks endocarditis
Arteriovenous malformation
Aneurysm
Hemoglobinopathy (sickle-cell disease)

Table 11.4. Syndromes with Major Vessel Occlusion

Middle cerebral artery
Contralateral weakness (arm and face weaker than leg)
Contralateral sensory loss (largely in arm)
Nonfluent (expressive) aphasia when dominant hemisphere
Gaze preference initially toward hemisphere infarcted
Homonymous hemianopia
Dementia
Anterior Cerebral Artery
Contralateral weakness (leg weaker than arm)
Contralateral sensory loss (largely in leg)
Affective disorder
Urinary incontinence
Dementia
Posterior Cerebral Artery
Contralateral visual field cut (homonymous hemianopia)
Reading difficulty when dominant hemisphere
Memory impairment
Brainstem signs

Relatively young patients with cerebrovascular accidents often have a reactive depression soon after the appearance of neurologic deficits or during the recovery from the stroke. Speech problems are especially likely to frustrate the patient, at least partly because the stroke victim feels more isolated by his inability to communicate than by any sensory or motor deficits that may have occurred with the stroke. Strokes involving the frontal lobes in front of the motor cortex, such as occur with occlusion of branches of the anterior cerebral artery, may cause affective changes characterized by marked apathy and loss of initiative. Right cerebral hemisphere damage often produces denial of the neurologic deficits as one of the stroke phenomena. Patients who will not or cannot recognize their deficits are difficult to rehabilitate.

GENERALIZED WEAKNESS

The type of weakness usually referred for psychiatric evaluation is generalized, rather than focal, weakness. Patients who fatigue easily, who develop muscle cramps with the slightest exertion, or who have inconsistent strength are often considered hysterics or malingerers and, in fact, may be. Unfortunately, there are many neuromuscular disorders that can produce diffuse weakness, variable strength, and painful muscle cramps. Some of these are treatable; and diagnosis of a neuromuscular disorder is valuable in any case since it spares the patient considerable misunderstanding and inappropriate treatment. Alternatively, patients with no 'energy' who seek medical attention and have no discernible organic problem should be given the benefit of psychiatric intervention.

Myasthenia Gravis and Myasthenic Syndromes

Patients with myasthenia gravis typically complain that they fatigue easily, feel most energetic when they first awaken in the morning, and occasionally note blurred or double vision. Most of the patients affected by the disease are young or middle-aged women (8). Marital or job-related problems develop in many of these cases because the spouse or employer doubts the authenticity of the complaint. There is no focal weakness or abrupt deterioration, and the patient's overall appearance does not change at all despite the chronic complaints of weakness and easy fatigability. The myasthenic patient does not develop painful muscle cramps or distal limb weakness. The muscles most often involved early in the disease are head and neck muscles. Extrinsic ocular muscles, that is, those that move the globe of the eye, are affected in more than ninety percent of cases (9). This ocular motor involvement explains the routine complaint of double vision or blurred vision. Fatigue is involved in the disturbed functioning of these muscles as well as skeletal muscles; the patient often notices that his vision deteriorates after he reads for a few minutes. Speech may become more nasal or slurred as the day progresses, and the patient's posture may appear to deteriorate as the day passes because of a progressive head droop (10).

Myasthenia gravis is a neuromuscular disorder only affecting voluntary muscles. Swallowing may be impaired, but only because the initial third of the esophagus has voluntary skeletal muscle. The involuntary lower part of the esophagus functions normally. Heart muscle is never affected, and bladder and bowel function are intact. The fundamental defect in the involved muscles is a reduction of available acetylcholine receptors on the muscle at the neuromuscular junction (8). Acetylcholine triggers the shift in ions at the neuromuscular junction that initiates the muscle contraction. The damage to the acetylcholine receptors is caused by an autoimmune disorder that involves the production of antireceptor antibodies in most, if not all, myasthenic patients (8,9).

The diagnosis is usually established by an edrophonium test and electromyographic studies. Edrophonium inhibits the enzyme cholinesterase that destroys acetylcholine at the neuromuscular junction. By inhibiting this enzyme, the edrophonium allows excess acetylcholine to accumulate at the neuromuscular junction and act on the damaged receptors. If myasthenia is responsible for the weakness, most patients will transiently become stronger when they are given intravenous edrophonium. The response lasts only a few seconds or minutes, but, if the response is dramatic, the diagnosis is established. Some patients with myasthenia gravis have ambiguous or negative edrophonium tests. To help establish the diagnosis, electrical activity in a skeletal muscle can be recorded while the nerve to that muscle is repetitively stimulated. The action potential of the muscle will rapidly decline to 70 or 80 percent of the initial voltage with this repetitive stimulation. If both of these tests are equivocal, more dangerous investigations are available for establishing the diagnosis. The simplest and most commonly performed is the curare test, in which a minute dose of curare is injected into the patient. The dose is calculated to be well below that which should cause any weakness in normal individuals. Because curare acts to block the acetylcholine receptor at the neuromuscular junction, patients with myasthenia gravis are extremely sensitive to the drug. Even a minute dose of curare given to a myasthenic patient will cause a substantial increase in weakness.

The treatment of myasthenia gravis has evolved steadily over the past 2 decades (10). Drugs to block the breakdown of acetylcholine at the neuromuscular junction were in clinical use even before the physiologic block was recognized to be on the muscle side of the junction. Corticosteroids were initially abandoned in treatment regimens when it was observed that patients became weaker when they were started on these drugs, but over the past few years the usefulness of long-term steroids in the treatment of myasthenia has been well established. The early observation that about 10 percent of patients with myasthenia gravis had thymic tumors led to investigations of this organ in all patients with myasthenia (8). Seventy-five percent of patients with myasthenia gravis have abnormal thymic glands, and, although the relationship between thymic disorders and myasthenia gravis is still controversial, there is general agreement that thymectomy is a valuable and relatively safe adjunct to the treatment of myasthenia (10). Thymectomy plays a major role in reducing the severity of the neuromuscular disease years after weakness first appears.

Rare diseases resemble myasthenia gravis clinically and must be considered in any patient under investigation for neuromuscular disease. Poisons can produce a myasthenic picture; but, unless foul play is involved, ingestion of the poison is usually reported in the clinical history. Botulism poisoning can occasionally mimic a severe myasthenic crisis, and so the patient and family must be questioned regarding food habits (10). Improper canning techniques are usually responsible for development of the responsible bacteria in preserved foods. The most common causes of myasthenic syndromes are tick paralysis and Eaton-Lambert syndrome. Tick paralysis is nothing more than poisoning by a tick that has burrowed into the victim's skin and discharged a toxin. Children occasionally pick these ticks up from their pets, and a careful search of all surfaces must be performed on any child with progressive weakness. Eaton-Lambert syndrome is a myasthenic syndrome associated with neoplasms, especially with carcinomas of the lung. The victims of this disease are usually older than the typical myasthenic patient at onset of the illness, and the electromyographic pattern found on repetitive stimulation of the muscle is dramatically different from that observed in myasthenia gravis. The action potential of the stimulated muscle increases in amplitude by three- to fourfold when rapid stimulation rates are used. Treatment of Eaton-Lambert syndrome is generally directed toward treatment of the underlying carcinoma.

Myopathies

Weakness may develop from disease of the muscle itself. Indications that the patient's problem is a myopathy, that is, an intrinsic disease of the muscle, include muscle tenderness, painful cramps, muscle swelling, and discolored urine. Inflammatory disease of the muscle usually causes muscle swelling and tenderness; this polymyositis is most commonly from parasites on a worldwide basis, but in the United States idiopathic disease is the usual cause (Figure 11.2). Parasites, such as *Taenia solium*, the organism responsible for cystecercosis, occasionally produce calcifications in the damaged muscle, a structural change that helps in the identification of the inflammatory basis for the muscle disease. Idiopathic myositis often shares features with the collagen vascular diseases. Generalized weakness may precede all other symptoms by weeks or months, and recognition of the specific type of myositis exhibited by the patient may necessarily wait several months before the evolution of the disease reveals the precise nature of the disease. The appearance of a violaceous discoloration about the eyes (heliotrope rash) will define the muscle disease as dermatomyositis. Longstanding Raynaud's phenomenon and newly appearing tightening of facial skin indicate scleroderma, another collagen vascular disease, as the basic process.

Sarcoidosis, a multisystem inflammatory disease characterized by non-caseating granulomas in many different organs, occasionally produces chronic fatigue and weakness on the basis of skeletal muscle damage (11). Women are more often affected by this myositis than are men, but an hysterical conversion reaction is rarely suspected, because of the proximal weakness and muscle tenderness that suggest a myopathy. The women

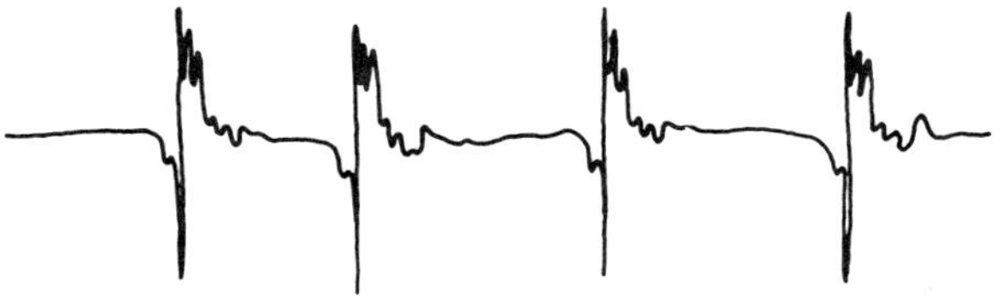

Figure 11.2. These bizarre, repetitive, spontaneous discharges from a resting muscle are called pseudomyotonic discharges. This type of involuntary muscle activity is usually seen on the electromyographic recording from a patient with polymyositis or other primary muscle disease.

usually developing a sarcoid myopathy are elderly, the mean age of presentation being 65 years (11). If a psychiatric problem is suspected in a woman suffering from this myopathy, it is usually endogenous depression. This affective disorder can cause chronic weakness and easy fatigability. An electromyogram will help establish the organic basis for the symptoms, by revealing electrical activity consistent with primary muscle damage (11). A muscle biopsy with demonstration of the granulomas in the muscle is the only reliable way to prove the diagnosis. Establishing the diagnosis is important primarily to spare the patient further investigations. Corticosteroids have been used to treat this muscle disease, but the results of treatment have been fairly inconsistent (11).

Middle-aged or elderly men developing diffuse muscle pain and stiffness, chronic fatigue, and some muscle tenderness may have polymyalgia rheumatica, an inflammatory disorder histologically similar to temporal arteritis (12). Men with this disorder are often treated for depression before the organic character of their complaints is recognized. Most of the pain and stiffness suffered by these individuals involves the proximal musculature, especially about the hip girdle. After the symptoms have been present for several months, muscle wasting may occur (13). An obvious depression does develop in many victims of the disease, a symptom which may delay recognition of the primary process (13). This is caused by a giant cell arteritis, and its onset may be either insidious or abrupt. Biopsy of the temporal artery will reveal inflammatory changes indistinguishable from those of temporal arteritis in half the patients suffering from polymyalgia rheumatica (12). As in temporal arteritis, the erythrocyte sedimentation rate will be markedly elevated. The active disease usually lasts months to years, and it will remit spontaneously if it is left untreated. The profound discomfort experienced by the patient militates against leaving this disease untreated. Corticosteroids dramatically relieve the symptoms of the disease and may prevent vascular complications of the polymyalgia rheumatica, such as cranial artery occlusions.

Metabolic problems can cause weakness with no apparent structural changes in the muscles. Severely depressed serum potassium levels will produce a muscle dysfunction severe enough to leave the patient paralyzed until the electrolyte abnormality is corrected (14). Such profound hypokalemia is usually the result of kidney disease. Patients with hepatolenticular degeneration (Wilson disease) often develop renal tubular acidosis, a metabolic problem associated with severe hypokalemia. This is of some relevance to the psychiatrist since patients with hepatolenticular degeneration frequently present with psychotic behavior as the earliest sign of their brain disease. This is usually a depressive psychosis, occasionally with suicide attempts; and so when a severely depressed patient develops generalized weakness that is associated with a low serum potassium, Wilson disease should be considered. Some patients with recurrent episodes of generalized weakness have spontaneous remissions without any therapy to correct their hypokalemia. Obviously, patients with this "periodic paralysis" are not extensively investigated because the weakness clears as inexplicably as it begins. The underlying hypokalemia is unrecognized unless electrolyte studies are obtained at the time of the weakness. This explains why most patients with hypokalemic periodic paralysis are presumed to have a conversion reaction and are referred for psychiatric evaluation (14). Periodic paralysis also occurs with transiently elevated serum potassium concentrations, but this is a much rarer disorder than hypokalemic periodic paralysis.

Thyroid disease can also cause generalized weakness, but precisely how this occurs is controversial (15). In some cases, the thyrotoxic patient will have transient changes in serum potassium levels and develop a hypokalemic periodic paralysis. Attacks of weakness with this periodic paralysis last minutes to days, and proximal limb muscles are usually more affected than distal muscles (15). Because there is high correlation between the development of myasthenia gravis and the occurrence of hyperthyroidism, any patient with weakness and apparent thyroid disease should be evaluated for myasthenia gravis (9). Presumably, these two disorders coexist so commonly because they both develop from autoimmune disorders. Thyroid disease alone can also produce weakness, whether the thyroid is hyperactive or hypoactive.

Several hereditary disorders cause weakness and muscle cramps in association with few or no other neurologic signs (16–18). Patients with these hereditary myopathies may have weakness from childhood that remains fairly stable or progresses during early adult life. Symptoms often include painful muscle cramps with relatively mild exertion and discolored urine after exercise. The change in the color of the urine is from myoglobin released from damaged muscle fibers; this protein has a brownish color. Some of the more common hereditary myopathies involve metabolic blocks in the handling of glycogen, a carbohydrate used to fuel muscle activity. Two of the better understood hereditary myopathies are McArdle disease and phosphofructokinase deficiency (17,19).

McArdle disease is a defect in muscle phosphorylase deficiency, an enzyme critical to glycogen metabolism (18). Patients with this disorder complain of pain and weakness with light activity. Chewing and talking can cause a dull, aching pain in the jaw, and more strenuous activity will routinely produce myoglobinuria. The discomfort and weakness increase when the patient is depressed, and so the disease can be easily misconstrued as functional. Electrical studies and routine muscle biopsy may reveal little abnormality, another factor leading to misdiagnosis of these patients (19). Enzyme studies on the muscle will reveal the defect.

Phosphofructokinase deficiency is clinically identical to McArdle disease. Patients with this disorder have lifelong weakness, muscle cramps, exercise intolerance, contractures following ischemic exercise, and episodic myoglobinuria (17). Eye movements and swallowing are not affected. Without special enzyme studies on a muscle biopsy, the diagnosis is easily missed. A glycogen metabolism disorder that is more easily diagnosed is acid maltase deficiency, in which case there is obvious accumulation of glycogen in the muscle fibers (17). All of these glycogen metabolic disorders are suggested by a failure to increase serum lactate levels when the patient does exercise with a limb that has decreased blood flow to it. This ischemic exercise test will produce marked increases in serum lactate in normal individuals, because lactate is the breakdown product in the metabolism of carbohydrate when oxygen is not available for other metabolic pathways (17).

Neuropathies

Disease of the nerves proximal to the neuromuscular junction can also produce weakness. Neuropathies rarely produce weakness independent of sensory deficits, but damage to the nerve must be considered in any patient with progressive weakness. Lead poisoning is one of the rare situations in which peripheral nerve disease causes a strictly motor deficit, but even with this poison peripheral neuropathy is a major problem in relatively few affected individuals.

That peripheral nerve damage is responsible for the weakness will be suggested by the absence of tendon reflexes. Tendon reflexes are preserved in neuromuscular junction disorders and myopathies. Unfortunately, many normal individuals have absent deep tendon reflexes. An electromyogram and nerve conduction study will establish that nerve damage is responsible for the disordered strength. A nerve biopsy may provide a specific diagnosis.

Peripheral neuropathy often produces focal weakness, rather than generalized weakness. Compression of the median nerve in the carpal tunnel of the wrist will produce wasting and weakness of some of the intrinsic muscles of the hand. Lead poisoning often produces a wrist-drop in adults exposed to the toxin as part of their work. Traumatic damage to the deep peroneal nerve at the head of the fibula produces a foot-drop. Many systemic diseases, such as amyloidosis, hypothyroidism, leprosy, diabetes mellitus, and systemic lupus erythematosus, may produce focal or diffuse neuropathy, but sensory disturbances accompany the motor deficits in virtually all of these. The treatment of the neuropathy is determined by the underlying disease responsible for the nerve damage.

Guillain-Barré Syndrome

Progressive paralysis that starts in the legs and subsequently involves the arms, the face, and the diaphragm is often from the Guillain-Barré syndrome (20). By the time the patient stops breathing, there is little doubt that an organic lesion is responsible for the weakness. Most of the diagnostic difficulties occur early in the evolution of signs and symptoms. The patient may have little more than generalized weakness or difficulty walking. The gait disturbance assumes no characteristic pattern, and the erratic, inconsistent gait that develops is easily confused with the astasia abasia of hysteria. Because the weakness progresses to its most severe stage within 2 to 3 weeks of the appearance of any symptoms, the authenticity of the problem is not in doubt for long.

Although this disorder is called a polyradiculopathy, that is, a disorder of the spinal nerve roots, it involves the peripheral nerves, the spinal roots, and the spinal cord (Figure 11.3). The signs and symptoms are almost exclusively limited to problems with strength. Patients occasionally have pins and needles or pain about their ankles at the onset of the disease, but prominent sensory abnormalities are characteristically absent. The autonomic nervous system is involved to some extent, causing a rapid heart beat and mild elevation of blood pressure in most severely affected patients. Patients usually have respiratory infections preceding the paralysis by several days or weeks, but at the time of the progressive weakness the patient will have no fever or other evidence of infection. The cause or causes of Guillain-Barré syndrome are unknown.

In its most severe form, this disorder interferes with breathing. The patient may require assisted ventilation for days or weeks before his diaphragm exhibits enough voluntary movement to sustain effective breathing. Facial strength, swallowing, and speech are all invariably impaired, but eye movements are rarely affected despite the significant involvement of other cranial nerves. Bladder function is also spared, and so the patient has the unlikely combination of paraplegia or quadriplegia with good bladder control. Tendon reflexes are impaired or lost.

The diagnosis is fairly certain if the cerebrospinal fluid has a markedly elevated protein content with little or no increase in the number of white blood cells. This so-called cytoalbuminemic dissociation was useful in differentiating the syndrome from poliomyelitis when that disease was common in the United States. Poliomyelitis produces a cerebrospinal fluid

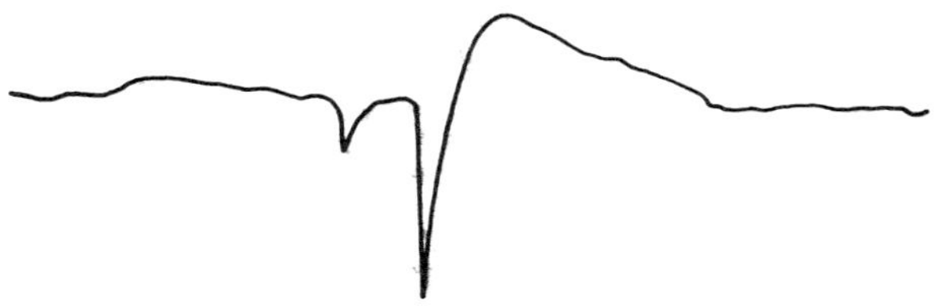

Figure 11.3. This abnormal muscle potential was recorded from a patient with denervation. The sharp downward deflection followed by a long upright wave is called a positive wave because the electromyograph is designed so that positive voltage changes are registered as downward deflections. This kind of electrical activity often appears in weakness from spinal cord or spinal root disease.

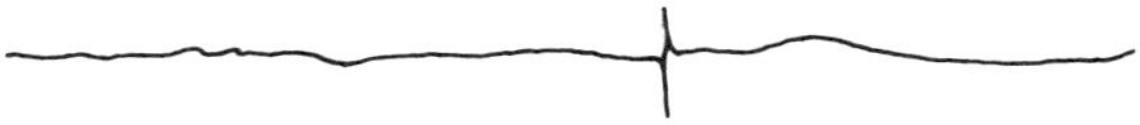

Figure 11.4. This low-voltage, short-duration potential recorded from a limb muscle is a typical fibrillation. The entire potential consists of a brief downward deflection, followed by an equally brief upward deflection. Fibrillations usually indicate anterior horn cell disease. Finding fibrillations in a middle-aged man with progressive weakness suggests amyotrophic lateral sclerosis.

profile more characteristic of a meningoencephalitis with a mildly elevated protein associated with a markedly elevated white blood cell count. Nerve conduction studies performed when the Guillain-Barré syndrome is at its worst will be abnormal. The markedly elevated cerebrospinal fluid protein occasionally produces a hydrocephalus, presumably by partly obstructing flow, and this increase in ventricle size can be easily seen on computed tomography of the head if it is present.

All deficits subside to varying extents over the course of several weeks or months. The first deficits to appear are usually the last to subside, and occasionally the weakness initially appearing with the illness does not resolve. Victims of this disease may be left with paraparesis. High dose corticosteroids have been used in many therapeutic trials, but these drugs have shown no consistent effect on the deficits. The best treatment currently available for this disorder is intensive respiratory care.

Amyotrophic Lateral Sclerosis

Degenerative disease of the motor neurons in the brain or in the spinal cord will produce progressive weakness that usually causes premature death. If there is evidence of both anterior horn cell disease and corticospinal tract disease, the condition is called amyotrophic lateral sclerosis and is usually fatal within months or a few years. Because the anterior horn cell of the spinal cord is the lower end of the motor system, disease of these cells alone is called lower motor neuron disease. Lower motor neuron disease generally causes death more quickly than upper motor neuron disease. The upper motor neurons are responsible for the integrity of the corticospinal tracts, and diseases in this system usually produce severe spasticity, as well as weakness.

Patients with amyotrophic lateral sclerosis often notice fine twitching or writhing movements in the weak muscles. This involuntary muscle activity is called a fasciculation; it represents the contraction of one motor unit, that is, the contraction of all the muscle fibers innervated by a single nerve fiber. These gross muscle phenomena are thought to indicate aberrant discharges by sick anterior horn cells. Progressive anterior horn cell disease is most consistently associated with small, abnormal muscle potentials, called fibrillations, appearing in resting muscles (Figure 11.4). No subcutaneous

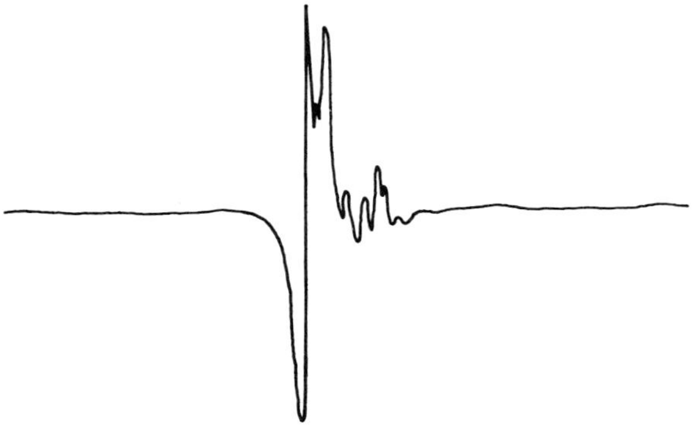

Figure 11.5. The patient exhibiting this polyphasic, long-duration, voluntary motor potential had chronic lower motor neuron disease.

movement appears with the fibrillation potential. With more chronic spinal cord disease, a variety of abnormal muscle potentials will appear on the electromyogram (Figure 11.5).

This kind of degenerative disease causes few psychiatric phenomena other than labile affect and depression. The labile affect is often associated with dysarthria and is called pseudobulbar palsy. The victim of this emotional incontinence has excessive emotional displays, such as laughing and crying, without the feelings normally triggering these displays. Depression develops as a reaction to the progressive disability and lethal character of the disease.

SPASTICITY

Changes in tone often accompany changes in strength. If weakness is from damage to a peripheral nerve, the affected muscles will have decreased tone. This flaccid weakness can also develop with damage to the spinal cord or to motor pathways coming from the brain, but an even more common pattern of weakness developing with a lesion in the motor sytem above the level of the anterior horn cell is spastic weakness. The patient may have no voluntary movement in the weak limb, but the tone in the limb is so greatly increased that it often cannot be moved passively. Moving the limb slowly will produce less resistance to movement, but in some patients the degree of spasticity is so great that even the slowest manipulation of the limb will produce no change in the position of the limb.

Spasticity develops with strokes, brain tumors, demyelinating disease, degenerative diseases, trauma, and a variety of other central nervous system problems. Occasional patients have severe spasticity with relatively mild weakness. Leg pain developing at rest may be an early sign of

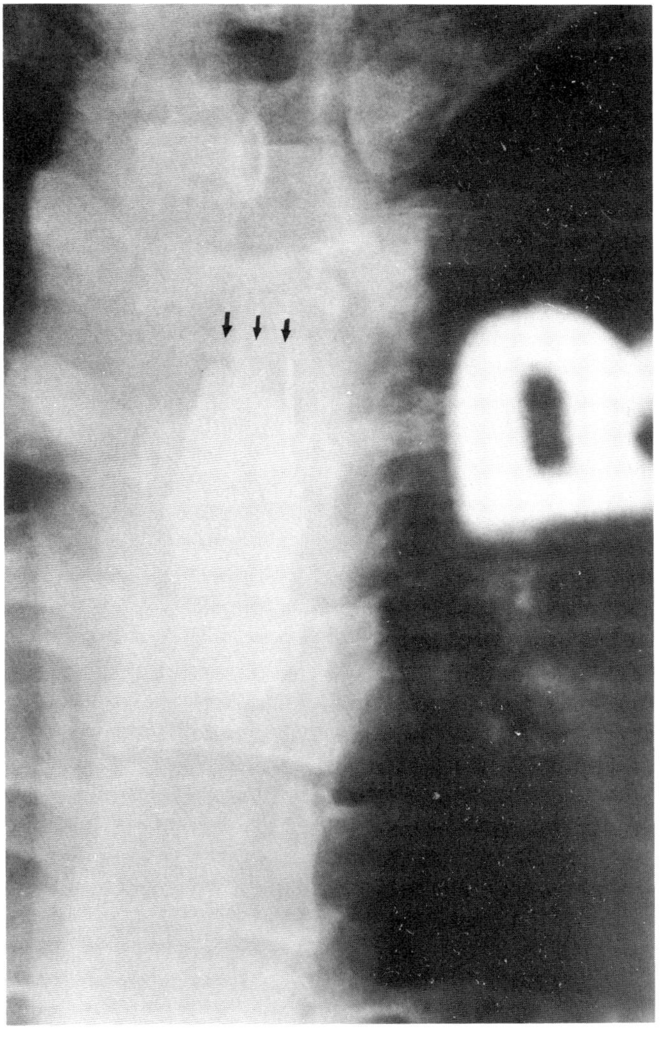

Figure 11.6. This myelogram shows a complete extradural block (arrows) at the level of the fourth thoracic vertebra in this 29-year-old woman with metastatic stromal uterine sarcoma. She complained of a rapidly progressive paraplegia. The spinal cord compression resulting from this kind of lesion will usually interfere with normal bladder and bowel function, but patients occasionally have weakness limited to the legs. The subarachnoid dye at the level of the block has a typical "paintbrush" appearance routinely seen with obstruction from a mass outside the spinal cord.

spasticity, and changes in gait may be obvious before even the patient realizes that there is a problem. Spasticity is often a sign of a progressive central nervous system disease, and its basis should be clearly established before the patient is told to live with the problem. Physicians often dismiss progressive spasticity as multiple sclerosis even though this is an exceedingly unusual pattern for the motor deficits appearing with multiple sclerosis

Investigations of the head and spine are appropriate in most cases of spasticity. If an electromyogram reveals widespread fibrillations in a middle-aged man with progressive spasticity and weakness, the diagnosis is almost certainly amyotrophic lateral sclerosis; but, even in this situation, a myelogram to study the spinal cord and foramen magnum is essential to rule out a treatable lesion below the level of the brain (Figure 11.6). Intracranial lesions are best seen with computed tomography of the head.

Spasticity is a chronic problem for many patients. There are several drugs available, including baclofen, dantrolene, and deanol, that often decrease the severity of spasticity, but this provides little help for many patients who discover that without the spasticity their limbs are too unstable because of the underlying weakness to be of much use. The victim of multiple sclerosis who had a spastic gait while off all medication may be unable to walk at all while on antispasticity drugs. Patients with chronic limb pains may profit from use of these drugs if the strength in their limbs is substantial despite the spasticity.

REFERENCES

1. Beal MF, Williams RS, Richardson EP Jr, et al: Cholesterol embolism as a cause of transient ischemic attacks and cerebral infarction. *Neurology (NY)* 31:860, 1981.
2. Toole JF, Yuson CP, Janeway R, et al: Transient ischemic attacks: A prospective study of 225 patients. *Neurology (NY)* 28:746, 1978.
3. Cartlidge NEF, Whisnant JP: Carotid and vertebral-basilar transient cerebral ischemic attacks. *Mayo Clin Proc* 52:117, 1977.
4. Caplan LR: Occlusion of the vertebral or basilar artery. *Stroke* 10:277, 1979.
5. Naritomi H, Sakai F, Meyer JS: Pathogenesis of transient ischemic attacks within the vertebrobasilar arterial systems. *Arch Neurol* 36:121, 1979.
6. McNamara JO, Heyman A, Silver D, et al: The value of carotid endarterectomy in treating transient cerebral ischemia of the posterior circulation. *neurology (NY)* 27:682, 1977.
7. Barnett HJM: Delayed cerebral ischemic episodes distal to occlusion of major cerebral arteries. *Neurology (NY)* 28:769, 1978.
8. Drachman DB: Myasthenia gravis (first of two parts). *N Engl J Med* 298:136, 1978.
9. Snead OC, Benton JW, Dwyer D, et al: Juvenile myasthenia gravis. *Neurology (NY)* 30:732, 1980.

10. Engel WK, Festoff BW, Patten BM, et al: Myasthenia gravis. *Ann Intern Med* 81:225, 1974.
11. Gardner-Thorpe C: Muscle weakness due to sarcoid myopathy. *Neurology (NY)* 22:917, 1972.
12. Lance JW: Headache. *Neurology (NY)* 10:1, 1981.
13. Hamilton CR Jr, Shelley WM, Tumulty PA: Giant cell arteritis: Including temporal arteritis and polymyalgia rheumatica. *Medicine (Baltimore)* 50:1, 1971.
14. Webb WL Jr, Gehi M: Electrolyte and fluid imbalance: Neuropsychiatric manifestations. *Psychosomatics* 22:199, 1981.
15. Engel AG: Neuromuscular manifestations of Graves' disease. *Mayo Clin Proc* 47:919, 1972.
16. Lazaro RP, Rolinson RD, Fenichel GM: Familial cramps and muscle pain. *Arch Neurol* 38:22, 1981.
17. Layzer RB, Rowland LP, Ranney HM: Muscle phosphofructokinase deficiency. *Arch Neurol* 17:512, 1967.
18. Rowland LP, Fahn S, Schotland DL: McArdle's disease. *Arch Neurol* 9:325, 1963.
19. McArdle B: Myopathy due to a defect in muscle glycogen breakdown. *Clin Sci* 10:13, 1951.
20. Guillain G, Barré JA, Strohl A: Sur un syndrome de radiculonévrite avec hyperalbuminose du liquide céphalo-rachidien sans reaction cellulaire. Remarques sur les caractères cliniques et graphiques des réflexes tendineux. *Bull Mém Soc Méd Hôpital Paris* 40:1462, 1916.

12 Sensory Abnormalities

Sensation is the most subjective of all neurologic functions. When a patient complains of pain, loss of sensitivity, or abnormal sensation, the existence of his problem and the extent of his problem are established by his complaints alone. Objective signs will substantiate the complaints infrequently, but, when these objective signs occur, they are usually quite dramatic. A patient with total loss of feeling in his feet may develop ulcers that penetrate to the bone in the anesthetic areas. Chronic complaints of low back pain radiating down one leg may be accompanied by progressive wasting of the calf muscles. Of course, the subjective elements of the sensory complaint are important. The pattern of pain or impaired sensation that the patient describes is often helpful in establishing whether or not there is a structural basis for the complaint, as well as what the structural basis is. Impaired sensation conforming precisely to a dermatomal pattern is too complicated to be contrived or hysterical, and a sensory disturbance with that pattern indicates that there is a lesion of the spinal root, rather than the peripheral nerve. Unfortunately, some of the most distressing disorders of sensation, such as the pain developing with lumbar disc disease, may never evolve into a distinctive pattern or be accompanied by power and coordination problems. In such instances, familiarity with the patient's personality and circumstances is more valuable than consistent neurologic signs in deciding what course of investigation and treatment to pursue.

PAIN

Pain is an unpleasant sensation, which often, but not invariably, signals an injury to some part of the body and directs the victim's attention to that injured part. Much more is involved in the experience of pain than the simple registration of a noxious stimulus by receptors that relay the information to the brain along sensory nerves and tracts. Sensory receptors certainly play a role in the perception of destructive or dangerous stimuli, but the information they provide is modified by both psychologic and physiologic factors that enhance or minimize the experience of pain. Precisely how pain is perceived and processed by the nervous system is still controversial (1,2). Melzack and Wall's brilliant "gate theory" of pain inspired considerable research into central nervous system mechanisms for registering noxious stimuli, but it did not explain many of the phenomena uncovered by the research it prompted (1). What can be said of pain is that it reflects more a body state than a focal condition. It is more akin to hunger or thirst as a sensory phenomenon than to vision or hearing (2). Pain impels the body to take some action to terminate the sensation. If the noxious stimulus is a lion gnawing at one's leg, the appropriate course for minimizing the intensity and duration of the pain is obvious: the lion's jaws must be disengaged from the leg. If the source of the pain is not at all obvious, as is often the case with chronic low back pain, seeking the correct course for abrogating the pain may become the focus of all the patient's activities (2).

Abnormal Sensations Interpreted as Pain

Dysesthesia is the neurologic term for the discomforting sensation experienced by the patient who complains of pain arising from a specific area of the body. The unpleasant sensation is usually elicited by irritation of or contact with the troublesome part, but dysesthesias may arise spontaneously. If the skin is unduly sensitive to minor stimuli, it is called hyperpathic. With hyperpathia, there is usually a slight delay between the application of the stimulus and the appearance of the pain. Once the pain develops, it is excessive, protracted, and relatively independent of the initial stimulus (3). Peripheral nerve disease, such as that developing with thiamine deficiency, commonly produces hyperpathia. The stimulus provoking the pain need not be noxious if a peripheral neuropathy is responsible for the hyperpathia. Stroking the bottom of the foot with a feather can elicit an intolerable burning sensation in the alcoholic patient with vitamin-deficiency neuropathy. Hyperpathia can develop with lesions in the central or peripheral nervous system, with neuronal destruction or demyelination (3). Multiple sclerosis, nerve root compression, limb amputation, arachnoiditis, midbrain infarction, and carcinomatous invasion of a peripheral nerve can all produce hyperpathia (3).

Abnormal sensations are not necessarily painful, but chronic abnormal sensations will often be described as a pain (Table 12.1). Total loss of sensation over part of the face is quite uncomfortable; and patients who have trigeminal nerve destruction to relieve the pain of trigeminal neuralgia (tic douloureux) frequently report that the anesthesia developing with the nerve destruction (anesthesia dolorosa) is worse than the pain experienced before treatment was attempted. Paresthesia is the pins-and-

Table 12.1. Sensory Abnormalities

Type	*Symptoms*
Anesthesia	Loss of all sensory modalities
Hypesthesia	Impaired perception of pain and touch
Paresthesia	Pins-and-needles sensation
Dysesthesia	Pain with all kinds of stimuli
Hyperpathia	Delayed, protracted pain with tactile stimuli

needles sensation commonly experienced when an individual inadvertently compresses a nerve. The affected limb or body surface is usually described as being "asleep." Paresthesias are annoying when they are transient, but if they persist the affected individual will complain of them as a 'pain' or intolerable sensation. Patients with meralgia paresthetica, a peripheral nerve disorder associated with paresthesias over the upper outer thigh that may last months, occasionally demand a nerve block to end the constant paresthesias they feel.

The variety of terms used by patients to describe their pain reflects the diversity of the sensations that can be intolerably distracting and discomforting. Some pain syndromes involve two or more distinct types of pain. A patient with lumbar disc disease may have a chronic dull ache in the small of the back, as well as a stiff drawing sensation in the muscles of one leg, which is periodically interrupted by transient sharp or electrical sensations that shoot down the back of the leg. With the form of neurosyphilis called tabes dorsalis, the patient has electric shocklike pains radiating down the legs, as well as paresthesias and loss of pain perception in the ankle joints (4). The varieties of head and facial pain are so extensive that they are discussed in a separate chapter.

Factors Influencing the Intensity of Pain

The perception of pain is influenced by several factors that include: (*1*) the attention given the pain, (*2*) the degree of associated anxiety, (*3*) the degree of associated depression, (*4*) the secondary gain derived from the suffering, and (*5*) the cultural tolerance of individuals who expand upon the discomfort they are experiencing (5). An individual faced with a direct threat to his life is less likely to have severe pain associated with an injury than is the individual faced with no persistent danger after the injury is inflicted. If the victim of the pain is aware of the cause and the implications of the pain he is perceiving and recognizes that he is not in grave danger, he will also experience less pain. Obviously, if enduring the pain spares the individual from participating in something more disagreeable than the pain, the victim of the sensory disturbance will be plagued by the discomfort for a longer time than he would be if resolution of the pain led to an unequivocal improvement in his life. Where social mores discourage the exhibition of pain and encourage more stoic approaches to the discomfort, the duration of the complaint is likely to be shorter than in societies where excessive sympathy and special privileges are accorded the pain victim.

Phases of Pain

There are at least three distinct phases of pain, immediate, acute, and chronic (2). In the immediate phase, the stimulus directs defensive activities. When the pain is registered, the individual will try to escape the noxious element or ward it off by fighting back. Conscious perception of the pain may be quite limited, but the activity it motivates is apparent. Acute pain develops as the patient attends to protecting the injured element. Anxiety is invariably a prominent element in acute pain as the victim assesses the damage done and considers various options for recovery (2). Chronic pain directs the patient's behavior to allow a rapid and complete recovery from the injury. Clearly, there are many instances in which recovery from the injury is not at all likely, either because the nature of the injury is obscure or the patient's disease is progressive. In these open-ended situations, the pain becomes intractable (2).

Depression and lassitude are common with chronic pain. The affected individual becomes obsessed with his condition and seeks one solution after another. The more obscure the cause of his pain, the more protracted and all-consuming will be the search for a solution (2). The intensity of the pain does not correlate with the degree of disability or even with the apparent suffering experienced by the patient (6). How a patient suffers and to what extent he appears to suffer is affected by secondary gain in many cases. Financial compensation, drug dependency, and work avoidance play major roles in the suffering of many chronic pain victims (6). When structural, inflammatory, or metabolic problems are clearly the basis for the discomfort, treatment is greatly simplified. Curing or treating the primary disease often reverses or palliates the associated pain. When the disease is not treatable, as is often the case with metastatic cancers, narcotic analgesics are a reasonable treatment option for relieving the intractable pain. Treatment is considerably more complicated and difficult when the patient has no organic lesion responsible for the chronic discomfort.

Chronic pain is, occasionally, the presenting complaint in patients with unrecognized depression (7). The pain provides a distracting issue for both the patient and his or her family. Marital maladjustment and problems in assuming responsibility in the family may be obscured by the undiagnosable complaint (8). All efforts at treating the problem fail or produce even more pain. The chronic pain endured by one member of the family becomes a scapegoat for the entire family; which member of the family develops the problem and assumes the sick role often seems arbitrary (8).

Failure and frustration are routinely tied to the pain problem. Sexual problems develop between marital partners in most conditions involving chronic pain, but this is especially true when the chronic pain has no apparent organic basis (8). The family consensus is that if the pain could be eliminated there would be no problems for the sufferer and for those burdened by him. Pain tolerance, the manner in which the pain appears, the pattern complaints about the pain assume, and the behavior exhibited by the victim of the pain are determined, at least in part, by the concurrent behavior of the family and by past family experiences (7). There is a higher incidence of chronic pain problems in the relatives and spouses of chronic pain sufferers with depression than in the relatives and spouses of depressed patients not complaining of somatic pain (7). Even the location of the chronic pain is remarkably consistent for each family. Individuals with unexplained chronic low back pain often come from families with several other members afflicted by unexplained chronic low back pain.

Patients with acute pain are rarely referred for psychiatric evaluation unless the acute episode is one of many recurrent episodes that have been unexplained by objective deficits. It is the patient with chronic pain who is most likely to seek psychiatric help because of depression and is most likely to be referred for a psychiatric opinion to assess the possible psychological bases for the intractable pain. There is, in fact, objective evidence that individuals complaining of chronic pain more commonly have psychiatric bases for their discomfort than individuals suffering from acute pain. The Minnesota Multiphasic Personality Inventory (MMPI) scores for patients with acute pain are unremarkable, but those for patients with chronic pain have elevated hysteria, depression, and hypochondriasis scores (5). Obviously, there are many organic causes of chronic pain, but intractable pain is often the product of psychologic problems.

FOCAL PAIN SYNDROMES

The site involved by the discomfort and the evolution of sensory changes in the part of the body affected by the pain can clarify the cause of the pain. Limb pain need not have a neurologic basis, and, in fact, when it does have an organic basis it usually arises from rheumatoid, vascular, or muscular disease. When there is no obvious joint disease and blood flow through the extremity appears to be adequate but not excessive, a neuromuscular problem should be considered. Obviously, pain radiating down the left arm of an elderly man after exercise must be considered cardiac in origin until proven otherwise. A child with dull pain in the thigh that shifts to intolerably sharp pain when a single point on the bone is pressed upon should be investigated for a bone lesion, such as osteomyelitis. Pain over the trunk, with the exception of that arising in the spine, usually does not have a purely neurologic basis. Severe, burning, right-sided chest pain is not likely to be from spinal root problems, but, occasionally, the problem proves to be a radicular *Herpes zoster* infection. When there has been structural damage to the central nervous system or the peripheral nervous system, it is reasonable to assume that the pain is a sequela of the damage. Commonly encountered situations are the limb pain of peripheral neuropathy and the unilateral discomfort following thalamic infarction.

Peripheral Neuropathy

Peripheral nerve disease from diabetes mellitus, thiamine deficiency, or insecticide poisoning may all produce burning in the feet or intolerance of pressure on the surface of the legs. Such pain may be so severe that the patient cannot stand on his feet or tolerate garments touching his legs. The discomfort arising with a peripheral neuropathy occasionally can be alleviated by correcting the underlying problem. Replacing a vitamin deficient in the diet may reduce the burning pains in the limbs; identifying and eliminating a neurotoxin the patient was exposed to will allow the nerves to recover, at least partially. Unfortunately, many of the common causes of peripheral nerve damage are not so easily treated. Controlling diabetes mellitus does not reverse peripheral nerve injury, and so the pain associated with this metabolic neuropathy will persist or evolve into hypesthesia (decreased sensation). Patients with severe pain from diabetic neuropathy may get some relief with a combination of the neuroleptic fluphenazine and the antidepressant amitriptyline (9). The basis for the analgesic action of this combination is unknown. The lightninglike pains characteristic of tabes dorsalis, a form of neurosyphilis, may disappear when the patient is given carbamazepine (10). The mechanism of action of this anticonvulsant in such paroxysmal pain disorders is also unknown.

Causalgia

Burning pains in a hand or foot occasionally develop with major nerve injuries in the limbs. The nerve damaged is invariably partly intact, and the cause of the injury is often a high speed projectile (11). S. Weir Mitchell described this pain syndrome in many soldiers wounded during the Civil War and popularized the term "causalgia" to specify this post-traumatic syndrome (12,13). The burning pain is usually worst in the digits and on the palm if the arm is injured or on the sole if the leg is injured. Skin over the affected limb is exquisitely sensitive to minor stimuli. The lightest contact, changes in ambient temperature, and even loud noises may trigger paroxysms of pain in the sensitive limb (12). The dysesthesias are commonly described as deep in the arm and persistent despite the absence of a constant stimulus, and the pain is felt in the distribution of the damaged nerve. Changing the position of the limb can worsen the abnormal sensory perception (11). Despite the excessive pain, the perception of touch and pain in the area of the dysesthesias is impaired (11).

Sweating in the distribution of the pain is also abnormal. Although the skin is usually warm and moist shortly after the injury, it usually becomes scaly and cool after weeks or months (12). Much of the altered perfusion and sympathetic activity in the limb may be secondary to its relative immobility. The victim of causalgia will exert considerable effort to avoid moving the affected limb.

The etiology of causalgia is unknown. Current opinion favors a disturbance in the sympathetic nerve supply to the injured limb, which results in the transmission of sympathetic impulses intended for the distal limb to afferent pain fibers (11,12,14). This mechanism would at least help explain why emotional factors affect the severity of the pain so profoundly. Consistent with this sympathetic rerouting model is the observed improvement with sympathectomy (11). Procaine block of the sympathetic ganglia proximal to the injury may be equally effective (12).

Meralgia Paresthetica

Damage to the lateral femoral cutaneous nerve of the thigh is a common and confusing cause of paresthesias and dysesthesias (12). A hysterical conversion reaction is often suspected with this disorder because there are no objective findings and the patient complains bitterly of annoying tingling or burning over the superior anterior and lateral thigh. This lateral femoral cutaneous neuropathy is also called meralgia paresthetica. Touch and pinprick may be substantially reduced over the affected area. The knee jerk is normal and strength in all leg muscles is intact. Contributing to the impression that this is a conversion reaction is the patient's report that the discomfort subsides if he is allowed to sit. Standing and walking exacerbate the symptoms, and so the patient is inclined to be quite inactive. Eighty percent of cases are unilateral (12).

Entrapment or other types of injury to the lateral femoral cutaneous nerve cause meralgia paresthetica. It usually occurs in the setting of obesity, pregnancy, or diabetes mellitus. The dysesthesias will resolve on their own if left untreated for weeks or months. A nerve block of the lateral femoral cutaneous nerve will relieve the dysesthesias in patients with disabling pain.

Shoulder-Hand Syndrome

Chronic pain similar to causalgia appears in patients with immobilizing injuries to a limb and with diseases that produce pain in a limb even though it is not injured (14,15). Cervical spine disease pressing on spinal roots to the arm and myocardial infarction with referred pain to the left arm can produce this idiopathic syndrome. The pain that develops with immobilization of the uncomfortable limb persists long after the initial limb injury or discomfort subsides. This differs from causalgia in that the patient has no apparent nerve injury in the limb affected by the chronic pain. A problem in sympathetic nerve function develops with this syndrome, and, consequently, it is often referred to as reflex sympathetic dystrophy or the shoulder-hand syndrome (14).

Early in the evolution of symptoms vascular changes develop in the immobilized limb. Vasomotor tone is impaired, and venous congestion is prominent. The limb becomes swollen, tender, and discolored. Because of the discomfort produced by these vascular changes, the patient's reluctance to move the limb voluntarily is reinforced. In days or weeks, the skin will exhibit changes in sweating and other autonomic functions and will eventually become atrophic. Contractures develop in joints of the affected limb, and strength may be profoundly impaired. After months of disabling pain, the patient will have some resorption of bone distally in the limb.

Individuals who refuse to use a limb for purely psychologic reasons will develop the changes characteristic of the shoulder-hand syndrome, and what started as a functional complaint will evolve into an unequivocally organic problem. About one-fifth of the patients developing the shoulder-hand syndrome have no apparent cause for the initial restriction of limb movements (14,15). Once immobilization of the limb occurs, whether it is because of a wrist fracture, a myocardial infarction, or no apparent reason, the vascular changes and associated pain will progress through the characteristic stages of reflex sympathetic dystrophy in some individuals. The severity of the shoulder-hand syndrome is unrelated to the seriousness of the initiating event. Profound joint contractures can develop in patients with idiopathic dystrophy, as well as in those with trauma-related dystrophy.

Sympathetic ganglion blocks are often helpful in alleviating the pain that develops with this syndrome, but physical activity, however painful it may be initially, is the best way to reverse the signs and symptoms of this syndrome (15). The earlier the physical therapy is begun, the simpler will be the restoration of normal function to the arm or leg involved. Corticosteroids and analgesics are also very helpful in resolving the signs and symptoms of reflex sympathetic dystrophy, but the most important factor in any successful treatment is starting soon after the limb pain first appears. The pain may subside spontaneously after several months, but the vasomotor problems and subsequent joint problems will progress if the patient is not treated.

LOW BACK PAIN

Low back pain is the most common chronic pain syndrome developing in patients with no evidence of systemic disease (8). The discomfort is often an isolated symptom, in which case its validity is difficult to establish. Occasionally, the patient's description of the pain will help differentiate between the pain from strictly organic disease and that from a conversion reaction or compensation neurosis. The patient generally describes pain with a structural or inflammatory basis in consistent and specific terms (Figure 12.1). Low back pain with no demonstrable organic basis prompts the complaining patient to use vague or variable terms to convey the nature of the discomfort (16). One curious result of this descriptive dichotomy is that low back pain is described as a much more intolerable and disabling sensation by the patients exhibiting no apparent organic basis for the pain than by the patients with unequivocal structural disease (16). Patients without apparent organic disease stress the superficial and deep qualities of the pain. There is often a notable component of pain in the skin that is exacerbated by light pressure. The obvious implication is that qualitative features of the low back pain are much less important than more quantifiable features, such as the duration of the pain, the context of its onset, the pattern of pain radiation, and the periodicity of pain recurrences (16).

Low back pain can be totally disabling despite the absence of any motor or sensory deficits. There need not be a history of local trauma or strain, and the symptom may be unchanging for weeks or months. Pain resulting from a back injury may be experienced initially in the leg or buttock, rather than the back, but as the discomfort evolves most patients will complain of problems in their backs.

Compensation Neurosis

Low back pain is ideal for someone eager to appear disabled but unable to show objective deficits (8). Some patients with authentic, but minor, back injuries, fail to return to normal activity for weeks or years because of chronic pain that cannot be explained by any organic lesion. What is initially an authentic disability becomes protracted when recovery proves disadvantageous. When litigation is pending for an accident during which a back injury was sustained, the pain may show no sign of resolving until the case is settled. This is not necessarily malingering. Pressures on the patient to remain disabled may be so substantial that patients ordinarily eager to overcome any disability find they cannot rid themselves of the discomfort that has resulted in an enormous investment of time and energy. Accusing the refractory patient of malingering will not hasten the recovery, but discussing the likelihood of such a "compensation neurosis" with the patient may produce resolution of some of the symptoms.

Quite often the patient is not alone in his obsession with the disabling back discomfort. The spouse or the entire family may play an important role in reinforcing the "sick role" that the patient has assumed (7,8). Refractory back pain allows the husband and wife to avoid sexual contact, regardless of which partner is suffering from the pain. A major sexual

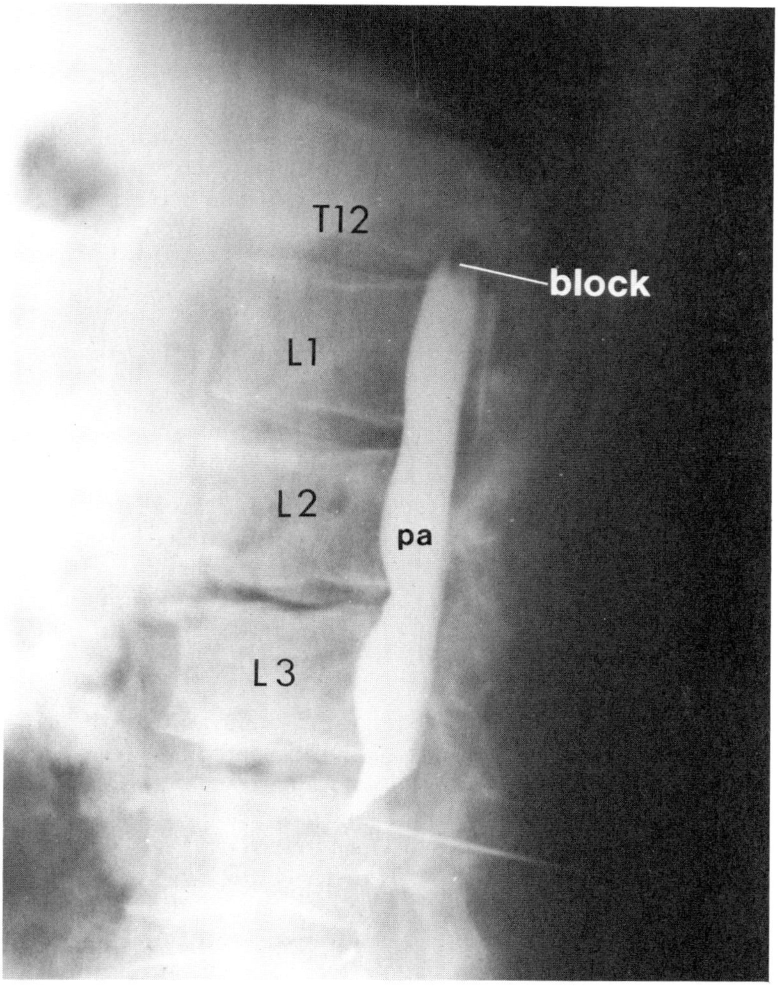

Figure 12.1. A 65-year-old man complained of back pain for about 3 weeks before this myelogram was performed. The pain radiated into his left leg, and the patient became most concerned when he developed myoclonic jerks in the legs. Bladder function was normal. The myelogram with lipid-soluble dye revealed an almost complete block at T12. The block stops the column of dye (pa) from flowing into the thoracic area. The patient was lying on his stomach with his head inclined down more than 20 degress when this film was obtained. T12, L1, L2, and L3 are labeled. The white line extending out from the back at the bottom of the photograph is the lumbar puncture needle. The extradural block was caused by a malignant growth of multiple myeloma tissue.

problem can be ignored or denied by introducing the "illness" between the reluctant sexual partners.

Ascertaining whether or not the patient has contrived pain or a conversion reaction, rather than structural disease in the back, is more than just a search for honesty. The kinds of intervention appropriate in cases of chronic back pain carry substantial risks. Refractory back pain is an acceptable reason to investigate and operate on a patient even when the back discomfort is not accompanied by any objective signs. Myelograms are routinely performed for chronic back pain complaints, and an equivocal disc herniation will justify surgery if the patient has intractable pain. A careful history and examination usually help define patients with pain from nerve compression and those with discomfort prolonged by a compensation neurosis.

Patterns of Pain with Low Back Pain Syndrome

Low back pain often results from lumbar disc disease causing spinal root compression. Alternative causes, such as degenerative arthritis of the spine or metastatic cancer, usually produce changes in the bone seen on plain spine films. Pelvic disease, especially in women, may produce severe pain referred to the lumbosacral area. Obviously every patient should have a complete physical examination, and this includes a careful gynecologic evaluation for all women with low back pain. An ovarian cyst or uterine tumor should be sought especially vigorously when the discomfort is atypical. Noninvasive studies, including ultrasonography of the pelvis, are justifiable for women with this complaint and should be utilized early in the investigation of the symptom. For those patients with diseased lumbar discs, the pain typically radiates down one leg. The path it follows and the point at which the radiating pain terminates will be dictated by the dermatome of the spinal root that is being compressed. Compression of the first sacral root (S1) will produce pain radiating down the back of the leg to the lateral aspect of the heel. Compression of the fifth lumbar root (L5) will produce pain extending into the meial malleolus or the great toe. The discomfort may be shooting or aching, but it will be fairly circumscribed. Pain from a radiculopathy will not radiate to all of the toes or progress down both the anterior and posterior aspects of the thigh.

The diagnosis of lumbar disc disease relies upon myelography. Although an electromyogram, which demonstrates denervation changes in a radicular pattern, is highly suggestive of spinal root compression, establishing compression of a lumbar or sacral spinal root requires a myelogram. With this radiographic study, an extradural mass arising in the intervertebral space is outlined by the dye placed in the subarachnoid space around the cauda equina and spinal cord. Occasionally, a mass will appear intradurally. This may be a tumor, especially if the patient has other evidence of neurofibromatosis, such as café-au-lait spots. Other tumors appearing in this region include meningiomas and ependymomas. An alternative explanation for root compression is spinal stenosis, a condition in which the spinal canal is too narrow to accommodate the spinal cord. The cord compression will obstruct the flow of the radiographic dye in the subarachnoid space.

Treatment

Myelography is a preoperative study. If the patient insists that he will refuse surgery regardless of what is found on the myelogram, this radiographic study is unjustifiable. Before myelography, patients with intractable pain are wise to try at least 2 weeks of strict bed rest in a recumbent position. Sitting propped up in bed on pillows only exacerbates the stress on the lumbar spine. Pelvic traction of 10 to 15 pounds is often helpful in limiting the patient's movements in bed. The traction does not serve to pull the vertebrae apart and reduce forces on the herniated disc, but it does reduce irritating movement of the vertebrae most likely to have the intervertebral disc herniation. If the pain persists despite 2 weeks at rest on a hard flat surface or if focal weakness or sensory loss appears, a myelogram is warranted.

Once a reasonable lesion has been identified on myelography, the surgeon can alleviate the source of root compression. Ordinarily, the lamina of the vertebra nearest the herniated disc is removed, and the herniated disc is resected. Obviously, considerable damage to the involved nerve root can develop during this procedure even in the most competent hands. A permanent foot drop or extensive sensory loss over the lower leg are risks of the procedure and are good reasons to delay surgery in a patient with a minor disc herniation that does not explain the symptoms exhibited.

Patients with no demonstrable structural lesion should be approached through a multidisciplinary program, with stress on increasing independence (6). Biofeedback, psychotherapy, occupational therapy, and family counseling all have a place in dealing with patients with unexplained low back pain. When the pain is refractory to all such reasonable intervention, the wisest course is to periodically reexamine the patient to look for an evolving lesion that was simply too small to be found when the pain began.

THALAMIC SYNDROME

Patients with pure sensory strokes, presumably on the basis of thalamic infarction, commonly have persistent pain on the side of the body exhibiting the acute sensory loss (Figure 12.2). Sensation in this thalamic syndrome may return largely to normal, but minor stimuli over the previously impaired side may elicit excruciating paroxysms of pain apparently arising from the area of contact. There will be no weakness or problem in coordination of the affected limbs (17). Infarcted brain tissue

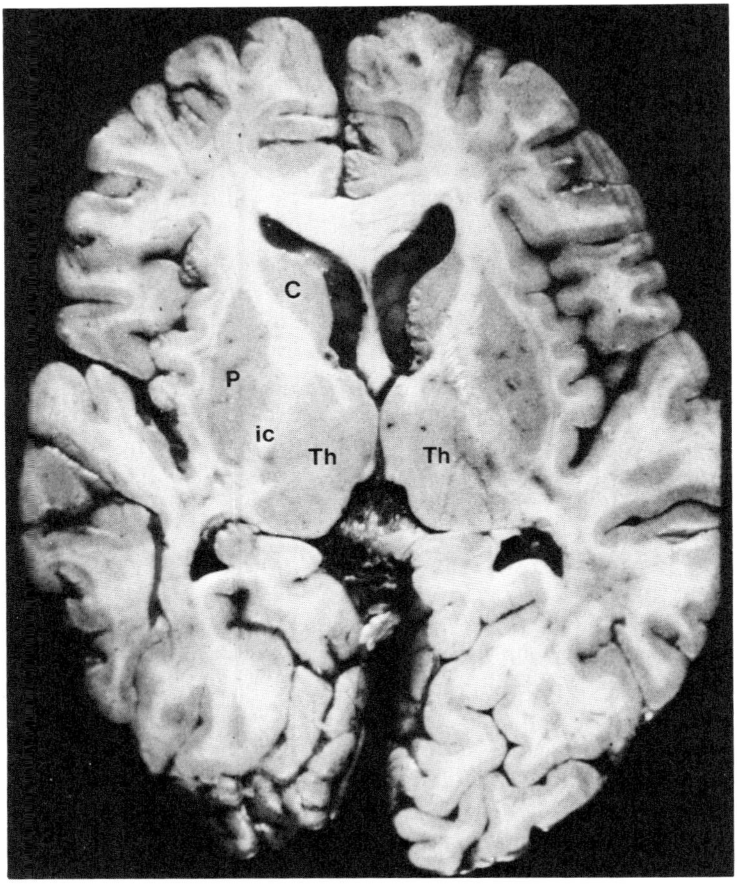

Figure 12.2. This horizontal section of a normal brain reveals the thalamic nuclei (Th) lying deep in the subcortical structures of both hemispheres. The head of the caudate nucleus (C) is anterior to the thalamus in this plane, and the thalamic nuclei are separated from the putamen (P) and, at a lower level, the globus pallidus of the basal ganglia by the internal capsule (ic). Vascular disease in the thalamus may produce a syndrome of intractable pain called the thalamic syndrome.

cannot be salvaged, but the pain of the thalamic syndrome can be dealt with symptomatically. The tricyclic antidepressant imipramine often relieves much of the discomfort without increasing the sensory impairment typical of the thalamic syndrome.

Central nervous system damage producing chronic problems with pain need not be limited to the thalamus or even to the brain. Spinal cord lesions commonly produce intractable or intermittent pain, presumably because of damage to pain fibers destined for the thalamus. Paroxysmal pains appear in some patients with multiple sclerosis. These are distinct from the electrical sensations that run up and down the spine on flexion of the neck (Lhermitte's sign), but both Lhermitte's paresthesias and the paroxysmal dysesthesias of multiple sclerosis may be abolished by carbamazepine, the anticonvulsant (10). Baclofen, a neurotransmitter agonist, may be useful in pain syndromes developing in multiple sclerosis and other disorders affecting the spinal cord (18). It certainly helps relieve the pain of flexor spasms that develop with cord injuries (18).

PHANTOM LIMB PAIN

Pain felt to be arising in a limb that has been amputated develops at least transiently in most individuals after loss of the limb (19). This phantom limb pain occurs less frequently when an arm or a leg has been denervated, rather than severed; and it occasionally develops when there has been spinal cord transection with loss of all sensory input from the limb (19). The patient complains of persistent searing or dull pain in the absent or deafferented limb and frequently will observe that the phantom limb feels as if it were abnormally large, abnormally small, or contorted (19,20). The cause of this phenomenon is unknown, but a reasonable hypothesis is that cortical images of the arm or leg are released when the brain obtains no sensory information from the absent limb (19).

This is a complex hallucination for which there is currently no good treatment. Traditional therapies have included revision of the amputation stump, sympathectomy, transcutaneous electrical stimulation, and psychotherapy. Temporary relief of the pain does occur, but none of these provides results that last more than a year or two (20). Biofeedback and relaxation techniques have been applied to this problem with allegedly better results than those obtained with other treatments (20). These methods were applied because patients developing phantom limb pain seemed to have rigid personalities with considerable resistance to accepting help. The pain and anxiety experienced by these individuals were directly related to each other. Assuming that at least part of the phantom limb pain was musculoskeletal tension induced by stress, biofeedback was used to block the musculoskeletal activity in the stump. The good results with biofeedback techniques presumably stem from the modulation of anxiety, rather than the elimination of irritation to the amputation site.

TREATMENT OF CHRONIC PAIN

Pain may persist despite the removal of an element irritating a nerve, such as a tumor pressing on a spinal root, or because of treatment that produces irreversible nerve injury, such as amputation of a limb. Treating chronic pain, whether it is from structural disease or psychiatric problems, is one of the most frustrating problems for neurologists and psychiatrists. Recently acquired insights into pain systems in the nervous system have suggested a variety of approaches to chronic pain, some of which have produced dramatic results in specific cases. The most important finding over the past few decades was the discovery of an intrinsic system for analgesia. Opiate-like substances in the central nervous system, called enkephalins and endorphins, can modulate the perception of pain (9). An endorphin mediated analgesia system, which controls pain signal transmission in the central nervous system, can be activated by exogenous opiates and nonopiate drugs, by electrical stimulation of central nervous system sites, and by a variety of peripherally acting stimuli, including acupuncture, electrical stimulation of the skin, and even placebo administration (9).

Placebo

Traditionally, a placebo has been viewed as an inactive substance given to a suggestible patient to relieve his imagined problem. This traditional view is inaccurate. Thirty-five percent of patients with structural causes of severe pain experience marked relief from the pain when they are given a placebo, that is, a medication with no intrinsic analgesic activity (9). Who will respond to the placebo is, in fact, quite unpredictable. Patients who are highly suggestible and easily hypnotized show no more consistent responses to placebo medication than other victims of chronic pain (9). Factors showing some correlation with a good response to placebo include excessive anxiety and an active basis for chronic pain (9). This means that patients with unequivocal lesion-related pain, such as that following surgery or with progressive cancer, have better placebo responses than less critically ill patients. The relief of pain is presumably activated by the central nervous system mechanisms utilizing endorphins. Naloxone, an opiate antagonist, abolishes placebo analgesia, a phenomenon consistent with the hypothesis that placebo given to a receptive patient can mobilize endogenous opioids (9).

Transcutaneous Electrical Nerve Stimulation

Stimulating a peripheral nerve by means of an electrical current transmitted transcutaneously does relieve pain, especially that associated with peripheral nerve injuries, in some patients (5,9). The theoretic bases leading to trials with transcutaneous nerve stimulation have been largely discarded and current views on this method implicate the endorphin system in the central nervous system. Naloxone, an opiate antagonist, blocks the analgesic effect of transcutaneous stimulation. The stimulation is most effective if it is applied proximal to the site of nerve injury, but it is also helpful in relieving chronic pain in patients with spinal cord injuries. Similar in effect and character is direct stimulation of the posterior columns of the spinal cord by electrodes introduced into the epidural space. This type of electrical stimulation relieves the chronic pain of some patients with causalgia, phantom limb pain, and other posttraumatic neuralgias (9). Dorsal column stimulation has many disadvantages, including decreasing effectiveness with time, increasing risk of infection, and progressive reactions to the electrodes. Some neurosurgeons have implanted electrodes directly into the brain to deal with chronic pain in terminally ill patients (9). Direct electrical stimulation of the thalamus may provide dramatic relief of the pain from central nervous system lesions or peripheral nerve injuries, but obviously this technique is appropriate in very few patients.

Acupuncture

The effects of acupuncture are similar to those of transcutaneous electrical stimulation, especially if the puncture is combined with electrical stimulation along the needle (9). Acupuncture is most effective if it is applied along the same dermatomal surface as that involved by the chronic pain. Chronic pain especially responsive to acupuncture is that from musculoskeletal damage, degenerative osteoarthritis, and several types of headache (5). The endorphin system in the brain is implicated in this technique: cerebrospinal fluid endorphin rises with acupuncture, and naloxone blocks the analgesic effect of acupuncture.

Medications for Chronic Pain

Narcotic analgesics are effective and reasonable for the chronic pain associated with metastatic cancer or other terminal illnesses. The addiction potential of these drugs limits their application in patients with painful, but curable, lesions. Intrathecal or epidural application of small doses of morphine may produce dramatic relief of severe pain, but its main disadvantage is that it requires some skill for safe application (21). The phenothiazine methotrimeprazine may be an effective analgesic despite its extrapyramidal side effects (21). The methylated tricyclic antidepressants, amitriptyline, imipramine, and doxepin, have analgesic effects especially in patients with migraine and some types of peripheral neuropathy (21). Amitriptyline combined with fluphenazine may relieve the chronic pain of postherpetic neuralgia and diabetic peripheral neuropathy (9). A combination of tricyclic antidepressants with butyrophenones may be even more effective in dealing with the hyperpathia and dysesthesias that develop with peripheral nerve injuries (22).

Biofeedback

Biofeedback provides visual or auditory cues that alert the patient to autonomic changes that he may then modify (5). This technique has been used with some success in alleviating migraine headache and controlling skeletal muscle spasm. The feedback is sometimes dependent upon electromyographic activity when the object is control of the striated muscle responses, a common objective in efforts to relieve tension. "Alpha wave training" techniques in patients monitoring their own electroencephalographic activity provide little relief from anxiety and pain, but hypnotic training has been effective against these problems. Distraction, anxiety reduction, suggestion, and sense of control all probably play roles in patients who relieve their chronic pain with self-hypnosis (5).

ANESTHESIA

Complete loss of sensation with no obvious impairment of strength or coordination in a limb is generally an hysterical symptom or a contrived complaint. The currently uncommon tabetic form of neurosyphilis could produce anesthesia in the ankle joints and lead to disorganization of the entire joint, but this cause of focal anesthesia is easily recognized by the typical pattern of joint involvement and positive serologic tests for syphilis (4). The other common organic cause of anesthesia is diabetes mellitus, but in this disease as well the anesthesia is focal, usually over the feet, and the diagnosis is easily established with fasting and postprandial blood sugars.

Spinal cord damage may produce unconventional patterns of anesthesia, but the sensory deficit with this kind of lesion is usually associated with a border zone of hyperpathia and with focal weakness. Syringomyelia, a cystic dilatation of the spinal cord, causes the most confusion because the deficits associated with this structural lesion take several different forms (Figure 12.3). Patients often discover anesthesia in their fingers or hands with this disorder only after they have burnt themselves or developed ulcers over the anesthetic areas. Weakness and wasting of the intrinsic muscles of the hands usually accompany these sensory problems, but associated problems range from ocular abnormalities to gait difficulty. The sensory impairment is described as a dissociated sensory loss, because pain and temperature perception may be completely absent while vibration and position sense are normal.

The syrinx or cyst extends several spinal cord levels in symptomatic individuals, and the fluid in the cyst will shift about as the patient's position is changed (Figure 12.4). This produces the characteristic myelographic picture of a swollen cervical cord when the patient is head down and a collapsed ribbon of spinal cord when the patient is upright. The cervical spinal cord can be seen in the collapsed state by introducing air into the subarachnoid space and allowing the air to rise by slowly tilting the prone patient upright.

Syringomyelia is usually a slowly progressive cause of anesthesia in the limbs. The patient will lose more sensation as the lesion enlarges, and focal weakness will also progress. Instilling contrast material into the cyst

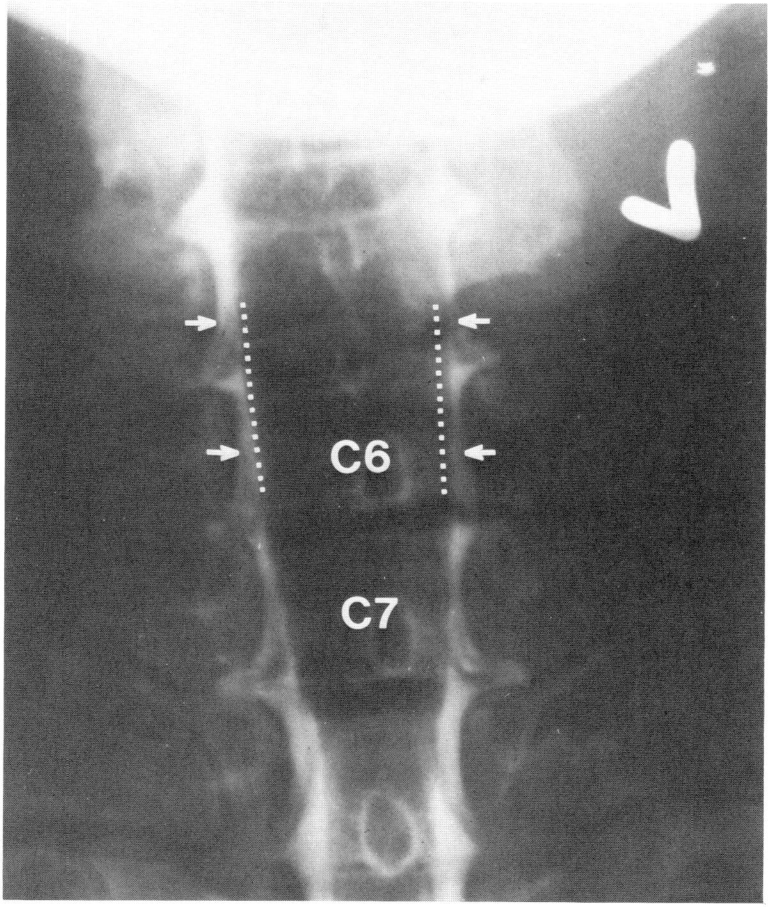

Figure 12.3. A 38-year-old woman complained of decreased sensation in her right arm and burning pain in her left hand. Because of complete loss of sensation over some fingertips, she had small burns on her fingers. Neurologic examination revealed impaired pain perception over both arms, spasticity in the left arm and leg, and an extensor plantar response on the left. This myelogram revealed a wide cervical spinal cord. An air myelogram revealed a syrinx in the cord (syringomyelia). The margins of the spinal cord are outlined by the dotted lines. The arrows indicate the limits of the subarachnoid space, delineated by the lipid-soluble dye. The sixth and seventh cervical vertebrae are labeled (C6, C7). The cyst dilating the cervical spinal cord collapsed when the patient was turned right side up; the fluid in the cyst simply shifted to a lower segment of the spinal cord.

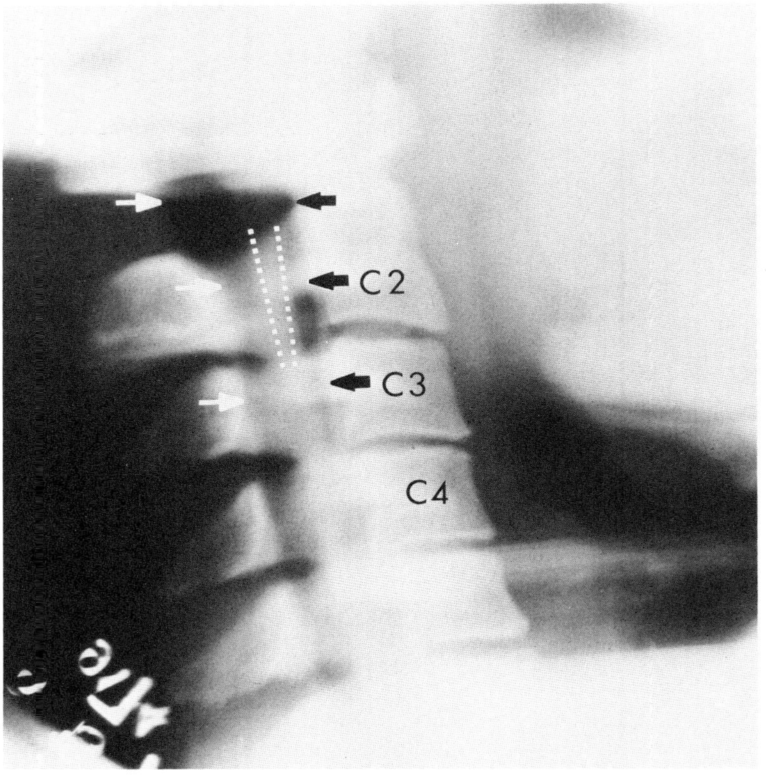

Figure 12.4. This is an air myelogram of the cervical spinal cord performed on the patient described in Figure 12.3. A thin ribbon of spinal cord was outlined by the air that rose around it as the patient was tilted into a more upright position. The cord is slightly wider than the space between the rows of white dots. The second, third, and fourth cervical vertebrae are labeled (C2, C3, C4). The column of air in the subarachnoid space is between the arrows and the outer margin of the spinal cord.

to scar the cavity or puncturing the cyst and drawing off some fluid occasionally delays the progression of the disease.

Hysterical anesthesia usually assumes nonphysiologic patterns, with the sensory deficit abiding by arbitrary anatomic boundaries, such as the midline of the body or the middle of a joint. The entire side of the body may be equally involved from the crown of the head to the foot. Even stimuli that should be transmitted across the midline, such as a vibrating tuning fork placed on one side of the frontal bone, are not perceived if they are placed on the factitiously anesthetic side of the body. Hemianesthesia on a clearly hysterical basis occurs most often on the left side of the body (23). One might speculate that this is a subconscious expression of psychologic disability by the nonverbal right cerebral hemisphere. This may cast the right hemisphere in an inappropriately mystical light, but the marked divergence between the two cerebral hemispheres in appreciating sensory disturbances when they are damaged suggests that they may evoke different perceptions of sensory integrity when they are undamaged.

IMPAIRMENT OF SPECIAL SENSORY FUNCTIONS

Damage to the nondominant cerebral hemisphere can produce disturbed perceptions of the contralateral body parts. The patient may deny paralysis of his arm; but, even more remarkably, he may deny that the arm connected to his shoulder is his. Despite only minor sensory deficits in the affected limb, he may report a stimulus on only the dominant limb when both are struck or touched simultaneously. Failing to recognize impairment on one side of the body is anosognosia. It appears with right cerebral hemisphere damage four to five times as often as with left hemisphere damage (23,24). There are numerous structural and infectious lesions which can produce anosognosia. An infarct of the nondominant hemisphere, a tumor of the right parietal lobe, or even a Herpes simplex encephalitis with considerable nondominant hemisphere involvement can all produce anosognosia as a prominent early sign (25).

Some sensory deficits develop rather exclusively with parietal lobe damage. The inability to recognize objects placed in the hand usually indicates contralateral parietal lobe damage. This astereognosis rarely develops with damage lower in the neuraxis than the cerebral cortex (26).

Barognosis is perception of weight differences. Patients with cerebellar hemisphere lesions will have defective barognosis, as well as other signs of cerebellar damage (27,28). The ataxic limb will usually perceive objects as heavier than they actually are (27). All other sensory functions are generally unaffected with cerebellar disease.

VISCERAL PAIN AND VOMITING

Pain is not necessarily limited to external surfaces. Much chronic pain involves the gastrointestinal tract, genitourinary tract, or respiratory tract. Patients with seizure disorders, especially complex partial seizures, frequently complain of abdominal discomfort, nausea, vomiting, borborygmi, and excessive salivation as seizure phenomena (29). These visceral complaints need not be followed by convulsions, but they often are, if the underlying problem is epilepsy. Paroxysmal pain in the abdomen is associated with altered consciousness in a kind of epilepsy occasionally seen in children, called abdominal epilepsy (29). Cyclical vomiting routinely occurs with this seizure disorder, and the child usually falls asleep after an acute attack. The electroencephalogram will be abnormal, the most common findings being spikes or sharp waves in the temporal lobes (29). Phenytoin suppresses the seizure activity and the abdominal discomfort that accompanies it.

Cramps or an obsession with defecation often occur during the aura of a complex partial (temporal lobe) seizure, but these complaints also develop during migraine headache attacks. Distinguishing between the conditions is usually simple because of the altered consciousness appearing with the epileptic disorder. The distinction is less simple in complicated migraine because of the focal neurologic deficits that may appear with this disorder. Both headaches and seizures can be produced by intracranial masses that increase the intracranial pressure and produce vomiting as an associated phenomenon. If a previously asymptomatic patient develops headache, seizures, nausea, and vomiting, an intracranial tumor or infection must be suspected (30). Posterior fossa tumors in children often present with little more than violent episodes of vomiting, often called projectile vomiting because of the force and abruptness of the vomiting (28, 30).

Pain on swallowing or unexplained vomiting are two of the commonest visceral problems likely to prompt a psychiatric evaluation. Obviously, vomiting need not be associated with any pain; it is a common symptom of central nervous system disease and may occur independently of other neurologic signs. Problems with esophageal peristalsis can cause either pain or vomiting. This may be an early sign of a collagen vascular disease, such as scleroderma, Seventy-five percent of patients with progressive systemic sclerosis have esophageal problems (31). Typically, mobility is lost at the distal end of the esophagus and a functional block, called achalasia, develops. The dull substernal pain that develops with achalasia is indistinguishable from chest pain induced by psychologic stress. Nervous system lesions producing achalasia include damage to the dorsal vagal nuclei in the brainstem, damage to the vagus nerve itself, and degeneration of the myenteric plexus of the esophagus (31).

Vomiting from strictly psychologic disturbances is usually seen in individuals in their late twenties or early thirties (32). These patients have no nausea and usually vomit only after meals. They can control the urge to vomit until they are in a bathroom or other appropriate facility, and if the symptom leads to their being hospitalized, the vomiting usually subsides. Self-induced vomiting is occasionally used as a method of weight control without dieting; patients with bulimarexia will eat to great excess periodically and force themselves to vomit to avoid obesity (32,33). Patients with anorexia nervosa also will force themselves to vomit to reduce their weight even when they are far below their normal weight for height. Fortunately, most individuals with self-induced vomiting do not have serious psychiatric disease (32). The developmental histories of these vomiters usually reveal adjustment problems, lack of assertiveness, and problems with setting limits on burdens and activities (32).

REFERENCES

1. Melzack R, Wall PD: Pain mechanisms: A new theory. *Science* 150:971, 1975.
2. DeJong RH: Prof. Wall's three phases of pain. *N Engl J Med* 301:1129, 1979.
3. Loh L, Nathan PW, Schott GD, et al: Effects of regional guanethidine infusion in certain painful states. *J Neurol Neurosurg Psychiatry* 43:446, 1980.
4. Lishman WA: *Organic Psychiatry*. London, Blackwell, 1980.
5. Hendler N, Fernandez P: Alternative treatments for chronic pain. *Psychiatr Ann* 10:495, 1980.
6. Newman RI, Seres JL, Yospe LP, et al: Multidisciplinary treatment of chronic pain: Long-term follow-up of low-back pain patients. *Pain* 4:283, 1978.
7. Mohamed SN, Weisz GM, Waring EM: The relationship of chronic pain to depression, marital adjustment, and family dynamics. *Pain* 5:285, 1978.
8. Maruta T, Osborne D, Swanson DW, et al: Chronic pain patients and spouses: Marital and sexual adjustment. *Mayo Clin Proc* 56:307, 1981.
9. Fields HL: Pain II: New approaches to management. *Ann Neurol* 9:101, 1981.
10. Tomson T, Tybring G, Bertilsson L, et al: Carbamazepine therapy in trigeminal neuralgia. *Arch Neurol* 37:699, 1980.
11. Bernard PG, Perlo VP: Horner syndrome with causalgia. *Neurology (NY)* 30:534, 1980.
12. Adams RD, Victor M: *Principles of Neurology*. New York, McGraw-Hill, 1977.
13. Mitchell SW, Morehouse GR, Keen WW Jr: *Gunshot Wounds and Other Injuries of Nerves*. Philadelphia, JB Lippincott, 1864.
14. Steinbrocker O: The shoulder-hand syndrome: Present perspective. *Arch Phys Med Rehabil* 49:388, 1968.
15. Bayles TB, Judson WE, Potter TA: Reflex sympathetic dystrophy of the upper extremity (hand-shoulder syndrome). *J Am Med Assoc* 144:537, 1950.
16. Leavitt F, Garron DC, D'Angelo CM, et al: Low back pain in patients with and without demonstrable organic disease. *Pain* 6:191, 1979.
17. Fisher CM: Pure sensory stroke involving face, arm, and leg. *Neurology (NY)* 15:76, 1965.
18. Young RR, Delwaide PJ: Spasticity. *N Engl J Med* 304:96, 1981.
19. DeVaul RA, Hall RCW: Hallucinations, in Hall RCW (ed): *Psychiatric Presentations of Medical Illness*. New York, SP Medical and Scientific Books, 1980, p 91.
20. Sherman RA, Gall N, Gormly J: Treatment of phantom limb pain with muscular relaxation training to disrupt the pain—anxiety—tension cycle. *Pain* 6:47, 1979.
21. Jacobs L, Karpik A, Bozian D, et al: Auditory-visual synesthesia. *Arch Neurol* 38:211, 1981.
22. Brown-Séquard CE: Lectures on the diagnosis and treatment of the various forms of paralytic, convulsive, and mental affections, considered as effects of morbid alterations of the blood, or of the brain or other organs. *Lancet* 2:515, 1861.
23. Galin D: Implications for psychiatry of left and right cerebral specialization. *Arch Gen Psychiatry* 31:572, 1974.
24. Valenstein E, Heilman KM: Emotional disorders resulting from lesions of the central nervous system, in Heilman KM, Valenstein E (eds): *Clinical Neuropsychology*. New York, Oxford University Press, 1979, p 413.
25. Raskin DE, Frank SW: Herpes encephalitis with catatonic stupor. *Arch Gen Psychiatry* 31:544, 1974.
26. Feinsod M, Bentin S, Moscovitch M, et al: Brainstem tumor presenting with unilateral astereognosis. *Neurology (NY)* 8:191, 1980.

27. Angel RW: Barognosis in a patient with hemiataxia. *Ann Neurol* 7:73, 1980.
28. Gilman S, Bloedel JR, Lechtenberg R: *Disorders of the Cerebellum.* Philadelphia, FA Davis, 1981.
29. Babb RR, Eckman PB: Abdominal epilepsy. *J Am Med Assoc* 222:65, 1972.
30. Parker SW: Case records of the Massachusetts General Hospital: Case 2-1981. *N Engl J Med* 304:100, 1981.
31. Cohen S: Motor disorders of the esophagus. *N Engl J Med* 301:184, 1979.
32. Rosenthal RH, Webb WL, Wruble LD: Psychogenic vomiting: Diagnosis and management. *Psychosomatics* 21:722, 1980.
33. Task Force on nomenclature and statistics, American Psychiatric Association: *Diagnostic and Statistical Manual of Mental Disorders* (*Third Edition*). Washington, DC, American Psychiatric Association, 1980.

13
Headaches and Facial Pain

Headaches may signal psychologic stress, progressive intracranial damage, transient vascular phenomena, or bone and joint disease. Whether the headache is a true pain or just an abnormal sensation and whether the head or just the face is involved by the discomfort are distinctions headache victims often find difficult to make. An estimated 80 percent of the population in the United States has at least one headache each year, and half of these are severe enough to interfere with normal activity (1). Tension headaches, vascular syndromes, and structural lesions in the brain are usually distinguishable on the basis of the history alone. A daily headache, lasting hours and appearing with equal severity on every day for several months is likely to be from tension or a brain tumor. Sharp, retro-orbital pain waking the patient on several successive nights suggests a type of vascular headache called cluster headache. If the patient hears a rushing sound synchronous with his pulse, an arteriovenous malformation may be responsible. Pain over the face and temple worsening with chewing suggests temporal arteritis or temporomandibular joint disease. Caffeine withdrawal can produce dull headaches, presumably on a vascular basis, that last hours or days (2). If there are no consistent physical findings, the history will direct the investigation of the headache. When, in fact, a structural lesion in or about the brain is responsible for the headache, neurologic signs of focal disease will usually be present.

The severity of the headache is unrelated to the seriousness of the lesion or condition responsible. Dull, chronic headaches associated with bitemporal visual field cuts develop with pituitary or parasellar masses. Thirty-five percent of undifferentiated pituitary adenomas present this way (3). Sharp, unilateral eye pain, lid ptosis, and pupillary dilatation commonly appear with an enlarging posterior communicating artery aneurysm. Intense feelings of pressure on the inside of the head, beginning abruptly and increasing in severity over the course of minutes, may signal the rupture of an aneurysm, with a resulting hemorrhage into the subarachnoid space (Figure 13.1). Equally severe pain develops with a similarly explosive onset in patients with cluster headache, a type of vascular headache not associated with structural damage to the central nervous system. The character and course of the headache is often informative in determining its etiology, but the intensity of the pain reported by the patient is not very helpful.

How extensive the investigation of an individual headache sufferer will be is related to the seriousness of the headache type suspected. An electroencephalogram and skull x-ray are reasonable and sufficient laboratory tests when the patient has signs and symptoms typical of tension headache; but a computed tomogram is essential when a brain tumor is suspected, and an arteriogram will be needed to rule out a suspected arteriovenous malformation or aneurysm. The clinician's initial impression, an impression reached after carefully discussing the character of the headache with the patient and thoroughly examining the patient, is central to the investigation and treatment of the headache or facial pain. Determining the cause of the headache is important in limiting the progression of a destructive lesion and also in limiting the patient's exposure to inappropriate treatment. Treatment ranges from mild analgesics and emotional support to chemotherapy and neurosurgery, depending upon the final diagnosis.

The brain has no pain fibers, and so, masses in the brain and structural damage to the brain cause discomfort by irritating structures adjacent to the nervous tissue. Pain sensitive structures in the skull include the venous sinuses; the dural arteries; fibers of the trigeminal (V), glossopharyngeal (IX), and vagus (X) cranial nerves; parts of the dura mater at the base of the skull; the upper cervical nerves; and the proximal 20 percent of the large arteries in the circle of Willis (4). Distention, displacement, and inflammation of pain-sensitive vascular structures are the usual causes of headaches not of purely psychologic origin. Areas outside the cranial vault likely to cause pain indistinguishable from the pain of strictly intracranial disease include the orbits, sinuses, mouth, and temporomandibular joints. Cervical spine disease also causes headache in some individuals, not because cervical nerves to the head are trapped or irritated, but because the pain from damaged synovial joints on the upper cervical vertebrae is referred to the back of the head (5). Confusion arises in the evaluation of head and face pain because the location of the pain does not necessarily correspond to the site of the pathology. A lesion irritating pain fibers along the posterior half of the sagittal sinus or the upper surface of the transverse sinus will be perceived as a pain in the eye or about the forehead on the same side as the intracranial lesion. The pain is referred anteriorly, because the first (ophthalmic) division of the trigeminal nerve (V) supplies both the area of the face over the eye and the venous structures damaged

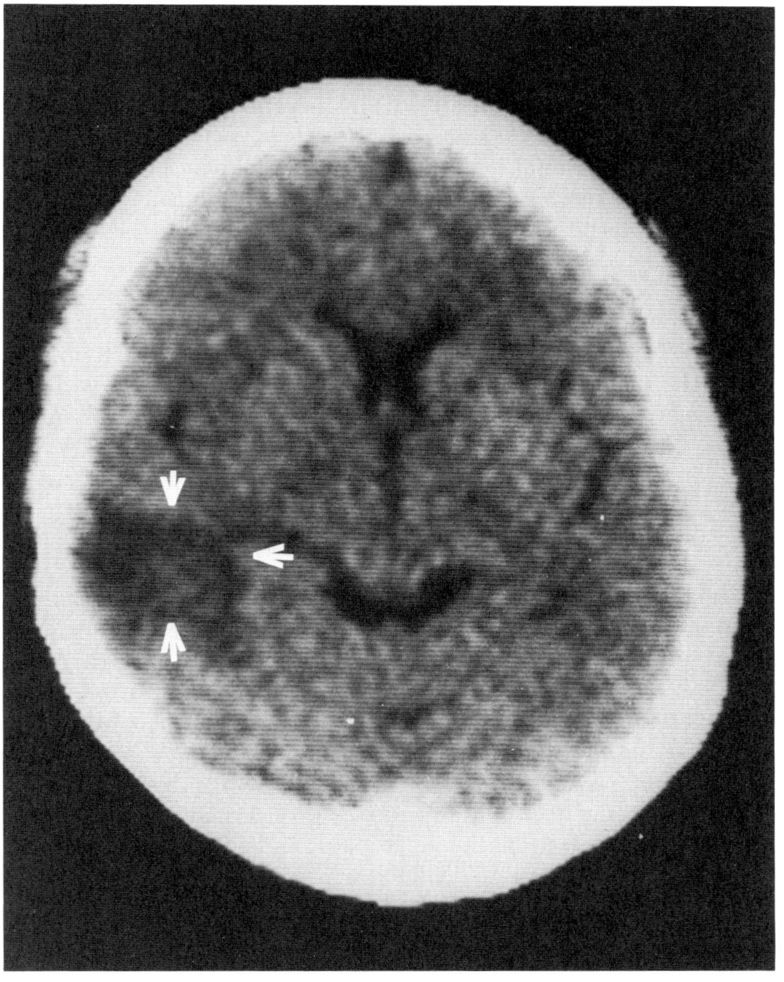

Figure 13.1. After several years of recurrent right-sided migraine headaches, this 40-year-old woman complained of progression of the headache pain over the course of 3 months. Although there were no premonitory neurologic signs, she abruptly developed a stiff neck and an extremely painful headache. A lumbar puncture revealed bloody cerebrospinal fluid, and physical examination revealed a left homonymous quadrantic field defect. No vascular abnormalities appeared on arteriography. The computed tomogram of the head obtained a few weeks after the acute episode showed a right hemisphere infarction (arrows) (courtesy of Drs. J. Loh and W. Hotson).

by this type of lesion. Whether the irritation is on the face or about the posterior fossa vascular sinuses, the pain is felt in the eye or face.

Fortunately, most headaches and facial pains are not from destructive intracranial lesions. Vasodilation of intracranial or extracranial blood vessels and sustained muscle contraction associated with anxiety, stress, or tension produce the majority of headaches. Extracranial disease and irritation of cranial nerves cause most problems with facial pain. Regardless of the severity of the pain, headaches and facial pains caused by these phenomena are benign. Depression plays a role in many different types of head and face discomfort, but signs of depression associated with headache or facial pain should not be overrated. Sleep disorders, chronic fatigue, loss of appetite, and other signs of anxiety or depression routinely develop in the patient suffering from sustained or progressive head pain (2). The somatic signs of depression are simply a product of the chronic pain, rather than the cause of that pain in many patients.

TENSION HEADACHE

Chronic headache complaints provide a socially acceptable escape from stressful demands or depressing conflicts. The headache may distract both the patient and those he complains to from the anxiety or depression that underlies the "functional" complaint, Anger, loss, frustration, embarassment, or inadequacy may all be the setting for a transient or constant headache that develops in the absence of a central nervous system lesion (4). Because there is no apparent organic substrate, this is often called a "psychogenic" headache. Included in this group of headaches are muscle contraction headaches, psychotic head pain, and conversion headaches (6). Migraine and other vascular headaches may be triggered by psychologic stress, and in some individuals they develop along with the more typically anxiety-related muscle contraction headache. Even though the patient with tension or psychogenic headache may have a discrete source of head or facial pain, such as dental malocclusion or minor facial trauma, the course of the psychogenic headache will be independent of any changes in the painful lesion that may have initiated it. In fact, in most cases the headache develops and persists without any apparent organic basis for the pain (6).

Including muscle contraction headaches with psychogenic headaches is somewhat misleading. Muscle contraction headaches develop with local irritation or strain of the neck, jaw, or scalp muscles. Cervical arthritis, temporomandibular joint disease, periodontal disease, and even eye strain can elicit muscle contraction headaches. All these organic problems must be considered before muscle contraction headache is ascribed to psychologic stress. Finding a physiologic abnormality, such as altered blood flow, does not diminish the likelihood of a psychogenic basis for the headache in patients with obvious psychologic conflicts. All psychogenic headaches may be mediated by local physiologic changes that accompany a repressed affect (7). Individuals with muscle contraction headaches have somewhat distinctive personality profiles on systematic evaluation (8). They characteristically somatize and exhibit borderline depressions. Men who frequently develop muscle contraction headaches tend to be more self-righteous than individuals who suffer from other types of headache (8). Patients with vascular headaches are less depressed and anxious than patients with muscle contraction headaches, but this may be because the vascular headache patient has longer pain-free intervals than the muscle contraction headache patient (8).

That tension headaches are usually from chronic muscle contraction is probably wrong (5). Objective evidence of excessive activity in the muscles about the head and face in patients with "muscle contraction" headaches is very limited. Certainly, patients under stress with a malocclusion may develop headache as they nervously clench their jaws, but most patients without such obvious structural problems have chronic tension headaches with persistently normal muscle activity (5). Alternative explanations offered to explain chronic tension headaches include vascular abnormalities similar to those suspected in migraine and impaired inhibition of pain perception. Whatever the cause of most chronic tension or muscle contraction headaches, it is clear that psychologic factors play a central role. More strictly psychogenic headaches develop in hypochondriacal or depressed individuals: in these individuals the pain may have no structural or physiologic basis, but distinguishing between these delusional psychogenic headaches and chronic tension headaches is impossible. Rather than making arbitrary distinctions between chronic tension headaches, nonstructural muscle contraction headaches, and delusional psychogenic headaches, it is reasonable to discuss these problems together as psychogenic headaches, with the understanding that psychogenic headaches may have a few different etiologies.

Characteristic of the psychogenic headache is the flamboyant description usually provided by the patient. The headache usually has no consistent frequency, location, duration, or character. A band of pressure or a feeling of neck tightness will be described bilaterally in 90 percent of patients with such headaches (4). Most patients with psychogenic headaches have poorly localized pain. Dramatic terms, such as "a flaming belt" or "a hammer with spikes on it," may be used to describe the type of pain. When chronic anxiety or tension is the apparent basis for the pain, the patient may complain that the nonpulsatile discomfort persists for days or weeks or even months with no spontaneous decrease in the pain and little relief from strong analgesics. Women have psychogenic headaches three times as often as men (1).

For many patients the headache is a straightforward symptom of a conversion reaction, many of these patients exhibiting hysterical personality types (7). The hysterical patient may smile throughout his description of the pain he is experiencing (9). This conversion reaction can occur in both men and women, and it will produce social or occupational incapacity in both (7). If the conversion of anxiety into an intractable headache is complete, the anxiety may be inapparent (6). Mild to moderate depression with somatization features will be found on psychologic testing of these patients with typical conversion headaches (10). A profoundly disabling chronic tension headache is frequently a symptom of a severe depressive illness (2).

Psychogenic headache is rare in frankly psychotic patients, even though patients with manic-depressive affective disorders and middle-life psychotic depressions have a higher incidence of headaches than nonpsychotic patients (4,6). Despite this greater than normal incidence of headache in psychotically depressed patients, the association of headache and psychosis should be viewed as suspiciously as the association of psychosis and seizures. The schizophrenic patient complaining of chronic headache should be investigated more thoroughly than the neurotic patient. This means a computerized tomogram soon after the appearance of the symptom and a lumbar puncture if the computerized tomogram is negative and the complaints are still evolving. Skull x-rays and an electroencephalogram are appropriate for all psychotic patients developing headaches.

Although patients with psychogenic headaches are usually eager to submit to extensive diagnostic tests and treatments, invasive tests are usually unnecessary and most treatments are consistently ineffective. Anyone with longstanding headaches should have a careful neurologic examination to look for evidence of a progressive lesion; but, failing to find evidence of organic disease, the physician should treat the patient with mild analgesics, such as aspirin and acetaminophen, and follow the evolution of the symptoms. More than 40 percent of headache victims will respond well to placebo alone (1). Medication effective against anxiety or depression may relieve the headache, as well as the other more obvious signs of depression (2,5). Noninvasive studies, including skull x-rays and an electroencephalogram, are appropriate at some time in the evaluation of the patient with chronic headache, but they are not a high priority if the patient's symptoms point to psychogenic headaches. Most patients want careful follow-up and frequent medication changes, and this demand for attention provides the physician with ample opportunity to repeatedly reevaluate the patient as part of his search for a destructive lesion. Unfortunately, many patients with psychogenic headaches are quite manipulative. Disordered sleep, altered bowel habits, and constantly shifting aches and pains justify the patient's demands for an assortment of drugs to deal with his symptoms. Many of the patients suffering from psychogenic headaches will vigorously resist psychiatric intervention even when that is suggested by a physician who has developed rapport with the steadfastly "ill" patient over the course of months.

The treatment of psychogenic headache, whether it is presumed to be from muscle contraction, tension, or psychosis, is primarily through psychiatric intervention. Formal psychotherapy may be unnecessary in most cases, but some assistance in developing strategies for dealing with the stressful elements in the chronic headache sufferer's life is appropriate. Biofeedback techniques have been used with inconsistent results, but this is a viable approach to relaxation for some patients. Any local structural problems, such as temporomandibular joint dysfunction, sinusitis, or cervical arthritis, must be dealt with separately even if there is no evidence that these problems are contributing to the psychogenic headache. Amitriptyline relieves the headache in some individuals, even when there is no associated depression (5).

VASCULAR HEADACHE

Vascular headaches include migraine, cluster, hypertensive, and vascular malformation headaches. Of these four, migraine and cluster are the most likely to occur on a chronic basis (Table 13.1). As much as 15 percent of the general population suffers from some type of vascular headache, one-third to one-half of that group complaining of migraine (1,11). About one-quarter of the affected patients develop their first headaches in childhood (1). There is a three to one female preponderance amongst patients with vascular headaches, if patients with cluster headaches are excluded (1,12). Twenty to 70 percent report other family members with the same problem, and the headache is often first noted at puberty (1,9).

Table 13.1. Common Features of Vascular Headaches

Type	*Prodrome*	*Pain*	*Duration*
Classic migraine	Scintillating scotomas Focal neurologic signs	Throbbing or sharp Unilateral Frontal, temporal, or parietal	1–6 hours
Common migraine	Altered mood (withdrawn) Disorientation	Throbbing or sharp Unilateral Frontal, temporal, or parietal	1–48 hours
Cluster headache	Sharp pain in eye or no prodrome	Stabbing, throbbing, or dull Unilateral Supraorbital or orbital	30–90 minutes
Complicated migraine	Focal neurologic signs or no prodrome	Sharp, throbbing, or dull Unilateral	Hours to days

Menstrual periods, menopause, pregnancies in adolescence, and oral contraceptive use may trigger headaches in some women (12). Some chemical agents, such as alcohol, monosodium glutamate, and nitrites may trigger vascular headaches in patients not ordinarily burdened by them (13). Fever, carbon dioxide retention, and hypoglycemia can induce headaches, but, again, susceptibility is important. Headaches induced by these abnormal conditions or provocative agents are often called toxic headaches.

Vascular dilatation is responsible for the pain in migraine, cluster, and toxic vascular headaches, that dilatation probably being accompanied by a sterile inflammatory reaction immediately about the susceptible blood vessels (13). Central nervous system activity probably triggers the dilatation, but the initial event in vascular headache is controversial and probably varies with the type of vascular headache (9). Although vascular dilatation is generally accepted as an integral part of the painful episodes in these vascular headaches, arteriography during the headache reveals no change in the blood vessels at a gross level (14). Cerebral blood flow studies do show changes in focal blood flow, especially with migraine, and that this is a systemic, rather than a local, disorder is emphasized by the reduced cutaneous blood flow in these patients (14).

Headache as a consequence of high blood pressure is very unusual; and, when it does occur, the diastolic blood pressure is generally greater than 120 to 140 millimeters of mercury (5,13). Hypertensive headaches are most often seen in the context of hypertensive encephalopathy, a malignant elevation of the systemic blood pressure associated with seizures, focal neurological deficits, or coma (13). Vasoactive substances are presumed to play a role in all of the vascular headaches, except those associated with structural anomalies, but the specific vasoactive substances responsible for inducing pain in various headache disorders is controversial.

Migraine

Migraine typically develops between 15 and 22 years of age in both men and women (11). The pain usually involves only one side of the head at a time and affects one side more often than the other. One temple or one side of the forehead is an especially common site for the pain. The pain is throbbing or stabbing, does not migrate, and may be preceded by visual abnormalities or focal weakness (14,15). Signs of an impending headache often develop at night or on awakening (9). These premonitory symptoms are called the aura, and they are presumed to develop with ischemia to the brain at the beginning of the migraine attack (9,14,15). Decreased blood flow preceding the headache can be reversed by having the patient inhale amyl nitrite, a vasodilating agent, and, consistent with the notion that vasoconstriction causes the aura, amyl nitrite may clear the aura (14).

Aura

About 65 percent of patients with migraine have focal neurologic symptoms before or during the headache (4). Fully one-third of these auras are visual distortions (4). Visual field cuts surrounded by an illusion of sparkling lights, called hemianopic scintillating scotomas, are especially common in the full-blown, or classic, migraine syndrome. These scintillating blind spots may be associated with electroencephalographic slowing over the affected occipital lobe, a prodromal change that continues for 10 to 20 minutes before the onset of the headache (4). Some patients complain of showers or stationary flecks of light, called photopsias, and others will see lines of light arranged in geometric patterns, called fortification scotomas. Unilateral weakness, local sensory disturbances, aphasia, confusion, and altered mood may all be part of the aura. Even patients who do not have these dramatic neurologic signs during the aura will exhibit affective or cognitive disorders in 40 percent of cases (9). The unilateral headache with less neurologic and more psychologic features to the aura is called common, rather than classic, migraine, but these are not distinctly different headache types. The visual changes, hemiparesis, or hemisensory deficits resolve as the headache begins and these are replaced by nausea, vomiting, and an aversion to light or noise during the headache (4). The prodrome occasionally develops without any subsequent headache, but such transient neurologic deficits without an associated migraine should be ascribed to migraine very reluctantly (9). Sensory seizures or transient ischemic attacks are more likely than migraine to cause these neurologic phenomena.

Migraine Pain

The unilateral head pain often centers about the temple after being ushered in by diffuse discomfort about the entire head. The pain is usually throbbing and routinely affects the same side of the head with almost every attack. Patients clearly recall attacks affecting the contralateral temple on rare occasions, but this switch is a fairly constant feature of the headache. With classic migraine, the pain subsides after several hours, most episodes lasting less than three hours. Throughout the headache the patient complains of a constant throbbing pain, often synchronous with the pulse, associated with nausea, vomiting, diarrhea, polyuria, excessive sweating, and cold limbs (9). This obviously, uncomfortable patient usually retires to bed in a dark, quiet room and lies still until the pain subsides.

Precipitating Factors

Migraine headaches are provoked or affected by a wide variety of substances. Menstruation is especially effective in susceptible women, and oversleeping can induce headaches in both men and women (9). Contraceptive pills increase the incidence of migraine and may increase the risk of fixed deficits in migraine sufferers (12). The precise role played by hormones in this disorder is unknown. Migraine usually remits during pregnancy as serum estradiol levels rise (13). Experimental infusion of some prostaglandins will also trigger a migraine in susceptible individuals, and norepinephrine will abort attacks (13).

The vasoactive substances tyramine and phenylethylamine occur in certain foods, such as chicken livers, pickled herrings, aged cheese, canned figs, and bean pods, and can evoke a migraine in a susceptible individual (7). This is not an allergic reaction to the food substances. This sensitivity to vasoactive substances and the tendency to suffer with migraine headaches are familial traits (9). The physiologic basis for this inherited susceptibility is probably tied to abnormal blood vessel reactivity to the vasoactive agents histamine, serotonin, plasma kinins, and related substances (13).

Neurotransmitter disorders may play a role in initiating migraine attacks, but there is no consensus on which neurotransmitters are most important and why they are disturbed in migraine headache sufferers (5). Gamma aminobutyric acid levels are elevated in the cerebrospinal fluid as much as 48 hours before the onset of the headache (13). This amino acid may be the earliest sign of the ischemia or may, in fact, play a role in triggering the headache. Cause and effect is also unclear in the abnormal platelet aggregation seen in migraine patients.

Psychologic Factors

Traditionally, migraine headaches have been ascribed to individuals with rigid, ambitious, obsessive-compulsive personality types, but this has been overstated (7). Clearly, migraine severity and frequency are affected by stress. Fear, anxiety, rage, and just prolonged mental strain can all precipitate recurrent migraines (9). These phenomena appear in patients with almost any personality type and are not distinctly more common in any particular personality type. Minnesota Multiphasic Personality Inventory (MMPI) profiles for both men and women suffering from migraine are unremarkable (8).

Although there is no consistent personality profile for the migraine patient some features do appear frequently (9). Quite often the patient is an intense, overly conscientious individual who becomes easily immersed in a morass of details (4). His expectations of others are often impossible to satisfy, and reviewing his early life will usually uncover an excessive concern with approval from those around him. Some speculate that the migraine patient never learned to handle aggressive energy (4). Headaches appear as the patient's energy, which is constantly called upon to order and control the elements in his life, is exhausted (4).

Part of the problem in assessing the importance of psychologic factors in migraine is the skewed population routinely studied. The only migraine sufferers closely examined have been those seeking medical or psychiatric assistance for their headaches. Forty-six percent of patients with the typical features of classic migraine never seek attention or conventional treatment for their headaches (11). In contrast, patients in psychotherapy for whatever reason complain of migraine headache two to three times more often than those in the general population (11). This disproportionate contribution to the routinely studied sample may have produced the view that migraine sufferers usually have repressed anger (11). What is clear is that patients in psychotherapy are more likely to seek attention for their migraines.

Investigation

The investigation of migraine headaches is largely directed by the history. Years before the headache appears, the patient may have problems with cyclic vomiting and motion sickness (9). Once headaches develop, they usually become stereotyped, predictable. With all the classic signs of migraine, including the aura, photophobia, nausea, vomiting, and unilateral head pain, developing over the course of years, attempts to control the headache without further investigation are appropriate if the neurologic examination is negative. Unfortunately, fewer than 30 percent of patients with migraine have these "classic" features (1).

Confusion understandably arises in the patients with substantial field cuts, limb weakness, and major sensory deficits as part of the aura. These signs are likely to be misconstrued as transient ischemic attacks from structural disease of the major vessels to the brain or from valvular heart disease. This misinterpretation is especially likely in patients over 50 years of age, a group that has a high incidence of both transient ischemic attacks and visual symptoms of migraine. Patients with both of these disorders will have visual changes involving areas of visual loss, but the appearance of typical fortification patterns or scintillations about the blind spots often helps to differentiate the migraine from the transient ischemic attack.

When the migraine does not have the classic features, but is still largely unilateral, throbbing, and associated with nausea and vomiting, the diagnosis is less certain. This "common" migraine merits closer follow-up than the classic form simply because the diagnosis is less certain. In the absence of any focal neurologic signs, attempts at control are more appropriate than further investigation. Common migraine has the same type of pain as classic migraine, but the pain persists for many hours or even a few days. Behavior during the attacks is withdrawn, and avoidance of noise, light, and personal contact is as prominent as in classic migraine. If the headache always occurs on the same side of the head, a computed tomogram of the brain is appropriate since this may be the first sign of a large arteriovenous malformation. Indeed, migraine of even the classic type may develop with occipital lobe arteriovenous malformations, but these vascular anomalies are usually large enough to be seen on computed tomography of the brain with contrast enhancement (16). An arteriogram is more helpful in diagnosing an arteriovenous malformation, but the additional risk cannot be justified unless the computed tomogram is suspicious or a bruit can be heard over the head (16). The headache caused by a vascular malformation will resolve with resection of the abnormality.

The transient deficits appearing with migraine will persist for disturbingly long intervals in some individuals and fixed deficits may even appear (13). These attacks are called "complicated" migraine and should prompt studies of the patient's blood coagulation and platelet functions. A deficit still apparent several hours after its onset and persisting through the headache is worrisome, but reversible hemiplegia or opthalmoplegia does occur as a benign feature of complicated migraine and may even persist for hours after the headache has ended (9). An arteriogram is often needed to evaluate the patency of cerebral vessels in these patients; but such a diagnostic study is hazardous in patients with migraine because of the reactivity of the blood vessels. Fixed deficits occasionally develop during the arteriogram, and so this type of invasive procedure should only be used when there is a high level of suspicion of a structural lesion. Some types of complicated migraine are associated with wide-ranging neurologic deficits (Figure 13.2). Familial hemiplegic migraine is associated in some instances with nystagmus, retinal degeneration, deafness, and clumsiness. The headaches, as well as the other signs of central nervous system disease, are inherited in an autosomal dominant pattern and clearly represent a degenerative disorder of multiple systems (17).

Treatment

Common and classic migraine remit spontaneously with age in all patients and transiently with pregnancy in 80 percent of female patients (9). Waiting and pregnancy are not acceptable to most patients suffering with these recurrent headaches, and so numerous methods have been used to stop or prevent the headaches. Medication, biofeedback, and relaxation training, and electrical counterstimulation have all had claims of success that are difficult to reproduce. With each technique, a psychotherapeutic component was probably as important in the observed effect as the other elements used.

Aside from techniques for dealing with stress, effective treatment and prevention of migraine headaches rely upon the use of agents that interfere with chemical mediators of excessive vasomotor activity and inflammation (13). Because of the abnormality in platelet function in many patients with migraine, agents that interfere with normal platelet activity, such as aspirin and sulfinpyrazone, have been used prophylactically with some reported decrease in migraine intensity and frequency (13). Although serotonin has long been considered an important element in the production of migraine, agents that simply block peripheral serotonin formation and action have not been successful in preventing migraine (13). Methysergide, a serotonin antagonist that also interferes with histam-

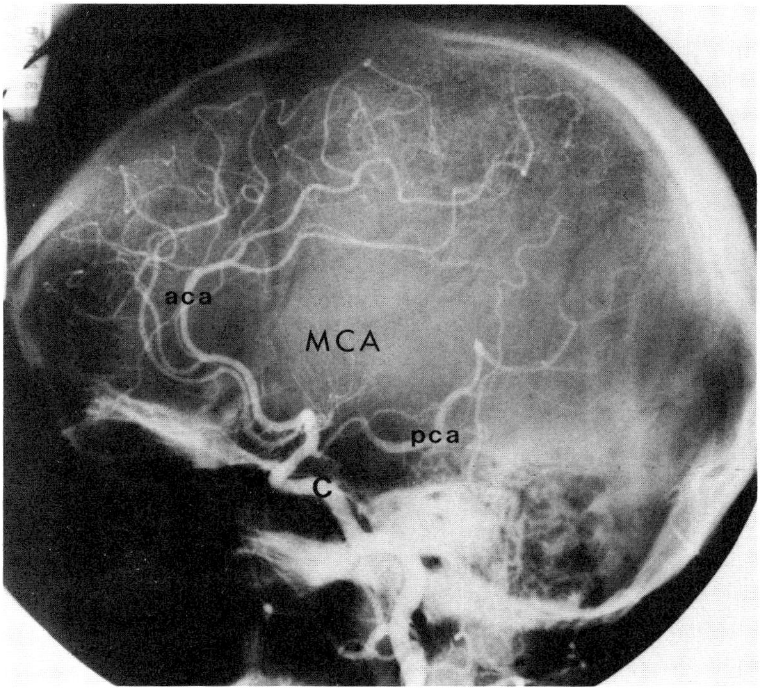

Figure 13.2. A 37-year-old woman with a long history of migraine headaches abruptly developed weakness of her left side. The left arm was completely paralyzed, and the left leg was substantially weaker than normal. An arteriogram revealed no filling of the middle cerebral artery. The patient had a massive infarction in the area of cortex (MCA) supplied by the middle cerebral artery branches. The anterior cerebral artery (aca) and the posterior cerebral artery (pca) were obvious from their origins off the internal carotid artery (C) to their terminal branches. This stroke in the setting of recurrent migraine headaches suggests complicated migraine.

ine liberation and acts as a vasoconstrictor, is effective when taken daily, but its disadvantages include retoperitoneal fibrosis and fibrotic changes in the heart valves with protracted use.

Traditional migraine treatment has focused on vasoconstrictor agents used at the onset of symptoms. Ergot derivatives have been used with considerable success, but their main disadvantage is that they will not prevent the headaches from occurring: they will only abort the headache once it has begun (13). Ergotamine tartrate, the most commonly used ergot derivative, also causes peripheral vasoconstriction in the recommended dose of 6 milligrams per 24 hours or up to 16 milligrams per week (1,18). Oral ergotamine is effective against classic and common migraine in only 40 to 50 percent of individuals, but it is more consistently effective when given rectally or intravenously (9). The vasoactive drug propranolol is effective in the prophylaxis of migraine headache. One-third of the patients with common migraine will have an excellent response to this beta-adrenergic blocking agent (18). These highly responsive patients have more than a 50 percent reduction in the number of migraine attacks, and another third of the headache patients taking propranolol show some reduction in headache frequency (18). Adverse effects of propranolol include fatigue, depression, hypotension, bradycardia, nausea, diarrhea, and, rarely, hypoglycemia or palpitations (18). It is inadvisable for use in patients with heart disease even though the effective dose range for treatment of migraine (80 to 240 milligrams) is relatively low. A more selective beta-blocking agent, metoprolol, used in doses of 50 milligrams three times daily, may prove safer than propranolol and equally effective (19). Metoprolol acts selectively on beta-1 adrenoceptors and thereby avoids many of the side effects induced by propranolol (19).

Cluster Headache

Cluster headaches are stabbing, burning, or boring pains over one side of the head, usually centered about or behind the eye with radiation of the pain to the temple or forehead on the same side as the affected eye (1). These headaches, also known as Horton histamine cephalgia or migrainous cranial neuralgia, develop in less than 1 percent of the population and over 90 percent of the individuals affected are men (1,20). Headaches begin during the second or third decade of life in most individuals (21). The pain is usually paroxysmal, lasting 30 minutes to 2 hours and is accompanied by excessive tearing, conjunctival injection, pupillary constriction (miosis), and eyelid droop (ptosis) over the painful eye (22,23). Other signs occasionally seen during a cluster headache include nasal congestion, nasal discharge (rhinorrhea), and slowing of the pulse rate.

Some patients have pain more limited to the lower part of the face. The pain is usually burning in these cases and seems to center about the cheek or the jaw (22). A partial Horner's syndrome (ptosis of the ipsilateral eyelid and miosis of the ipsilateral pupil) with increased sweating over the forehead ipsilateral to the pain occurs in about one-fourth of cases of this type of cluster headache (22). Victims of this lower facial cluster headache or migrainous neuralgia develop their symptoms later in life than most victims of cluster, and they exhibit a higher incidence of peptic ulcers as a chronic problem (22). A family history of migraine is occasionally found in patients with cluster headache pain affecting the upper face, but it is usually absent when the lower face is primarily affected (22).

Psychologic changes during the headache are striking. The patient becomes extremely agitated and destructive. He invariably paces, rocks, complains, and otherwise exhibits considerable irritability (20). Customarily, even-tempered individuals become extremely abusive. Unfortunately, there is usually little warning of an impending headache: from the onset to the peak of the headache is usually just 5 minutes (9). Most of the pain will subside within 30 to 90 minutes.

Headache Frequency

Attacks often develop 90 minutes after sleep-onset and are associated with rapid eye movement (REM) sleep. One third of cluster headache sufferers describe an "ice-pick-like pain" at the start of the headache or awakening them from sleep (15). The same eye is affected in each cluster of headaches, although the pain may shift to the other side of the head with the development of a new cluster (1). The pattern of occurrence of the headaches falls into one of two categories in most cases: episodic and chronic. Episodic or periodic cluster headache is the more typical pattern with attacks occurring one to five times daily for several weeks or months (22,23). After this discrete episode the attacks stop, at least for most of the remaining year and occasionally the attack will not recur for years at a time (20,23). Spring and autumn are the seasons favored by the headaches, but episodes may occur when the patient is unusually relaxed, such as on holiday (20). Asymptomatic intervals get longer as the patient gets older (22). Drinking alcohol may also trigger an attack. Unlike the situation in migraine headache, there is no evidence of a familial pattern to the occurrence of episodic cluster headache (1). If the headache cluster lasts longer than 4 months, the patient is suffering from chronic, rather than periodic or episodic, cluster headaches (22).

Chronic Cluster Headache

Chronic cluster headache, or chronic migrainous neuralgia, as it is also known, need not ever totally remit; in some cases it will occur year round. Patients with chronic cluster headaches form a distinct population of headache sufferers, not at all similar to the population susceptible to periodic cluster headache. The first attack will occur between the third and sixth decades of life (22). Many of the affected individuals are middle-aged women, and some of the headache episodes respond to aspirin or indomethocin (20). Only about 10 percent of cluster headache sufferers have the chronic form, and an even smaller number have headaches with features of both cluster and common migraine (20).

The pattern of the headaches is so stereotyped with cluster headaches that there is little opportunity to confuse this problem with more malignant lesions. Arteriovenous malformation may produce similar signs, but fixed deficits or a seizure disorder usually evolve with this vascular lesion. Pheochromocytoma, a tumor of the adrenal gland, can cause similar clusters of headaches, but patients with this problem will have pain on both sides of their head and will exhibit tachycardia and hypertension in association with the headache (20).

Etiology

The cause of cluster headaches is unknown. Whole blood histamine increases at the onset of the attacks, an observation that prompted the name "histamine headaches" (13). Histamine is a potent vasodilator, and there is evidence that orbital and nearby extracranial arteries are dilated during the headache (1). Abnormalities in the fine structure of the extracranial blood vessels persist between attacks, but clear-cut changes in regional cerebral blood flow are more apparent with migraine than with cluster headaches (14). There is no phase of decreased blood flow (ischemia) in the cluster headache, but an arteriogram performed during the attack will reveal narrowing in the internal carotid as it emerges from the carotid canal of the skull (21). The edema in the wall of the internal carotid artery causing this narrowing may be responsible for some of the autonomic features of the cluster headache. The sympathetic nerve fibers to the eye may be damaged by pressure from the carotid artery swelling as the fibers ascend along the outer wall of that artery (14). This would explain the partial Horner's syndrome seen in some patients with cluster headache. The ophthalmic artery ipsilateral to the side of the retro-orbital pain is dilated during the acute attack, and this may account for the high incidence of this location for the pain in cluster headaches (21). That blood vessels near the painful area are preferentially disturbed during a cluster headache is supported by the thermographic picture obtained during the attack. There are spotty areas of coolness over one eye (21).

Treatment

The early view that histamine was of central importance in this headache disorder prompted trials of the histamine antagonist methysergide. Methysergide is effective in 75 percent of patients with cluster headache, even though the role of histamine in this disorder is controversial (1). This drug also acts as a serotonin antagonist and as a vasoconstrictor, and this may account for its effectiveness (13). Unfortunately, methysergide also causes retroperitoneal and cardiac valve fibrosis with long-term use, and few physicians are comfortable using this drug for more than 2 or 3 months at a time (1). It is also not very effective against the chronic form of cluster headache (22). Other medications used to prevent the development of the headaches include chlorpromazine and propranolol. The phenothiazine, chlorpromazine, is effective in up to 90 percent of patients with cluster, as well as migraine, headaches at doses of 100 to 700 milligrams daily; the risk of parkinsonism and tardive dyskinesia with this drug make it unattractive (1,2). Propranolol, the beta-adrenergic receptor blocker, has shown considerable promise as a prophylactic drug, the required dose ranging from 100 to 300 milligrams daily. Patients with cardiac disease should be treated with considerable caution because of the risk of myocardial damage if the drug is stopped abruptly. Corticosteroids will also suppress cluster headaches. Prednisome at 40 milligrams daily is highly effective in middle-aged individuals (30 to 45 years old) with refractory headache (5,20). Unfortunately, obesity, osteoporosis, hypertension, and diabetes mellitus may develop as side effects of the prednisone even at this dose. Ergotamine tartrate 2 milligrams orally before the attack occurs may abort the cluster headache in individuals with the periodic form, but this is feasible only if the headache occurs with such regularity that its onset can be predicted within an hour or two of its occurrence (20).

As many as half the patients with chronic or episodic cluster have relief with lithium carbonate (22,23). Patients over 45 years of age are especially likely to respond to this drug at a dose of 600 to 1200 milligrams daily (20). A bout of headaches may subside within a week of starting treatment with the drug, and individuals with chronic cluster headache may see relief within 1 or 2 weeks even if they have had the headaches for several months. The therapeutic level in the serum is usually 1.0–1.5 milliequivalents per liter, but even at that level the patient may be toxic with nausea, fatigue, tremor, thirst, weight gain, and confusion (23). Rare patients develop hypothyroidism or a goiter on lithium, and patients with unsuspected renal disease may develop nephrogenic diabetes insipidus (23). The mode of action of lithium in the relief of cluster headaches is unknown.

Other Causes of Retro-orbital Pain

Pain behind the eye is not necessarily from cluster or migraine headaches. A structural lesion in or behind the eye should be the principal concern in any patient with eye pain, whether or not there is any change in vision (Figure 13.3). If a careful eye examination reveals no ocular pathology, several uncommon conditions must be considered. These include intracranial aneurysms and periorbital infections. The diagnosis is simpler if the patient has impaired eye movements associated with the eye pain. An aneurysm on the posterior communicating artery usually produces pupillary dilatation, as well as ophthalmoplegia associated with the retro-orbital pain. A similar picture develops with a carotid-cavernous fistula, a vascular problem in which a connection develops between the carotid artery and the cavernous sinus at the point where the artery courses through the sinus. The fistula forms when an aneurysm sitting in the cavernous sinus bursts and "bleeds" into the sinus, rather than into the brain or the subarachnoid space (Figure 13.4). With fistula formation, the painful eye will usually be injected, often bulging, and occasionally pulsatile. One of the more common and more puzzling causes of painful ophthalmoplegia is the Tolosa-Hunt syndrome (24,25). Pain behind the eye in the Tolosa-Hunt syndrome may precede the ophthalmoplegia by days; and, although the pain and weakness may persist days or weeks, a spontaneous remission will usually occur (24). The pain is a gnawing or boring pain that seems to originate directly behind the eye. There is

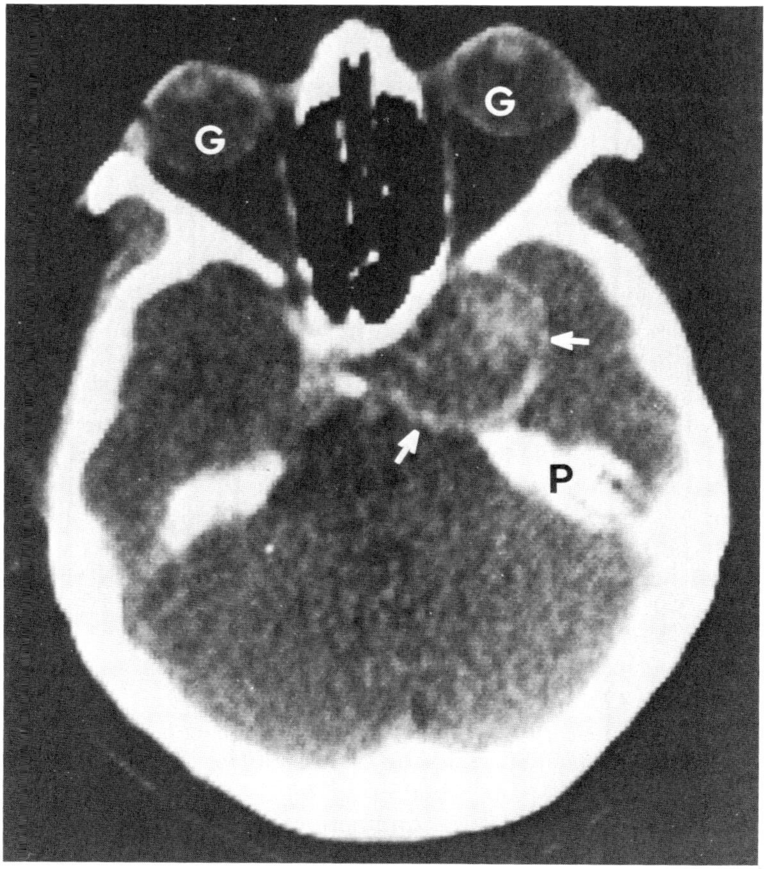

Figure 13.3. This computed tomogram with contrast enhancement reveals why the 70-year-old woman examined had persistent retro-orbital pain. Her skull radiograms were slightly abnormal in the area just posterior to the globe of the eye. The superior orbital fissure was widened, and the sella turcica was asymmetric. This slightly calcified mass was a giant aneurysm (arrows) in the cavernous sinus. The petrous pyramid of the left temporal bone is labeled P, and the globes of the eyes are labeled G.

occasionally some vomiting associated with the pain, and the pupil in the affected eye may be dilated (24). The transient character of the symptoms suggests cluster headache or ophthalmoplegic migraine to most physicians dealing with the problem. Attacks recur at intervals of months or years. The responsible lesion in the Tolosa-Hunt syndrome is probably an inflammatory lesion in the cavernous sinus (25). The cranial nerves responsible for eye movements travels through the cavernous sinus on their way to the eye and are vulnerable at this point. The pain usually responds to high dose steroid treatment.

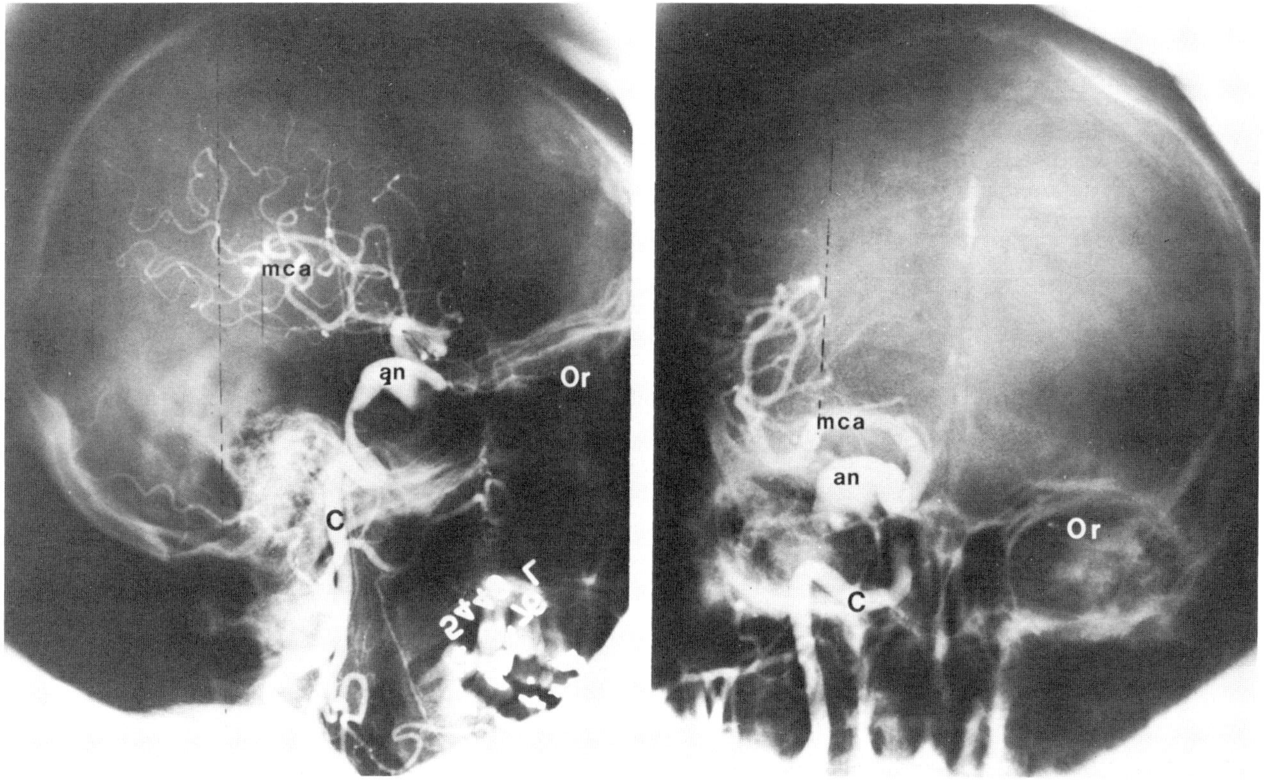

Figure 13.4. This arteriogram (lateral and anteroposterior views) reveals a giant aneurysm (an) in the cavernous sinus of the patient whose computed tomogram is shown in Figure 13.3. The internal carotid artery (C), the middle cerebral artery (mca), and the orbit (Or) are labeled.

Hypertensive Headache

High blood pressure is an extremely common problem in the United States, and many of the patients suffering from this disorder complain of episodic or chronic headaches. Examination of the blood pressure at the time of the headache will often reveal a greater than normal elevation of the mean blood pressure. Some physicians have interpreted this as evidence that transient elevations in blood pressure can cause headaches. Others see this as simply an exacerbation of the hypertension by a headache or exacerbation of both the hypertension and a chronic headache disorder by stress. Profound elevations of blood pressure with resultant seizures, focal neurologic deficits, and altered consciousness (hypertensive encephalopathy) will usually be associated with a headache, but this does not prove that mild elevations of blood pressure can produce headache. Patients treated with monoamine oxidase inhibitors for depression may have severe headaches developing acutely in association with sudden increases in their blood pressure. This occurs when they eat a tyramine-containing food. Similar headaches develop in patients with pheochromocytoma, a tumor of the adrenal gland, when their blood pressures abruptly increase. Regardless of whether or not the patient with hypertension has a headache, the blood pressure must be controlled. The real risks to the hypertensive patient are cardiovascular and cerebrovascular disease, not headache (Figure 13.5).

An unusual, but particularly disturbing, setting for hypertension-related headaches is sexual intercourse. Susceptible individuals complain that they develop diffuse, dull headaches during some sexual encounters, with the headache achieving its greatest intensity at orgasm (5). This type of headache not only disturbs normal sexual function, but it also may produce focal neurologic signs that do not resolve. Brainstem infarction is apparently responsible when the headache leaves the hypertensive individual with focal deficits. Patients with these sexual headaches are wise to avoid sexual excitement if they have a low grade headache.

Temporal Arteritis

Vascular disease occasionally produces headache as the principal symptom of the disorder. One of the more common vascular diseases typically producing head pain is temporal arteritis. The victim of this disease will complain of sharp pain at the temple or a dull pain about the top of the head with focal tenderness over the temples (15). Additional complaints include pain in the jaw with chewing or prolonged talking and generalized malaise with depression and loss of interest in all activities (26). A sudden loss of vision in one eye is, unfortunately, one of the most common early symptoms. Without treatment, more thaa 50 percent of patients with this disease will become blind in one or both eyes (26). Additional ocular

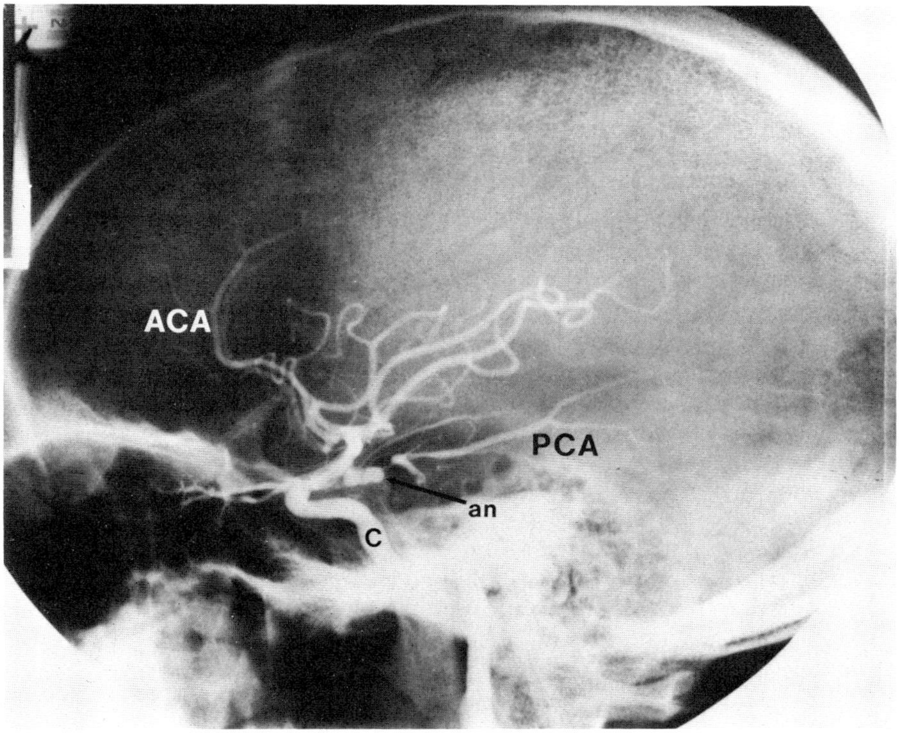

Figure 13.5. This arteriogram was performed on a 37-year-old man who developed headache, neck stiffness, and diffuse weakness while he was defecating. Although there were no focal deficits, he had blood in his spinal fluid. The arteriogram revealed a large aneurysm (an) of the posterior communicating artery. There is a segment of the artery connecting to the posterior cerebral artery (PCA) that is narrowed by spasm. The anterior cerebral artery (ACA) is normal. The bleeding from the aneurysm was presumably triggered by an acute rise in intracranial blood pressure associated with defecation.

symptoms include blurred vision, transient loss of vision (amaurosis fugax), conjunctivitis, scintillating scotomas, photophobia, and transient ophthalmoplegia. Fever, loss of appetite, weight loss, and a mild elevation in the peripheral white blood cell count all suggest a chronic infection, but a diligent search for infection will reveal nothing (26). Women are affected four times as often as men (5).

Headache is the most common initial complaint in victims of temporal arteritis (26). The typical headache is abrupt in onset and centered on the temples with radiation to the scalp, face, occiput, or jaw. The pain may be worse at night and discrete spots on the scalp may have extraordinary sensitivity. Admittedly, the precise pattern the headache assumes is quite variable (26). Examination of the temporal arteries will often reveal tender, pulseless threads of tissue where the superficial artery would ordinarily run. The headache may be chronic or episodic, and many victims of temporal arteritis are treated for tension headache before the seriousness of their condition is appreciated.

This is an inflammatory disease that produces obliterative changes in the large and medium-sized vessels of the head. Branches of the external carotid and ophthalmic artery are especially vulnerable to this disease, but the vertebral artery and the posterior ciliary artery of the eye are also routinely inflamed (5,15). Claudication pain in the jaw develops with obliteration of branches of the facial artery, and blindness occurs because there is occlusion of branches of the ophthalmic artery (26). The damage to the eye is primarily in the optic nerve, rather than the retina. Damage to other cranial vessels can cause cerebral symptoms, including dementia, confusion, hallucinations, depression, convulsions, hemiparesis, cranial nerve palsies, and coma (26).

Victims of temporal arteritis are invariably over 55 years of age, and the diagnosis is usually suspected when the erythrocyte sedimentation rate is discovered to be over 60 or 70 millimeters per hour. A normal sedimentation rate does not rule out this inflammatory disease, but only 30 percent of biopsy-proven cases of temporal arteritis have sedimentation rates below 40 millimeters per hour (5). Aside from a mild hypochromic anemia and a slight elevation in the cerebrospinal fluid protein content, there will be little objective evidence to confirm the diagnosis without biopsy of the temporal arteries. Some patients have joint pain and proximal muscle tenderness, but even in these individuals electrical studies on the muscles will be normal and biopsy of tender muscles will be unrevealing (26).

Any elderly person complaining of severe headache should be investigated for this disease. If the sedimentation rate is elevated and there is no other obvious explanation for the discomfort, treatment should be started immediately. Blindness is a very real risk in individuals left untreated. If the diagnosis is suspected, but not established, a biopsy of the temporal artery will help. The inflammatory changes with typical giant cell infiltrates are easily identified.

The treatment is high dose steroids. Prednisone started at 100 milligrams daily and tapered as the sedimentation rate falls provides some protection against complications of this disease. Unfortunately, victims of temporal arteritis are invariably elderly, and high dose steroids pose special problems in this group. Latent diabetes is easily unmasked and osteoporosis will quickly develop. Left untreated, patients will have remission of their symptoms in weeks or months, but the problem will recur and the next exacerbation may be heralded by the sudden onset of irreversible blindness (26). Even with corticosteroid therapy, vision will be impaired in 13 percent of affected individuals (5). Patients with temporal arteritis must be monitored for neurologic and medical complications of both the disease and the treatment.

Vascular Malformations

Unilateral headaches indistinguishable from migraine on clinical grounds often develop with vascular malformations. These malformations are congenital abnormalities that increase in size or influence as the patient gets older. They may involve just venous, just arterial, or both venous and arterial structures. Early indications of the malformation may include little besides the dull, unilateral headache and transient neurologic deficits typical of a migraine headache. Left untreated, the malformation may bleed or enlarge. In either case there will be damage to the brain, and the patient will suffer a stroke. Neurologic deficits can evolve slowly over the course of years with a vascular malformation, and patients so affected usually have seizures associated with the malformation.

Diagnosis of the malformation depends upon arteriography. If the malformation is very large, it may be apparent on computed tomography of the brain with contrast enhancement, but in many cases computed tomography will not positively identify the lesion. An electroencephalogram also may point to the location of the structural lesion, but not define its nature. A clue to the existence of the vascular malformation can occasionally be obtained during the physical examination by listening to the head. Auscultation over the temples or over the orbits may detect a bruit produced by the high volume of blood flowing through the malformation.

Treatment of vascular malformations is surgical. If the lesion is superficial, a complete resection should be attempted. If the lesion is too deep for surgery, occlusion of some of the involved blood vessels with silicon balls or glue may reduce the long-term complications of the malformation. Unfortunately, just occluding the feeding vessels does not protect the patient from an intracerebral hemorrhage.

STRUCTURAL AND INFECTIOUS CAUSES OF HEADACHE

Structural causes of headache are often overlooked in patients with apparent psychologic problems. A compensation neurosis after severe head injury is more easily embraced as the explanation for an intractable headache than is structural brain disease, especially if the physician responsible for the patient has been frustrated in all his efforts to treat the headache. Physicians more personally involved with their patients may have a natural disinclination to entertain a more malignant etiology for an intractable headache, such as chronic subdural hematoma, chronic central nervous system infection, or brain tumor. Increased intracranial pressure is easily overlooked when the patient is a young, otherwise healthy woman with no obvious neurologic signs or symptoms. The real problem for the physician in any of these situations is deciding how vigorously to pursue the patient's complaints. At some point, a headache with no obvious organic etiology must be dealt with as a psychologic problem.

Posttraumatic Headache

Headache is common after any head injury. The pattern of headache is extremely variable, and the duration of the complaint is entirely unpredictable. If the patient suffered an obvious cerebral contusion with persistent neurologic signs months after the injury, it is reasonable to expect the headache to persist for months, if not years (Figure 13.6). Dealing with this type of protracted pain is often frustrating for both the physician and the patient. Mild analgesics usually provide no relief, and narcotic medications lead to the unavoidable conflicts of dependence that develop with use of any addictive drug. Complicating the management of any patient with posttraumatic headache is the posttraumatic depression that lasts weeks to months after serious head injury. This depression certainly may exacerbate the headache, but it should not be judged the sole cause of the headache. A reasonable approach to posttraumatic headache includes treatment of the depression with tricyclic antidepressants or with psychotherapeutic support or both and treatment of the headache with analgesics.

Any patient with significant head injury, progressive affective changes, and chronic headache should be investigated for a chronic subdural hematoma. A computed tomogram of the brain without contrast is usually sufficient to dismiss this potentially lethal complication of head injury. Meningitis may develop in patients with fractures extending into the sinuses or the ears, but these infections are usually rapidly progressive, even if they develop several months after the fracture. Whenever there is a question of meningitis, the cerebrospinal fluid should be examined.

Most posttraumatic headaches are idiopathic and transient. The mild analgesic most effective for the patient should be systematically sought. Propoxyphene, acetaminophen, aspirin, or a combination of one of these with a small dose of codeine is occasionally effective against the chronic headache. There may be a delay of days between the trauma and the appearance of the headache, in which case it is usually helpful to warn the patient that he will probably have discomfort in the near future, and that this is not necessarily a grave sign.

Intracranial Tumors

Patients with chronic headaches are often concerned that they might have a brain tumor. Fortunately, intracranial neoplasia is rarely the cause of headaches. When a tumor is present, there are usually other signs of neurologic damage besides the headache. The brain itself is insensitive to destructive lesions in its substance, and headache will develop with brain

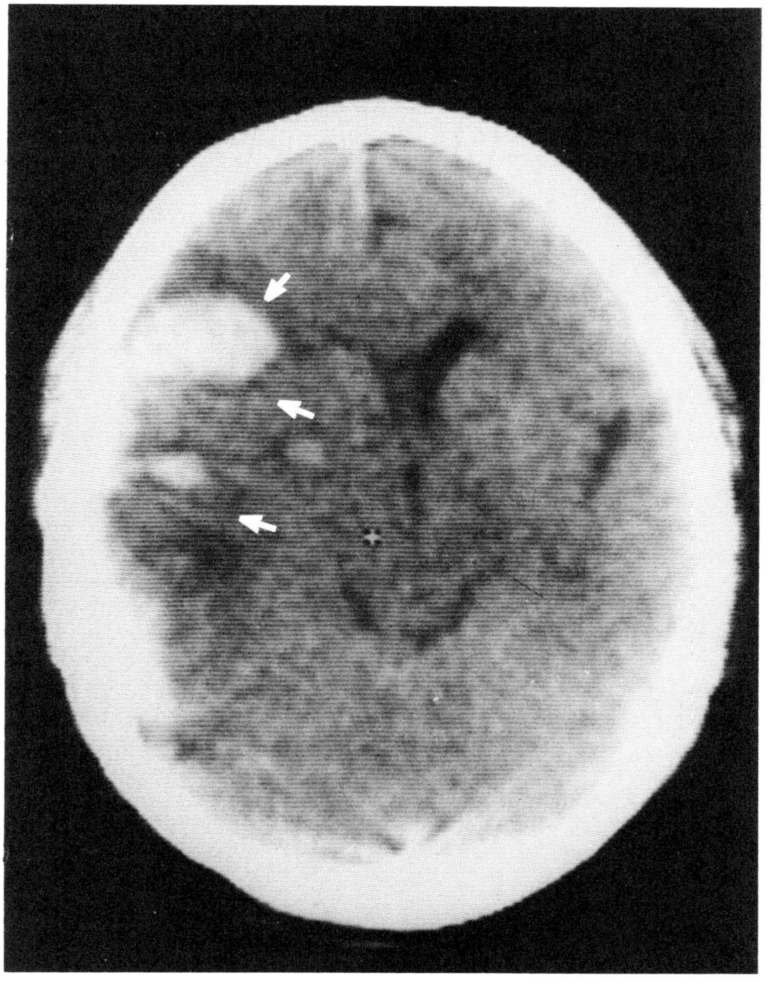

Figure 13.6. A 59-year-old man fell from the second-floor window of his apartment and was lethargic for 2 days after the fall. Acutely, he was described as having left facial weakness and impaired intellectual function. The computed tomogram of his brain revealed an extensive contusion (indicated by the arrows) extending from his right frontal lobe into his right temporal and parietal lobes. The white collection just beneath the skull is fresh blood. One year after the head injury, this man still had severe headaches every morning (courtesy of Drs. J. Loh and W. Hotson).

tumors only if there is stretching of vascular structures or irritation of some meningeal surfaces. The discomfort may, in fact, develop from a lesion extending from the skull irritating the meninges (Figure 13.7). Even with obstructive hydrocephalus, headache is generally a fairly late symptom of the increased intracranial pressure.

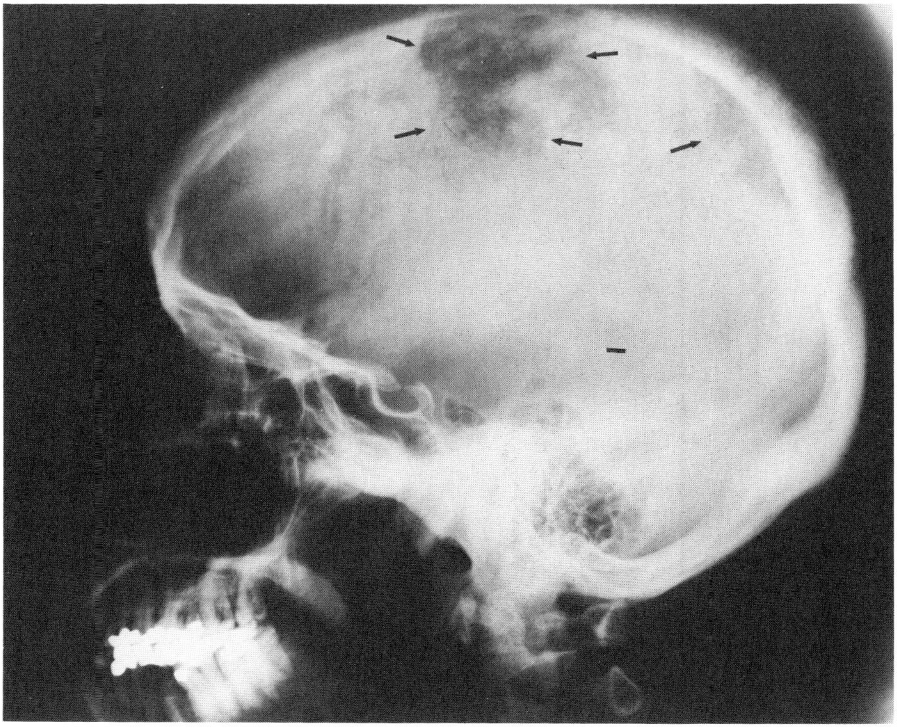

Figure 13.7. A plain skull film revealed multiple areas of eroded bone (arrows) in this 29-year-old woman with stromal uterine sarcoma. Multiple bone lesions were also apparent on radionuclide bone scan. The skull erosions were from metastatic uterine sarcoma.

The location of head pain with intracranial lesions is variable. Posterior fossa lesions may produce pain at the base of the skull by stretching the meninges innervated by the upper cervical spinal roots, but just as often the patient with a posterior fossa lesion complains of pain behind or above the eye. Anatomically, this is understandable because the inferior surface of the tentorium cerebelli, the fold of meninges separating the cerebellum from the cerebrum, is innervated by the first division of the trigeminal nerve, the same nerve that innervates the skin of the face over the eye and forehead.

If the patient is concerned that his discomfort is from a malignant intracranial lesion, he may get some reassurance from a negative electroencephalogram and skull radiogram. Patients obsessed with the possibility of a brain tumor usually have problems requiring more attention than is feasible during an initial evaluation by any physician. Most doctors will refer the patient to a psychiatrist or psychologist as soon as the preliminary tests to check for a structural lesion are completed.

Pseudotumor Cerebri

Young women, often obese and occasionally on sex hormone supplements, are especially prone to develop the poorly understood syndrome of benign intracranial hypertension, which is also known as pseudotumor cerebri (27). The patient appears to have a cerebral tumor because she complains of severe headache of recent onset and has unequivocal papilledema. This swelling of the optic nerve does reflect increased intracranial pressure, but the intracranial hypertension is not from a tumor or cerebrovascular hypertension. The increased pressure is apparently from increased fluid in the head. There is no hydrocephalus, and, in fact, computed tomography of the brain will reveal relatively small ventricles or even slitlike ventricles (27). There is swelling in the brain substance itself, producing extremely high intracranial pressures and reducing the ventricles to remarkably small volumes. The headaches are diffuse, dull, and occasionally throbbing, and they may increase with abrupt changes in head position. If the increased intracranial pressure persists for more than a few weeks, the patient will develop impaired vision as swelling of the optic nerve enlarges the physiologic blindspot. Prolonged intracranial hypertension can lead to permanent loss of much central vision.

The diagnosis is made by excluding the possibility of an underlying tumor. Computed tomography of the brain with and without contrast enhancement will suggest the diagnosis if the typical configuration of the ventricles is observed. Once the physician is fairly confident that there is no intracranial mass lesion, he is obliged to check the cerebrospinal fluid pressure and content. The pressure will be greater than 200 millimeters of water for most patients with pseudotumor cerebri, and it will exceed 400 millimeters of water in some. The cerebrospinal fluid examination not only documents the increased intracranial pressure, but also helps eliminate the possibility of an unsuspected chronic infection or meningeal carcinomatosus. Unfortunately, many young women presumed to have pseudotumor cerebri prove to have intracranial tumors.

The clinical picture of pseudotumor cerebri develops after several well-defined problems, but in most patients the etiology is never found. Head trauma occasionally precedes the appearance of the increased intracranial pressure, but metabolic problems are more commonly implicated. Excessive exposure to vitamin A, ingestion of tetracycline or nalidixic acid, and hypoparathyroidism are all occasionally followed by pseudotumor cerebri (27). Patients who have been on corticosteroids for a long time may develop this benign intracranial hypertension when the steroids are stopped (5).

The diagnostic spinal tap is also therapeutic. If enough cerebrospinal fluid is removed to bring the pressure close to the normal range (up to 150 millimeters of water), the patient usually experiences considerably less headache and may have improved visual acuity. Spinal taps traditionally have been the treatment of choice for this disorder, at least from the physician's point of view. Repeated spinal taps in experienced hands carry little morbidity and may produce a complete remission of all signs and symptoms within a few weeks or months. Visual fields must be followed closely, and the papilledema may provide a simple guide to the required frequency of the spinal taps. Some patients will have resolution of the disorder after just one or two spinal taps; others will require weekly spinal taps over the course of months. Salt restriction and diuretic medication are also routinely used to treat this disorder.

The alternative to repeated spinal taps is high dose corticosteroid treatment. Prednisone given at 60 to 100 milligrams daily may decrease the intracranial pressure quickly and reliably, but the adverse effects of the corticosteroid weigh heavily against its prolonged use. Most of the patients with this disorder are extremely obese, a problem that presumably increases their susceptibility to the disease. Corticosteroids will increase the obesity and may precipitate the additional problem of diabetes mellitus. There is little alternative to corticosteroids in extremely obese patients. Lumbar puncture without fluoroscopic assistance may be impossible in these individuals, and weight reduction is usually unsuccessful in individuals chronically distracted by the severe headache.

Remissions may be permanent or transient. Each attack must be dealt with just as vigorously to prevent loss of vision. If more conservative measures fail to keep the intracranial pressure at a tolerable level, a ventricular shunt may be necessary. This type of drastic intervention is a last resort, not only because it involves introduction of a tube into the brain itself but also because it is a technically difficult procedure in a patient with small ventricles.

Central Nervous System Infection

Meningitis or encephalitis often presents with a headache, but the cause of the diffuse head discomfort is usually obvious within a few hours or days when the patient develops a stiff neck and fever. The headache with such infections may be limited to the base of the skull or to the supraorbital area, but it is usually not well localized. Subtle personality changes may precede both the headache and the fever, and focal neurologic signs often develop once the infection is well established. Chronic infections are more misleading than acute infections. A chronic cryptococcal meningitis may produce little more than headaches for weeks before focal neurologic signs develop. Susceptible individuals are usually immunosuppressed because of chemotherapy or hematologic disease, and so they may never mount a fever or they may even become hypothermic. Anyone complaining of headache and stiff neck should be examined for the possibility of meningitis. With meningococcal meningitis the patient often develops small red spots in the skin, known as petechial hemorrhages. Patients with chronic tuberculous meningitis usually have progressive cranial nerve signs. Whenever there is any suspicion of meningitis as the cause of a headache, the physician is obliged to obtain cerebrospinal fluid for analysis and culture.

Subdural Hematoma

A chronic subdural hematoma may develop days, weeks, or months after head trauma. Patients on hemodialysis for renal failure occasionally develop subdural hematomas even with no history of head trauma. Elderly patients may suffer minor head trama before developing a subdural hematoma, but they frequently cannot recall any event that would explain the development of the blood clot overlying the brain. Symptoms of a chronic subdural hematoma may include little more than headache and confusion, but most patients will develop focal neurologic signs before the subdural collection progresses to the point where the patient slips into coma. This lesion is lethal because it will lead to herniation of the brain either across the falx cerebri or through the tentorium cerebelli. Because the clinical signs developing in patients with chronic subdural hematomas are not very specific, suspicion that a patient has a subdural collection must rest upon evaluation of the type of patient developing the neurologic signs and symptoms prompting medical attention. A dialysis patient with confusion and headache is certainly a more reasonable candidate for a chronic subdural hematoma than a middle-aged business man with depression and chronic headache. When there is reason to entertain a chronic subdural hematoma, the patient should have a computed tomogram of the head. If a subdural collection is found, it should be removed. Some physicians have attempted dealing with chronic subdural hematomas by giving the patient high dose corticosteroids, but the experience with this approach has been disappointing. A chronic subdural hematoma should be viewed as a surgical emergency.

Increased Intracranial Pressure

Increased intracranial pressure for any reason can cause headache. The type of head pain is variable, but it is generally not unilateral and is often associated with nausea and vomiting. Hydrocephalus is the usual cause of increased intracranial pressure. Obstruction to the flow of cerebrospinal fluid causes hydrocephalus in patients with brain tumors or other lesions interfering with the free flow of the cerebrospinal fluid. Hydrocephalus can occur with no obstruction to the flow of the fluid, in which case the problem is almost invariably a defect in the reabsorption of the cerebrospinal fluid. Diagnosis of increased intracranial pressure requires measurement of cerebrospinal fluid pressure, but that may be a dangerous procedure when the increased pressure is from a space-occupying lesion, such as a brain abscess or tumor. If there is no apparent mass lesion to explain the increased pressure, a ventricular shunt may be necessary to relieve the pressure. If a mass is present, it should be dealt with by surgery or radiation, depending upon its nature.

FACIAL PAIN

Facial pain occasionally develops as a symptom of depression and commonly leads to depression when it is intractable. Determining whether depression caused the symptom or the facial pain caused the affective disorder is often not at all simple. There are several neurologic disorders producing facial pain as the initial symptom or the only symptom, and establishing which is responsible is of considerable practical importance. Most facial pain syndromes are treatable, and treatments are not similar for different syndromes. The two most commonly encountered forms of facial pain are "typical" and "atypical." Typical facial pain is sharp, paroxysmal, and very brief. The discomfort is felt in a well-circumscribed area, that area often following the pattern of innervation of one division of a cranial nerve. Cranial nerves V, VII, IX, and X are those usually involved. No fixed neurologic deficits accompany typical facial pain, but destruction of the nerve responsible will eliminate the pain. Atypical facial pain is not at all paroxysmal and follows no anatomic pattern. Severe depression may be found when this type of pain is investigated. Both types usually affect the lower face, but the character of the pain is so different in each that there is usually no problem distinguishing between the two.

Other types of facial pain develop with local tissue damage about the face, in the sinuses, or about the teeth. Temporomandibular joint dysfunction can produce chronic facial discomfort, and intracranial lesions may produce pain referred to the face. All these structural bases for facial pain should be thoroughly investigated before treatment for typical or atypical facial pain is started.

The pattern of pain will suggest neurologic disease in some cases and masked depression in other cases; this will direct therapeutic approaches to the pain. Unfortunately, facial pain may be misleading, and what appears to be a classic case of trigeminal neuralgia may prove to be an atypical case of nasopharyngeal carcinoma. Most important in the assessment of any patient with facial pain is attention to changes in the character of the pain and to the appearance of signs of local tissue damage. The elimination of facial pain often has a dramatic effect on the sufferer's personality and behavior, but this largely affective change does not imply a psychologic basis for the observed disorder. On the contrary, patients with depressive disorders underlying their facial pain may exhibit little symptomatic relief or psychologic improvement despite numerous therapeutic approaches to their complaint.

Tic Douloureux (Trigeminal Neuralgia)

Paroxysmal shooting or stabbing pain in the face arises with disease of the sensory nerve of the face, the trigeminal or fifth cranial nerve (28). Because of the tic-like brevity of the pain and the extraordinary intensity of the discomfort with trigeminal neuralgia, this cranial nerve dysfunction is called tic douloureux. Although it has been recognized as a distinct entity for over 200 years, its cause is still unknown. Most patients complain of a burning or electrical pain lasting less than a second and distributing to a relatively restricted area of the face. The intense pain will evoke an involuntary contraction of the face in some patients. Most victims of this disorder will recognize an area on the face or in the mouth that will trigger the pain when it is touched. If this trigger point is in the mouth, the patient usually seeks dental attention and commonly has several teeth removed before the neurologic basis for this pain is recognized. Trigger points in the mouth can be especially disabling because they will interfere with eating or at least with chewing. If the sensitive area is on the face, the patient will take extraordinary precautions to avoid stimulating it. These include avoiding close contact with other people who might inadvertently touch the area.

The trigeminal nerve has three main divisions, the ophthalmic (V1), the maxillary (V2), and the mandibular (V3) (28). The pain of tic douloureux is almost always limited to only one or two of these divisions, and these are usually V2 and V3, the maxillary and mandibular divisions (21). The pain may shoot into the eye or into the cheek, but it generally does not affect both of these areas together. If the ophthalmic division is involved, a more malignant basis for the pain should be considered. Retro-orbital tumors or chronic infections may be responsible for sensory abnormalities in this division of the nerve. Facial weakness is never a complaint with tic douloureux; and, in fact, involvement of any other cranial nerve usually indicates a lesion in the brain. Patients with facial pain and impaired external rotation of the eye have an osteomyelitis or a tumor at the tip of the petrous pyramid, the segment of the temporal bone that both the fifth and sixth cranial nerves pass as they travel to the front of the skull (28). The combination of facial pain over the ophthalmic division of the trigeminal nerve and a lateral rectus palsy is called Gradenigo's syndrome, a problem most often seen in patients with infections extending into the petrous bone from the mastoid air cells in the temporal bone (Figure 13.8). Careful neurologic examination will reveal no objective sensory or motor deficits about the face and head in true trigeminal neuralgia. Despite years of paroxysmal pain, the patient with tic douloureux always has intact facial sensation.

Seasonal changes may affect the severity of the pain substantially. Many patients find they have the most bouts of pain during cold weather. Moving to a warm climate occasionally eliminates the pain with no other

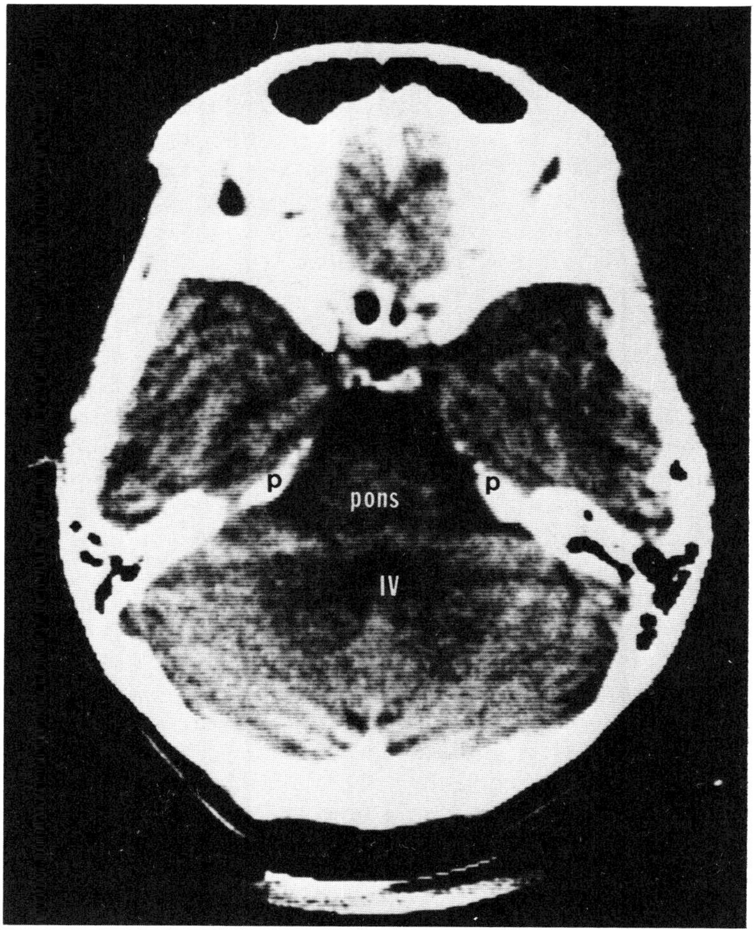

Figure 13.8. Gradenigo's syndrome develops when an infection or tumor in the tip of the petrous pyramid (p) damages the sixth cranial nerve, which is arising in the pons, and irritates the fifth cranial nerve. The first division of the trigeminal nerve is most often affected, resulting in pain above the eye. The damage to the abducens nerve causes the eye on the painful side to turn inward. The fourth ventricle (IV), which lies between the pons and the cerebellum, can also be seen on this computed tomogram.

treatment. The pain is invariably unilateral, and the acute stabbing pain may be followed by a more prolonged dull or burning discomfort over the same area of the face. This dull component of the pain may radiate to the ipsilateral ear. Most patients are affected when they are over 50 years of age, and women are more vulnerable than men by a ratio of three to one (21).

The cause of this facial pain is unknown. Although disease of the trigeminal nerve is the presumed basis for the sensory dysfunction, the most common cause of that dysfunction is still controversial. Current theories favor a viral basis for the dysesthesias. *Herpes simplex* has been implicated by a few investigators. Some neurosurgeons believe that compression of the nerve as it enters the brainstem by the superior cerebellar artery causes the damage that leads to the facial pain (5). No theory is universally accepted.

Typical trigeminal neuralgia occasionally develops with intracranial lesions that press on the nerve. Acoustic neuromas, cholesteatomas, basilar artery aneurysms, and angiomas can all produce facial pain in the distribution of the trigeminal nerve. Occasionally, patients with a long-standing history of tic douloureux prove to have multiple sclerosis (5). If a mass or a demyelinating lesion is responsible for the trigeminal nerve dysfunction, the patient should eventually develop other signs of intracranial disease.

Several kinds of treatment are available despite the uncertainty surrounding the etiology of this disorder. Carbamazepine, an anticonvulsant, in doses of 600 to 1200 milligrams per day will relieve the pain completely in 70 to 80 percent of patients (29). This drug is usually effective within 24 hours of its introduction and may completely abolish the pain at very low serum levels (29). It acts by interfering with conduction in the brainstem sensory tracts. Those who cannot tolerate this drug because of allergic, gastrointestinal, or hematologic reactions may respond to phenytoin, another anticonvulsant, at doses of 200 to 400 milligrams daily (30). Like carbamazepine, phenytoin depresses excitatory synaptic transmission in the trigeminal nucleus (30). With both of these drugs, the patient may be kept pain-free on a dose lower than that initially necessary to eliminate the pain.

A nonanticonvulsant that is effective in some patients who fail to respond to carbamazepine or phenytoin is baclofen, a derivative of the inhibitory neurotransmitter gamma-aminobutyric acid (31). Relatively high doses (60 to 80 milligrams per day) are needed in most patients before baclofen will be effective. The problem patients are those unresponsive to all of these oral medications.

The severity of the pain makes the patient very accommodating, and a number of surgical approaches have been developed as a result of this patient cooperation. The techniques currently used include alcohol injection into the trigeminal nerve or the gasserion ganglion and radiofrequency damage to the ganglion (5,32). Positioning an electrode in the ganglion and using radiofrequency waves to damage the nerve has the advantage of producing little, if any, facial anesthesia when it is successful. Cutting the nerve or destroying the gasserion ganglion from which the three divisions originate will produce permanent facial anesthesia, a disturbance of facial sensation that may be as aggravating for the patient as the tic douloureux. Working on the assumption that compression of the nerve by the anterior inferior or superior cerebellar artery is the problem, some neurosurgeons have treated the disorder by placing cushioning material between the artery and the nerve. All of these techniques have had some success, but the pain may recur months or years after the surgical intervention regardless of the approach.

Atypical Facial Pain

Atypical facial pain usually arises with minor nerve trauma and major psychologic problems. The nerve damage may be equivocal, but the psychologic problems are invariably obvious. The facial pain is dull, but constant; it usually does not respond to analgesics or nerve blocks (21). Attacks of the pain start episodically, but evolve into an unremitting complaint. A dental procedure or facial injury may "trigger" the initial episode of atypical facial pain, but the constant aching sensation will persist long after the initiating trauma has passed (21). This type of pain is usually unilateral and limited to the lower half of the face (9). The patient often complains of an aching or crushing pain in the cheek, at the angle of the jaw, to one side of the nose, or diffusely over the lower half of the face (21,33). The severity of the pain usually waxes and wanes for no apparent reason; at its worst, it may radiate into the neck or into other parts of the head. Occasionally, the patient complains of nasal stuffiness, excessive tearing, blocked ears, and even ringing in the ears when the pain is most severe (33). Shooting pains, electric shocklike sensations, and trigger points for the pain are invariably absent (33). The changes in the severity of the pain show no diurnal pattern: the discomfort is no worse at night than during the day.

Years before the appearance of the atypical facial pain, many of these patients have long-term problems with common migraine (9). Women complain of atypical facial pain much more than men, and the usual age of onset is 30 to 50 years of age. Before they seek neurologic attention, they often submit to numerous dental, medical, or surgical procedures (21).

This type of facial pain generally indicates an underlying depression, anxiety state, or related psychologic problem. Repressed rage, feelings of failure or frustration, sexual conflicts, or intense disappointment may all surface when the patient is questioned about circumstances coincident with the atypical facial pain (21). These patients routinely insist on discussing the facial pain and resist efforts to connect other problems to the pain (21). It is apparent in some patients that the symptoms of pain represent repressed anger or rage, which may elicit considerable guilt (21). The history may reveal an important figure in the patient's life who suffered with a similar pain and toward whom the patient has many conflicting feelings. Occasionally, the symptom is a "reprisal response" to a coincidental emotional trauma, the patient directing his complaint of pain to those involved in his emotional trauma (21). Obviously, the psychologic setting for the facial pain can be complex, and extensive probing into the background of the symptom is best delayed until a fairly stable bond is established between the physician and the patient. The pain cannot be dismissed as just a manifestation of depression, but a cautious approach to extensive medical tests is advisable.

Antidepressant treatment is the most effective approach to this disorder. Tricyclic antidepressants are effective after 1 to 2 weeks of therapeutic doses. Younger patients may have some improvement with muscle relaxation techniques alone, but this is best linked to psychotherapy (33). A psychotic depression is a real danger in patients with this disorder, and psychiatric intervention should be begun as soon after the diagnosis as is feasible (9).

The cause of atypical facial pain is unknown (21). Some investigators believe it has a physiologic basis and is not solely a conversion reaction. They attribute the discomfort experienced by the patient to dilatation in the extracranial blood vessels centering about the division of the maxillary artery that supplies the sphenopalatine region (21). Presumably, cerebrocortical activity triggers this local vascular reaction.

Temporomandibular Joint Dysfunction

Pain seeming to arise in the jaw or in the temporomandibular joint is often secondary to temporomandibular joint dysfunction or, as it is also called, the myofascial pain dysfunction syndrome (33). This type of facial pain is invariably just in front of the ear, but is occasionally referred to the forehead or teeth. The patient will complain of tenderness in the preauricular area and, occasionally, over the muscles of mastication, specifically the masseter and temporalis muscles. There is no bone or joint damage initially, but in time osteoarthritic changes appear at the temporomandibular joint, presumably as a result of trauma to the joint with excessive muscle activity (33). Mandibular movements may be restricted, and crepitus may be felt at the temporomandibular joint with jaw movement. The pain is usually dull, almost always unilateral, and invariably progressive. Chronic anxiety or acute stress may precipitate this pain syndrome. Techniques to relax the jaw muscles, as well as tricyclic antidepressants, are sometimes effective in alleviating the pain.

Raeder's Syndrome

An inflammatory or granulomatous reaction of unknown cause in the middle cranial fossa may produce complaints similar to those seen in atypical facial pain. The patient has chronic, dull, often severe, facial pain over the distribution of part or all of the trigeminal nerve. Distinguishing this inflammatory problem from the syndrome of atypical facial pain is the partial Horner syndrome that accompanies the pain. The patient has a small pupil (miosis) and a drooping eyelid (ptosis) on the same side of the face as the pain (22). Sweating is normal in this partial Horner syndrome because the fibers responsible for sweating leave the main sympathetic supply before the inflammatory lesion is encountered. Postganglionic fibers of the sympathetic system are specifically affected in this syndrome, and this means that the pupil will exhibit responses to dilating substances characteristic of denervation sensitivity of peripheral origin (22).

Postherpetic Neuralgia

Herpes zoster infection of the face always produces severe pain acutely, but when the superficial viral infection subsides, the patient may be left with chronic facial pain. This is a problem primarily affecting the elderly. The obvious etiology is viral damage to the trigeminal nerve, but despite this obvious basis it is exceedingly refractory to treatment. The ophthalmic division of the trigeminal nerve is most often affected, and the patient commonly has discoloration or scarring over the area previously involved by the cutaneous lesion (28). Tricyclic antidepressants, neuroleptics, and carbamazepine have all been used in the treatment of this chronic pain disorder with unsatisfactory results. This is discussed further in the chapter on sensory abnormalities.

REFERENCES

1. Caviness VS, O'Brien P: Current concepts: Headache. *N Engl J Med* 302:446, 1980.
2. Caviness VS, O'Brien P: Headache. *N Engl J Med* 303:223, 1980.
3. Martinez AJ, Lee A, Moossy J, et al: Pituitary adenomas: Clinicopathological and immunohistochemical study. *Ann Neurol* 7:24, 1980.
4. Friedman AP: Nature of headache. *Headache* 19:163, 1979.
5. Lance JW: Headache. *Neurology (NY)* 10:1, 1981.
6. Weatherhead AD: Headache associated with psychiatric disorders: Classification and etiology. *Psychosomatics* 21:832, 1980.
7. Packard R: Psychiatric aspects of headache. *Headache* 19:168, 1972.
8. Sternbach RA, Dalessio DJ, Kunzel M, et al: MMPI patterns in common headache disorders. *Headache* 20:311,1980.
9. Graham JR: Migraine headache: Diagnosis and management. *Headache* 19:133, 1979.
10. Kudrow L, Sutkus BJ: MMPI patterns specificity in primary headache disorders. *Headache* 19:18, 1979.
11. Schnarch DM, Hunter JE: Migraine incidence in clinical vs nonclinical populations. *Psychosomatics* 2:314, 1980.

12. Martin JB, Reichlin S, Brown GM: *Clinical Neuroendocrinology*. Philadelphia, FA Davis, 1977.

13. Dalessio DJ: Classification and mechanism of migraine. *Headache* 19:144, 1979.

14. Edmeads J: Vascular headaches and the cranial circulation—Another look. *Headache* 19:127, 1979.

15. Raskin NH, Schwartz RK: Icepick-like pain. *Neurology (NY)* 30:203, 1980.

16. Kattah JC, Luessenhop AJ: Resolution of classic migraine after removal of an occipital lobe AVM. *Ann Neurol* 7:93, 1980.

17. Zifkin B, Andermann E, Andermann F, et al: An autosomal dominant syndrome of hemiplegic migraine, nystagmus, and tremor. *Ann Neurol* 8:329, 1980.

18. Propranolol for prevention of migraine headaches. *Med Lett Drugs Ther* 21:77, 1979.

19. Ljung O: Treatment of migraine with metoprolol. *N Engl J Med* 303:156, 1980.

20. Kudrow L: Cluster headache: Diagnosis and management. *Headache* 19:142, 1979.

21. Freidman AP: Atypical facial pain. *Trans Pac Coast Oto-Ophthalmol Soc* 58:155, 1977.

22. Pearce JMS: Chronic migrainous neuralgia. A variant of cluster headache. *Brain* 103:149, 1980.

23. Lithium for cluster headache. *Med Lett Drugs Ther* 21:78, 1979.

24. Hunt WE, Meagher JN, LeFever HE, et al: Painful ophthalmoplegia. *Neurology (NY)* 9:56, 1959.

25. Tolosa E: Periarteritic lesions of carotid siphon with clinical features of carotid infraclinoidal aneurysm. *J Neurol Neurosurg Psychiatry* 17:300, 1954.

26. Hamilton CR Jr, Shelley WM, Tumulty PA: Giant cell arteritis: Including temporal arteritis and polymyalgia rheumatica. *Medicine (Baltimore)* 50:1, 1971.

27. Donaldson JO: Pathogenesis of pseudotumor cerebri syndromes. *Neurology (NY)* 31:877, 1981.

28. Brodal A: *The Cranial Nerves*, ed 2. Oxford, Blackwell, 1965.

29. Tomson T, Tybring G, Bertilsson L, et al: Carbamazepine therapy in trigeminal neuralgia. *Arch Neurol* 37:699, 1980.

30. Rushton JG: Medical treatment of trigeminal neuralgia. *Med Clin North Am* 52:797, 1968.

31. Fromm GH, Terrence CF, Chattha AS, et al: Baclofen in trigeminal neuralgia. *Arch Neurol* 37:768, 1980.

32. Auger RG, Piegras DG, Laws ER Jr, et al: Microvascular decompression of the facial nerve for hemifacial spasm: Clinical and electrophysiologic observations. *Neurology (NY)* 31:346, 1981.

33. Gessel AH: Tension control for musculospastic pain. *Psychosomatics* 21:913, 1980.

14 Disturbed Vision, Hearing, and Balance

VISUAL ABNORMALITIES

Vision may be lost or altered as a fairly isolated symptom. When an individual complains of blindness, the physician generally has little trouble determining whether the deficit is real or not, regardless of the cause of the blindness. The evaluation of the patient is more complicated when he complains of altered, rather than absent, vision. Altered vision is an essentially subjective complaint. Highly complex visual phenomena are easily mistaken for hallucinations, and an individual with such visual abnormalities with no prior history of mental illness may be thought psychotic and inappropriately referred for psychiatric evaluation and treatment. If the patient's description of his visual disturbance suggests structural disease, it often will also indicate the site and nature of the structural lesion. Quite often an individual with severe visual impairment will not admit that he sees bizarre phenomena, even if these are handicapping him, for fear that such an admission would make him appear insane. Encouraging the patient to explain in as much detail as possible the basic features of his disturbed vision usually simplifies the evaluation of these patients.

TEMPORARY BLINDNESS

Vision in one eye or part of one visual field may be completely lost for minutes or weeks. With demyelinating disease, such as multiple sclerosis, an acute inflammation of the optic nerve, optic neuritis, often impairs or temporarily eliminates vision in one eye. This is a relatively common cause of transient blindness in young adults, and it usually produces subtle

Table 14.1. Causes of Transient Blindness in One Eye

Optic neuritis (multiple sclerosis, infection)
Transient ischemia (amaurosis fugax)
Trauma to the eye
Optic nerve compression

objective findings (Table 14.1). The patient will have pain in the affected eye, but the fundus will appear unremarkable, especially if the optic nerve is inflamed somewhat posterior to its exit from the eye, a condition called retrobulbar neuritis. Vision in that eye will lose color and clarity, but light perception is usually preserved. Even when the eye appears completely normal, objective evidence of a lesion can be gathered from functional tests, such as the afferent pupillary response, a phenomenon dependent upon the consensual pupillary response as already discussed in the section on diagnostic tools. After an acute attack of optic neuritis, vision recovers over the course of days or weeks, but complete restoration of visual acuity is unlikely.

When visual loss in one eye is much more fleeting, the condition is called amaurosis fugax. Vision in one eye becomes obscured and is restored over the course of seconds or minutes. This is a painless monocular visual loss usually resulting from vascular disease (1). Emboli from the internal carotid artery or from diseased heart valves can temporarily occlude the ophthalmic artery and produce ischemia of the retina, which, in turn, leads to blindness. A vasculitis or just pressure on the vessels to the retina may also cause this transient loss of vision (1). When vision is restored, it is generally at the level of acuity present before the attacks, but with every episode of visual loss, there is the possibility that vision will not return and that permanent damage to the retina will occur (Table 14.1).

More common than complete loss of vision in an eye is loss or obscuration of vision in part of one visual field (Table 14.2). These blindspots, or scotomas, are characteristic of classic migraine. Half of the patients with

Table 14.2. Causes of Transient Visual Field Abnormalities

Migraine
Transient ischemic attacks
Glaucoma
Focal seizures
Brain tumor
Arteriovenous malformations
Optic chiasm compression
Conversion reaction

neurologic symptoms occurring before their headaches will complain of disturbed vision (2). The blindspot in migraine may be surrounded by sparkling lights, in which case it is called a scintillating scotoma. When these appear as the prodrome to a migraine headache, they usually persist 10 to 20 minutes before resolving. Vision returns to normal after the headache prodrome, and most patients recognize that the transient disturbance in vision involved both eyes. The blindspot frequently has angular margins, reminiscent of ancient fortifications, but whether the scotoma is surrounded by scintillations or fortifications, the blindspot will subside before the headache begins (2). Scintillating scotomas rarely develop with arteriovenous malformations or tumors in the occipital lobes; but whenever a persistent field cut or other fixed neurologic deficit appears with the transient scotoma, a progressive structural lesion of the brain must be suspected. A more uncommon pattern of visual disturbance in migraine is photopsia, which is a shower of lights or stationary flecks of light (2,3). All of these visual disturbances characteristic of migraine can appear independently of the headache. The scotomas or photopsias may follow the evolution typical of a migraine prodrome, but a headache may fail to develop. Obviously, these isolated symptoms warrant more careful observation than the visual phenomena appearing as part of a classic migraine, but in most cases no structural brain lesion ever develops.

Visual loss that starts out as a transient phenomenon associated with poorly formed images, like scintillations, is more serious when the visual loss becomes fixed, even if only in part. Tumors of the optic nerve and optic chiasm often evoke transient visual phenomena described by patients as stars, sparkles, and rockets (Figure 14.1). The optic chiasm is the bundle of nerve fibers formed by the junction of the two optic nerves; some fibers cross the midline in this structure and, along with uncrossed fibers, course to the geniculate bodies as the optic tracts. Well-formed hallucinations do not occur with disease of the retina, optic nerve, or optic chiasm. Pathology other than migraine should always be sought when the visual disturbance is at all atypical (Figure 14.2). Transient loss of vision in one visual field is a common complaint developing with transient ischemic attacks, that is, temporary impairment of brain perfusion. When transient field cuts appear in young adults, systemic lupus erythematous, a cause of arteritis in the brain, should be suspected (4). Multiple sclerosis, an arteriovenous malformation, or a brain tumor may also be responsible, but all of these usually produce more extensive symptoms if a visual field cut is apparent.

Transient loss of all vision in both eyes is uncommon, but there are a few neurologic conditions that can produce this symptom (Table 14.3). An unusual form of migraine, which is presumed to involve the basilar artery, and so is called basilar migraine, can produce transient blindness and sudden loss of consciousness (5). Basilar migraine is obviously a diagnosis made by excluding more serious causes of these symptoms. Basilar impression, a deformity of the base of the skull likely to compromise

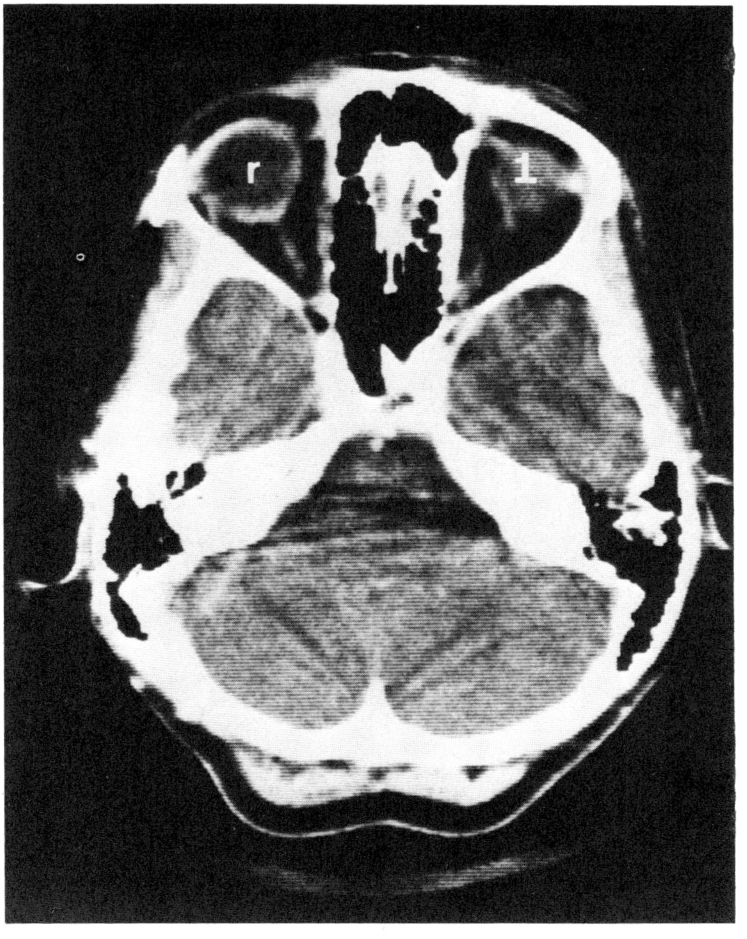

Figure 14.1. A routine computed tomogram of the head can reveal abnormalities in and around the eye. This normal computed tomogram cut through the globe of the right eye (r) and glanced across the upper surface of the globe of the left eye (l). The optic nerve is apparent on both sides, and individual extraocular muscles are well defined for the part of their course running through the section of this scan. The superior oblique muscle can be seen trailing obliquely from the top of the medial half of the left globe. The lateral rectus muscle is attached to the lateral aspect of the right globe. The walls of the orbits provide sharp contrast with the orbital contents.

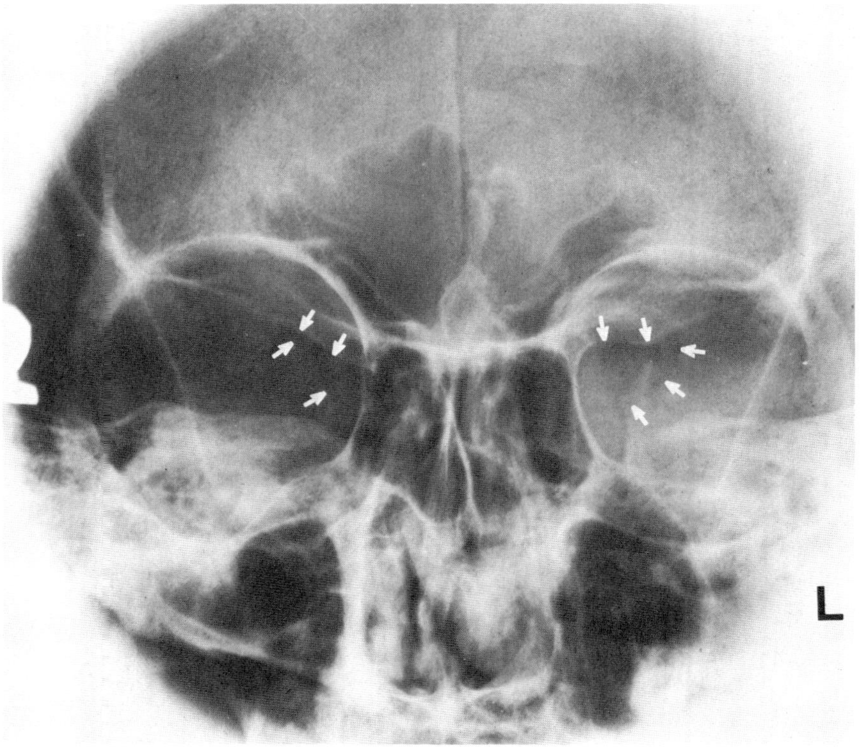

Figure 14.2. This x-ray film of the skull led to the discovery of a giant aneurysm in the 70-year-old woman studied. The patient had severe pain behind the left eye. The radiogram reveals a widened superior orbital fissure (arrows) on the left (L). Calcification in the aneurysm makes the walls of the left orbit appear thicker (whiter) than those of the right orbit.

blood flow through the vertebral arteries, occasionally produces loss of vision or dimming of vision along with of other focal neurologic signs, such as unilateral weakness, vertigo, and altered consciousness (6). This skeletal abnormality may also produce the illusion of yellow vision (6). Intraocular pressures should be checked in any patient complaining of

Table 14.3. Causes of Transient Blindness in Both Eyes

Basilar migraine
Vertebrobasilar insufficiency
Basilar impression
Hysterical blindness
Optic neuritis

fleeting visual loss; early treatment of glaucoma will limit the subsequent loss of vision. Patients with glaucoma often complain of halos around lights and eye pain associated with the increased intraocular pressure.

PARTIAL LOSS OF VISION

Hysterical blindness is rarely confused with true loss of vision, but partial visual loss is more difficult to assess. At least partially intact vision is needed to elicit optokinetic nystagmus with a striped cloth or visual pursuit with a mirror moving in front of the face. Feigned blindness can be readily established with these simple tests. The patient who admits to seeing some objects but fails to see others may have a field cut, that is, a loss of vision limited to part of the visual field. This blindspot is called a scotoma if it affects only one eye. Sickle-shaped blindspots frequently develop in patients with untreated glaucoma. Everyone has a physiologic blindspot just lateral to the point of central vision, but in some disorders this blindspot enlarges and extends into central vision. This type of blindspot is called a centrocecal scotoma, and it accounts for those instances when the patient has excellent peripheral vision but denies all perception of items directly in front of him. This disorder was routinely ascribed to sexual promiscuity until the twentieth century. The notion that reckless sexual activity can lead to this type of blindness has been generally abandoned, but some ophthalmologists now blame alcohol or tobacco abuse. The cyanide produced by burning tobacco, especially pipe tobacco, may injure the optic nerve. The causes of this kind of visual loss are still controversial. Certainly, some vitamin deficiencies, such as vitamin B_{12} deficiency, can cause centrocecal scotomas. Most common of all causes of centrocecal visual loss in young and middle-aged adults is a retinal infection by histoplasmosis (7). The average age of onset for centrocecal visual loss in that instance is 44 years of age. Patients with this infection may complain initially of microscopia, that is, the misperception of items in the environment as smaller than they really are (7). The underlying lesion is hemorrhagic detachment of the retina.

Enlargement of the physiologic blindspot without involvement of central vision is routinely seen with increased intracranial pressure (8). Young women with pseudotumor cerebri (benign intracranial hypertension) may develop considerable visual impairment by this route. The increased intracranial pressure is reflected in papilledema and probably causes ischemia of the optic disc because of disc swelling (8). Increased intracranial pressure may cause recurrent attacks of transient visual blurring and, occasionally, permanent blindness (8).

The pattern of permanent visual loss may provide considerable insight into the cause of the visual loss (Table 14.4). Tubular vision or tunnel vision suggests hysteria. With this symptom, the patient has peripheral

Table 14.1. Visual Field Defects

Pattern	*Name*	*Common Causes*
Half of visual field impaired on same side in both eyes	Homonymous hemianopia	Stroke Brain tumor Brain abscess
Lateral half of visual field impaired in both eyes	Bitemporal hemianopia	Mass on optic chiasm
Medial half of visual field impaired in both eyes	Binasal hemianopia	Glaucoma
One-quarter of visual field lost on same side in both eyes	Homonymous quadrantanopia	Temporal lobe or parietal lobe lesion

vision that is increasingly impaired as the distance from objects increases. A normal field of vision, regardless of the defects included in it, will expand in size as it gets farther away from the patient. This is simply because the eye is the vertex of a cone of vision with a necessarily larger diameter at points more remote from the vertex. The hysterical patient ignores this rule and acts as if he is looking into a tunnel of constant diameter. A bitemporal field cut suggests a lesion pressing on the optic chiasm. In adults, this is most likely to be a pituitary adenoma (9). In children, an optic glioma, meningioma, or craniopharyngioma would be more likely. A binasal field cut usually results from glaucoma. Peripheral field cuts that progress during the examination are invariably due to hysteria.

PSYCHIC BLINDNESS: VISUAL AGNOSIA

An individual may clearly see an object or picture and yet fail to perceive its nature or significance. This failure in recognition is called psychic blindness or visual agnosia. The term agnosia was introduced by Sigmund Freud in 1891, and since that time there has been considerable controversy over whether or not this is a real entity. Some neurologists who deal with visually impaired patients on a regular basis believe that the fundamental problem in patients with alleged visual agnosia is a defect in the visual field, interfering only partially, but crucially, in the perception of complete forms (10). Most neurologists, however, are convinced that patients with normal visual activity may exhibit disturbed visual recognition. These problems with recognition may assume several forms, ranging from an inability to name an object presented visually to a problem with viewing any object as a single entity, rather than as a collection of parts. The most extreme example of this psychic blindness occurs in the Klüver-Bucy syndrome, in which the patient explores all objects with his mouth regardless of their unpleasantness or danger (11–14).

Strictly defined, visual agnosia is an inability to recognize objects by sight, which cannot be explained by a concurrent sensory impairment, dementia, aphasia, inattention, or alteration in consciousness (10,15,16). The affected individual may have a right visual field cut or inattention to his left side, but these deficits should not account for his recognition problem. The patient with visual agnosia sees the object, but he does not appreciate what it is or what it does unless he examines it with an alternative sensory system. A key can be identified after it is held, and a radio will be correctly named after it is played. Without the additional sensory information, the impaired individual will deny any idea of what the object is and will deny ever having seen a similar item, regardless of how familiar the object is (15).

The problem is not with finding the name (17). Offered a multiple choice of names, the patient will not choose the correct one. Despite this inability to name the object, he can accurately draw it in some cases. Once the object is recognized by holding or touching, naming it will be speedy and accurate. Associated impairments in recognition seen with visual agnosia include problems with color recognition. The patient can readily recall the color of familiar objects, such as an apple or a fire engine, and he can accurately match color cards of various hues, but he cannot point to a card of a specific color and name the color (15,18).

More likely to arouse suspicion of a psychiatric basis for the "psychic blindness" is prosopagnosia, a selective deficit in recognition of familiar faces (16,19). The affected individual will deny knowing or ever having seen before family members and close friends. Each time the familiar individual arrives, the patient will exhibit no recognition of his face, although the patient will quickly recognize and accurately identify the visitor's voice, mannerisms, or perfume. The patient does not relearn the faces of his friends or relatives. Rather than there just being an amnesia for previously learned faces, there is a static problem in processing visual information. The patient's explanation for his disability is usually that there is a cloud in front of his eyes, that his acuity is faulty. Objective tests of acuity will reveal no impairment adequate to explain the recognition problems. Problems with facial recognition often can be tied to damage in the right parietotemporal area, although impaired facial recognition can develop with lesions in either cerebral hemisphere and is often seen in patients with impaired language comprehension (19). The problem in recognition may be limited to accurately perceiving the emotion conveyed by a facial expression (20). This limited perceptual defect is invariably associated with a right hemisphere lesion, a clinical finding supporting the notion that the nondominant hemisphere plays an important role in the elaboration and perception of emotions. A left visual field defect is usually apparent in patients with prosopagnosia, another indication that right parieto-occipital damage is involved in the appearance of the syndrome.

Psychic blindness may extend to a remarkably fine level of perceptual difficulty, such as the recognition of an entity formed from component parts. The patient can identify the wheels, axles, metal panels, and windows of a train, but fails to realize the item he is looking at is a train. This problem is called simultanagnosia and it is usually associated with damage to the occipitotemporal cortex of the left hemisphere (21). The name for this agnosia stresses the patient's limited ability to perceive the simultaneous form or aggregate produced by the component parts (17). The basic defect seems to be in the interpretation of complex perceptions (21).

Psychic blindness usually appears with damage to the dominant (left) occipital lobe with the lesion extending from the inner face of the occipital cortex into the posterior segment (splenium) of the corpus callosum, the massive, fiber bundle connecting the two hemispheres (15,17). Because this same lesion occurs in patients with the much less complex reading difficulty called pure word blindness, some investigators have suggested that the occipital cortex must also be disconnected from visual memories in the nondominant hippocampus to produce the typical picture of psychic blindness (16,22). Patients with visual agnosia invariably have infarctions in the occipital lobe, corpus callosum, and hippocampal connections caused by occlusion of the posterior cerebral artery. A right homonymous hemianopia is routinely associated with the visual agnosia. Presumably, this type of lesion prevents images from the intact left visual field from being associated with memories of visual patterns stored in the nondominant hemisphere or with names and verbal descriptions of objects stored in the dominant hemisphere.

That a structural lesion is responsible for psychic blindness can be easily established by computed tomography and electroencephalography. Lesions too small to be resolved by the computed tomogram will still produce focal changes on the electroencephalogram. Patients with no defects apparent on either of these studies usually have a psychogenic basis for their problems with recognition. Specifically, if the patient cannot recognize the faces of family members, but quickly learns to recognize individual members of the medical staff, a psychiatric problem must be assumed responsible. The perceptual difficulty characteristic of visual agnosia does not discriminate between items of varying importance in the environment.

There is no treatment for visual agnosia. The severity of the impairment may subside if infarction is responsible for its appearance, but the deficit is usually permanent to some degree once it occurs. Patients with this kind of residual deficit often appear much more perceptually intact than they are, because they do not have obvious blindness or confusion. Misunderstandings often arise with family members or employers who do not realize that the apparently well patient cannot function at simple tasks requiring object recognition.

DOUBLE VISION: DIPLOPIA

Double vision is a common complaint in patients with either neurologic or psychiatric problems. The most common cause of diplopia in patients seeking general medical attention for the acutely appearing symptom is hysteria (Table 14.5). Men and women under excessive psychologic strain may abrubtly perceive that items close to their faces appear double. In most cases they actually do see a double image of some objects, but this is because they are fixing their gaze on remote objects and attending to near objects. This failure to converge visually on the object of interest will produce a double image of the near object in all normal individuals, but this unavoidable double image is ordinarily ignored. The patient's own description of what he is perceiving is usually enough to establish the diagnosis. When there is doubt over the functional nature of the diplopia, a red glass test, as described below, will help clarify the nature of the defect. With hysteria, the results will usually be remarkably inconsistent. Patients complaining of double vision that persists when they close one eye are almost invariably hysterical. Diplopia usually requires visual input from both eyes. Rare monocular lesions, such as lens dislocations and retinal detachments, may cause double vision limited to the damaged eye, but in these instances the defect in the damaged eye is apparent on ophthalmoscopic examination of the eye.

The setting for the diplopia often simplifies finding its cause. Severe

Table 14.5. Causes of Diplopia

Hysteria
Trauma
Diabetes mellitus
Brainstem infarction
Multiple sclerosis
Intraocular masses
Myasthenia gravis
Posterior fossa tumors
Nasopharyngeal carcinoma
Meningitis
Meningeal carcinomatosus
Thyroid disease
Narcoleptic sleep attacks
Drug effects

head trauma may evoke transient or persistent diplopia by damaging the extraocular muscles or the ocular motor nerves. Damage to the trochlear nerve (cranial nerve IV) is especially common with deceleration injuries to the head or face of the sort that occur with automobile accidents. The impaired intorsion of the eye that results from injury to this nerve will oblige the patient to tilt his head away from the side of the injured eye to avoid having double vision. Diabetes mellitus is the most common nontraumatic cause of authentic diplopia. The oculomotor (III) nerve is infarcted by vascular complications of the diabetes, and, as a result, the patient acutely develops impaired adduction of the affected eye. Because the parasympathetic nerve fibers of the oculomotor nerve, going to the pupil, have a vascular supply different from that to the ocular motor fibers, the diabetic patient will have normal pupillary reactions despite the impaired extraocular movements. This is important because a similar defect will arise with an aneurysm on the posterior communicating artery in the circle of Willis pressing on the oculomotor nerve. The pupil is persistently dilated in that instance because the parasympathetic fibers on the oculomotor nerve are crushed along with the ocular motor fibers.

Any lesion interfering with the function of the ocular motor cranial nerves (III, IV, VI) may cause double vision or blurred vision. Common lesions include vascular damage from brainstem hemorrhage or infarction, demyelinating lesions from multiple sclerosis, and pressure effects of posterior fossa tumors. With increased intracranial pressure, the abducens nerve (VI) is especially vulnerable to injury. The patient will have impaired abduction on the involved side. Papilledema will usually appear with this ocular sign of increased pressure, and attention will be directed away from the eye by this combination of signs. A tumor in the eye itself can also interfere with extraocular muscle activity, but this type of lesion is usually associated with protrusion of the eye, so-called proptosis (Figure 14.3).

A nonstructural cause of double vision is intrinsic muscle disease or neuromuscular junction disease affecting the extraocular muscle. Myasthenia gravis presents with diplopia in many of the affected individuals, and several types of hereditary ophthalmoplegia may induce at least transient double vision. Drugs interfering with ocular coordination, a function sensitive to many sedatives, must be sought in all patients complaining of transient diplopia.

Red glass testing will help establish precisely which muscle or muscles are functioning improperly. Covering one eye with a red glass filter, the examiner asks the patient whether he sees a bright penlight held about 1 meter away as one light or two. If the patient sees a red light distinctly separate from the white light, his convergence is faulty; two separate lights are seen because the light source is falling on unrelated areas of the retina in the two eyes. If the red filter is over the eye with the weak muscle, the red light perceived by the patient will be displaced in the direction in which his eye would be pulled by the weak muscle if it were functioning

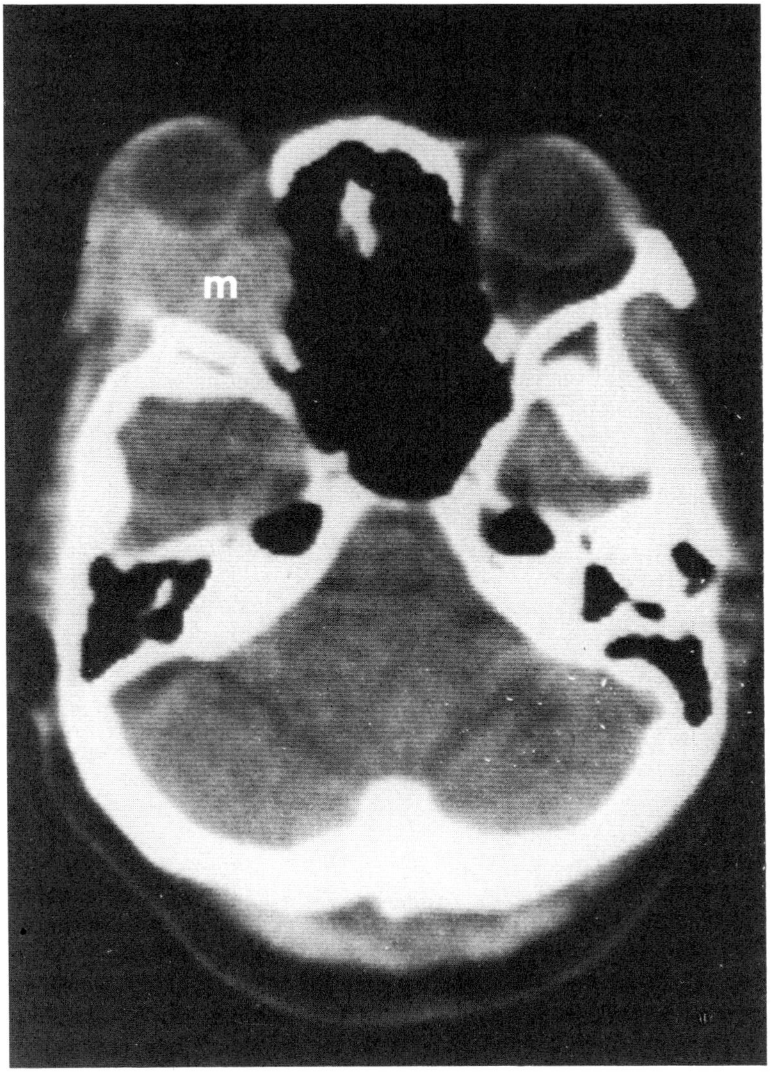

Figure 14.3. A 64-year-old woman noticed that her right eye was protruding. An orbital computed tomogram revealed that the proptosis was caused by a mass (m) behind the globe of the eye. Eye movements are usually disturbed by a mass of this size, and the loss of coordinated eye movements would cause double vision or blurred vision in most cases (courtesy of Drs. J. Loh and W. Hotson).

normally. Moving the bright source toward the normal extremes of ocular excursion will help define the full set of extraocular muscles that are weak. The red glass test will uncover diplopia in some patients with no complaints of double vision. These patients have esophorias or exophorias, tendencies for an eye to wander medially or laterally when it is allowed to move independently of the other eye. With the introduction of the red filter, conjugate gaze is undermined because the brain sees different images coming from the two eyes, even though the only difference in the images is the color.

Double vision or poor alignment of the images arising in the two eyes occasionally develops with extensive field cuts. One patient with a prominent bitemporal hemianopia secondary to chiasmatic compression by a pituitary tumor complained of occasional double vision, but he had even more disturbing problems with accurate alignment of his residual visual fields. While studying betting forms that designated racing horses by letters in one column and by names in the adjacent column, he noticed that he was consistently picking the wrong letters for the horses on which he wished to bet. Presumably, his compromised visual fields did not provide enough overlap in visual images to prevent the images from sliding past each other. This would be even more likely with a binasal hemianopia.

Any patient with fairly convincing evidence of diplopia should be checked for local disease in or around the eye. A nasopharyngeal carcinoma extending from the sphenoid sinus into the orbit may damage the innervation to an extraocular muscle. Hyperthyroidism may induce non-neoplastic material to collect behind the globe and limit movement of one or both eyes. Thyroid disease also causes an ocular myopathy with fibrosis in selected extraocular muscles, limiting full extraocular movements. If local disease is not apparent or implied by simple screening tests, such as skull x-rays and thyroid function tests, then a closer assessment of the orbits and orbital contents is appropriate. Computed tomography and orbital sonography are the safest and most accurate methods for accomplishing this. Computed tomography will also allow examination of the intracranial contents. A sphenoid wing meningioma or an intracerebellar tumor will be revealed with contrast enhancement of the computed tomogram. In the absence of any structural disease, the patient should be checked for diabetes mellitus, although diplopia is unlikely as the first symptom of this metabolic disease. A fasting blood sugar and 2-hour postprandial sugar should adequately establish whether diabetes is a legitimate concern. Myasthenia gravis can usually be diagnosed with an edrophonium test. This fast acting cholinesterase inhibitor will usually alleviate the diplopia if neuromuscular junction disease is the problem. A provocative curare test is rarely necessary to establish the diagnosis of myasthenia gravis, but it is helpful in equivocal cases. Electromyography is valuable in diagnosing primary muscle disease and neuromuscular junction disease. Patients will rarely need a cerebrospinal fluid evaluation, but, if there is any reason to suspect a chronic meningitis, such as tuberculous meningitis, is involved in the visual problem, a lumbar puncture should be performed. If the pupil is dilated in the eye with limited motion, an arteriogram will be needed to rule out an aneurysm as the cause of the diplopia.

Diplopia is a symptom easily relieved by patching one eye. Elimination of the symptom, however, requires treatment of the underlying condition. Traumatic injuries usually produce a transient ocular motor dysfunction that requires no intervention. If the diplopia persists, surgical adjustment of the muscles may be necessary. Local neoplasms may leave permanent ocular motor problems even if the tumor can be successfully treated. Diabetic ophthalmopathies usually remit over the course of several months regardless of the diabetic control, and myasthenic ocular palsies will remit only as long as the patient is treated with cholinesterase inhibitors or corticosteroids. An aneurysm on the posterior communicating artery that is large enough to cause oculomotor signs is likely to bleed; this vascular problem can only be approached with surgery.

VISUAL NEGLECT

Patients with nondominant hemisphere strokes commonly neglect the left side of their bodies and may neglect elements in their left visual fields (23). This visual inattention characteristically appears with parietal lobe lesions, but it also develops with lesions in the pulvinar nuclei and the superior colliculi, both elements of the subcortical gray matter (24). Visual attention depends on two distinct systems. The first visual system depends upon pathways between the lateral geniculate nucleus of the diencephalon and the striate cortex of the occipital lobe. This system simply identifies objects that are in the visual field (24). The second system depends on pathways between the superior colliculus, the pulvinar nuclei, and the parietal lobe cortex. This second visual system detects events occurring in the visual field, establishes their location, and directs visual attention to them for recognition and identification by the first system (24). Events occurring peripherally, that is at more than 20 degrees from the center of vision, are the main concern of this second system (24). With a parietal lobe lesion, the patient is inattentive to the contralateral visual field even when no field cut is apparent (25). Targets in this neglected field are completely overlooked if there is any sort of distraction in the ipsilateral visual field. Even shifting gaze from one object to another in the defective field is more halting and indecisive than in the unaffected field (24).

Men are more likely than women to exhibit this functional asymmetry in the parietal lobes with structural damage to this part of the cerebral cortex, but both men and women with right cerebral hemisphere injuries will have more problems with visuospatial tasks than patients with left hemisphere injuries (25,26). The left visual field is apparently of special importance in visuospatial tasks because men are better at these tasks than women and they exhibit a left visual field superiority or "dominance" on manipulating or perceiving spatial relationships; women do not exhibit this right hemisphere dominance on testing for visuospatial tasks as consistently as men (26). This functional asymmetry makes men more vulnerable to dramatic deficits in visuospatial perception after right hemisphere damage (26).

HALLUCINATIONS

Numerous neurologic disorders produce visual hallucinations indistinguishable from those experienced by psychotic patients. The classical definition of an hallucination is that it is the perception of an object that is not there, and it is distinct from an illusion in that the perception is not instigated by the misinterpretation of a real object (27). Occasionally, the patient will realize that his visual perception is not real, and this is sometimes called a pseudohallucination to distinguish it from the phenomenon that occurs without any associated insight (27).

There are many causes of visual hallucinations. Sensory deprivation, sleep deprivation, intense emotional conflict, overt psychosis, and central nervous system disease can all cause this visual disorder (27). Hallucinations are common, but benign, phenomena in patients with narcolepsy, the visual phenomena occurring when the patients awaken or fall asleep (27). The most common organic causes of hallucinations are toxic confusional states, such as those seen with alcohol abuse, uremia, hepatic failure, and drug abuse (28). Several over-the-counter sleep preparations have atropinic drugs that may elicit florid hallucinations in susceptible individuals with no history of hallucinogen use. Central nervous system tumors and infections can cause hallucinations, but this rarely happens. Irritation of the lateral surface of the nondominant temporal lobe will usually produce visual hallucinations (27). Lesions in the occipital lobe produce more geometric hallucinations. The visual phenomena in cases of diffuse or focal central nervous system disease probably reflect irritation of the visual association cortex by the disease process. Associated neurologic signs may indicate the organic nature of these visual phenomena, but more frequently only the patient's history and course will suggest a nonfunctional etiology.

Alcohol-Related

Delirium tremens, the acute confusional state developing with alcohol withdrawal in the chronic alcohol abuser, often involves vivid persecutory hallucinations (29). The affected patient will be tormented by visions of insects, monsters, and human figures, all intent upon killing or maiming him. Alcohol or the vitamin deficiencies associated with alcoholism need not act directly on the central nervous system to elicit bizarre visual perceptions. Hallucinations develop in some alcoholic patients secondary to hepatic encephalopathy.

Drug-Induced

Drug-induced hallucinations may develop with drugs that are nervous system poisons, as well as some not ordinarily considered neurotoxins, such as ibuprofen, an anti-inflammatory drug. Well-formed visual delusions will appear with exposure to the poison thallium (30). With levodopa treatment of Parkinson disease, about one-third of the patients will complain of hallucinations after they have been on the drug for more than 2 years (31). These are usually recurrent, nocturnal illusions, and they are characteristically not threatening. The parkinsonian patient is awake and alert at the time of the hallucinations, but he will usually note remarkably vivid dreams during the weeks that the hallucinations are occurring (31). Temporary discontinuation of the levodopa may be necessary to stop the hallucinations.

Structural Causes

A mass pressing on the optic tract or a lesion producing ischemia in the occipital lobe occasionally produces peduncular hallucinosis. This is a visual disturbance involving impaired visual acuity, dizziness, vertigo, and frank hallucinations (29). The patients see well-defined, brightly colored people and animals, appearing in miniature and moving about excitedly. Rather than being threatened by these hallucinations, the patient is likely to express curiosity (29). This is distinct from micropsia, a visual delusion arising with irritative lesions over the occipital or parietal cortex and, rarely, with retinal damage (7). The patient with micropsia sees real people and objects markedly reduced in size. This may appear intermittently as the aura for a seizure (28,29). The miniature objects are real; only the scale is delusional. Well-organized hallucinations with recognizable characters performing familiar activities probably originate in the visual association cortex rather than the primary visual cortex (28).

Patients with visual field cuts occasionally complain of well-formed hallucinations in the part of the visual field with no true vision. These images may cross into the intact field of vision, but, more commonly, they stay in the blind field. This is probably just a seizure phenomenon in many patients with irritative lesions producing their field cuts, but these highly structured hallucinations also develop with strictly parietal or occipital lesions that produce no clinical seizures. The images are usually of people, animals, body parts, and building elements moving in stereotyped ways. These hallucinations are in full color with all the clarity and symmetry of real objects. Sometimes the images appear in miniature, but there are no auditory hallucinations associated with the visual phenomena. Real faces, indeed familiar faces, may appear out of the blind visual field, but they will not say anything. The figures may nod and pass in procession or even act threateningly, but the patient rarely feels threatened by them. The field cut associated with these hallucinations is invariably a homonymous hemianopia (28).

These visual phenomena usually subside over the course of days or months, but rare patients have persistent hallucinations. Anticonvulsants, such as phenobarbital, help most of the patients with field cut hallucinations suppress the images. The effectiveness of anticonvulsants in this disorder supports the hypothesis that these images arise from irritation of the visual association cortex by a destructive lesion. The hallucinations developing with homonymous hemianopias are not as complex as well integrated visual memories. They may be simply elements used by visual memory that are inadvertently activated by irritative lesions near the visual association cortex (28).

Phosphenes

More poorly formed hallucinations called phosphenes also develop with structural lesions in or over the visual cortex. These are flashes of colored or white light appearing as spots, lines, or swirls that may move across the visual field (29). These flashes of light are seen in the absence of a visual stimulus (32). Retinal and optic nerve lesions also commonly elicit these elementary visual phenomona. Twelve percent of patients with tumors of the optic nerve or optic chiasm report seeing stars, spots, rockets, rotating wheels, bubbles, or balloons (28). These illusions are commonly experienced as the "stars" seen when someone is struck in the eye. Ionizing radiation and traction on the retina by the vitreous can also evoke phosphenes (32). The patient with optic neuritis may see phosphenes each time he moves his eye. Patients with substantial visual loss may have phosphenes evoked by sharp sounds; these phenomena subside as vision returns (32). Unless there is an obvious pathologic condition in the retina or optic nerve, a structural lesion over the occipital lobe, such as a tumor, arteriovenous malformation, cerebral infarction, or cortical scar, must be suspected in the patient with these visual illusions (32).

Phosphenes are not at all suspicious when they appear with narcolepsy. Patients with this sleep disorder often have these flashes and swirls of light as hypnagogic hallucinations. More typical hypnagogic or hypnopompic hallucinations occur in the interval between deep sleep and wakefulness and usually consist of scenes with people and animals, rather than just flashes of light. Characteristically, phosphenes are seen only when the narcoleptic patient is lying quietly in a dark room. This is not the only visual disturbance seen with narcolepsy. Double vision and vision limited by bilateral ptosis are fairly common at the onset of sleep attacks (33).

Visual phenomena indistinguishable from phosphenes may develop in temporal lobe epilepsy, but the affected patient will invariably have altered consciousness at about the time of the visual abnormality (34). This occasionally leads to difficulty in distinguishing between a seizure disorder and narcolepsy, but that difficulty is resolved with an electroencephalogram (34). Visual phenomena, such as phosphenes and more complex hallucinations, are not unexpected with temporal lobe lesions. The inferior temporal cortex plays an important role in processing visual information (35). Information on colors and patterns seem to be integrated in the inferior temporal lobe. Visual recognition is impaired in experimental animals when the inferior temporal cortex is removed, especially when the right temporal lobe is damaged (35). Complex visual hallucinations also occur in patients with temporal lobe tumors (36).

Localization of Visual Phenomena

Lesions in several areas of the brain are associated with their own particular kinds of hallucinations. Patients with parietal lobe lesions may perceive distortions in their own bodies. They complain that one limb is shorter than its fellow or that an extra limb is present (36). This is distinct from the denial of ownership of a limb that appears with nondominant hemisphere strokes. With occipital lobe lesions, the range of hallucinations is fairly extensive. In addition to the unstructured phosphenes, the patient may experience distortion of objects in one visual field. Colored figures in procession, polyopic hallucinations, may march from the peripheral field of vision to central vision. Obviously, patients reporting such experiences are easily misdiagnosed as schizophrenic before the structural lesion in the occipital lobe is discovered. This is also true for the patient with structural occipital lobe damage who sees a doubling of figures in only one quadrant of vision or sees upper visual field objects in the lower visual field (36). Occasionally, patients describe multiple images of a real person involved in a delusional activity. Patients may also see persistent images when they redirect their gaze (28). An old image presents like the ghost on a television picture tube after the patient looks away. This perseveration of an image is called palinopsia. Less dramatic is the distortion of images called metamorphopsia that is also associated with occipital lobe damage. Both of these visual phenomena subside with phenobarbital treatment if they are from irritative lesions in the occipital cortex. All of these hallucinations should arouse suspicion of an occipital lobe tumor, abscess, or arteriovenous malformation (3). With resection of the lesion, the patient will have a field cut, generally free of visual hallucinations.

Subcortical lesions may also produce visual hallucinations (37,38). Damage to the hypothalamus, pons, and midbrain have all been associated with simple and complex hallucinations, but a lesion in these areas is rarely the explanation for hallucinations. With cerebellar or brainstem damage, the patient may experience oscillopsia, which is rhythmic, illusory movement of the environment from side-to-side or up-and-down. Even with profound nystagmus, oscillopsia is rarely reported, and so this is much more than an ocular motor disorder. Damage to the optic nerve or chiasm, such as that developing with the demyelinating lesions of multiple sclerosis, occasionally produces hallucinations triggered by noises. This auditory-visual synesthesia involves perceptions ranging from flashes of white light to complicated colored hallucinations (38). The sound necessary is usually similar to that needed to elicit a startle reaction, and the hallucinations developing always occur in the most defective part of the disturbed visual field (38). The auditory stimulus seems to be misdirected to the visual association cortex.

Extensive occipital cortical destruction, resulting in blindness, may evoke the hallucinatory syndrome of Anton (28,39). The cortically blind patient may report seeing clearly scenes that are entirely delusional. Despite his obvious inability to manage independently in his environment, the patient with Anton's syndrome denies that he is blind. These hallucinations develop from the sensory deprivation associated with the cortical blindness.

PSYCHIC GAZE PARALYSIS

Gaze paralysis can develop with no apparent weakness in ocular muscles and no damage to the ocular motor nuclei. In most cases this is the result of a progressive degenerative disease of the central nervous system, such as Parkinson disease or progressive supranuclear palsy (40,41), disorders in which vertical gaze is primarily impaired. A much less common, but much more peculiar, disturbance of voluntary gaze is psychic gaze paralysis or Balint's syndrome (42). There are three major features of psychic gaze paralysis (17). The patient cannot voluntarily look toward objects at the periphery of central vision; efforts to point at a target or otherwise respond to visual stimuli will be extremely clumsy and inaccurate; and attention to items in the peripheral field will be profoundly defective. Formal visual fields will often reveal tunnel vision resulting from this neglect of all peripheral visual stimuli.

Involuntary eye movements will be normal. Caloric stimulation of the labyrinth will elicit full extraocular movements, and doll's eye movements will be prominent despite the patient's apparent alertness. The patient's response to items in his center of vision indicates that he does not perceive more than one object or part of an object at one time (17). These patients seem to have bilateral visual neglect as the basis for their ocular motor abnormality.

This rare syndrome usually develops only in the context of bilateral parietal lobe lesions. Metastatic tumors to several parts of the brain could produce such bilateral lesions, but a brain lesion would be obvious with such multifocal disease. Psychiatric disease may be suspected in the patient who suffered a parietal lobe infarction in the remote past and appears with psychic gaze paralysis with a new lesion on the opposite side.

This disorder is distinct from the oculogyric crisis that may develop in patients taking phenothiazines. Peripheral vision is not disturbed with oculogyric crisis, and the involuntary deviation of the eyes is often quite painful. Abnormal limb or neck postures may be associated with oculogyric crises, and the episodes can usually be terminated with intravenous diphenhydramine injection.

AUDITORY ABNORMALITIES

Hearing and balance are the principal functions of the ear. Problems with both develop with disease in the ear, in the brain, or in the connections between the two. Auditory hallucinations and dizziness are the symptoms arising with disease of the ear or its connections that most often pose problems in diagnosis. Either of these abnormalities may arise with purely psychiatric or purely neurologic disorders. The context of the symptom often clarifies its etiology. A patient with a long history of epilepsy is more likely to have an auditory hallucination as the aura of a seizure than as the first sign of an acute psychosis. A hypochondriacal patient who complains of intractable dizziness is probably having a conversion reaction, unless the subjective problem is associated with vomiting and nystagmus. The objective neurologic signs increase the likelihood of structural brain or ear disease, rather than of an hysterical balance disorder (Figure 14.4). Obvious problems develop with psychotic patients who are taking medications that can induce balance or hearing disorders, but who also have psychiatric disorders that frequently evoke these symptoms. Depressed patients occasionally complain of dizziness, but the depressed patient on lithium carbonate may have vertigo, nausea, vomiting, and nystagmus as side effects of the drug. The schizophrenic patient with auditory hallucinations may have the hallucinations as a reaction to anticholinergic medication, such as benztropine, given to relieve the parkinsonism induced by neuroleptic drugs. Whatever the psychiatric problem or drug history, a careful neurologic evaluation is appropriate whenever a patient complains of altered hearing or disturbed balance. Conversely, the absence of a psychiatric history does not substantially alter the likelihood that purely subjective complaints, such as dizziness and auditory hallucinations, are from structural nervous system disease.

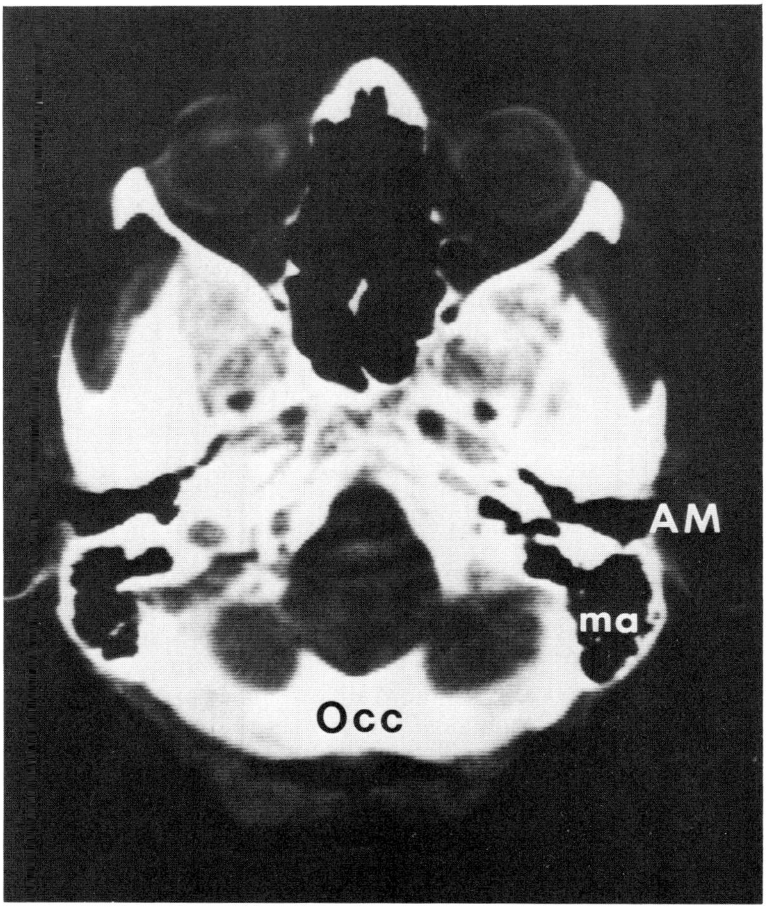

Figure 14.4. Computed tomogram sections through the base of the skull can reveal obvious abnormalities in or around the auditory meatus (AM), but x-ray films of the skull are generally more informative, especially if special tomographic techniques are used. The computed tomogram of the posterior fossa is valuable in the investigation of hearing abnormalities because it will reveal masses on the auditory nerve or abutting the brainstem. This computed tomogram is normal and provides an excellent view of the mastoid air cells (ma) in the temporal bone and of the inferior aspect of the occipital bone (Occ). The faint densities in the anterior thirds of the optic globes are the lenses.

VERTIGO AND DIZZINESS

Vertigo is distinct from dizziness in character, but not necessarily in severity. With vertigo the patient perceives movement of the environment and often feels forcibly thrown to one side. Nausea and vomiting are common with vertigo, regardless of the cause of the symptom. Dizziness is a less discrete sense of instability in space. The patient may have some nausea associated with the dizziness, but vomiting is unlikely unless it is self-induced. Stumbling and falling may occur with dizziness, but they are less likely than with vertigo. Inner ear, cerebellar, and brainstem disease are the most common causes of both vertigo and dizziness (43,44). Although stress may evoke complaints of dizziness more often than of vertigo, that a patient complains only of dizziness should not lessen suspicions that an organic lesion is responsible.

Vertigo associated with ringing in the ears (tinnitus) and progressive hearing loss is usually from disease of the inner ear. One idiopathic disorder causing this triad of problems, which presumably arises from disease of the inner ear, is Ménière's syndrome. This syndrome is characterized by intermittent bouts of severe vertigo, often with nausea, vomiting, and nystagmus, associated with hearing loss and tinnitus that persist between the acute attacks of vertigo (45). The attacks of vertigo may last a few minutes or several hours and recur several times a day for weeks or only a few times a year. Although some patients have ear infections or trauma before the development of Meniere's syndrome, most have no antecedent injuries to the ear or to the central nervous system (46). About two-thirds of the individuals who develop this idiopathic vertigo and hearing loss are in their fifth or sixth decade of life (46). Antihistamines may be effective against the severe attacks of vertigo in some individuals, but it will not prevent the progressive loss of hearing. Patients with frequent attacks of severe vertigo may profit from surgical destruction of the labyrinth or of the nerves to the labyrinth. Many patients have spontaneous remissions.

Other causes of vertigo include inflammatory lesions of the labyrinth (labyrinthitis) and of the nerve from this balance organ (vestibular neuronitis). Attacks of vertigo with these diseases are often days or weeks long. This is also true when there is a tumor in the posterior fossa at the cerebellopontine angle (Figure 14.5). Common tumors in this location are schwannomas and meningiomas. Hearing loss and other cranial nerve lesions will evolve with a mass lesion in this location, but dizziness or vertigo may be the principal problem for months or years (44). Patients complaining of vertigo or chronic dizziness should be examined for large, brownish patches on their skin, called café-au-lait spots. These appear in hereditary neurofibromatosis (von Recklinghausen's disease) and are associated with a high incidence of bilateral cerebellopontine angle schwannomas (Figure 14.6).

Individuals with cerebrovascular disease occasionally develop dizziness or vertigo because there is an inadequate supply of blood to the posterior fossa. The blood vessels supplying this area are the vertebral and basilar arteries, and so the condition is called vertebrobasilar insufficiency. A distinct episode of vertigo, lasting minutes or hours, caused by inadequate perfusion to this part of the brain is a transient ischemic attack, that is, a

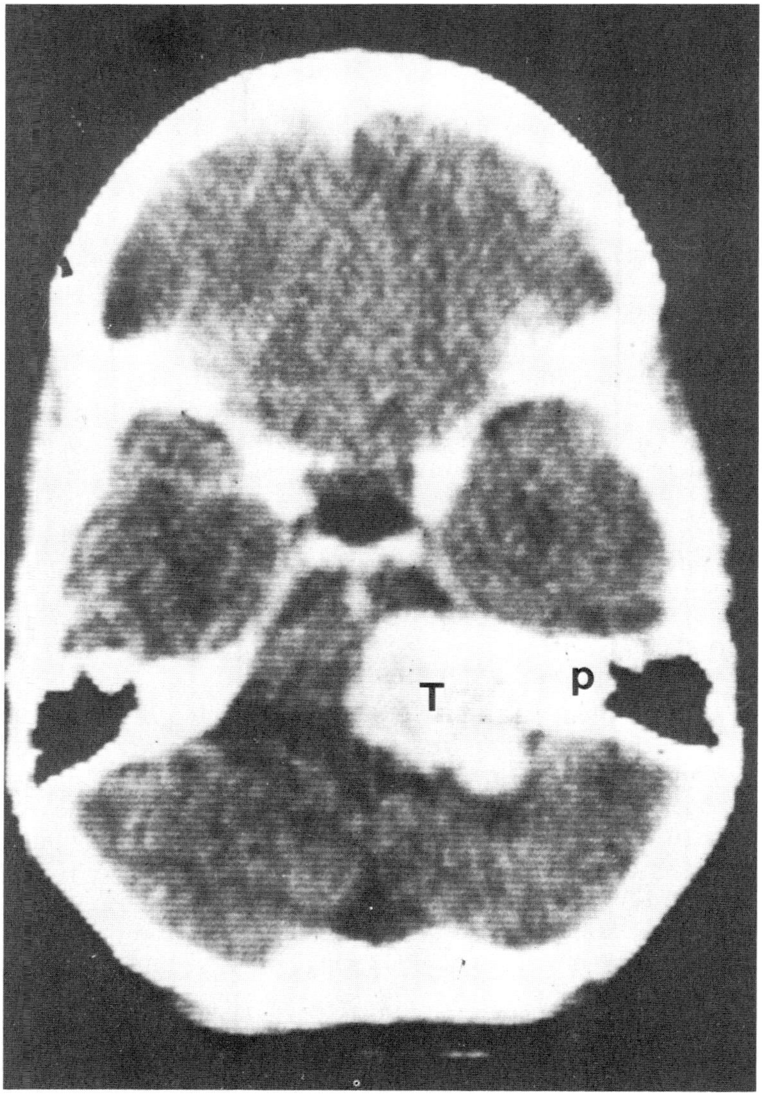

Figure 14.5. A computed tomogram of the brain with contrast enhancement revealed a large mass (T) in the posterior fossa of this 8-year-old girl. The mass was growing out of the petrous pyramid (p) of the temporal bone and impinging upon both the pons and the cerebellum. At surgery, this was found to be a tumor of the lining of the eighth cranial nerve, called a schwannoma (courtesy of Dr. S. Kreps).

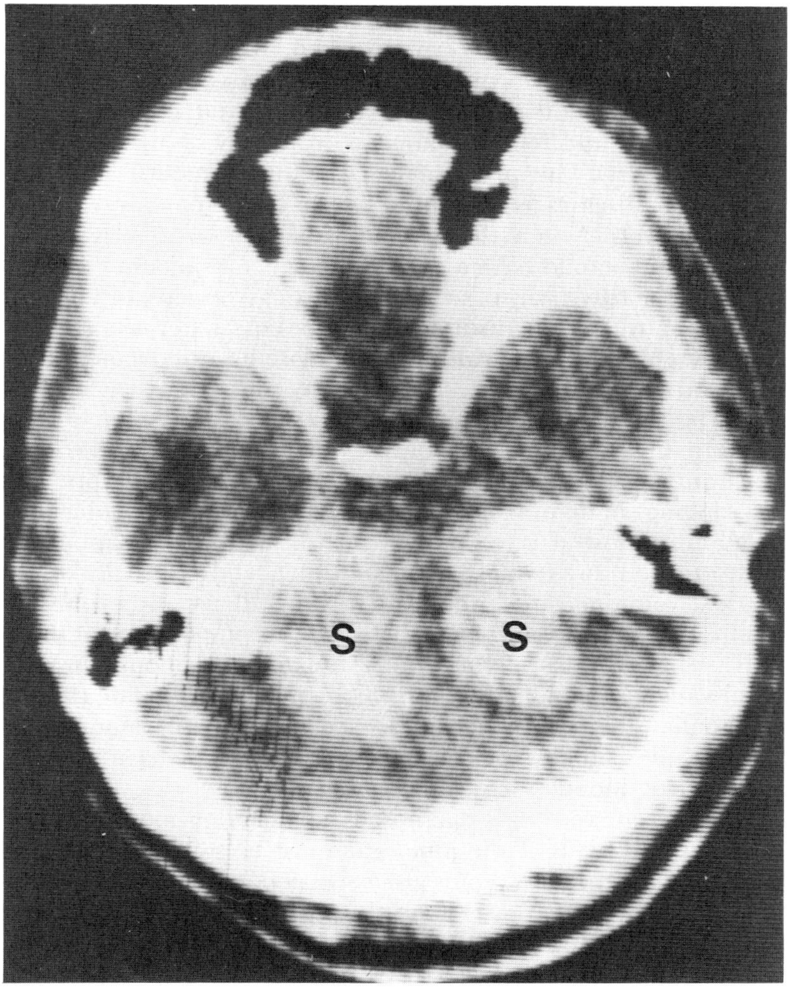

Figure 14.6. A computed tomogram with contrast enhancement revealed bilateral acoustic schwannomas (S) in the posterior fossa of this 16-year-old boy with von Recklinghausen's neurofibromatosis. These tumors produce progressive hearing loss and are often bilateral when this hereditary disease of the nervous system is responsible. Other types of intracranial tumors develop less frequently than schwannomas in this disease, but they are fairly common. This child had a meningioma arising from the right temporal bone and had hydrocephalus as a complication of his multiple intracranial tumors.

reversible neurologic deficit developing with poor blood flow but associated with no permanent damage. Vertigo caused by vertebrobasilar insufficiency is rarely an isolated symptom. Most patients will have other signs of brainstem dysfunction during the attack. Slurred speech, staggering gait, double vision, and focal weakness all routinely occur with vertebrobasilar insufficiency. The problem in evaluating patients with many of these structural diseases is that most of the symptoms are difficult to evaluate objectively. When there is any question of a nervous system lesion, the patient should have a careful otologic examination with caloric stimulation of the labyrinths to see if there is an asymmetry or abnormality in response to a well-defined stimulus. Hot or cold water sets up currents in the endolymph of the labyrinth that simulate head movements.

Some neurologic or otologic causes of vertigo are very difficult to distinguish from anxiety or hysteria. Benign recurrent vertigo is one such condition. In this disorder, episodes of vertigo occur with varying frequencies, ranging from once daily to once yearly, are more prevalent in females ranging in age from 7 to 55 years old, and coincide with menstruation in most affected individuals (5). The vertigo appears quite abruptly, often on awakening in the morning, and is usually associated with nausea, vomiting, and excessive sweating. It usually evolves into a positional vertigo, that is, one exacerbated by certain positions of the head; and it invariably subsides spontaneously after minutes, hours, or days (5). Emotional stress, alcohol, and lack of sleep may all precipitate the attacks. In some families, this type of vertigo is associated with migraine headaches, but even in these families, the affected individuals may have headache or vertigo occurring independently of each other.

Benign recurrent vertigo is diagnosed by excluding more lethal conditions. Structural disease of the inner ear must be sought conscientiously even when the patient's symptoms are associated with predictably stressful events, such as air travel (43). Even during the vertiginous attacks, the patient has no other focal neurologic signs, although the electroencephalogram may show some slow activity over both temporal areas, even between attacks (5). Caloric tests of labyrinthine function will reveal no abnormalities between attacks of vertigo (5).

Although this is not a symptom of depression, benign recurrent vertigo may be prevented by regular tricyclic antidepressant use. Amitriptyline taken daily will prevent the attacks. Permanent remissions often occur.

HEARING LOSS

Hearing loss develops with hysterical conversion reactions, as well as with damage to the ear, the brainstem, or the cerebral cortex. Loud noises (acoustic trauma), impact trauma, otosclerosis, otitis media, degenerative cochlear disease, and many other problems affecting the ear directly can produce impaired hearing or loss of hearing. Injuries to the eighth cranial nerve and tumors at the cerebellopontine angle also impair hearing by disturbing the connection between the inner ear and the brainstem. Structural lesions in the central nervous system commonly cause hearing impairment, but generally do not produce deafness. The most common causes of hearing impairment at the level of the brainstem are multiple sclerosis, vertebrobasilar insufficiency, and malignant tumors (47). Less common causes of deafness include syringobulbia, angiomas, abscesses, encephalomyelitis, collagen vascular disease, familial degenerative disorders, and tuberculosis (47). Obviously, with most hearing disorders arising on the basis of brainstem disease there will be other cranial nerves involved besides the eighth nerve. Cerebellar connections, sensory systems, and motor tracts will be caught up in the disease if it involves a substantial part of the brainstem. Hearing loss is bilateral in 73 percent of the patients who have hearing loss because of a brainstem lesion (47). In some brainstem disorders, such as vertebrobasilar insufficiency, the hearing impairment will be both bilateral and fairly symmetric in more than 80 percent of cases (47). The one brainstem disorder producing a relatively high incidence of unilateral hearing loss when hearing loss is at all present is multiple sclerosis (47). This is not to say that multiple sclerosis is a common cause of deafness: it is, in fact, a rare cause of substantial hearing loss (48). With objective tests, the hearing impairment can be detected in many patients with multiple sclerosis who have no symptoms of hearing impairment.

Some patients with difficulty hearing complain that loud noises or voices sound disturbingly loud or are simply irritating. This is caused by a phenomenon called recruitment, and it is often seen with damage to the acoustic end-organ, the cochlea. Recruitment also may appear with brainstem disease, but it is much less common in disease outside the ear (47). It develops least often when impaired hearing is on the basis of cerebral cortical damage. The contradictory character of the deficit raises questions about the authenticity of the patient's hearing complaints. Objective audiologic tests can determine whether recruitment is from an organic lesion or a psychologic disorder. Recruitment is occasionally confused with aphasia and other receptive problems because the patient complains of impaired word perception.

Pure Word Deafness

There is, in fact, a condition arising with cerebral cortical damage in which the patient cannot understand spoken words, regardless of the loudness of the speech, even though he clearly perceives the sound. This is called pure word deafness: the patient acts deaf to verbal stimuli, but responds briskly and appropriately to nonverbal sounds (49). These patients have not lost their language abilities completely. They can still speak normally, but they have a selective inability to understand spoken words; reading and writing are entirely intact (17). Repetition of spoken words is lost. The patient often complains that he hears voices, but he cannot make out the words. People seem to be speaking in a foreign language (17). The affected individual may discover that his comprehension of words improves when people speak more slowly and when he uses lip-reading as an adjunct to listening. This disorder is often confused with psychogenic deafness, simply because the deficit is so unusual and so slight (49). The site of cerebral damage is probably in the first temporal convolution, near the primary auditory cortex and Wernicke's area. Distinctive features in the cerebral lesion necessary to produce pure word deafness probably include a subcortical location and bilateral temporal lobe involvement (22,49).

Cerebrovascular disease is the usual cause of pure word deafness. Patients who have had strokes that produced a typical Wernicke's (receptive) aphasia may develop pure word deafness after they have partly recovered from the initial language disorder. Auditory hallucinations and paranoid delusions commonly occur during this recovery period, phenomena reinforcing the impression that the patient has a functional psychosis precipitated by the stress of his illness (17).

Auditory Agnosia

Pure word deafness is a problem with the recognition of verbal sounds, but there are other types of recognition problems or auditory agnosias that do not involve language. Patients with normal pure tone audiometry and speech discrimination thresholds may be unable to recognize common sounds (17). Although language comprehension will be normal in these individuals, they lose all ability to recognize musical tones and fail to respond to threatening noises. This problem is extremely rare, but much of its rarity is probably apparent, rather than real, because patients with this kind of complaint will often be dismissed as confabulatory or eccentric.

Cortical Deafness

Deafness rarely develops from a lesion in the cerebral cortex. Even with bilateral destruction of the primary auditory cortices, there is usually no substantial, permanent loss of hearing (17). When auditory function is impaired, the type of hearing problem manifest is inconsistent and usually leads to the diagnosis of psychogenic deafness. This type of problem develops with strokes in most cases, but it may also develop with encephalitis or head trauma. The temporal lobes are the principal sites of damage.

Disturbed Musical Function

The left hemisphere is vital to the comprehension of verbal material in most individuals, but the perception and recognition of music is a right hemisphere function in individuals who are not professional musicians (35). Patients with extensive left hemisphere damage may be able to sing the lyrics of a song, even when they are totally unable to use the same words in unmelodic language (25,50). Problems with musical function are obviously less likely to be recognized than problems with language, but formal testing of the ability to recognize melodic items fairly consistently suggests right hemisphere dominance for this skill (17).

The brain does not divide systems for musical production and perception in the unambiguous manner it does for language (51). The simplest acoustic features of either speech or music are dealt with equally well by either the right or the left hemisphere in left hemisphere dominant individuals, but more complex elements of music, such as harmonies, are perceived more readily by the right cerebral hemisphere (35). Complaints of problems with musical recognition or appreciation are difficult to interpret because central nervous system mechanisms for dealing with music are so poorly understood. Any patient complaining of musical difficulties should be evaluated for language problems and other signs of cerebral cortical damage.

AUDITORY HALLUCINATIONS

Auditory hallucinations are most common in schizophrenia and complex partial seizures. Other psychiatric and neurologic conditions can exhibit auditory hallucinations, but they are less consistently a feature. With delirium tremens, the patient withdrawing from alcohol will experience threatening visual and auditory hallucinations. Intense affective disorders, such as a psychotic depression, can elicit delusional, critical voices (27). With schizophrenia, the hallucinated sound is more likely to be distinct voices and is more likely to involve complex sentences than the hallucinations of individuals with strictly neurologic disease (27). Schizophrenic patients also describe the phenomenon of echo de pensée, a hallucination in which the patient hears his own thoughts spoken aloud (27).

If the auditory hallucinations are clearly associated with a drug withdrawal, as is the case with delirium tremens, little investigation of the disorder is appropriate. When the hallucinations appear without a prior psychiatric history, a critical examination of the brain is essential. This will include encephalographic studies with nasopharyngeal leads to better record from the inner face of the temporal cortex, a likely site of origin for epileptogenic activity that could trigger complex partial seizures. If the patient sleeps during the electroencephalogram, the likelihood of detecting an abnormality will be increased substantially. This may be induced by using chloral hydrate. A computed tomogram of the brain, with and without contrast enhancement, will reveal a structural lesion, such as a tumor or arteriovenous malformation, responsible for the cortical irritation. If the hallucinations are progressing over the course of days and a typical schizophrenic cognitive disorder is not emerging, the patient should be further evaluated with a lumbar puncture to obtain cerebrospinal fluid for examination. Chronic infection or an unsuspected subarachnoid hemorrhage could account for the auditory hallucinations.

TINNITUS

Tinnitus is a simply structured sound heard for an interval of from minutes to years as an isolated problem or in association with other neurologic or psychiatric symptoms. The patient usually complains of a ringing or hissing noise arising in an ear or from within his skull. This noise is usually loudest when the environment is quietest. It may be adequately annoying to produce severe sleep deprivation. Common causes of tinnitus include aspirin overdose, acoustic nerve injury, brainstem disease, cochlear disorders, and organic psychoses (27,52). Considerations in any patient with complaints of unremitting noise inside the head should include the possibility that the patient has just what he complains of, that is, a structural lesion in the head that is producing noise (Table 14.6). Arteriovenous malformations can produce pulsating or continuous noises associated with the high volume of blood flow through them. The patient hears a bruit from the blood flow, and the physician can often hear this noise if he puts a stethoscope over the patient's temples or eyes.

Atypical noises should be viewed even more suspiciously. One patient complaining of a ticking noise in his ear had myoclonic jerks in a muscle near the anterior wall of the external auditory meatus, and with every contraction the patient heard a snapping noise. Tinnitus is rarely a complaint in functional psychoses, but the patient may develop severe psychiatric problems because of the tinnitus. These include suicidal ideation. Personality changes are common in patients suffering from sleep deprivation caused by the constant noise.

Treatment of the tinnitus includes masking of the sound with a matched frequency and suppression of the noise with antihistamines or benzodiazepines. Recent trials with intravenous lidocaine suggest that this may be an effective way to reduce the tinnitus in patients profoundly depressed by the noise and the sleep deprivation caused by the noise (52).

Table 14.6. Causes of Tinnitus

Causes of Tinnitus
Aspirin overdose
Cochlear disease
Acoustic nerve injury
Brainstem disease
Arteriovenous malformation
Posterior fossa tumor

BILATERAL DEAFNESS

Complete, bilateral hearing loss occasionally develops as a hysterical complaint. Before an extensive otologic investigation of the deafness is begun, the authenticity of the complaint should be established. Patients with well-established psychiatric problems, such as schizophrenia and psychotic depressions, may develop apparent deafness with no associated organic lesions. Such psychiatric reactions are usually quite transient, with protracted episodes rarely lasting more than 1 or 2 weeks. Objective tests of acoustic reflexes, such as the stapedial reflex, help to clarify whether or not the patient has truly lost hearing (53).

Obviously, even psychotic patients may be exposed to ototoxic drugs or may develop bilateral ear infections. Recurrent subarachnoid hemorrhage can produce episodic personality changes and lead to bilateral hearing loss. This disorder is called subpial siderosis because of the iron deposits that develop along the central nervous system under the pial lining. A careful audiologic examination is usually sufficient as a first step in the evaluation of these patients with questionable hearing loss. If deafness is authentic, further otologic and neurologic studies will be dictated by the patient's other symptoms or the course of the disease.

REFERENCES

1. Troost BT, Sufit RL, Grand MG: Sudden monocular visual loss in pseudotumor cerebri. *Arch Neurol* 36:440, 1979.
2. Friedman AP: Nature of headache. *Headache* 19:163, 1979.
3. Kattah JC, Luessenhop AJ: Resolution of classic migraine after removal of an occipital lobe AVM. *Ann Neurol* 7:93, 1980.
4. Bennett R, Hughes GRV, Bywaters EGL, et al: Neuropsychiatric problems in systemic lupus erythematosus. *Br Med J* 4:342, 1972.
5. Moretti G, Manzoni GC, Caffarra P, et al: "Benign recurrent vertigo" and its connection with migraine. *Headache* 20:344, 1980.
6. Taylor AR, Chakravorty BC: Clinical syndromes associated with basilar impression. *Arch Neurol* 10:475, 1964.
7. Meredith TA, Aaberg TM: Hemorrhagic peripapillary lesions in presumed ocular histoplasmosis. *Am J Ophthalmol* 84:160, 1977.
8. Hayreh SS: Optic disc edema in raised intracranial pressure. VI. Associated visual disturbances and their pathogenesis. *Arch Ophthalmol* 95:1566, 1977.
9. Martinez AJ, Lee A, Moossy J, et al: Pituitary adenomas: Clinicopathological and immunohistochemical study. *Ann Neurol* 7:24, 1980.
10. Bender MB, Feldman M: The so-called "visual agnosias." *Brain* 95:173, 1972.
11. Poeck K: Pathophysiology of emotional disorders associated with brain damage, in Vinken PJ, Bruyn GW (eds): *Handbook of Clinical Neurology*. New York, American Elsevier, 1969, vol 3, p 343.

12. Klüver H, Bucy PC: An analysis of certain effects of bilateral temporal lobectomy in the rhesus monkey, with special reference to psychic blindness. *J Psychol* 5:33, 1938.
13. Klüver H, Bucy PC: Psychic blindness and other symptoms following bilateral temporal lobectomy in rhesus monkeys. *Am J Physiol* 119:352, 1937.
14. Marlowe WB, Mancall EL, Thomas JJ: Complete Klüver-Bucy syndrome in man. *Cortex* 11:53, 1975.
15. Rubens AB, Benson DF: Associative visual agnosia. *Arch Neurol* 24:305, 1971.
16. Benson DF, Segarra J, Albert ML: Visual agnosia-prosopagnosia. *Arch Neurol* 30:307, 1974.
17. Rubens AB: Agnosia, in Heilman KM, Valenstein E (eds): *Clinical Neuropsychology*. New York, Oxford University Press, 1979, p 233.
18. Geschwind N, Fusillo M: Color-naming defects in association with alexia. *Arch Neurol* 15:137 1966.
19. Hamsher K deS, Levin HS, Benton AL: Facial recognition in patients with focal brain lesions. *Arch Neurol* 36:837, 1979.
20. Valenstein E, Heilman KM: Emotional disorders resulting from lesions of the central nervous system, in Heilman KM, Valenstein E (eds): *Clinical Neuropsychology*. New York, Oxford University Press, 1979, p 413.
21. Warrington EK, Shallice T: Word-form dyslexia. *Brain* 103:99, 1980.
22. Geschwind N: Neurological foundations of language, in Myklebust HR (ed): *Progress in Learning Disabilities*. New York, Grune & Stratton, 1968, vol I, p 182.
23. Albert ML: A simple test of visual neglect. *Neurology (NY)* 23:658, 1973.
24. Zihl J, Cramon D von: The contribution of the "second" visual system to directed visual attention in man. *Brain* 102:835, 1979.
25. Galin D: Implications for psychiatry of left and right cerebral specialization. *Arch Gen Psychiatry* 31:572, 1974.
26. McGlone J, Kertesz A: Sex differences in cerebral processing of visuospatial tasks. *Cortex* 9:313, 1973.
27. DeVaul RA, Hall RCW: Hallucinations, in Hall RCW (ed): *Psychiatric Presentations of Medical Illness*. New York, SP Medical and Scientific Books, 1980, p 91.
28. Lance JW: Simple formed hallucinations confined to the area of a specific visual field defect. *Brain* 99:719, 1976.
29. Sherwin, I, Geschwind N: Neural substrates of behavior, in Nicholi AM (ed): *The Harvard Guide to Modern Psychiatry*. Cambridge, Belknap Press, 1978, p 59.
30. Prick JJG: Thallium poisoning, in Vinken PJ, Bruyn GW (eds): *Handbook of Clinical Neurology*. New York, American Elsevier, 1979, vol 36, p 239.
31. Klawans HL: Levodopa induced psychosis. *Psychiatr Ann* 8:447, 1978.
32. Lessell S, Cohen MM: Phosphenes induced by sound. *Neurology (NY)* 29:1524, 1979.
33. Zarcone V: Narcolepsy. *N Engl J Med* 288:1156, 1973.
34. Hecker A, Andermann F, Rodin EA: Spitting automatism in temporal lobe seizures. *Epilepsia* 13:767, 1972.
35. LeDoux JE, Barclay L, Premack A: The brain and cognitive sciences. *Arch Neurol* 4:391, 1978.
36. Teuber HL: Prospects for research on schizophrenia: Effects of focal brain lesions. *Neurosci Res Program Bull* 10:381, 1972.
37. Balasubramaniam V, Ramamurth B: Stereotaxic amygdalotomy in behavior disorders. *Confin Neurol* 32:367, 1970.
38. Jacobs L, Karpik A, Bozian D, et al: Auditory-visual synesthesia. *Arch Neurol* 38:211, 1981.

39. Anton G: Über die Selbstwahrnehmungen der Herderkrankungen des Gehirns durch den Kranken bei Rindenblindheit und Rindentaubheit. *Arch Psychiatr Nervenkr* 32:86, 1899.

40. Steele JC: Progressive supranuclear palsy. *Brain* 95:693, 1972.

41. Steele JC, Richardson JC, Olszewski J: Progressive supranuclear palsy. *Arch Neurol* 10:333, 1964.

42. Balint R: Seelenlähmung des "Schauens", optische Ataxie, räumliche Störung der Aufmerksameit. *Monatsschr Psychiatr Neurol* 25:57, 1909.

43. Jaffe BF: Vertigo following air travel. *N Engl J Med* 301:1385, 1979.

44. Gilman S, Bloedel JR, Lechtenberg R: *Disorders of the Cerebellum.* Philadelphia, FA Davis, 1981.

45. Ménière P: Sur une forme particulière de surdité grave dépendant d'une lésion de l'oreille interne. *Gaz Med Paris* 16:29, 1861.

46. Merritt HH: *A Textbook of Neurology,* ed 5. Philadelphia, Lea & Febiger, 1973.

47. Luxon LM: Hearing loss in brainstem disorders. *J Neurol Neurosurg Psychiatry* 43:510, 1980.

48. McAlpine D, Lumsden CE, Acheson ED: *Multiple Sclerosis. A Reappraisal.* Baltimore, Williams & Wilkins, 1972.

49. Albert ML, Sparks RW, Helm NA: Melodic intonation therapy for aphasia. *Arch Neurol* 29:130, 1973.

50. Shoumaker RD, Ajax ET, Schenkenberg T: Pure word deafness. *Dis Nerv Syst* 38:293, 1977.

51. Oscar-Berman M, Goodglass H, Donnenfeld H: Dichotic ear-order effects with non-verbal stimuli. *Cortex* 10:270, 1974.

52. Shulman A, Seitz MR: Central tinnitus. *Laryngoscope* (in press).

53. Shallop JK: The measurement of middle ear function, in Singh S (ed): *Measurement Procedures in Speech, Hearing, and Language.* Baltimore, University Park Press, 1975, p 279.

Index